Diagnostic Pathology: Neuropathology

Diagnostic Pathology: Neuropathology

Edited by Josh Vaughan

AMERICAN
MEDICAL PUBLISHERS
www.americanmedicalpublishers.com

American Medical Publishers,
41 Flatbush Avenue,
1st Floor, New York,
NY 11217, USA

Visit us on the World Wide Web at:
www.americanmedicalpublishers.com

ISBN: 978-1-63927-291-4

Cataloging-in-Publication Data

Diagnostic pathology : neuropathology / edited by Josh Vaughan.
p. cm.
Includes bibliographical references and index.
ISBN 978-1-63927-291-4
1. Nervous system--Diseases--Diagnosis. 2. Nervous system--Diseases--Pathogenesis.
3. Nervous system--Diseases. I. Vaughan, Josh.
RC348 .D53 2022
616.804 75--dc23

Table of Contents

Preface

Neuropathology is a subspecialty of anatomic pathology that is concerned with the study of the diseases of nervous system tissue, with the aid of surgical biopsies and autopsies. This field is closely associated with the clinical domains of neurology and neurosurgery which refer to neuropathological results for making a diagnosis. If a neuropathy is suspected and less invasive methods cannot deliver a diagnosis, a biopsy of nervous tissue from the brain or spinal cord is taken to aid in the diagnosis. When a mass is detected by medical imaging, a biopsy is generally requested. The post-mortem diagnosis of dementia and other conditions of the central nervous system is also within the scope of this field. This book includes some of the vital pieces of work being conducted across the world, on various topics related to neuropathology. While understanding the long-term perspectives of the topics, the book makes an effort in highlighting their impacts as a modern tool for the understanding of neuropathy. It will serve as a valuable source of reference for graduate and post graduate students in diagnostic pathology.

Significant researches are present in this book. Intensive efforts have been employed by authors to make this book an outstanding discourse. This book contains the enlightening chapters which have been written on the basis of significant researches done by the experts.

Finally, I would also like to thank all the members involved in this book for being a team and meeting all the deadlines for the submission of their respective works. I would also like to thank my friends and family for being supportive in my efforts.

Editor

Preface

1

Brainstem tau pathology in Alzheimer's disease is characterized by increase of three repeat tau and independent of amyloid β

Miho Uematsu[1,2,3], Ayako Nakamura[1], Momoko Ebashi[1,4], Katsuiku Hirokawa[5], Ryosuke Takahashi[2] and Toshiki Uchihara[1*]

Abstract

Introduction: Alzheimer-type neuropil threads (NTs) and neurofibrillary tangles (NFTs) are comprised of either 4 repeat (4R)-tau, 3 repeat (3R)-tau, or a mixture of both. In the hippocampus, the number of NFTs, and the proportion of 3R tau progressively increases. If this preferential accumulation of 3R tau also occurs in the brainstem, it may be fundamentally related to progression of Alzheimer pathology.

Methods: Midbrain and pontine sections of brainstems from 23 cases (Braak-NFT stages I/II: 8, III/IV: 8, and V/VI: 7) were double immunofluorolabeled for 4R and 3R tau. High-resolution (0.645 μm/pixel), in-focus snapshots were tiled to cover entire brain sections using a virtual slide system. Each lesion was classified by size (NT < 200 μm^2 < NFT) and staining profile (3R/4R). In addition, the localization and quantity of amyloid β (Aβ) deposits were examined in adjacent sections for comparison with tau.

Results: The data sets obtained from approximately 286 gigabytes of image files consisted of 847,763 NTs and 7859 NFTs. The proportion of 3R tau-positive NTs and NFTs in the midbrain, and 3R tau-positive NTs in the pons gradually increased with advancing NFT stages, while the proportion of 3R tau-positive NFTs in the pons was already elevated at early stages. Aβ deposits were absent at NFT stages I/II, and when present at later stages, their regional distribution was different from that of tau. These observations suggest that a progressive increase in the proportion of 3R tau occurs independently of Aβ deposits.

Conclusions: This is the first quantitative analysis of NFTs and NTs in the human brainstem. We demonstrate that the proportion of 3R tau in the brainstem neurofibrillary changes increases with disease progression. Because this phenomenon is shared between the brainstem and the hippocampus, this increase may be fundamental to the pathogenesis of Alzheimer disease.

Keywords: Alzheimer disease pathology, Tau isoform, Human brain, Virtual slide imaging, Brainstem

* Correspondence: uchihara-ts@igakuken.or.jp
[1]Laboratory of Structural Neuropathology, Tokyo Metropolitan Institute of Medical Science, 2-1-6 Kamikitazawa, Setagaya-ku, Tokyo 156-8506, Japan
Full list of author information is available at the end of the article

Introduction

Neurofibrillary tangles (NFTs) and neuropil threads (NTs), collectively called the neurofibrillary changes, are pathological hallmarks of Alzheimer disease (AD), which exhibit a stereotypical pattern of hierarchical progression initiated around the hippocampus [5]. The extent of neurofibrillary changes correlates with the severity of dementia in AD [56]. Subcortical nuclei also exhibit Alzheimer-related neurofibrillary pathology [24, 29]. Probably prior to the limbic area, subcortical nuclei such as the dorsal raphe nucleus (DRN) and locus coeruleus (LC) develop neurofibrillary changes much earlier, because they are sometimes detectable under 30 years of age in subclinical phases [6, 19, 46]. However, it is not known how these brainstem lesions change along disease progression [2]. This prompted us to examine how neurofibrillary changes in the brainstem are similar to and different from those in the limbic areas with special attention to tau isoforms.

Neurofibrillary changes are immunoreactive mainly toward the hyperphosphorylated form of tau protein [20, 25]. Exon 9–12 of the tau gene, each containing imperfect repeat, encode a microtubule-binding domain, and inclusion or exclusion of exon 10 via alternative splicing generates isoforms with four repeats (4R tau) or three repeats (3R tau), respectively [17].

Paired helical filaments (PHFs) from the brains of AD consist of both 4R and 3R tau [18]. Neurofibrillary changes of neurofibrillary tangle-predominant dementia are also comprised of both 4R and 3R tau [31]. However, participation of each isoform is not random. At cellular level, each NFT is considered to undergo morphological changes from pretangles, NFTs, to the ghost tangles, and this morphological maturation has been shown to coincide with the transition from 4R tau predominant pretangles to 3R tau predominant ghost tangles. [21, 28, 34, 35, 54]. Interestingly, regional extent of each isoform is differently regulated; for example, 3R tau-positive lesions are abundant in the areas in which tau deposition begins early, such as parahippocampal area and subiculum, while 4R tau-positive lesions are dominant in the areas in which tau deposition begins later, such as CA4 [21, 28, 34, 35]. This regional gradient of isoform is maintained from the early to late stages of AD [21]. It is then hypothesized that chronological change of tau isoform, 4R for early pretangles vs. 3R for late ghost tangles, is orchestrated to generate regional gradient of tau isoforms throughout disease progression. If such orchestrated regulation of tau isoforms is fundamental to AD, it is plausible that similar phenomena are also at work in the brainstem.

Comprehensive quantitative analysis on the double immunofluorolabeled brainstem sections for 4R and 3R tau may clarify the tau isoform distribution in the brainstem lesions including the assessment of their colocalization. However, single-plane fluorescence image may suffer from unclear boundaries due to inaccurate focusing, which is highly problematic when quantifying the lesion sizes or morphologies. To overcome these problems, we changed conventional imaging strategy by introducing "extended focus imaging (EFI)", which extracts pixels with maximal local contrast from multiple vertical planes and reconstructs a single in-focus image. With this strategy incorporated in the virtual slide system, it was possible to delineate even minute lesions such as NTs at whatever depth in the vertical planes of the section. While virtual slide imaging has been scarcely employed for quantitative analysis [47], it was only after these technical refinements that we were finally successful in extracting all the immunofluorolabeled lesions within the full range and depth of the section with clear contours, enrolling them all in the comprehensive quantitative analysis. Using this new method, we counted all the NTs and NFTs with different tau isoform profiles on postmortem brainstem sections from cases with different stages of neurofibrillary pathology in the present study.

With the advent of the same virtual slide system, we also attempted to map amyloid β (Aβ) deposits, another hallmark of Alzheimer-related pathologies, in the sections adjacent to those used for tau isoform quantification for direct comparison. Aβ deposition exhibits a hierarchical distribution from neocortex, gradually involving the brainstem after Thal amyloid phase 3 [51]. Aβ deposition plays a role in early-onset familial AD, caused by mutation of genes such as *APP* and *PSEN1* [16, 45]. Moreover, reports suggest that Aβ is essential for the initiation of synaptic and neuronal tau pathology [32, 60]. However, the correlation between the severity of dementia and degree of the Aβ accumulation is much weaker than that of neurofibrillary pathology [56]. Because few reports are available on the topographical distribution of Aβ in the brainstem [27] and no data are available on their possible relation to tau deposits in the brainstem, our novel approach may clarify possible relation between tau and Aβ deposition in the brainstem.

Here, our comprehensive quantitative analysis on double-immunofluorolabeled midbrain and pontine sections for 4R and 3R tau has demonstrated that the preferential increase of the proportion of 3R tau-positive neurofibrillary changes occurs with disease progression in the brainstem, but independently of Aβ deposition. Because this is a shared phenomenon between brainstem and hippocampus, it is fundamental to the progression of Alzheimer-related tau pathology.

Materials and methods

Subjects

Twenty three autopsied brains with different cortical NFT stages (Table 1, Braak and Braak's NFT stages I/II:

8 cases, III/IV: 8 cases, V/VI: 7 cases) were enrolled in this study with informed consent and the approval of the ethics committee of Tokyo Metropolitan Institute of Medical Science and Nitobe-Memorial Nakano General Hospital. These cases have previously been anonymized and subjected to standardized neuropathological assessment at Tokyo Metropolitan Institute of Medical Science, including silver impregnations by Gallyas and Campbell-Switzer method, and DAB immunohistochemistry with anti-phospho-tau (Ser202, Thr205) antibody AT8 (Thermo Fisher Scientific K.K., Tokyo, Japan) of representative brain regions. The brainstem sections of all cases, and cortical sections of selected cases underwent DAB immunohistochemistry with anti-alpha-synuclein phospho (Ser129) monoclonal antibody (1:10,000, Clone pSyn#64, Wako, Japan). Diagnosis of NFT stage, Consortium to Establish a Registry for Alzheimer's Disease (CERAD) neuritic plaque score, and the evaluation of Lewy body distribution and frequency were performed following the published criteria [5, 37, 38]. Cases with non-Alzheimer-type tau deposits (e.g. progressive supranuclear palsy, corticobasal degeneration, argyrophilic grain disease and Pick body disease) were excluded. Concomitant Lewy pathology was observed in case 1, 9, 13 and 23 (Table 1, Additional file 1).

Distinction of 4R and 3R tau by double immunofluorescence

The autopsied brains were immersion-fixed in 4% formalin for 4 weeks. The brainstem was sliced perpendicular to the axis and embedded in paraffin. The levels of the sections were coordinated between cases by encompassing landmark anatomical structures (superior colliculus (SC) and red nucleus (RN) for the midbrain, and

Table 1 Characteristics of subjects

Case	Age at death	Sex	Braak's cortical NFT stages	Lewy pathology	Brainstem NFT							Comparison of 3R tau % with 4R tau%			
					Midbrain				Pons			Neuropil thread		NFT	
					Superior colliculus	Periaqueductal gray Ventral/Dorsal	Linear raphe nucleus	Substantia nigra Medial/Lateral	Locus coeruleus	Dorsal raphe nucleus	Median raphe nucleus	Midbrain	Pons	Midbrain	Pons
1	74	M	I/II	+ (B)	+	+ / +	+	+/+	+	+	+	<	<	<	<
2	81	M	I/II	–	+	+ / +	+	+/+	+	+	+	<	<	<	>
3	71	F	I/II	–	+	++/++	+	+/++	+++	+	++	>	>	<	>
4	77	M	I/II	–	+	+ / +	+	+/+	+	+	+	<	<	>	>
5	78	M	I/II	–	+	+ / +	+	+/+	++	+	+	<	>	<	>
6	87	M	I/II	–	+	+ / +	+	+/+	++	+	++	<	<	<	<
7	68	M	I/II	–	+	+ / +	+	+/+	+	+	+	<	<	<	<
8	63	M	I/II	–	+	+ / +	+	+/+	+	+	+	<	>	>	>
9	86	F	III/IV	+ (B)	+	++ / +	+	+/++	+++	+	++	<	>	>	>
10	93	M	III/IV	–	+	++ / +	+++	++/++	++	+	++	<	>	>	>
11	100	F	III/IV	–	+	++ / +	++	+/++	+++	+	++	>	>	>	>
12	83	F	III/IV	–	+++	++ / +	++	+/+	++	+	++	>	>	>	>
13	86	M	III/IV	+ (T)	+	++ / +	+	+/+	+	++	+++	>	<	<	<
14	92	F	III/IV	–	+	+ / +	+	+/+	+++	++	++	>	>	>	>
15	95	F	III/IV	–	+	+ / +	+	+/++	+	+	+++	<	>	>	>
16	80	M	III/IV	–	+	+ / +	+	+/+	+++	+	++	>	<	<	<
17	82	M	V/VI	–	+++	+++ / +	++	++/++	++	++	+++	>	>	>	>
18	93	M	V/VI	–	+	+++ / +	+++	++/+	+++	+++	+++	>	>	>	>
19	94	F	V/VI	–	++	+++ / +	+++	++/+	+++	+	+++	>	>	>	>
20	89	F	V/VI	–	+	+++ / +	+++	++/++	+++	++	+++	>	>	>	>
21	102	F	V/VI	–	++	+++ / +	++	+/++	+++	+	++	<	<	>	>
22	85	M	V/VI	–	++	+++ / +	+++	+++/++	+++	++	+++	<	<	<	<
23	88	F	V/VI	+ (N)	+++	++ / +	+++	+++/++	+++	++	+++	>	>	>	>

Concomitant Lewy pathology is described as brainstem-predominant (B), transitional (T) and neocortical (N), according to McKeith criteria [37]. The regional counts in the 1 mm^2 microscopic field with maximal neurofibrillary tangle (NFT) or well-defined compact Aβ deposition density is graded as follows; – (absent): none in the field, + (sparse): 1–9/field, ++ (mild) 10–19/field, +++ (moderate): 20- /field. For the comparison of 3R tau (%) with 4R tau (%), **>** indicates that the proportion of 3R tau is greater than that of 4R tau, while **<** indicates that the proportion of 4R tau is greater than that of 3R tau, on each section

Table 1 Characteristics of subjects *(Continued)*

Case	Formalin-fixed brain weight (g)	CERAD neuritic plaque score	Brainstem Aβ deposition										
			Midbrain					Pons					
			Total	Superior colliculus	Periaqueductal gray Ventral / Dorsal	Linear raphe nucleus	Substantia nigra Medial/ Lateral	Total	Locus coeruleus	Dorsal raphe nucleus	Median raphe nucleus	Reticular formation	Pontine nucleus
1	1310	0	–	–	–	–	–	–	–	–	–	–	–
2	1455	A	–	–	–	–	–	–	–	–	–	–	–
3	1240	0	–	–	–	–	–	–	–	–	–	–	–
4	1350	0	–	–	–	–	–	–	–	–	–	–	–
5	1410	A	–	–	–	–	–	–	–	–	–	–	–
6	1375	B	–	–	–	–	–	–	–	–	–	–	–
7	1390	0	–	–	–	–	–	–	–	–	–	–	–
8	1515	0	–	–	–	–	–	–	–	–	–	–	–
9	1190	B	–	–	–	–	–	–	–	–	–	–	–
10	1430	B	++	++	- / +	–	–	++	++	–	–	–	–
11	1150	A	–	–	–	–	–	+	+	–	–	–	–
12	1100	B	++	++	+ / ++	–	+/–	+	+	–	–	–	–
13	1270	B	+	+	–	–	–	+	+	–	–	–	–
14	1130	B	+	+	–	–	–	–	–	–	–	–	–
15	1260	C	++	++	- / +	–	+/–	–	–	–	–	–	–
16	1400	B	+	+	–	–	+/–	–	–	–	–	–	–
17	1185	C	+++	+++	+ / ++	+	+/–	+++	+++	+	++	+	+
18	1080	C	+	+	- / +	–	+/+	+++	+++	+	++	+	–
19	1350	C	+++	+++	- / +	–	++/+	+	+	–	–	–	–
20	1300	B	++	++	+ / ++	+	–	+	+	–	–	–	–
21	1140	0	–	–	–	–	–	–	–	–	–	–	–
22	1395	C	+++	+++	+ / ++	+	++/++	+++	+++	+	++	+	+
23	1170	C	+++	+++	+ /+++	–	++/+	+++	+++	+	+	+	+

LC and superior cerebellar peduncles for the pons) (Fig. 1a). The 6-μm thick sections were deparaffinized for double immunofluorolabeling with antibodies against isoform-specific anti-4R tau antibody (rabbit polyclonal, Cosmo Bio Co, Tokyo, Japan), raised against amino acids 275–291 of human 4R tau, which is deamidated at N279 [10, 22], and anti-3R tau antibody (RD3, mouse monoclonal, Merck Millipore, Germany) [11]. To reduce diffuse cytoplasmic staining with the RD3, the sections were pretreated with 0.25% potassium permanganate for 15 min, 2% oxalic acid for a minute, and >99% formic acid for 30 min at room temperature, and autoclaved in 0.05 M citrate buffer for 20 min at 120 °C [53]. This pretreatment also improved immunolabeling with polyclonal anti-4R tau (data not shown). Sections were washed with phosphate-buffered saline (PBS) with 0.03% polyoxyethylene (10) octylphenyl ether (Triton X-100), blocked for 30 min in 5% normal goat serum/0.05% NaN_3/PBS with 0.03% Triton X-100, and incubated with polyclonal anti-4R-tau antibody (1:3000) and RD3 (1:300), diluted in the blocking buffer at 4 °C for 4 days. To reduce autofluorescence of lipofuscin, sections were treated with Sudan Black B [44]. Quenching of the autofluorescence of lipofuscin was confirmed by spectral analysis (Additional file 2: Figure S1). Primary antibodies were labeled with Alexa 488 conjugated with anti-rabbit IgG (Molecular Probes, Oregon, USA, 1:200) and Alexa 568 conjugated with anti-mouse IgG (Molecular Probes, Oregon, USA, 1:200), respectively, diluted in PBS with 0.03% Triton X-100 overnight in the dark. Sections were mounted with buffered glycerol containing 0.1% *p*-phenylenediamine. For anatomical assessment, immediately adjacent sections were stained with Hematoxylin & Eosin and Klüver-Barrera (KB) methods.

Diaminobenzidine (DAB) immunohistochemistry

For precise comparison of Aβ with tau deposits, neighboring sections from the same tissue blocks used for tau immunohistochemistry were subjected to Aβ/DAB immunohistochemistry. For the confirmation of the observation of 4R and 3R tau double-immunofluorolabeling, representative sections were also subjected to RD4 (mouse monoclonal anti-4R tau antibody, Merck Millipore, Germany) or RD3/DAB immunohistochemistry

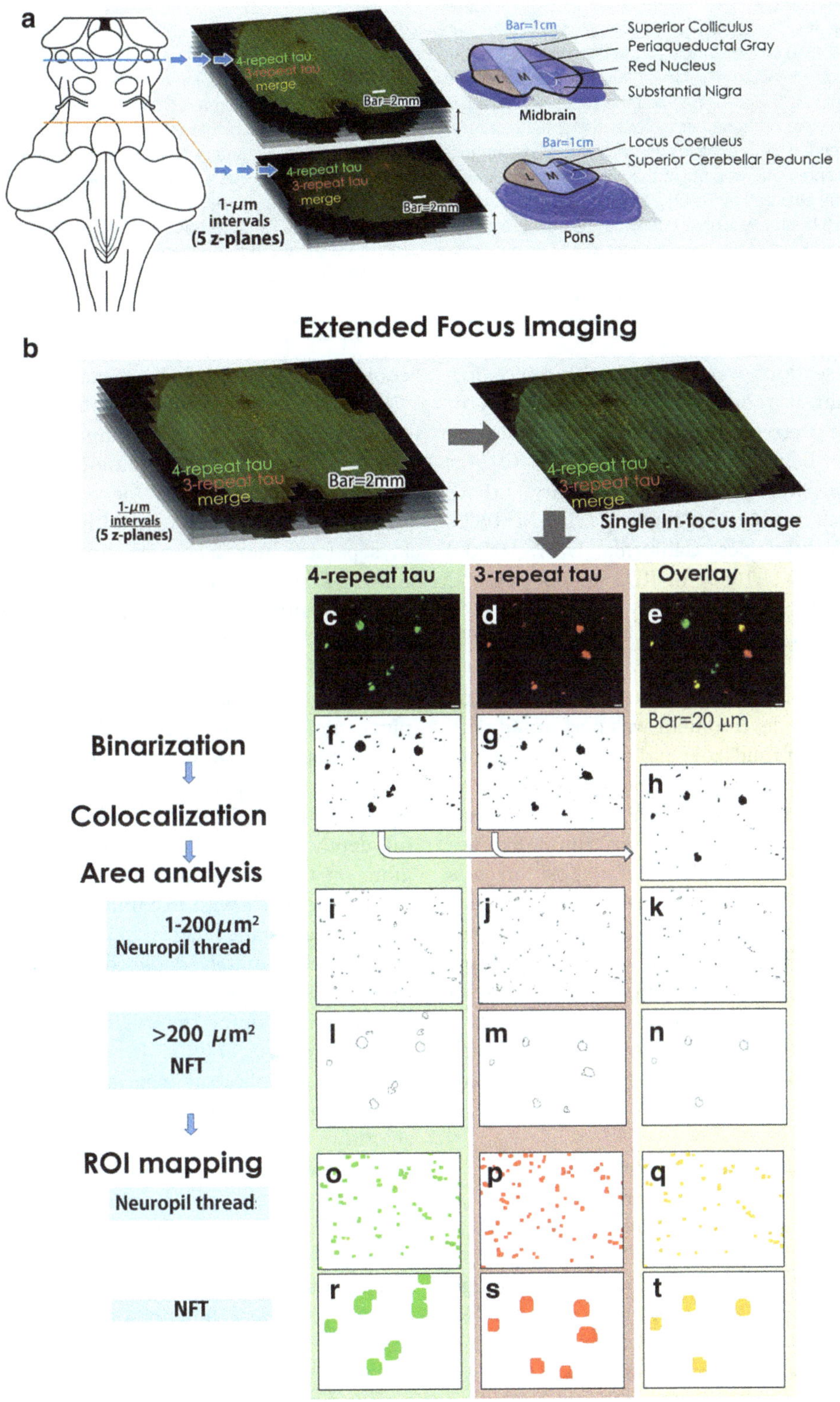

Fig. 1 (See legend on next page.)

(See figure on previous page.)

Fig. 1 CENSUS (Complete ENumeration and Sorting for Unlimited Sectors) via immunofluorescence to count all neurofibrillary changes and sort everything by a virtual slide system. Image acquisition by virtual slide system and subsequent quantitative analysis and ROI mapping. (**a**) Image capturing at the coordinated anatomical levels. Midbrain sections included the superior colliculus (SC) and red nucleus (RN), and the pontine sections included the locus coeruleus (LC) and the superior cerebellar peduncles. The snapshots captured with 10 times objective lens in separate fluorescence channels were put together to cover the entire tectum and tegmentum. 5 vertical planes at 1 μm intervals were simultaneously captured. (**b**) The extended focus imaging (EFI) module picked up pixels with maximum local contrast to make a single in-focus image from 5 vertical planes. (**c**-**e**) Representative parts of the separate channels of the extended-focused images and their overlays are shown. Bar = 20 μm. (**f**-**h**) These images were binarized by Triangle algorithm (**f**, **g**), followed by binary colocalization analysis on ImageJ (h). (**i**-**n**) Particle analysis program sorted all immunolabels by size, which we defined as neuroil threads (NTs, area 1–200 μm^2, **i**-**k**) and neurofibrillary tangles (NFTs, area > 200 μm^2, **l**-**n**), with retrospective inspection into the original counterpart for confirmation. Outlines are shown. (**o**-**t**) ROI mapping of the immunolabels. The outlines of the ROIs selected in area analysis are uniformly exaggerated and colored (4R tau/*green*, 3R tau/*red*, colocalization/*yellow*) on ImageJ to abstract the immunolabels of NTs (**o**-**q**) and NFTs (**r**-**t**), as automatic immunolabel mappings

[11]. For Aβ, the sections were treated with > 99% formic acid for 5 min at room temperature. For RD4 or RD3, sections were pretreated as described in the section above [53]. After being treated with 1% H_2O_2 for 30 min, the sections were incubated in primary anti-Aβ mouse monoclonal antibody (Clone 6F/3D, M 0872; DAKO, Agilent Technologies, California, USA, 1:1000) at 4 °C for 2 days, RD4 (1:1000), or RD3 (1:3000) at 4 °C for 4 days, and biotinylated secondary anti-mouse antibody (BA-2000, Vector, California, USA, 1:1000) for 2 h. After subsequent incubation with streptavidin biotinylated horseradish peroxidase complex (ABC Elite, Vector, California, USA), color development was performed with DAB in the presence of imidazole and nickel ammonium chloride. They were examined by light microscopy, and the same virtual slide system used for tau deposits. For semi-quantitative grading of Aβ deposition, only the number of well-defined, compact Aβ deposition was counted, while ill-defined, fleecy deposition and dot-like deposition (smaller than approximately 1μm^2) was not included in the count. The amount of well-defined, compact Aβ deposition in 1 mm^2 microscopic field with maximum deposition density was graded as follows; – (None): no amyloid deposition in the field, + (Sparse): 1–9/field, ++ (Mild): 10–19/field, +++ (Moderate): 20-/field (Table 1).

CENSUS (Complete ENumeration and Sorting for Unlimited Sectors) via immunofluorescence to count all neurofibrillary changes and sort everything by a virtual slide system (Fig. 1)

We obtained a virtual slide image covering full range and depth of the section at high resolution, and enrolled all the immunofluorolabels in the whole investigated area in comprehensive particle analyses. For this, we used a virtual slide system VS120 (Olympus, Tokyo, Japan) equipped with UPLSAPO 10 times objective lens (Olympus, Tokyo, Japan), a triple-band dichroic mirror unit (U-DM3-DA/FI/TX, Olympus), band path filter with peak emission wavelength at 518 nm (for 4R tau/Alexa 488) and 580 nm (for RD3/Alexa 568), a sensitive cooled charge-coupled device camera (ORCA-R^2 C10600-10B, Hamamatsu Photonics, Shizuoka, Japan), and VS-ASW software (Olympus, Tokyo, Japan). Serial snapshots of a double-immunofluorolabeled section (4R tau/Alexa 488 and RD3/Alexa 568) were captured by VS120 on motorized stage with 10 times objective lens in separate fluorescence channels, and put together to make a seamless broad image, covering the whole tectum and tegmentum (Fig. 1a, Additional file 3: Figure S2). The resolution of each snapshot was 1376 pixels (horizontal) × 1038 pixels (vertical) at 0.645 μm/pixel with 10 times objective lens (original 8 bit). After subtracting the overlapping margins, the area per snapshot reduced to approximately 1138 pixels × 834 pixels (0.398 mm^2/snapshot). 5 vertical planes at 1 μm intervals were simultaneously captured (Fig. 1a). To show all the immunolabels at full depth of the section with high accuracy, the EFI program on CellSens software (Olympus, Tokyo, Japan) extracted the pixels with maximum local contrast from the 5 vertical planes and made a single in-focus image (Fig. 1b, c-e), which minutely depicted even small threadlike lesions. These images were converted to big-tagged image file format, retaining the original resolution, to be further operated on ImageJ (NIH, Bethesda, Maryland, USA). The images were uniformly binarized in separate channels according to the threshold operationally defined by Triangle algorithm [59] on ImageJ (Fig. 1f, g). Colocalization analysis between binary images was subsequently performed with ImageJ plug-in (P. Bourdoncle, Institut Jacques Monod, Paris, France) (Fig. 1h). Particle analysis program of ImageJ showed particle size of each immunofluorolabel automatically, as well as X-Y coordinate, in separate fluorescence profiles. We defined particles with a 1–200 μm^2 area as NTs (Fig. 1i-k), and with an area larger than 200 μm^2 as NFTs (Fig. 1l-n). The results of the analyses were inspected against the original counterparts to ensure that each lesion was properly represented, and apparent contaminants (e.g. nonspecific staining of the vessel walls) were excluded from the count. For analysis of the regional differences, necessary parts were extracted from the virtual slide images. The regional counts in the 1 mm^2 field with maximal NFT density was graded as follows; – (absent): no NFTs in the field, + (sparse): 1–9/field, ++ (mild) 10–19/field, +++ (moderate): 20- /field (Table 1). The results of the particle analyses were highlighted as regions of interest (ROIs) on ImageJ. The outline width of ROI depiction was uniformly widened and flattened onto a blank image file with same pixel size as the original. These abstracted outlines served as immunolabel mappings of NTs (Fig. 1o-q) and NFTs (Fig. 1r-t) in different tau-isoform profiles. Also, the virtual slide images of Aβ/DAB immunohistochemistry were captured with 10 times objective lens, and underwent thresholding by RGB values (R: 0–110, G: 60–150, B: 60–150) on CellSens software (Olympus, Tokyo, Japan). This procedure separated black-brown DAB labeling from reddish-brown neuromelanin and particle analysis highlighted the former as ROIs. The outline widths of these ROIs were uniformly widened and simplified on ImageJ to serve as the immunolabel mapping of Aβ deposition. We propose this virtual-slide based quantitative analysis of multifluorolabeled specimen as "Complete ENumeration and Sorting for Unlimited Sectors (CENSUS)" via immunofluorescence.

Statistical analysis

All statistical analyses were performed using software R (version 3.2.3, R Foundation for Statistical Computing, Vienna, Austria.). $P < 0.05$ was considered significant. To find the differences in the means of data between cases, Fisher's exact test or paired t-test with Bonferroni correction was performed. The counts of NTs and NFTs in each tau isoform, and their proportion to the total counts on the entire section were obtained. The proportional data underwent arcsine transformation prior to further analysis to make the data distribution closer to normal. Since arcsine of 1 equals 1.57, axis for the plot of arcsine-transformed proportion ranged from 0 to 1.57. The characteristics of individual cases were stratified into 3 subgroups as follows; age at death: young-old (ages 63–80 years, $n = 7$), middle-old (81–90 years, $n = 9$), and very-old (91–102 years, $n = 7$), NFT stages: I/II ($n = 8$), III/IV ($n = 8$) and V/VI ($n = 7$), CERAD plaque score: 0/A ($n = 9$), B ($n = 8$), C ($n = 6$), and the formalin-fixed brain weight (g): above 1350 ($n = 8$), 1200–1350 ($n = 7$), and below 1200 ($n = 8$). To assess whether there is a significant orderly increasing or decreasing trend along these stratifications, Jonckheere's trend test was performed. To explore the best-fitting regression models of the plots, the model that yields the least Akaike's Information Criterion was searched from quadratic ($y = ax^2 + bx + c$), linear ($y = bx + c$ or $y = c$), exponential ($y = ab^x$), and power ($y = ax^b$) regression models (the formulas for all the regression models are available on request). The NFT stages (I/II, III/IV, V/VI), CERAD neuritic plaque score (0, A, B, C) and brainstem Aβ deposition (–, +, ++, +++) were converted to numeric variables from 0 to 3 [43]. Odds ratio and 95% confidence intervals for the percentages of sections with greater proportion of 3R tau than 4R tau during the advancement of cortical NFT stages (from I/II, III/IV to V/VI) were calculated by a univariate binomial logistic regression model (Additional file 1). In the box plots, the box represents the 25th and 75th percentiles, the horizontal line in the box represents the median, whisker show the 10th and 90th percentiles, and the white circles represent the outliers. Lines with asterisk indicate statistically significant differences.

Results

Topographical distribution is similar between NTs and NFTs, and between 4R and 3R tau (Fig. 2)

Midbrain and pontine sections from 23 cases with different NFT stages were double-immunofluorolabeled for 4R and 3R tau (Table 1). The neurofibrillary changes were present in midbrain and pons of all the investigated cases (Table 1). We captured 300,860 snapshots (approximately 0.398 mm^2 per snapshot after subtracting the overlapped area) of these sections in total, which were 30,086 snapshots on XY planes with 5 vertical planes in 2 fluorescence channels, by the virtual slide system (detailed in Additional file 1). The investigated area was approximately 120 cm^2 in total. We performed comprehensive quantitative analyses on these images as described above (Fig. 1). The data sets obtained from approximately 286 gigabytes of image files consisted of 847,763 NTs (602,839 in the midbrain, 244,924 in the pons) and 7859 NFTs (4948 in the midbrain, 2911 in the pons). Each data retained the information of the location and tau isoform profile of the particle. Based on the results of quantitative analyses, immunolabel maps of the NTs and NFTs in different tau isoform profiles were operationally drawn (representative maps in Fig. 2).

The topographical distribution was similar between NFTs and NTs (Fig. 2, bottom two rows of midbrain and pons), and between 4R and 3R tau (Fig. 2, left four columns). The neurofibrillary changes were accentuated at the periaqueductal gray (PAG, ventral half-dominant), linear raphe nucleus (LRN), ventral tegmental area, and substantia nigra (SN) of the midbrain, and the LC, DRN, median raphe nucleus (MRN), and parabrachial nucleus of the pons (Fig. 2). Immunolabel maps of Aβ were also operationally drawn (Fig. 2, right column). Aβ deposits were accumulated at the SC, PAG (dorsal half-dominant), SN (medial half-dominant), LC, reticular formation (RF), and MRN. Topographical differences between tau and Aβ deposits will be described later in detail.

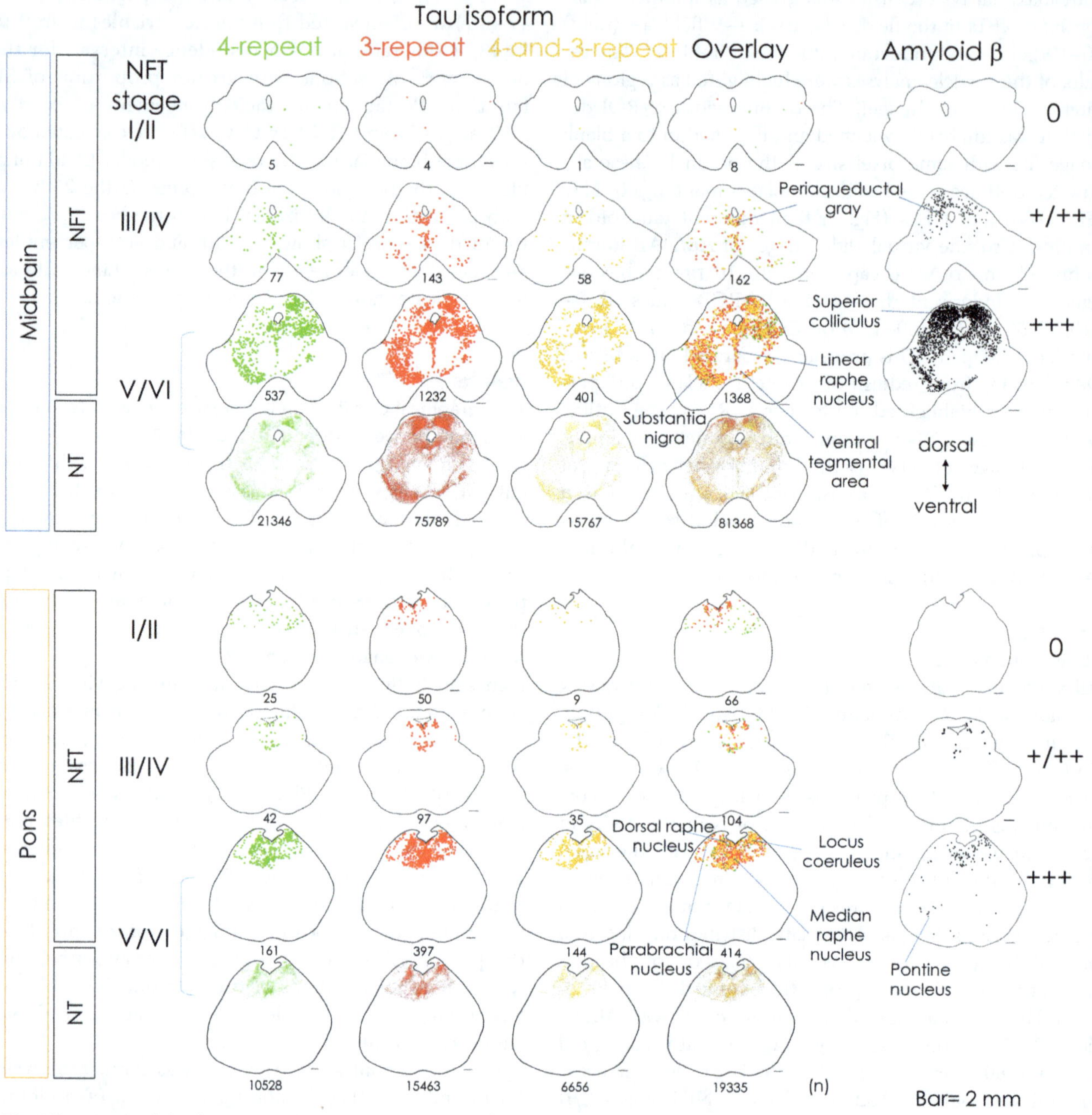

Fig. 2 Topographical distribution is similar between NTs and NFTs, and between 4R and 3R tau. Representative immunolabel mapping of the tau deposition in separate isoform profiles (4R tau-positive/*green*, 3R tau-positive/*red*, 4R/3R tau both-positive/*yellow*), overlays, and amyloid β (Aβ, *black*). The number indicates the sum of immunolabels on each section. From top to bottom: the midbrain of case 5, 10, and 23, and the pons of case 3, 10, 23, with cortical NFT stages I/II, III/IV, V/VI, and the amount of local Aβ deposition of 0, +/++, +++, respectively. Bar = 2 mm. The dot sizes are irrelevant to the scale. Topographical distribution did not differ considerably between NFTs and NTs, and between tau isoform profiles. However, tau and Aβ deposits were different in their distribution, i.e.; at the periaqueductal gray (PAG, ventral-half vs. dorsal-half dominance in case 10), linear raphe nucleus (LRN), and dorsal raphe nucleus (DRN) (abundant tau deposition vs. few Aβ in cases 10 and 23)

Total counts of neurofibrillary changes increase with disease progression (Fig. 3)

We assessed whether the total counts of neurofibrillary changes in the brainstem increase with disease progression (Fig. 3a *a-d*, b *a-d*). Jonckheere's one-sided test for increasing trend generally revealed significant increasing trends of the total counts of NTs and NFTs, with advancing age and Alzheimer-related cortical pathologies; i.e., cortical NFT stage, CERAD neuritic plaque score, and brain weight reduction (Fig. 3a *a-d*, b *a-d*, $p < 0.05$), apart from a minor exception (Fig. 3a *d*, the count of the midbrain

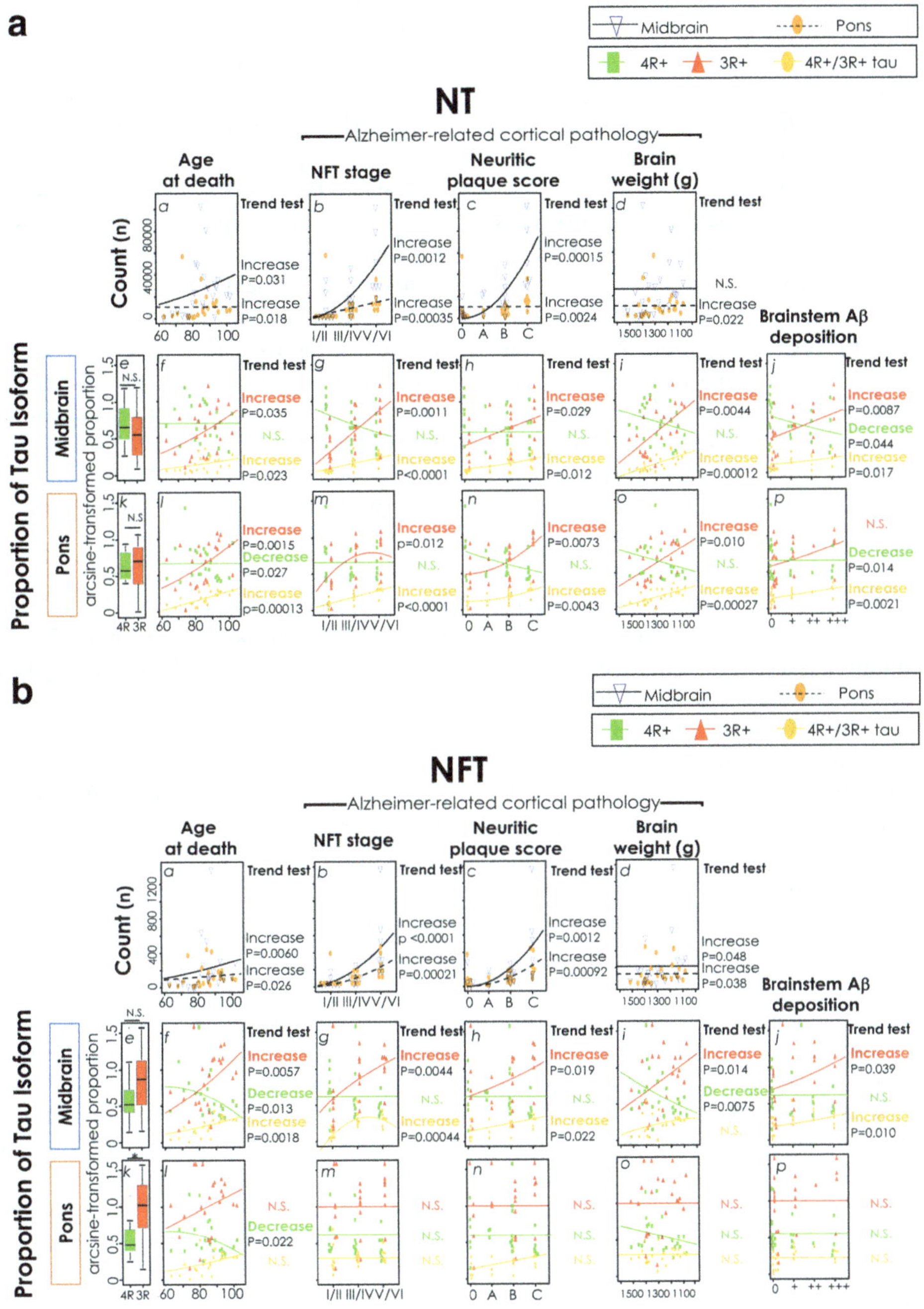

Fig. 3 The proportion of 3R tau-positive midbrain NFTs progressively increases with disease progression, while that of pontine NFT is persistently dominant over 4R tau. (**a** *a-d*, **b** *a-d*) The plots and best-fitted regression curves/lines of total counts of the NTs (**a** *a-d*) and NFTs (**b** *a-d*) against age at death, and Alzheimer-related cortical pathologies of the individual cases: i.e., cortical NFT stage, CERAD neuritic plaque score, and brain weight (descending order). Midbrain (*navy triangle*) and pons (*orange oval*). P-values of the Jonckheere's one-sided test for the orderly increasing or decreasing trend are indicated at the *right* side of the regression models when $p < 0.05$. N.S.: not significant. The total counts significantly increased with advancing age and Alzheimer-related cortical pathologies, with minor exception (**a** *d*, the count of the midbrain NTs against brain weight reduction, Jonckheere's trend test, $p = 0.054$). (**a** *e, k*, **b** *e, k*) *Box plots* of the arcsine-transformed proportion of 4R (*green*) and 3R (*red*) tau-positive lesions. Only pontine NFTs showed significantly higher overall mean of the proportion of 3R tau-positive lesions than that of the 4R tau ($p = 0.0093$ (*), paired t-test with Bonferroni correction). (**a** *f-j, l-p*, **b** *f-j, l-p*) Plots of arcsine-transformed proportion (4R tau/*green rectangle*, 3R tau/*red triangle*, 4R/3R tau both-positive/*yellow oval*) against age at death, cortical NFT stage, CERAD neuritic plaque score, brain weight (in inverse order), and the degree of local Aβ deposition at the midbrain and pons, with best-fitted regression models. *P*-values of Jonckheere's trend test are noted when $p < 0.05$ (from *top* to *bottom* on the *right side* of each panel; 3R tau-positive/*red*, 4R tau-positive/*green*, 4R/3R tau both-positive/*yellow*). The proportion of 3R tau-positive and/or 4R/3R tau both-positive lesions showed significant increasing trends with advancing age and Alzheimer-related cortical pathologies, as well as local Aβ deposition, except for those of pontine NFTs, which remained stably elevated (**b** *l-p*)

NTs against brain weight reduction, Jonckheere's trend test, $p = 0.054$).

The proportion of 3R tau-positive midbrain NFTs gradually increases to be dominant along disease progression, while that of pontine NFTs is persistently elevated (Fig. 3)

To see which of the tau isoforms contributes to the increase of total counts of neurofibrillary changes with disease progression, we calculated the proportion of 4R and 3R tau-positive neurofibrillary changes to the total, and compared their overall means by paired t-test (Fig. 3a *e, k*, b *e, k*). The overall mean of the proportion of 3R tau-positive pontine NFTs (Fig. 3b *k*, red box plot) was significantly higher than that of 4R tau (Fig. 3b *k*, green box plot, paired t-test with Bonferroni correction, $p = 0.0093$), while the difference was not significant for the NTs of the midbrain and pons (Fig. 3a *e, k*) and the NFTs of the midbrain (Fig. 3b *e*) (paired t-test with Bonferroni correction, $p = 1.0$, 1.0 and 0.68, respectively).

We next assessed whether the proportion of 4R and 3R tau-positive NTs and NFTs alter with disease progression at the midbrain and pons. Jonckheere's one-sided test for increasing or decreasing trend (detailed in method) revealed that the NTs of the midbrain and pons and the NFTs of the midbrain showed significant increasing trends in the proportion of 3R tau-positive lesion with advancing age (Fig. 3a *f, l*, b *f*), NFT stage (Fig. 3a *g, m*, b *g*), CERAD neuritic plaque score (Fig. 3a *h, n*, b *h*), and reducing brain weight (Fig. 3a *i, o*, b *i*). Furthermore, in the subgroups of very-old age (age 91-), advanced NFT stages (V/VI) and low brain weight (below 1200 g), paired t-test revealed that the mean of the proportion of 3R tau-positive midbrain NFT was significantly higher than that of 4R tau (paired t-test with Bonferroni correction, $p = 0.0017$, 0.033, 0.0017, respectively, detailed in Additional file 1), indicating that the proportion of 3R tau-positive midbrain NFTs progressively increases and dominates over that of 4R tau in the advanced phase. The proportion of 4R/3R tau both-positive lesion also showed significant increasing trend for NTs of the midbrain and pons (Fig. 3a *f-j, l-p*) and the NFTs of the midbrain (Fig. 3b *f-j*), with advancing age and Alzheimer-related pathologies, with a minor exception (midbrain NFT against brain weight reduction, Fig. 3b *i*, Jonckheere's trend test, $p = 0.061$).

On the other hand, the pontine NFTs did not show any increasing or decreasing trend for the proportion of 3R tau or 4R/3R tau both positive lesions (Fig. 3b *l-p*) on Jonckheere's trend test. Together with the result of paired t-test (Fig. 3b *k*), this result indicated that the proportion of 3R tau-positive pontine NFTs were persistently elevated from younger age and early phase of the disease.

Taken together, these findings indicated that, along the increase in the total count of neurofibrillary changes, the proportion of 3R tau-positive midbrain NFTs increased with disease progression and became significantly higher than that of 4R tau in advanced disease subgroups, while the proportion of 3R tau-positive pontine NFTs remained stably elevated from the early phase.

RD4 and RD3 DAB immunohistochemistry (Fig. 4)

The adjacent sections taken from the same tissue blocks as the representative sections depicted in Fig. 2 were subjected to single DAB immunohistochemistry with RD4 or RD3 antibodies to assess the reproducibility of the observation by immunofluorescence. DAB immunohistochemistry of these representative sections was in line with the finding based on immunofluorescence that the proportion of 3R tau positive NFTs in the midbrain increased with advancing NFT stages, while the proportion of 3R tau positive NFTs in the pons was high already in early stages.

Topographical distribution of neurofibrillary changes on the midbrain and pontine sections (Fig. 5)

We next aimed to clarify the topographical distribution of neurofibrillary changes on the midbrain and pontine sections from 23 cases (Table 1, Fig. 5). In 80% of the cases with NFT stages III-VI (Table 1, 12 out of 15 cases), neurofibrillary changes affected the ventral half of PAG more severely (Fig. 5a, b, open arrows) than the dorsal counterpart (Fig. 5a, b, solid arrows, $p = 0.000011$, Fisher's exact test). By comparison to KB-stained section (Fig. 5d, nearby section of Fig. 5b), the ventral predilection sites of neurofibrillary changes at the PAG were rich in large neurons of DRN (Fig. 5d, open arrow), while the dorsal counterparts were rich in smaller neurons (Fig. 5d, solid arrow). At the midbrain (Fig. 5a, Table 1), the neurofibrillary changes were also accentuated at the LRN (Fig. 5a, open arrowhead), ventral tegemental area, and SN (Fig. 5a, solid arrowhead). At the pons, the neurofibrillary changes were accentuated at the LC (Fig. 5c, open arrows), DRN (Fig. 5c, open arrowheads), MRN (Fig. 5c, solid arrowheads), and parabrachial nucleus (also Table 1).

Progressive accumulation of Aβ deposits is not topographically parallel to tau deposits (Fig. 6)

Next, we compared the topographical distribution of Aβ deposits to that of tau on neighboring sections at the midbrain and pons. Aβ deposits at the midbrain (Fig. 6a-d) and pons (Fig. 6e-g) showed various morphologies. Fleecy amyloid deposits [50] surrounded some of the capillary walls (Fig. 6d). The amount of Aβ deposits was associated with increasing trends of NFT stages (Jonckheere's trend test, $p = 0.00018$ and 0.00037, for midbrain and pons, respectively, Fig. 6h). However, only 57% of investigated cases showed Aβ deposits at either or both the

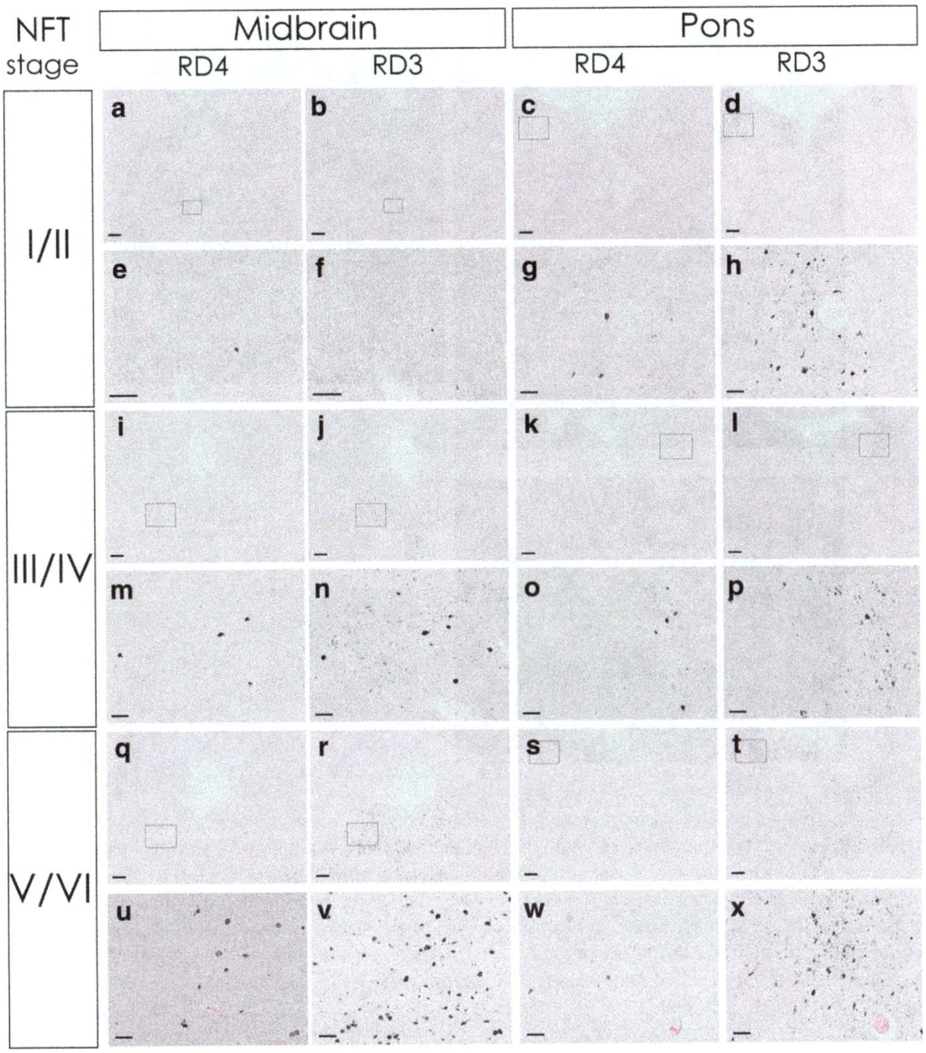

Fig. 4 RD4 and RD3 DAB immunohistochemistry. Representative adjacent sections of the same cases as those shown in Fig. 2 underwent DAB immunohistochemistry with RD4 or RD3. From top to bottom: the midbrain of case 5, 10, and 23, and the pons of case 3, 10, 23, with cortical NFT stages I/II, III/IV, V/VI, respectively. Insets in the images above (**a-d**, **i-l**, **q-t**) correspond to the area shown in the images below (**e-h**, **m-p**, **u-x**) for each section. The results of DAB immunohistochemistry were in line with the findings based on immunofluorescence that the proportion of 3R tau positive NFTs in the midbrain increased with advancing NFT stages while the proportion of 3R tau positive NFTs in the pons was high already in early stages. Scale bar = 500 μm (**a-d**, **i-l**, **q-t**), 100 μm (**e-h**, **m-p**, **u-x**)

midbrain and pons (Table 1, Fig. 6i, 0% of the cases with NFT stages I/II, 87.5% of stages III/IV and 86% of stages V/VI). For example, case 21, with cortical NFT stages V/VI and CERAD neuritic plaque score 0 (Table 1), exhibited AT8-positive neurofibrillary changes at the midbrain and pons (Fig. 6j, LC), but no Aβ deposits on the neighboring sections (Fig. 6k).

When present, the SC (Fig. 6l, m, open arrowheads) was the most severely affected region of all investigated areas by Aβ deposition (Table 1), and the predilection sites included the LC (Fig. 6n, open arrow), MRN (Fig. 6n, solid arrowhead), and RF (Fig. 6n). Lesions in RN and pontine base were only sparsely detected even in advanced cases. The subnucleus medialis of the PAG (Fig. 6l, m, solid arrowheads), which surrounds the aqueduct, did not show Aβ deposition in the investigated cases.

The predilection sites of Aβ deposition differed considerably from those of tau (Table 1, Fig. 2) at the PAG, DRN, LRN, and SN, as described below. The Aβ deposition affected the dorsal PAG more severely (Fig. 6l, solid arrow) than the ventral counterpart (Fig. 6l, open arrow) in 9 out of 9 cases with any deposition therein (p = 0.000041, Fisher's exact test). This dorsal predilection of Aβ at the PAG dissociated from the ventral predilection of tau deposits (Fig. 5a, b, open arrows). Also, at the DRN and LRN, where tau deposits were abundant, the Aβ deposits were rarely detected (Table 1). Finally, medial half of the SN was affected by the Aβ deposition more severely

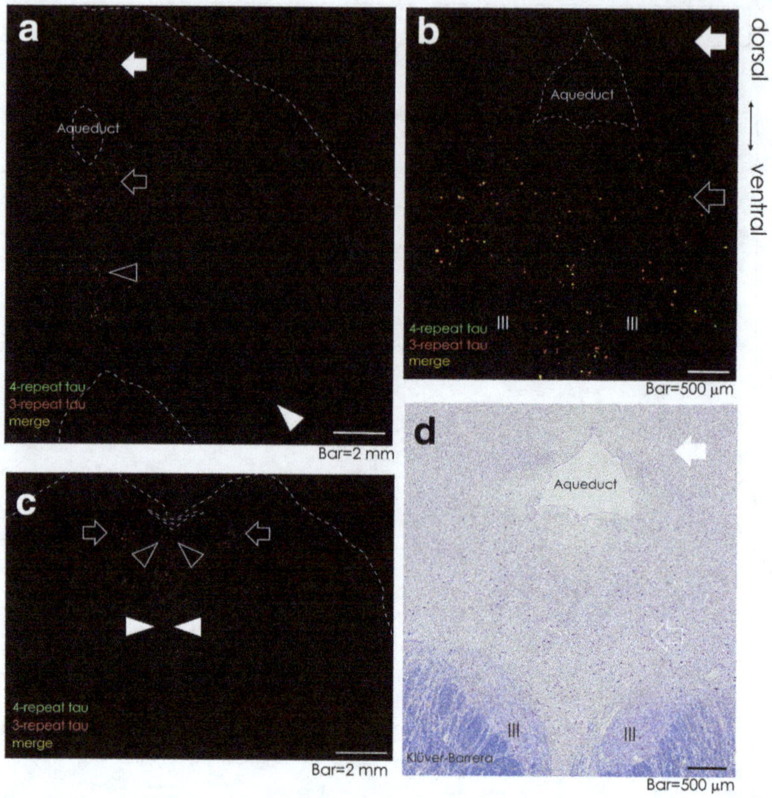

Fig. 5 Topographical distribution of neurofibrillary changes at the midbrain and pons. Representative virtual slide images double-immunofluorolabeled with anti-4R (*green*) and 3R (*red*) tau, with colocalization (*yellow*) on overlays, of the midbrain (**a**, **b**, case 18 and 10, respectively) and pons (**c**, case 18). At the midbrain, the neurofibrillary changes were accentuated at the ventral PAG (**a**, **b**, *open arrow*), LRN (**a**, *open arrowhead*), and substantia nigra (SN, **a**, *solid arrowhead*). The neurofibrillary changes often affected the ventral half of the PAG (**a**, **b**, *open arrows*) more severely than the dorsal half (**a**, **b**, *solid arrows*). By comparison to KB-stained section (**d**, case 10, nearby section to **b**), the lesions in the ventral PAG coincided with the area where the large neurons of DRN were present (**d**, *open arrow*). The oculomotor nuclei (**b**, **d**, III) were not involved with neurofibrillary changes. At the pons, the neurofibrillary changes were accentuated at the LC (**c**, *open arrows*), DRN (**c**, *open arrowheads*), and median raphe nucleus (MRN, **c**, *solid arrowheads*). Scale bar = 2 mm (**a**, **c**), and 500 μm (**b**, **d**)

than the lateral half in 6 out of 8 cases with any deposits therein (75%, $p = 0.0070$, Fisher's exact test), while the amount of tau deposits was not significantly different between medial and lateral SN ($p = 1.0$, Fisher's exact test).

Taken together, the Aβ deposition at the midbrain or pons was absent in all the cases with NFT stages I/II, although gradually increased to be present in 86% of stages V/VI. When present, the predilection sites of Aβ deposition included the SC, PAG (dorsal half-dominant), SN (medial half-dominant), LC, RF, and MRN. On the other hand, the ventral half of the PAG, DRN and LRN, which were the areas in which neurofibrillary changes were abundant, were much less intensely affected by Aβ deposition. These differences in distribution suggested that the tau and Aβ deposition may occur independently of one another at least to some extent.

Discussions

In this study, we performed virtual-slide based comprehensive quantitative analyses on double-immunofluorolabeled sections of midbrain and pons for 4R and 3R tau, and clarified that the proportion of 3R tau-positive midbrain NFTs progressively increased (Fig. 3b *e-i*) and dominated in the advanced disease phase, while that of pontine NFT persistently dominated over 4R tau (Fig. 3b *k-o*). The obtained results suggested a possibility that the dominant immunoreactive epitopes of tau isoform is changing along disease progression in neurofibrillary changes, even after their formation.

For tau-isoform specific immunolabeling, two monoclonal antibodies, RD3 and RD4, have been used as the standard. However, RD3 and RD4 are both monoclonal antibodies raised in mouse, which hampers their distinction if anti-mouse secondary antibodies are used for their fluorodetection. Double labeling with two unconjugated primary antibodies raised in the same host species is difficult to achieve, and requires unconventional procedures. To circumvent this cross talk, our group performed double immunofluorolabeling with RD3 and RD4 in the previous studies by a combination of

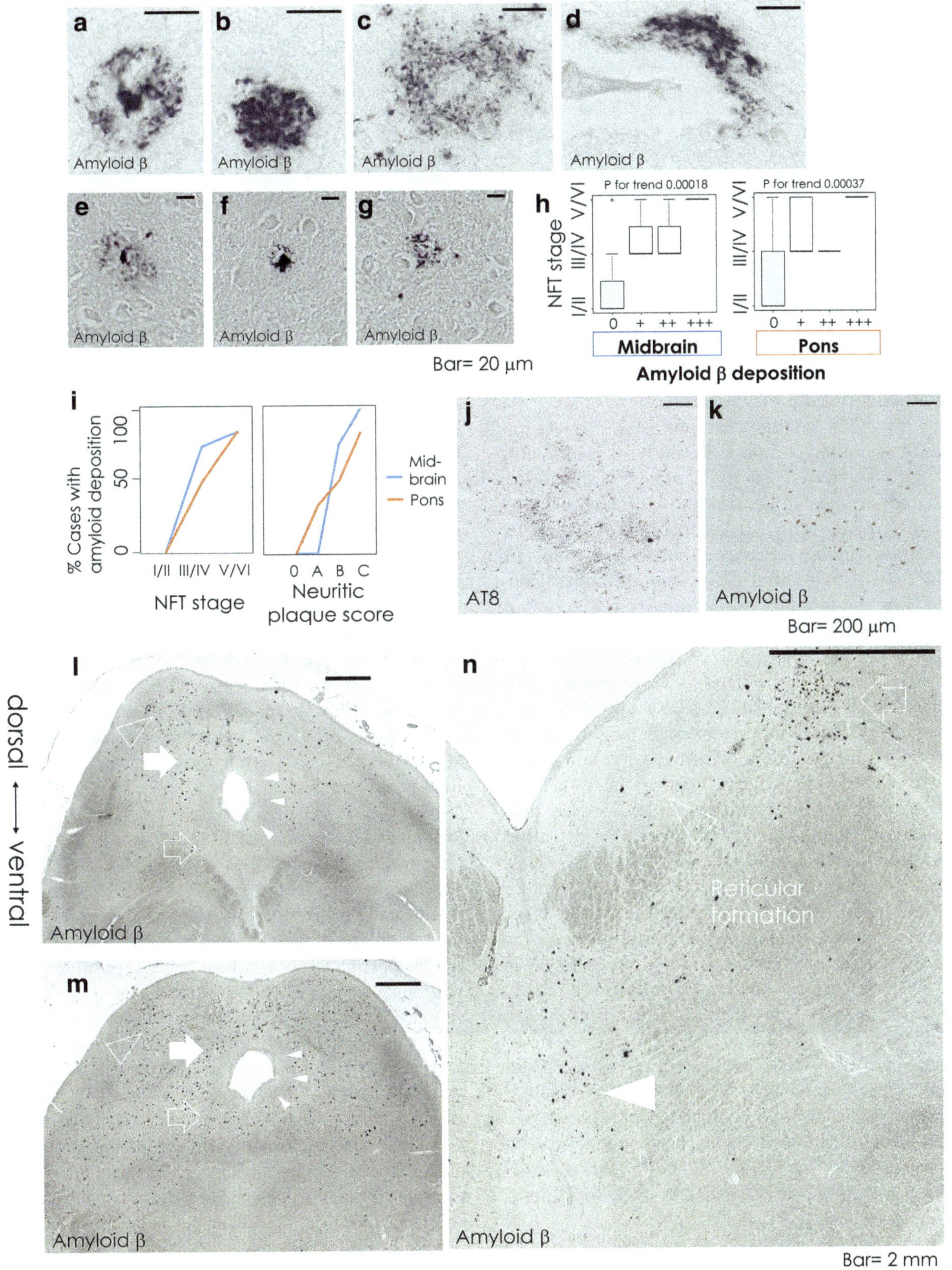

Fig. 6 (See legend on next page.)

(See figure on previous page.)

Fig. 6 Progressive accumulation of Aβ deposits is not topographically parallel to tau deposits. **a-g** Representative midbrain (**a-d**, case 23, SC) and pontine section (**e-g**, case 23, pontine nucleus), stained with Aβ/DAB. As Iseki et al. have described [27], Aβ deposits showed various morphologies; e.g., amyloid plaques type 1 (**a**, **e**, *'amyloid core with surrounding processes'*), type 2 (**b**, **f**, *'amorphous amyloid with surrounding processes'*), and type 3 (**c**, **g**, *'ill-defined aggregation of the fine processes'*). Fleecy amyloid deposits [50] surrounded a capillary wall (d). Scale bar = 20 μm. (**h**) Box plots of the cortical NFT stages in different degrees of local Aβ deposition at the midbrain (*left* panel) and pons (*right* panel). **i** Percentages of the cases with Aβ deposition at the midbrain (*blue*) and pons (*orange*) with advancing NFT stages (*left* panel) and CERAD neuritic plaque score (*right* panel). **j**, **k** DAB staining of AT8 (**j**) and Aβ (**k**) immunohistochemistry at the LC (case 21) showed absence of Aβ in the presence of tau deposition in this case. Bar = 200 μm. **l-n** Aβ/DAB-stained sections of the midbrain (**l**, **m**, cases 10 and 23, respectively) and pons (**n**, case 22) showed dorsal predilection of Aβ deposition at the PAG (l, *solid arrow*), which was dissociated from the ventral predilection of tau deposition (Fig. 5a, b, *open arrows*). The SC (**l**, **m**, *open arrowheads*) showed abundant Aβ deposition. The subnucleus medialis (**l**, **m**, *solid arrowheads*) was free of Aβ depositions. Bar = 2 mm. LC (**n**, *open arrow*), MRN (**n**, *solid arrowhead*) and reticular formation (**n**) showed involvement with Aβ deposition. Lesions in the DRN (**n**, *open arrowhead*) were only sparsely detected. Bar = 2 mm

tyramide signal amplification (TSA) of the hyper-diluted RD3, followed by conventional immunofluorolabeling of the RD4 [21, 54]. Although this double labeling by the TSA method enabled precise quantification of RD3/RD4 labeling on NFTs on hippocampus [21], the staining procedure is rather complex. Recently, a rabbit polyclonal antibody raised against 4-repeat tau, which is deamidated at asparagine residue 279, has been reported to strongly stain tau lesions in the Alzheimer's disease brain without cross reaction with 3R tau [10]. Introduction of this rabbit polyclonal antibody against 4R tau for the double immunofluorolabeling along with the mouse monoclonal antibody RD3 is much more simple and straightforward, because these antibodies are raised in different host species. The amount of DAB immunolabeling with polyclonal anti-4R tau (1:30,000) was equivalent to or slightly greater than the amount of immunolabeling with monoclonal RD4 (1:1000, Additional file 4: Figure S3).

The prevalence of each isoform can be precisely demonstrated by immunohistochemistry via brightfield chromogenic detection such as DAB [28, 34, 35]. However, DAB labeling is convincing if only single epitope (3R or 4R tau) is evaluated. Comparison of adjacent sections may identify double labeled lesion (3R and 4R tau) only if the targets are large enough as NFTs to be included in both sections. In this study, however, we also aimed to examine NTs for their sizes and isoform profiles (3R and 4R tau). Because the threads are much smaller than NFTs, exact identification of isoform profile (3R only, 3/4 R both positive, 4R only) on such small target is not feasible through comparison of adjacent sections, or bright-field dual-color chromogenic labeling. Thus, colocalization of 4R and 3R tau isoforms on the thread is accurately distinguishable only with multi-immunofluorolabeling [21, 23, 54].

Complete ENumeration and Sorting for Unlimited Sectors (CENSUS) via immunofluorescence

Because our CENSUS approach standardizes the acquisition condition of fluorescence microscopic images and operationally picks up all the immunopositive lesions contained in the histological sections (Fig. 1), the data sets, once obtained, can be arbitrarily processed for size quantification (Fig. 1), mapping based on XY coordinates (Figs. 1, 2), calculations of the proportion of isoform (Fig. 3), and their possible relation to disease progression can be demonstrated (Fig. 3). This CENSUS fundamentally changed conventional morphometric approaches, usually calculating local density of predefined ROIs, to test whether the results corroborate the predefined working hypothesis. Moreover, local density of a lesion may be influenced by the atrophy of the target structure and overall neuronal loss [52]. For example, an increase in the lesion density may be accentuated if the entire structure is atrophied, even when the count number remained relatively unchanged. Because CENSUS approach picks up all the lesions in the section, interpretation is much more straightforward than conventional ROI-based approach.

Progressive dominance of 3R tau lesions in the postmortem brainstem

Previous reports showed that the NFTs matures morphologically from 4R tau dominant pretangles to 3R tau dominant ghost tangles in the hippocampus, and that the proportion of 3R tau-positive neurofibrillary changes was higher in the hippocampal subregions with advanced neurofibrillary pathology than those involved in later stage [21, 28, 34, 35, 54]. Thus, it is hypothesized that this tau-isoform transition during the morphological maturation of the NFT is orchestrated to form the regional progression of 3R tau dominance in the hippocampus along the perforant path containing unidirectional hippocampal circuitry, beginning in the entorhinal and transentorhinal cortices, subsequently progressing to the subiculum and CA1, and further to CA 3–4 [21]. In the previous studies, however, the effect of disease progression on tau isoform prevalence was not fully evaluated [21, 28, 34, 35].

In this study, we enrolled sufficient number of samples to evaluate the effect of disease progression, and by employing CENSUS approach, we clarified that the proportion of 3R tau-positive NFTs in the midbrain and the NTs in the midbrain and pons gradually increased with advancing Alzheimer-related cortical pathology (Fig. 3a *f-i*, *l-o*, b *f-i*). This gradual increase in the proportion of 3R tau probably explain why there was not a significant difference between the overall means of the proportion of 4R and 3R tau in these neurofibrillary changes (Fig. 3a *e*, *k*, b *e*, paired t-test). On the other hand, the overall mean of the proportion of 3R tau-positive pontine NFT was significantly higher than that of 4R tau (Fig. 3b *k*) and it was stably elevated along disease progression (Fig. 3b *l-o*, Jonckheere's trend test), indicating that the proportion of 3R tau-positive NFTs was persistently dominant in the pons but not in the midbrain. This difference does not necessarily indicate that the mechanism of tau deposition is different between pons and midbrain. Rather, this difference is explained if pontine neurons are liable to develop neurofibrillary changes from earlier stage than midbrain neurons. It is then expected that similar progressive dominance in 3R tau may be detectable if pontine samples from younger individuals are included, which is a subject for future studies. If regional gradient of isoform around hippocampus is oriented along a defined major circuity such as performant path, what kind of circuitries in the brainstem are responsible for the gradient? Because neuroanatomical connections in the brainstem are much more complex [4, 39, 40, 42] than that of the hippocampus, it is practically impossible to identify possible candidate circuitries in the brainstem, if any, that may account for such gradient. It is also possible that isoform regulation could be independent of the circuit and each neuron may regulate tau isoforms independently of each other, which needs fundamental reconsiderations in the future studies. Although preceding studies have suggested that the earliest neurofibrillary lesions are detected in the brainstem [6, 19, 46], it is difficult to directly compare the extent of 3R tau dominance between different anatomical structures, because the densities and characteristics of the underlying neuronal population are quite different. Therefore, we focused on the trend of increase for the proportion of RD3 at the coordinated horizontal anatomical levels between cases, rather than direct comparison between the data of the midbrain and pons or between the data of the brainstem and the hippocampus (Additional file 5: Figure S4), and did not attempt to show that brainstem tau lesions develop prior to hippocampus in this study. Rather, we demonstrated that the progressive accumulation of 3R tau over 4R tau is shared between brainstem and the hippocampus.

Biochemical evaluation for 3R and 4R tau by immunoblotting may be potentially interesting and helpful in the future studies. However, considering the small number of NFTs in the AD brainstem, such experiment may require significant numbers and sufficient volume of precious frozen samples from the brainstem (at least midbrain and pontine tegmentum), which are not readily available.

What triggers the increase of the proportion of 3R tau-positive neurofibrillary changes with disease progression?

What are the possible mechanisms that regulate isoform-dependent deposition of tau in each neuron? If progressive increase of 3R tau in Alzheimer-type NFT mirrors relative abundance of 3R tau molecule or of its production, it is expected that the amount of mRNA is progressively upregulated in relevant areas. Although data on the brainstem have not been reported, mRNA of 3R tau is not upregulated in AD brains and in normal controls [8, 15, 26, 36, 58]. This raises a possibility that some post-translational modifications of 4R and 3R tau and their interactions may be responsible for such progressive representation of 3R tau over 4R tau. For example, in vitro assembly of 4R tau is significantly decreased by coincubation with 3R tau [1]. Another in vitro study has demonstrated that 4R and 3R tau monomers can grow onto the 4R/3R tau filaments and/or 3R tau filaments, while only 4R tau monomers can grow onto 4R tau filaments [12]. Do the aggregates composed of 4R and 3R tau exhibit corresponding immunoreactivity to both 4R and 3R tau? If an excess of one isoform over the other in the aggregates results in conformational alteration of tau molecules, epitope representation of each isoform could be skewed as if one of the two were absent, even if it is still integrated in the aggregates. Moreover, recent studies on mass spectrometric analyses of sarkosyl-insoluble and protease-resistant tau filaments from human brain with AD and cryo-electron microscopic analyses demonstrated that the protease-resistant cores of tau filaments contained abundant residues of the exon 11–12, which is proposed to adopt a combined cross- β/ β-helix structure with two identical protofilaments, as well as over a dozen of residues on the C-terminal side of exon 10 (4R tau) and exon 9 (3R tau), which exhibit unsharpened density on cryo-electron microscopy like a less ordered β-sheet [14, 48]. These results were compatible with the peptides identified in earlier studies, although there were some variations in the residue length [30, 57]. Still, it is unknown whether these C-terminal fragmentation of tau filaments occurs physiologically to the neurofibrillary changes in vivo. Even if the protease-resistant cores of tau filament are fundamental structures for neurofibrillary changes, how they are related to tau isoforms remains to be clarified because epitopes specific to tau isoforms were not included in the protofilament, a principal constituent of the protease-resistant cores. Because representation of each isoform is modified by aggregation, conformation and fragmentation, which epitopes of tau isoforms are involved in different tau filaments in the human brains may be crucial.

By taking advantage of the dual visibility of quantum dot (fluorescent nanocrystal identifiable also on electron microscopy) used as immunolabeling, we developed a method to correlate fluorescent microscopic images with their exact counterpart on immunoelectron microscopy [33, 49, 55]. This approach will clarify how either 4R or 3R tau epitope is involved in the formation of tau filaments at different stages of their formation in vivo. As double-immunofluorolabeling for 4R and 3R tau successfully demonstrated relationship between the isoforms at light microscopy level, we are now trying to improve this immunoelectron microscopy so that two different epitopes for 4R and 3R tau are visualized in relation to tau filaments of different morphologies and stages. It is expected that in vivo relation between 4R and 3R tau will be better understood if this double-labeling immunoelectron microscopy is successful for tau filaments.

Discrepancies in the topographical distribution of tau and Aβ deposition

In the present study, the neurofibrillary changes were present without nearby Aβ in 43% of the cases (Table 1). Such discrepancy between tau and Aβ deposition is attracting an increasing attention [3, 7, 9, 13]. Regional distribution of tau [41] and that of Aβ [27, 51] in the brainstem have also been described. Because these had been described separately, it was not clear how tau and Aβ deposits are spatially related. The present study is the first that compared distribution of tau and Aβ deposits directly in neighboring sections of the same cases at different stages of disease progression (Figs. 2, 5, 6). The neurofibrillary changes were frequent in the ventral half of the PAG (Fig. 5a, b, open arrows), while the Aβ deposition was frequent in its dorsal half (Fig. 6l, solid arrow). Although there was an increase in the proportion of 3R tau-positive midbrain neurofibrillary changes with advancing neuritic plaque score (Fig. 3a *h*, *n*, b *h*), Aβ deposition was not directly linked to this increase of neurofibrillary changes, because their distributions were discrepant in the brainstem (Figs. 2, 5, 6). The most striking example of such discrepancy was detected in a case of centenarian (102 years old, case 21, Table 1), which showed a clinical history of dementia, 3R tau-dominant brainstem NFTs, NFT stages V/VI, but neuritic plaque score 0 and the absence of Aβ deposition at the midbrain and pons (Fig. 6k). Taken together, our observations suggested that the tau deposition and the progressive dominance of 3R tau-positive lesions may occur independently of Aβ deposition in the human brainstem at least to some extent.

Conclusions

In conclusion, we have shown that a progressive increase in the proportion of 3R tau-positive lesions is extended to brainstem lesions as a fundamental to the pathogenesis of AD. The topographical differences between tau and Aβ deposits suggested that the formation of neurofibrillary changes and the increase in the proportion of 3R tau-positive lesions occur independently of regional Aβ deposition in the brainstem. In the future, ultrastructural localization of tau isoforms in relation to their filaments may clarify how changing proportion of isoforms are related to different stages of neurofibrillary changes, undertaking evolutionary changes from pretangles to ghost tangles.

Additional files

Additional file 1: This file contains additional description of the image acquisition, and concomitant Lewy pathology of the investigated cases. The file also contains the results of additional statistical studies, including the regional difference in the proportion of 3R tau positive neurofibrillary changes on the same horizontal levels of the brainstem. (DOCX 25 kb)

Additional file 2: Figure S1. Quenching of autofluorescence after Sudan Black B treatment. Autofluorescence of intraneuronal lipofuscin is known to be prominent in the brainstem when quenching treatment is not performed. To clarify the effect of Sudan Black B treatment, we measured fluorescence emission spectra of intraneuronal lipofuscin on formalin-fixed, paraffin-embedded midbrain sections using Zeiss LSM780 lambda mode with or without the Sudan Black B treatment. The fluorescence spectrum of lipofuscin with excitation at 488 nm was broad and gently sloping (a-e, emission peak at 591 nm). This very intense fluorescence with broad spectrum agreed with the preceding studies on the fluorescence of lipofuscin. Sudan Black B treatment eliminated this autofluorescence of the lipofuscin (f-j, adjacent section). The fluorescence spectrum of lipofuscin did not overlap with the fluorescence spectra of Alexa 488- and Alexa 568-conjugated secondary antibodies labeling anti-4R tau antibody and RD3, respectively, on the pontine section, which underwent the Sudan Black B treatment (k-o). The small peak around 600 nm with excitation at 488 nm corresponded to colocalized Alexa 568 signal, which was blocked by the dichroic mirror on image capturing of the Alexa 488 signal. Therefore, we concluded that the autofluorescence of lipofuscin was effectively quenched by Sudan black treatment and did not affect the result of our study. Em: emission, Ex: excitation. (TIFF 7768 kb)

Additional file 3: Figure S2. Representative partial virtual slide images of the midbrain and pontine sections double immunofluorolabeled for 4R (green) and 3R tau (red), with colocalization (yellow). From top to bottom; case 7, 9, 18, in NFT stages I/II, III/IV, and V/VI, respectively. Insets in the low power field images (left row) correspond to the magnified images (right row). Bar = 200 μm and 50 μm, respectively. (TIFF 2019 kb)

Additional file 4: Figure S3. Comparable tau immunolabeling with two antibodies RD4 (monoclonal) and 4R tau (polyclonal). DAB immunohistochemistry using rabbit polyclonal anti-4R tau (a, 1:30,000 dilution) and mouse monoclonal RD4 (b, 1:1000 dilution) on adjacent hippocampal sections showed that the amount of immunolabeling with rabbit polyclonal anti-4R tau was equivalent to or slightly greater than the amount of immunolabeling with mouse monoclonal RD4. (TIFF 6926 kb)

Additional file 5: Figure S4. Predominance of RD3+ NFTs over RD4+ NFTs is shared between brainstem and hippocampus. To see whether the same trend of RD3 dominance for the neurofibrillary changes over RD4 is also demonstrated by the conventional DAB immunohistochemistry, we performed quantification of the RD3 and RD4 levels on representative adjacent pontine and hippocampal sections. After thresholding of the DAB labeling by RGB values, the counts and sizes of RD3 and RD4 were calculated on CellSens software (Olympus). RD3/RD4 ratio of total NFT counts and area on the pontine section were 6.00 and 4.49, respectively, indicating more intense deposition of RD3-positive neurofibrillary changes than RD4 (a, c, case 17). While the difference in the methods used make direct comparisons difficult, this observation of RD3 dominance agreed with our double-immunofluorolabeling of the same case using anti-4R tau antibody and RD3. RD3/RD4 ratio of total NFT counts and area on the hippocampal sections were 25.6 and 34.3, respectively. Thus, the dominance of 3R tau was also detected for the neurofibrillary changes in the hippocampal area of the same case (b, d, case 17). (TIFF 3761 kb)

Acknowledgements
This work was supported by Grant-in-Aid for JSPS KAKENHI Grant Numbers 17H03555 (TU), 16 K14572 (TU) and 14 J04872 (MU, as DC1 fellow of JSPS). We are grateful to Dr. Junjiro Horiuchi (Tokyo Metropolitan Institute of Medical Science) for critically reading this manuscript, and to Professor Yasuo Ohashi, PhD (Statcom Co., Ltd., Tokyo, Japan, Department of Integrated Science and Engineering for Sustainable Society, Faculty of Science and Engineering, Chuo University, Tokyo, Japan) for the advice on statistical analyses.

Authors' contributions
MU and TU designed the experiments, interpreted the data and wrote the manuscript. MU performed the experiments and analyzed the data. AN and ME gave technical support and advice. KH provided patient samples and information. KH and RT critically read and revised the manuscript. All authors read and approved the final manuscript.

Competing interests
The authors declare that they have no competing interests.

Author details
[1]Laboratory of Structural Neuropathology, Tokyo Metropolitan Institute of Medical Science, 2-1-6 Kamikitazawa, Setagaya-ku, Tokyo 156-8506, Japan. [2]Department of Neurology, Kyoto University Graduate School of Medicine, Sakyo-ku, Kyoto, Japan. [3]The Japan Society for the Promotion of Science (JSPS), Chiyoda-ku, Tokyo, Japan. [4]Division of Neurology, Department of Medicine, Nihon University School of Medicine, Itabashi-ku, Tokyo, Japan. [5]Department of Pathology, Nitobe-Memorial Nakano General Hospital, Nakano-ku, Tokyo, Japan.

References
1. Adams SJ, DeTure MA, McBride M, Dickson DW, Petrucelli L (2010) Three repeat isoforms of tau inhibit assembly of four repeat tau filaments. PLoS One 5:e10810
2. Attems J, Thomas A, Jellinger K (2012) Correlations between cortical and subcortical tau pathology. Neuropathol Appl Neurobiol 38:582–590
3. Bancher C, Jellinger KA (1994) Neurofibrillary tangle predominant form of senile dementia of Alzheimer type: a rare subtype in very old subjects. Acta Neuropathol 88:565–570
4. Beckstead RM, Domesick VB, Nauta WJ (1979) Efferent connections of the substantia nigra and ventral tegmental area in the rat. Brain Res 175:191–217
5. Braak H, Braak E (1991) Neuropathological stageing of Alzheimer-related changes. Acta Neuropathol 82:239–259
6. Braak H, Del Tredici K (2011) The pathological process underlying Alzheimer's disease in individuals under thirty. Acta Neuropathol 121:171–181
7. Braak H, Del Tredici K (2015) The preclinical phase of the pathological process underlying sporadic Alzheimer's disease. Brain 138:2814–2833
8. Chambers CB, Lee JM, Troncoso JC, Reich S, Muma NA (1999) Overexpression of four-repeat tau mRNA isoforms in progressive supranuclear palsy but not in Alzheimer's disease. Ann Neurol 46:325–332
9. Crary JF, Trojanowski JQ, Schneider JA, Abisambra JF, Abner EL, Alafuzoff I et al (2014) Primary age-related tauopathy (PART): a common pathology associated with human aging. Acta Neuropathol 128:755–766
10. Dan A, Takahashi M, Masuda-Suzukake M, Kametani F, Nonaka T, Kondo H et al (2013) Extensive deamidation at asparagine residue 279 accounts for weak immunoreactivity of tau with RD4 antibody in Alzheimer's disease brain. Acta Neuropathol Commun 1:54
11. de Silva R, Lashley T, Gibb G, Hanger D, Hope A, Reid A et al (2003) Pathological inclusion bodies in tauopathies contain distinct complements of tau with three or four microtubule-binding repeat domains as demonstrated by new specific monoclonal antibodies. Neuropathol Appl Neurobiol 29:288–302
12. Dinkel PD, Siddiqua A, Huynh H, Shah M, Margittai M (2011) Variations in filament conformation dictate seeding barrier between three- and four-repeat tau. Biochemistry 50:4330–4336
13. Duyckaerts C, Braak H, Brion JP, Buée L, Del Tredici K, Goedert M et al (2015) PART is part of Alzheimer disease. Acta Neuropathol 129:749–756
14. Fitzpatrick AWP, Falcon B, He S, Murzin AG, Murshudov G, Garringer HJ et al (2017) Cryo-EM structures of tau filaments from Alzheimer's disease. Nature 547:185–190
15. Ginsberg SD, Che S, Counts SE, Mufson EJ (2006) Shift in the ratio of three-repeat tau and four-repeat tau mRNAs in individual cholinergic basal forebrain neurons in mild cognitive impairment and Alzheimer's disease. J Neurochem 96:1401–1408
16. Goate A, Chartier-Harlin MC, Mullan M, Brown J, Crawford F, Fidani L et al (1991) Segregation of a missense mutation in the amyloid precursor protein gene with familial Alzheimer's disease. Nature 349:704–706
17. Goedert M, Spillantini MG, Potier MC, Ulrich J, Crowther RA (1989) Cloning and sequencing of the cDNA encoding an isoform of microtubule-associated protein tau containing four tandem repeats: differential expression of tau protein mRNAs in human brain. EMBO J 8:393–399
18. Goedert M, Spillantini MG, Cairns NJ, Crowther RA (1992) Tau proteins of Alzheimer paired helical filaments: abnormal phosphorylation of all six brain isoforms. Neuron 8:159–168
19. Grinberg LT, Rüb U, Ferretti RE, Nitrini R, Farfel JM, Polichiso L et al (2009) The dorsal raphe nucleus shows phospho-tau neurofibrillary changes before the transentorhinal region in Alzheimer's disease. A precocious onset? Neuropathol Appl Neurobiol 35:406–416
20. Grundke-Iqbal I, Iqbal K, Tung YC, Quinlan M, Wisniewski HM, Binder LI (1986) Abnormal phosphorylation of the microtubule-associated protein tau (tau) in Alzheimer cytoskeletal pathology. Proc Natl Acad Sci U S A 83:4913–4917
21. Hara M, Hirokawa K, Kamei S, Uchihara T (2013) Isoform transition from four-repeat to three-repeat tau underlies dendrosomatic and regional progression of neurofibrillary pathology. Acta Neuropathol 125:565–579
22. Hasegawa M, Watanabe S, Kondo H, Akiyama H, Mann DM, Saito Y et al (2014) 3R and 4R tau isoforms in paired helical filaments in Alzheimer's disease. Acta Neuropathol 127:303–305
23. Hibbs AR, MacDonald G, Garsha K (2006) Colocalization. In: Pawley J (ed) Handbook of biological confocal microscopy, 3rd edn. Springer, New York, pp 667–669
24. Hirano A, Zimmerman HM (1962) Alzheimer's neurofibrillary changes. A topographic study. Arch Neurol 7:227–242
25. Ihara Y, Nukina N, Miura R, Ogawara M (1986) Phosphorylated tau protein is integrated into paired helical filaments in Alzheimer's disease. J Biochem 99:1807–1810
26. Ingelsson M, Ramasamy K, Russ C, Freeman SH, Orne J, Raju S et al (2007) Increase in the relative expression of tau with four microtubule binding repeat regions in frontotemporal lobar degeneration and progressive supranuclear palsy brains. Acta Neuropathol 114:471–479
27. Iseki E, Matsushita M, Kosaka K, Kondo H, Ishii T, Amano N (1989) Distribution and morphology of brain stem plaques in Alzheimer's disease. Acta Neuropathol 78:131–136
28. Iseki E, Yamamoto R, Murayama N, Minegishi M, Togo T, Katsuse O et al (2006) Immunohistochemical investigation of neurofibrillary tangles and their tau isoforms in brains of limbic neurofibrillary tangle dementia. Neurosci Lett 405:29–33
29. Ishii T (1966) Distribution of Alzheimer's neurofibrillary changes in the brain stem and hypothalamus of senile dementia. Acta Neuropathol 6:181–187
30. Jakes R, Novak M, Davison M, Wischik CM (1991) Identification of 3- and 4-repeat tau isoforms within the PHF in Alzheimer's disease. EMBO J 10:2725–2729

31. Jellinger KA, Attems J (2007) Neurofibrillary tangle-predominant dementia: comparison with classical Alzheimer disease. Acta Neuropathol 113:107–117
32. Jin M, Shepardson N, Yang T, Chen G, Walsh D, Selkoe DJ (2011) Soluble amyloid beta-protein dimers isolated from Alzheimer cortex directly induce tau hyperphosphorylation and neuritic degeneration. Proc Natl Acad Sci U S A 108:5819–5824
33. Kanazawa T, Adachi E, Orimo S, Nakamura A, Mizusawa H, Uchihara T (2012) Pale neurites, premature α-synuclein aggregates with centripetal extension from axon collaterals. Brain Pathol 22:67–78
34. Kitamura T, Sugimori K, Sudo S, Kobayashi K (2005) Relationship between microtubule-binding repeats and morphology of neurofibrillary tangle in Alzheimer's disease. Acta Neurol Scand 112:327–334
35. Lace G, Savva GM, Forster G, de Silva R, Brayne C, Matthews FE et al (2009) Hippocampal tau pathology is related to neuroanatomical connections: an ageing population-based study. Brain 132:1324–1334
36. Majounie E, Cross W, Newsway V, Dillman A, Vandrovcova J, Morris CM et al (2013) Variation in tau isoform expression in different brain regions and disease states. Neurobiol Aging 34:1922 e7-1922.e12
37. McKeith IG, Galasko D, Kosaka K, Perry EK, Dickson DW, Hansen LA et al (1996) Consensus guidelines for the clinical and pathologic diagnosis of dementia with Lewy bodies (DLB): report of the consortium on DLB international workshop. Neurology 47:1113–1124
38. Mirra SS, Heyman A, McKeel D, Sumi SM, Crain BJ, Brownlee LM et al (1991) The consortium to establish a registry for Alzheimer's disease (CERAD). Part II. Standardization of the neuropathologic assessment of Alzheimer's disease. Neurology 41:479–486
39. Pasquier DA, Kemper TL, Forbes WB, Morgane PJ (1977) Dorsal raphe, substantia nigra and locus coeruleus: interconnections with each other and the neostriatum. Brain Res Bull 2:323–339
40. Qi J, Zhang S, Wang HL, Wang H, de Jesus Aceves Buendia J, Hoffman AF et al (2014) A glutamatergic reward input from the dorsal raphe to ventral tegmental area dopamine neurons. Nat Commun 5:5390
41. Rüb U, Stratmann K, Heinsen H, Turco DD, Seidel K, Dunnen W et al (2016) The brainstem tau Cytoskeletal pathology of Alzheimer's disease: a brief historical overview and description of its anatomical distribution pattern, evolutional features, Pathogenetic and clinical relevance. Curr Alzheimer Res 13:1178–1197
42. Samuels ER, Szabadi E (2008) Functional neuroanatomy of the noradrenergic locus coeruleus: its roles in the regulation of arousal and autonomic function part I: principles of functional organisation. Curr Neuropharmacol 6:235–253
43. Sardanelli F, Di Leo G (2009) Variables and measurement scales. In: Biostatistics for radiologists. Springer-Verlag Italia, Milan, pp. 42-44
44. Schnell SA, Staines WA, Wessendorf MW (1999) Reduction of lipofuscin-like autofluorescence in fluorescently labeled tissue. J Histochem Cytochem 47:719–730
45. Sherrington R, Rogaev EI, Liang Y, Rogaeva EA, Levesque G, Ikeda M et al (1995) Cloning of a gene bearing missense mutations in early-onset familial Alzheimer's disease. Nature 375:754–760
46. Simic G, Stanic G, Mladinov M, Jovanov-Milosevic N, Kostovic I, Hof PR (2009) Does Alzheimer's disease begin in the brainstem? Neuropathol Appl Neurobiol 35:532–554
47. Takeda T, Uchihara T, Nakayama Y, Nakamura A, Sasaki S, Kakei S et al (2014) Dendritic retraction, but not atrophy, is consistent in amyotrophic lateral sclerosis-comparison between Onuf's neurons and other sacral motor neurons. Acta Neuropathol Commun 2:11
48. Taniguchi-Watanabe S, Arai T, Kametani F, Nonaka T, Masuda-Suzukake M, Tarutani A et al (2016) Biochemical classification of tauopathies by immunoblot, protein sequence and mass spectrometric analyses of sarkosyl-insoluble and trypsin-resistant tau. Acta Neuropathol 131:267–280
49. Tatsumi S, Uchihara T, Aiba I, Iwasaki Y, Mimuro M, Takahashi R et al (2014) Ultrastructural differences in pretangles between Alzheimer disease and corticobasal degeneration revealed by comparative light and electron microscopy. Acta Neuropathol Commun 2:161
50. Thal DR, Sassin I, Schultz C, Haass C, Braak E, Braak H (1999) Fleecy amyloid deposits in the internal layers of the human entorhinal cortex are comprised of N-terminal truncated fragments of Abeta. J Neuropathol Exp Neurol 58:210–216
51. Thal DR, Rüb U, Orantes M, Braak H (2002) Phases of a beta-deposition in the human brain and its relevance for the development of AD. Neurology 58:1791–1800
52. Tomonaga M (1983) Neuropathology of the locus ceruleus: a semi-quantitative study. J Neurol 230:231–240
53. Uchihara T, Nakamura A, Shibuya K, Yagishita S (2011) Specific detection of pathological three-repeat tau after pretreatment with potassium permanganate and oxalic acid in PSP/CBD brains. Brain Pathol 21:180–188
54. Uchihara T, Hara M, Nakamura A, Hirokawa K (2012) Tangle evolution linked to differential 3- and 4-repeat tau isoform deposition: a double immunofluorolabeling study using two monoclonal antibodies. Histochem Cell Biol 137:261–267
55. Uematsu M, Adachi E, Nakamura A, Tsuchiya K, Uchihara T (2012) Atomic identification of fluorescent Q-dots on tau-positive fibrils in 3D-reconstructed pick bodies. Am J Pathol 180:1394–1397
56. Wilcock GK, Esiri MM (1982) Plaques, tangles and dementia. A quantitative study. J Neurol Sci 56:343–356
57. Wischik CM, Novak M, Thøgersen HC, Edwards PC, Runswick MJ, Jakes R et al (1988) Isolation of a fragment of tau derived from the core of the paired helical filament of Alzheimer disease. Proc Natl Acad Sci U S A 85:4506–4510
58. Yasojima K, McGeer EG, McGeer PL (1999) Tangled areas of Alzheimer brain have upregulated levels of exon 10 containing tau mRNA. Brain Res 831:301–305
59. Zack GW, Rogers WE, Latt SA (1977) Automatic measurement of sister chromatid exchange frequency. J Histochem Cytochem 25:741–753
60. Zempel H, Thies E, Mandelkow E, Mandelkow EM (2010) Abeta oligomers cause localized ca(2+) elevation, missorting of endogenous tau into dendrites, tau phosphorylation, and destruction of microtubules and spines. J Neurosci 30:11938–11950

2

Poly-GR dipeptide repeat polymers correlate with neurodegeneration and Clinicopathological subtypes in *C9ORF72*-related brain disease

Nobutaka Sakae, Kevin F. Bieniek, Yong-Jie Zhang, Kelly Ross, Tania F. Gendron, Melissa E. Murray, Rosa Rademakers, Leonard Petrucelli and Dennis W. Dickson*

Abstract

Frontotemporal lobar degeneration (FTLD) is heterogeneous in clinical presentation, neuropathological characteristics and genetics. An expanded GGGGCC hexanucleotide repeat in *C9ORF72* is the most common genetic cause of both FTLD and motor neuron disease (MND). Dipeptide repeat polymers (DPR) are generated through repeat-associated non-ATG translation, and they aggregate in neuronal inclusions with a distribution distinct from that of TDP-43 pathology. Recent studies from animal and cell culture models suggest that DPR might be toxic, but that toxicity may differ for specific DPR. Arginine containing DPR (poly-GR and poly-PR) have the greatest toxicity and are less frequent than other DPR (poly-GP, poly-GA). A unique feature of arginine-containing DPR is their potential for post-translational modification by methyl-transferases, which produces methylarginine DPR. In this report, we explored the relationship of DPR and methylarginine to markers of neurodegeneration using quantitative digital microscopic methods in 40 patients with *C9ORF72* mutations and one of three different clinicopathologic phenotypes, FTLD, FTLD-MND or MND. We find that density and distribution of poly-GR inclusions are different from poly-GA and poly-GP inclusions. We also demonstrate colocalization of poly-GR with asymmetrical dimethylarginine (aDMA) immunoreactivity in regions with neurodegeneration. Differences in aDMA were also noted by clinical phenotype. FTLD-MND had the highest burden of poly-GR pathology compared to FTLD and MND, while FTLD-MND had higher burden of aDMA than FTLD. The results suggest that poly-GR pathology is associated with toxicity and neurodegeneration. It remains to be determined if dimethylarginine modification of poly-GR could contribute to its toxicity.

Keywords: C9ORF72, Dipeptide repeat polymers (DPR), Poly-GR, Neurodegeneration, Dimethylarginine

Introduction

Frontotemporal lobar degeneration (FTLD) is heterogeneous in clinical presentation, neuropathological characteristics and underlying genetic causes. Clinically, FTLD manifests in changes in behavior, personality and language, but it can also be associated with motor neuron disease (MND), including amyotrophic lateral sclerosis (upper and lower motor neurons affected), progressive muscular atrophy (lower motor neurons predominantly affected) and primary lateral sclerosis (upper motor neurons primarily affected) [8, 12, 13]. Hexanucleotide repeat expansions in chromosome 9 open reading frame 72 gene (*C9ORF72*) are the most common genetic cause of FTLD and MND [7, 24], which are collectively referred to as c9FTLD-MND. The neuropathological features of c9FTLD-MND include nuclear RNA foci, inclusions composed of repeat-associated non-ATG (RAN) translated dipeptide repeat polymers (DPR) and TDP-43 pathology. Of these features, DPR pathology and nuclear RNA foci are unique and highly specific to c9FTLD-MND. RAN translation can occur in both sense and antisense directions generating five different DPR: poly-(glycine-alanine/poly-GA), poly-(glycine-arginine/poly-GR) and poly-(glycine-proline/poly-GP) encoded by the sense strand, and poly-(proline-alanine/poly-PA), poly-(proline-arginine/poly-PR) and poly-(proline-glycine/poly-PG)

* Correspondence: dickson.dennis@mayo.edu
Department of Neuroscience, Mayo Clinic, 4500 San Pablo Road, Jacksonville, FL 32224, USA

by the antisense strand [1, 11, 21]. In human brains, DPR inclusions are detected predominantly in neurons as cytoplasmic inclusions, but nuclear inclusions and rare inclusions in glial cells are also found [26]. There is evidence that DPR inclusions are detected in presymptomatic individuals before significant neurodegeneration and TDP-43 pathology is detected [19, 32]. Recent progress in developing animal models of c9FTLD-MND suggests that toxicity of specific DPR polymers is variable. Several pathogenic mechanisms, not mutually exclusive, may be at play including nuclear dysfunction, altered RNA splicing, impaired nucleocytoplasmic transport, altered RNA granule dynamics, and disruption of proteostasis. Of the various DPR species, poly-PR and poly-GR are most toxic in Drosophila [20] and in cell culture models [9, 15, 30, 31, 33, 34]. The reasons that poly-PR and poly-GR are more toxic remain unknown, but given their high arginine content, one might hypothesize that methylarginine post-translational modification might contribute to their toxicity. Arginine residues in polypeptides can be modified by methyltransferases to conjugate one (monomethylarginine) or two (dimethylarginine) methyl groups. Dimethylarginine modifications have been reported in proteins in human plasma and urine, and their levels are increased in conditions associated with enhanced protein breakdown, such as tumor growth and neurodegenerative disorders [27]. There are two isomers of dimethylarginine, symmetric dimethylarginine (sDMA) and asymmetric dimethylarginine (aDMA). The biologic function of DMA is not well known; however, elevated levels of aDMA in plasma predict poor prognosis in many diseases, such as cerebrovascular disease and Crohn's disease, where DMA modification is considered toxic [29]. The presence of DMA modifications has not been specifically studied in c9FTLD-MND.

Several studies have reported clinicopathological correlates of DPR in brains of c9FTLD-MND, but most have been relatively small autopsy series and used mostly semiquantitative methods [6, 17, 26]. It remains to be determined if there are correlations of specific DPR with clinical or neuropathological subtypes of *C9ORF72*-related disease. To address this issue, we sought evidence to support our hypothesis that arginine-containing DPR, poly-GR in particular, might correlate with the severity of neuropathology and that DMA modification might be related to a gain of toxicity in poly-GR. To investigate this, we systematically evaluated sense strand DPR (poly-GA, poly-GP and poly-GR), as well as aDMA in 40 patients with FTLD, FTLD-MND or MND. We found that poly-GR pathology correlated with neurodegeneration and clinicopathologic subtype. Further, we detected a correlation between the distribution of poly-GR and aDMA pathologies. Taken together, our results suggest a possible mechanism of poly-GR toxicity that could be the basis of novel therapeutic approaches.

Material and methods

Case materials

Forty cases of FTLD or MND with C9ORF72 repeat expansion mutation were obtained from the Mayo Clinic brain bank. The C9ORF72 expansion carriers had pathological diagnoses of FTLD, MND or FTLD-MND. All cases were submitted to or autopsied by the brain bank for neurodegenerative disorders at the Mayo Clinic in Jacksonville, Florida. Clinical information (age at death, sex, clinical diagnosis, disease duration, and family history) was obtained from available medical records. The left hemibrain was fixed in 10% formalin, and the right hemibrain was frozen at − 80 °C. Formalin-fixed tissue was sampled with standardized dissection methods and embedded in paraffin blocks.

Genetic analyses

All cases had hexanucleotide repeat expansions in *C9ORF72* based on a repeat-primed polymerase chain reaction method that detects expansions of the GGGG CC hexanucleotide, and for most cases, the expansions was confirmed with Southern blotting. [7]

Diagnostic neuropathology

Gross and macroscopic neuropathological assessment was performed by standardized procedures. Formalin-fixed, paraffin-embedded tissue samples were cut at 5 μm thickness and mounted on glass slides for further study. The neuropathologic assessment included immunohistochemistry for phospho-TDP-43 (pTDP-43; mouse monoclonal; Cosmo Bio USA, Carlsbad, CA) and C9RANT antibody [1]. A TDP-43 pathologic subtype was assigned to each case using the harmonized classification scheme [18] based upon morphology and distribution of lesions in cortical and subcortical regions [14].

Immunohistochemistry and double-label immunofluorescence

Immunohistochemistry was performed on 5-μm thick sections from formalin-fixed paraffin embedded tissue. Glass-mounted sections were de-parafinized in xylene and rehydrated in ethanol and dH_2O. Rabbit polyclonal antibodies used for DPR immunohistochemistry were as follows: poly-GA (Rb9880), poly-GP (Rb5823), poly-GR (Rb7810) (Leonard Petrucelli, Mayo Clinic, Jacksonville, FL [1, 11]). A rabbit polyclonal antibody (ASYM24 07–414, MilliporeSigma, Burlington, MA) was used for immunohistochemistry for aDMA. Regions of interest were middle frontal gyrus (FCtx), motor cortex (MCtx) and hippocampus. Adjacent sections were immunostained for phospho-TDP-43 as above. All Immunoperoxidase sections were processed on a DAKO AutostainerPlus (Agilent/DAKO, Santa Clara, CA) with the DAKO EnVisionTM+ system-HRP with diaminobenzidine as the chromogen. Nonspecific antibody binding was blocked with normal goat serum (Sigma, St Louis, MO).

For double immunofluorescence staining, a rat monoclonal antibody was used to detect poly-GR (5H9, MilliporeSigma, Burlington, MA) and a rabbit polyclonal antibody was used to detect aDMA (MilliporeSigma, Burlington, MA). The fluorochromes were Alexa Fluor 568 and Alexa Fluor 488 conjugated to anti-rabbit or anti-rat IgG (Invitrogen/ThermoFisher, Waltham, MA).

Assessment of neurodegeneration

For assessment of neurodegeneration, H&E stained sections of FCtx, MCtx and hippocampus were evaluated. Degeneration was graded semiquantitatively as absent (0), mild (1), moderate (2) or severe (3) based on the presence of spongiosis, neuronal loss and gliosis. In FCtx, neurodegeneration was typically associated with superficial laminar spongiosis, while in the hippocampal dentate fascia, discontinuity in the density of granular neurons was used as an indicator of neuronal loss and neurodegeneration. In hippocampal subfields – CA4 and CA2/3 – degeneration was assessed by neuronal loss and astrogliosis (see Additional file 1: Figure S1).

Image analysis

Digital microscopy methods used in this study have been described previously [22]. Briefly, immunostained glass slides were scanned on an Aperio ScanScope XT slide scanner (Aperio Technologies/Leica Biosystems, Buffalo Grove, IL) producing high resolution digital images. The regions of interest in the hippocampus included the entire hippocampus, as well as delimited subregions of dentate fascia, CA4 sector and CA2/3 sector. In MCtx and FCtx, the region of interest was the entire thickness of the cortex where the pial surface was parallel to the cortical gray-white junction. Digital image analysis was performed using Aperio ImageScope software. A color deconvolution algorithm was used to count the number of pixels that were strongly immunostained by the chromogen. The output variable was percentage of strong positive staining relative to total pixels in the region of interest.

Analytic algorithms for poly-GA had to be adapted to exclude signals two standard deviations above and below the mean because some cases had unexplained background staining. Given this limitation, we also used manual counting methods for poly-GA, as well as for aDMA. In all cases, aDMA labeled not only cytoplasmic inclusions, but also many nuclei presumably due to detection of methylated histones or other nuclear proteins [10]. The poly-GA and aDMA manual counts were performed on digital images. In order to make comparisons between the various DPR, it was also necessary to perform manual counts for poly-GP and poly-GR. The number of inclusions detected from manual counts was assessed in the same area traced for image analysis. Manual counts and positive pixel burden from color deconvolution image analysis were highly correlated for both poly-GP and poly-GR (Additional file 2: Figure S2). Only the motor cortex had poor correlation between poly-GP manual counts and positive pixel burden, in part due to prominent cytoplasmic immunoreactivity in large neurons, including Betz cells. These did not represent inclusions in that they had diffuse cytoplasmic staining, instead of compact cytoplasmic inclusion bodies, which were manually counted. As with image analysis, manual counts were expressed as density per square millimeter by dividing the manual count by total area of the annotated region of interest.

Cell culture experiments

HEK-293 T cells were grown in Opti-Mem plus 10% FBS and 1% penicillin-streptomycin. To examine methylation of poly-GR proteins, HEK-293 T cells were grown in 12-well plates or on coverslips in 24-well plates. Cultures were transfected with 1 μg (12-well plates) or 0.5 μg (24-well plates) of an expression vector[GFP, GFP-$(GR)_{50}$ or GFP-$(GR)_{100}$ using Lipofectamine 2000 (Life Technology). Four hours after transfection, the cultured cells were treated with methylarginine transferase inhibitor, AdOx (A7154, Sigma), at concentration of 5 or 20 μM. DMSO was used as vehicle control. Twenty-four hours after treatment, the cultured cells were harvested for Western blot analysis or fixed for immunofluorescence staining.

Immunofluorescence staining

HEK-293 T cells were fixed with 4% paraformaldehyde in PBS for 15 min, and then permeabilized with PBS-0.5% Triton X-100 for 10 min. To examine aDMA, cells were blocked with 5% nonfat milk for 1 h at room temperature, and then incubated overnight at 4 °C with rabbit polyclonal anti-aDMA antibody (ASYM24, Millipore). After washing, cells were incubated with the corresponding Alexa Fluor 568-conjugated goat anti-rabbit secondary antibody (1:500, Molecular Probes) at room temperature for 2 h. After washing, they were mounted with Vectashield Mounting Media with DAPI (Vector Laboratories). Images were obtained on a Zeiss LSM 510 META confocal microscope. To quantify the number of cells positive for GFP and aDMA, microscopic fields were randomly selected at 40X magnification. For each field, the number of GFP-positive cells and aDMA-positive aggregates, as well as aggregates with double staining, were manually counted, blinded to condition. These counts were used to calculate the average percentage of aDMA aggregates in cells expressing GFP, GFP-$(GR)_{50}$ or GFP-$(GR)_{100}$.

Biochemical studies of cell lysates

Cell pellets were lysed in co-immunoprecipitation (co-IP) buffer (50 mM Tris–HCl, pH 7.4, 300 mM NaCl, 1% Triton X-100, 5 mM EDTA) plus 2% SDS, and both protease and phosphatase inhibitors, sonicated on ice, and then centrifuged at 16,000×g for 20 min. Supernatants were saved as cell lysates. The protein concentration of supernatants was determined by BCA assay (Thermo Scientific) prior to Western blot analysis. Cell lysates were diluted with 2 × SDS-loading buffer at a 1:1 ratio (*v*/v), and then heated at 95 °C for 5 min. Equal amounts of protein were loaded into 12-well 4–20% Tris-glycine gels (Novex). After transferring proteins to membranes, membranes were blocked with 5% nonfat dry milk in TBS plus 0.1% Tween 20 (TBST) for 1 h, and then incubated with rabbit polyclonal anti-GFP antibody (A-6455, 1:4000, Life Technologies), rabbit polyclonal anti-GR antibody (Rb7810, 1:2000), rabbit polyclonal anti-aDMA antibody (07–414, 1:1000, EMD Millipore), or mouse monoclonal or GAPDH antibody (H86504M, 1:10000, Meridian Life Science) overnight at 4 °C. Membranes were washed in TBST and incubated with donkey anti-rabbit or anti-mouse IgG antibodies conjugated to horseradish peroxidase (1:5000; Jackson ImmunoResearch) for 1 h. Protein expression was visualized by enhanced chemiluminescence treatment and exposure to film.

Statistical analyses

Sigma Plot Version 12 (Systat Software, San Jose, CA) was used for statistical analyses. Due to small sample sizes, non-parametric Kruskal-Wallis analysis of variance on ranks (ANOVA on Ranks) was performed on quantitative measures to assess differences between the groups. Post hoc pairwise comparisons were performed between each of the groups using Mann-Whitney rank sum test. For categorical data (e.g., sex and APOE genotype), a Chi-square test was used to compare groups. Fisher's exact test was used for comparison of pairwise categorical data if the counts were less than 5. Correlative analysis was performed using Spearman rank order correlation. A p-value < 0.05 was considered statistically significant.

Results

Demographics features of study cohort

The 40 patients with *C9ORF72* mutations included 13 with FTLD, 14 with FTLD-MND and 13 with MND. Demographic information is summarized in Table 1. Patients with FTLD had significantly longer disease duration than patients with MND. They were also significantly older at death compared to both FTLD-MND and MND. The median age at death was 74 for FTLD, 61 for FTLD-MND and 56 for MND. Median disease durations were 6.4 years for FTLD, 3.6 years for FTLD-MND and 2.4 years for MND.

Table 1 Demographics of clinicopathologic subgroups

Subgroup	N (F/M)	Age at death	Disease duration
FTLD	13 (2/11)	74 (71, 83)*	6.4 (4.4, 10)*
FTLD-MND	14 (7/7)	61 (60, 68)*	3.6 (2.2, 5.5)
MND	13 (9/4)	56 (50, 68)	2.4 (1.3, 3.5)

All variables analyzed with Kruskal-Wallis ANOVA on Ranks, and data are displayed as median (25th and 75th range), unless otherwise noted
*Statistically significant p-value ($p < 0.05$); all p-values for ANOVA on Ranks comparison of all three groups

Spectrum of poly-GA, poly-GP and poly-GR pathology

In this study, we limited neuropathological analyses to sense strand DPR (poly-GA, poly-GP and poly-GR) given the paucity of inclusions and the lack of good detection reagents for antisense DPR (poly-PA and poly-PR). We focused particularly on poly-GR pathology, and compared the pathology of poly-GR with poly-GP and poly-GA pathology as these have been shown by both our previous studies and those of others to be the most abundant DPR species in brain samples. Consistent with previous reports, we found that most of the DPR inclusions were neuronal cytoplasmic inclusions (Fig. 1); dystrophic neurites were less frequent [1, 11, 16, 17, 21, 26]. In contrast to poly-GP and poly-GA, we did not detect dystrophic neurites with immunohistochemistry for poly-GR. These results are consistent with a previous study that showed almost complete lack of poly-GR immunoreactive dystrophic neurites [26]. Glial cytoplasmic inclusions were also occasionally detected with poly-GA and poly-GP immunohistochemistry, but they were very rare with poly-GR immunohistochemistry.

Poly-GR inclusion distribution among clinicopathologic subgroups

To evaluate whether poly-GA, poly-GP or poly-GR pathology differs among different clinicopathologic subgroups, we quantified lesion burden with image analysis. Although there were no significant differences between the subgroups for burden of poly-GA and poly-GP, poly-GR was significantly different in the three clinicopathologic subgroups. While overall lesions were sparse, we found greater burden of poly-GR inclusions in the FCtx of FTLD-MND compared to MND, and significantly more poly-GR inclusions in specific hippocampal subfields (i.e. CA2/3) of FTLD-MND compared to FTLD, as well as a trend for increases in CA4 of FTLD-MND compared to FTLD (Additional file 3: Table S1). We found poly-GR density was significantly different in FTD/MND in frontal cortex and hippocampus.

Correlations between poly-GR pathology and neurodegeneration

We hypothesized that if poly-GR is neurotoxic, the density of poly-GR inclusions might be associated with

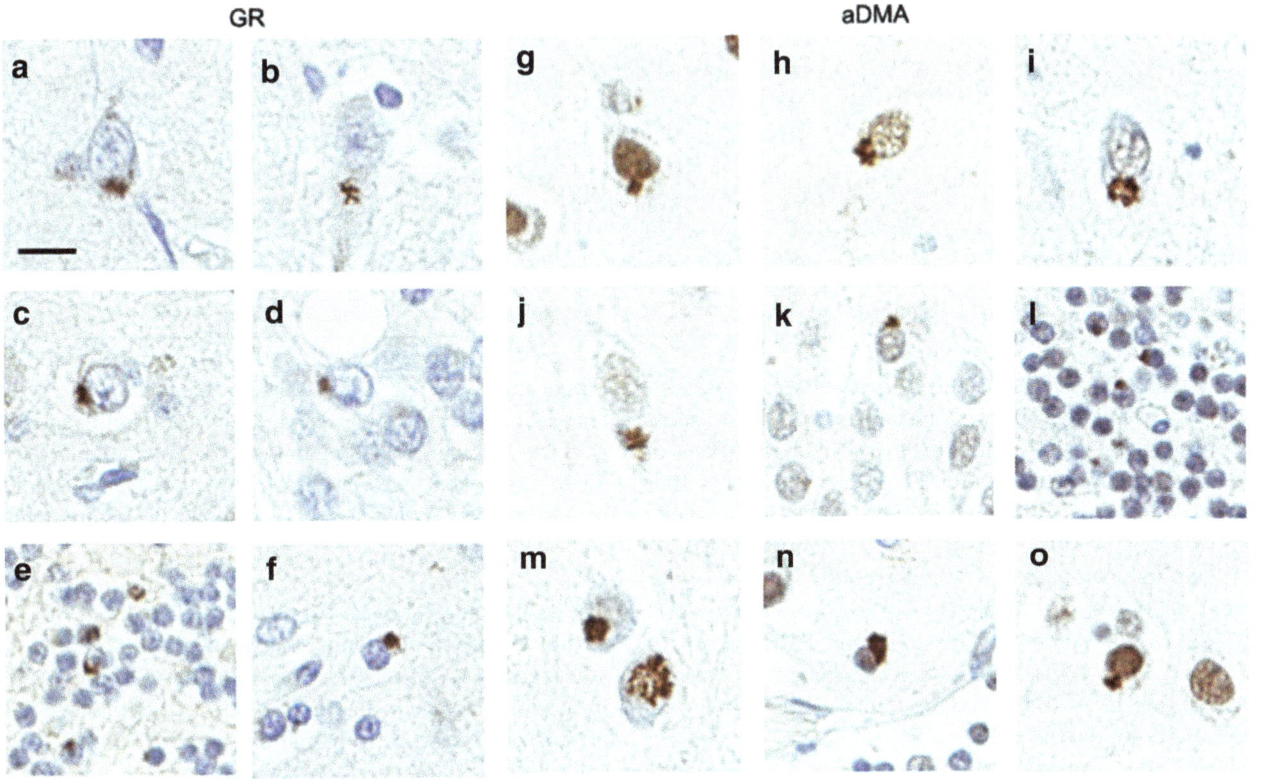

Fig. 1 Morphology of poly-GR and aDMA pathology. Immunohistochemistry for poly-GR reveals neuronal cytoplasmic inclusions in frontal cortex (**a**), CA2/3 (**b**), CA4 (**c**), DF (**d**), and cerebellar granular layer (**e**). Inclusions in glial cells were very rare (**f**). Immunohistochemistry for aDMA shows neuronal cytoplasmic inclusions, as well as variable nuclear immunoreactivity, which was dense in some neurons (**g**), moderate in others (**h**) and minimal in others (**i**); inclusions in CA2/3 (**j**), DF (**k**) and (**l**) cerebellar granular layer (**n**); neuronal nuclear inclusions (NII) (**m**); and rare glial cytoplasmic inclusions (**n, o**). Scale bar represents 20 μM. FCtx = frontal cortex, MCtx = Motor cortex, DF = dentate fascia, CA = hippocampal subfields, Cbl = cerebellar granular cell layer

neurodegeneration. We thus analyzed the burden of poly-GA, poly-GP and poly-GR, as well as pTDP-43 using a color deconvolution algorithm of digital images of regions of interest. In the same regions we scored the severity of neurodegeneration with semi-quantitative methods. As expected, there were strong correlations between density of pTDP-43 pathology and neurodegeneration in FCtx ($r = 0.46$, $p = 0.004$), hippocampal DF ($r = 0.40$, $p = 0.01$) and CA4 ($r = 0.61$, $p = 0.00006$) (see Additional file 4: Figure S3). Interestingly, we also found a strong correlation between poly-GR density and neurodegeneration in FCtx ($r = 0.45$, $p = 0.004$), but a less robust correlation between poly-GR density and neurodegeneration in the hippocampal DF ($r = 0.33$, $p = 0.04$) (Table 2). Representative images of poly-GR and neurodegeneration are illustrated in Fig. 2. In contrast to other sense-strand DPR (poly-GA and poly-GP), poly-GR showed correlation with neurodegeneration even though the density of lesions was far less for poly-GR compared with poly-GA and poly-GP.

Spectrum and distribution of poly-GR pathology and aDMA distribution

To assess our hypothesis that DMA modification may contribute to a possible toxic gain of function in poly-GR inclusions, we studied the morphology and distribution of inclusions immunoreactive for aDMA. We also quantified

Table 2 Correlations of phospho-TDP-43 and DPR burden with neurodegeneration

	FCtx	DF	CA4
poly-GA	$r = -0.19$	$r = 0.20$	$r = 0.10$
	$p = 0.28$	$p = 0.24$	$p = 0.57$
poly-GP	$r = -0.14$	$r = 0.26$	$r = 0.31$
	$p = 0.42$	$p = 0.12$	$p = 0.06$
poly-GR	$r = 0.45$	$r = 0.33$	$r = -0.01$
	$p = 0.004$	$p = 0.04$	$p = 0.96$
pTDP-43	$r = 0.46$	$r = 0.40$	$r = 0.61$
	$p = 0.004$	$p = 0.013$	$p = 0.00006$

P-values are from Pearson's test of correlation. Significant *p*-values (< 0.05)
FCtx frontal cortex, *DF* dentate fascia, *CA4 cornu ammonis* sector 4

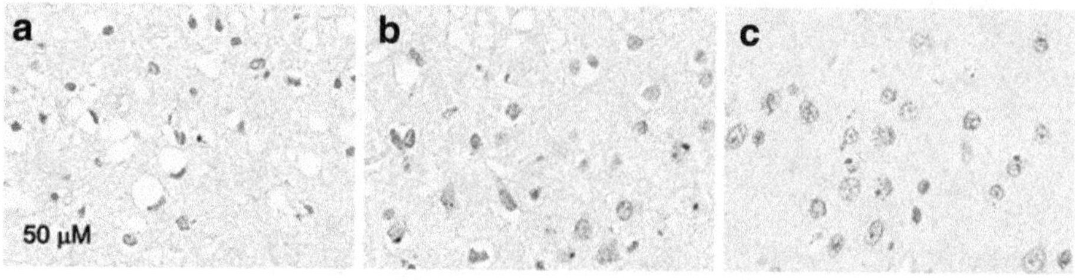

Fig. 2 poly-GR density and neurodegenerationpoly-GR density is associated with neurodegeneration in FCtx and DF. Representative images show neurodegeneration and poly-GR inclusions. Most severe neurodegeneration with spongiosis and gliosis, but sparse poly-GR inclusions in FTLD (**a**) Severe neurodegeneration with spongiosis and gliosis in FTLD-MND (**b**) Mild neurodegeneration in MND (**c**). Scale bar represents 50 µM

aDMA using western blot analysis in a subset of cases included in the larger immunohistochemical study. Blots were also probed with antibody to sDMA. The focus of this sub-analysis was on four FTLD-MND patients that had the most significant poly-GR pathology. Four FTLD-MND patients without *C9ORF72* mutations were included for comparison. We detected high molecular weight aDMA-immunoreactive species in brain lysates of c9FTLD-MND (Additional file 5: Figure S4), but not of sporadic FTLD-MND. We did not detect any differences between c9FTLD-MND and sporadic FTLD-MND for sDMA (Additional file 5: Figure S4).

Given these results, we focused only on aDMA in subsequent histopathologic studies. We characterized the spectrum of poly-GR and aDMA pathology in *C9ORF72* patients. As mentioned above, poly-GR neuronal inclusions were observed throughout the brain. Only a few glial inclusions and isolated neuronal intranuclear inclusions were detected, while no dystrophic neurites were detected (Fig. 1). Immunohistochemistry for aDMA labeled neuronal inclusions as well as many nuclei, the latter probably related to physiologic methylation of nuclear proteins such as histones (Fig. 1). As we observed for poly-GR, most of the inclusions immunoreactive for aDMA were neuronal cytoplasmic inclusions; glial inclusions were sparse, and no dystrophic neurites were found.

Similar distribution of poly-GR and aDMA immunoreactivities in c9FTLD-MND brains

We used double immunofluorescence labeling to determine what proportion of the poly-GR inclusions also had aDMA immunoreactivity. We found frequent colocalization of poly-GR and aDMA in neuronal inclusions of the DF and CA4 sector of the hippocampus (Fig. 3). We performed manual counts of poly-GR and aDMA immunoreactive inclusions because excessive nuclear signal of aDMA precluded use of image analysis methods. We foun that manual counts and image analysis results were highly correlated (Additional file 2: Figure S2). We found similar densities and distributions of poly-GR and aDMA immunoreactive inclusions in FCtx, MCtx and hippocampal DF (Fig. 4a-c). As expected, there was a strong correlation between poly-GR and aDMA (Fig. 3) and this was true for all brain regions analyzed (Additional file 6: Table S2). Taken together, these data suggest that a significant portion of poly-GR pathology may be methylated in *C9ORF72*-related disease.

Clinicopathological correlations of poly-GR and aDMA pathology based on manual inclusion counts

We investigated poly-GA, poly-GP, poly-GR and aDMA immunoreactive inclusions in clinicopathologic subgroups, as assessed from manual counts. Similar to results described above, the density of poly-GR and aDMA immunoreactive neuronal inclusions was greater in patients with FTLD-MND compared to FTLD or MND. In the hippocampus, density of poly-GR inclusions was significantly greater in the DF, CA4 and CA2/3 of FTLD-MND compared to FTLD (Table 3). In addition, the density of aDMA inclusions was significantly greater in CA4 of FTLD-MND compared to FTLD. In frontal cortex, the density of poly-GR inclusions in FTLD-MND was significantly greater than in both FTLD and MND (Table 3). These results were similar to those obtained by image analysis using color deconvolution algorithms (Additional file 3: Table S1).

In vitro evidence of poly-GR methylation

To obtain further insight into poly-GR pathology in c9FTLD-MND, we overexpressed GFP-tagged poly-$(GR)_{50}$ or poly-$(GR)_{100}$ and treated the cells with adenosine dialdehyde (AdOx), a global methyltransferase inhibitor, at two concentrations (5 µM and 20 µM). GFP-$(GR)_{50}$ accumulated only in the nucleus, whereas GFP-$(GR)_{100}$ was detected in both the nucleus and cytoplasm. The cytoplasmic aggregates resembled inclusion bodies (Fig. 5). These results suggest that formation of poly-GR aggregates might be determined, in part, by repeat length, with longer repeats forming cytoplasmic inclusions resembling those seen in human brain cells (Fig. 1). To study the relationship between poly-GR aggregation and aDMA modification, we performed double immunofluorescent staining. There was frequent colocalization of poly-GR and aDMA in

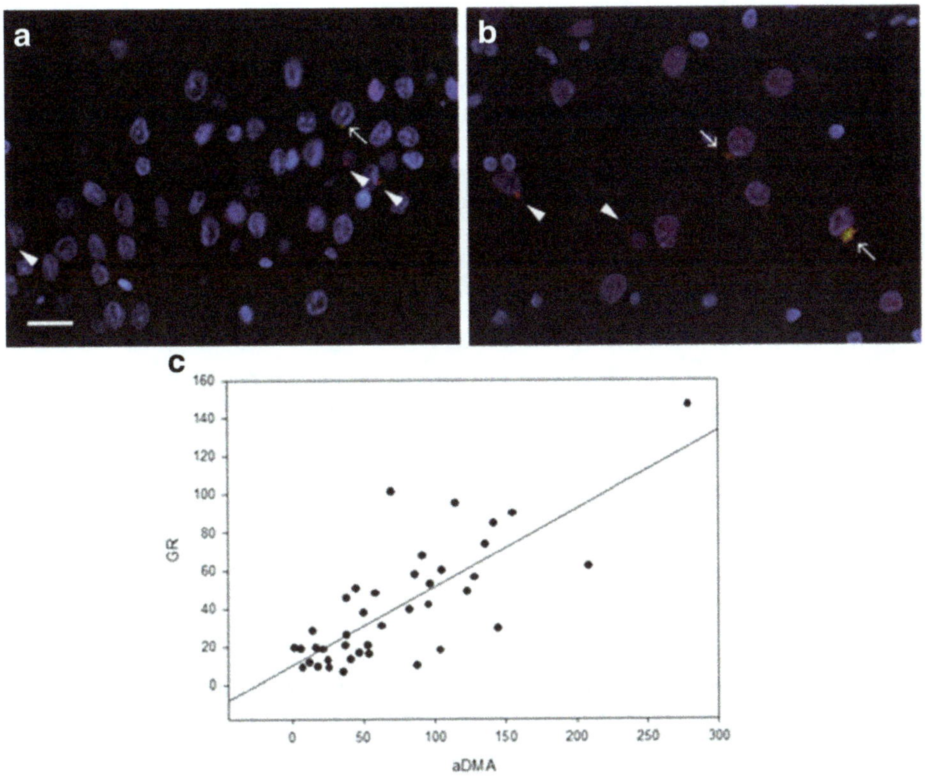

Fig. 3 Colocalization of poly-GR and aDMA. Poly-GR neuronal cytoplasmic inclusions in the dentate fascia and CA4 of the hippocampus. Sparse poly-GR inclusions in the dentate fascia show colocalization with aDMA (arrow). Note that not all poly-GR aggregates contain aDMA (arrowheads) (**a**). Moderate poly-GR inclusions show colocalization with aDMA in CA4 (arrows). Again, not all poly-GR aggregates contain aDMA (arrowheads) (**b**). Scale bars: 10 μm. Plot shows the association of poly-GR and aDMA neuronal inclusions in the dentate fascia. The line shows linear regression ($r = 0.77$) (**c**)

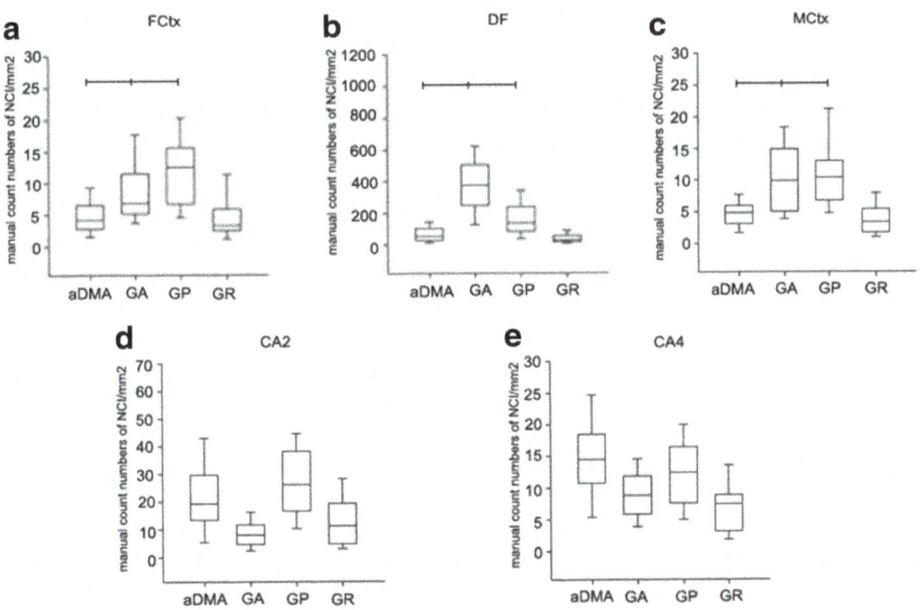

Fig. 4 Overall frequency of inclusions for sense strand DPR and aDMA. Quantitative analysis of poly-GA, poly-GR and aDMA density in frontal cortex, hippocampus and motor cortex. The total number of inclusions counted in each case and the density of inclusions were calculated by total numbers of inclusions/total stained area (mm^2). Frontal cortex (**a**), dentate fascia (**b**), motor cortex (**c**), CA2/3 (**d**), and CA4 (**e**). All variables analyzed with Kruskal-Wallis ANOVA on Ranks followed by Dunn's post hoc test and data are displayed as median (25th and 75th range). *Statistically significant p-value ($p < 0.05$); all p-value for ANOVA on Ranks comparison of all groups

Table 3 Burden of DPR and aDMA by region in clinicopathologic subgroups

	FCtx	DF	CA4	CA2/3	MCtx
	poly-GA				
FTLD	6.4 (3.8, 9.4)	310 (110, 470)	6 (4.1, 9.5)	5.6 (4.5, 8.3)	5.8 (3.7, 12)
FTLD-MND	7.5 (5.6, 15)	420 (320, 630)	9.5 (6.6, 13)	9.7 (4.7, 15)	14 (6.2, 17)
MND	7.4 (5.8, 13)	380 (280, 480)	10 (7.4, 14)	8.2 (3.0, 12)	9.3 (6.5, 13)
	poly-GP				
FTLD	9.7 (5.9,14)	120 (71, 262)	8 (6.7, 13)	19 (13, 33)	10 (6.7, 13)
FTLD-MND	13 (11, 18)	180 (98, 270)	13 (7.4, 18)	31 (19, 39)	10 (8.0, 14)
MND	10 (6.6, 16)	130 (86, 230)	13 (10, 17)	27 (16, 39)	11 (4.9, 18)
	poly-GR				
FTLD	3.0 (2.2, 4.2)	16 (9.5, 48)	3.0 (2.3, 5.6)	5.1 (3.3, 9.3)	2.6 (1.3, 5.5)
FTLD-MND	6.8 (3.7, 9.5)*	49 (26, 86)*	8.5 (6.8, 12)*	17 (11, 26)*	4.7 (3.1, 7.9)
MND	2.9(1.1, 3.4)	26 (18, 51)	7.5 (4.7, 8.8)	12 (3.7, 22)	2.6 (1.2, 4.9)
	aDMA				
FTLD	3.3 (2.8, 4.7)	83 (31, 100)	10 (6.8, 14)	16 (10, 37)	3.4 (2.1, 5.6)
FTLD-MND	5.5 (3.1, 8.2)	77 (21, 140)	17 (14, 22)*	25 (17, 36)	5.6 (4.6, 6.8)
MND	4.0 (2.1, 7.4)	53 (31, 81)	15 (12, 20)	15 (6, 29)	3.5(2.5, 5.6)

In frontal cortex, $p < 0.001$, FTLD vs. FTLD-MND, $p = 0.005$, FTLD-MND v.s MND. In DF, $p = 0.02$, FTLD vs. FTLD-MND. In CA4, $p = 0.002$, FTLD vs. FTLD-MND. In CA2/3, $p = 0.003$, FTLD vs. FTLD-MND. All variables analyzed with Kruskal-Wallis ANOVA on Ranks and data are displayed as median (25th and 75th range)
*Statistically significant p-value ($p < 0.05$); all p-value for ANOVA on Ranks comparison of all three groups
FCtx frontal cortex, *MCtx* Motor cortex, *DF* dentate fascia, *CA* (*cornu ammonis*)

cytoplasmic aggregates of GFP-$(GR)_{100}$ cells. Treating cells with AdOx decreased cytoplasmic aggregates in GFP-$(GR)_{100}$ cells, while having no effect on the number of cells expressing GFP (Fig. 5c and d). To confirm immunofluorescent findings, we performed western blot analysis. Consistent with the results of immunostaining, only GFP-$(GR)_{100}$ cells showed evidence of high molecular weight aDMA-immunoreactive species (arrows in Fig. 6). These results suggest that poly-GR aggregation may be modulated by arginine methylation.

Discussion

An expanded hexanucleotide repeat in *C9ORF72* is the most frequent cause of FTLD and MND. One consequence of the expanded repeats is formation of DPR polymers through unconventional RAN translation [1, 21]. Despite increasing evidence from animal and cell culture models suggesting individual DPR have different degrees of toxicity, the manifestations of this toxicity and pathomechanisms are poorly understood in the human brain. Moreover, the relationship of DPR-related neuropathology with various clinicopathologic subtypes of *C9ORF72*-related disease is not well understood. In this study, we focused on poly-GR and provide evidence that density of poly-GR inclusions correlates with neurodegeneration more robustly than other DPR, especially in individuals with the most severe clinicopathologic phenotype, FTLD-MND. In addition, we explored a possible association of poly-GR toxicity with post-translational modification by methylation. In clinicopathological analysis, we demonstrated differences in distribution of poly-GR inclusions compared with poly-GA and found that certain brain regions, such as the hippocampal DF, have abundant poly-GA inclusions, but very few poly-GR inclusions. Moreover, poly-GR inclusions are closely associated with histologic features of neurodegeneration, especially in the hippocampus and FCtx. We found a similar distribution of poly-GR and aDMA-positive inclusions, and co-localization of poly-GR with aDMA. Of the three clinicopathologic phenotypes of *C9ORF72*-related disease, the FTLD-MND subgroup had the most inclusions immunoreactive for poly-GR and aDMA, especially in the FCtx and in several subregions of the hippocampus.

Only a few studies have addressed possible differences in DPR species in clinicopathological subtypes of *C9ORF72*-related disease. A semiquantitative neuropathologic study by Mackenzie and coworkers of 8 cases of FTLD, 16 of FTLD-MND and 11 of MND, found no relationship between specific DPR species and clinicopathologic phenotype, except for moderate association of poly-GA-positive dystrophic neurites with histologic markers of degeneration in the frontal cortex [17]. In another semiquantitative study by Schludi and coworkers in a cohort of 3 FTLD, 4 FTLD-MND and 2 MND, poly-PR inclusions were more abundant in FTLD than MND in the hippocampus, while poly-GA inclusions were more abundant in cerebellar granular layer of

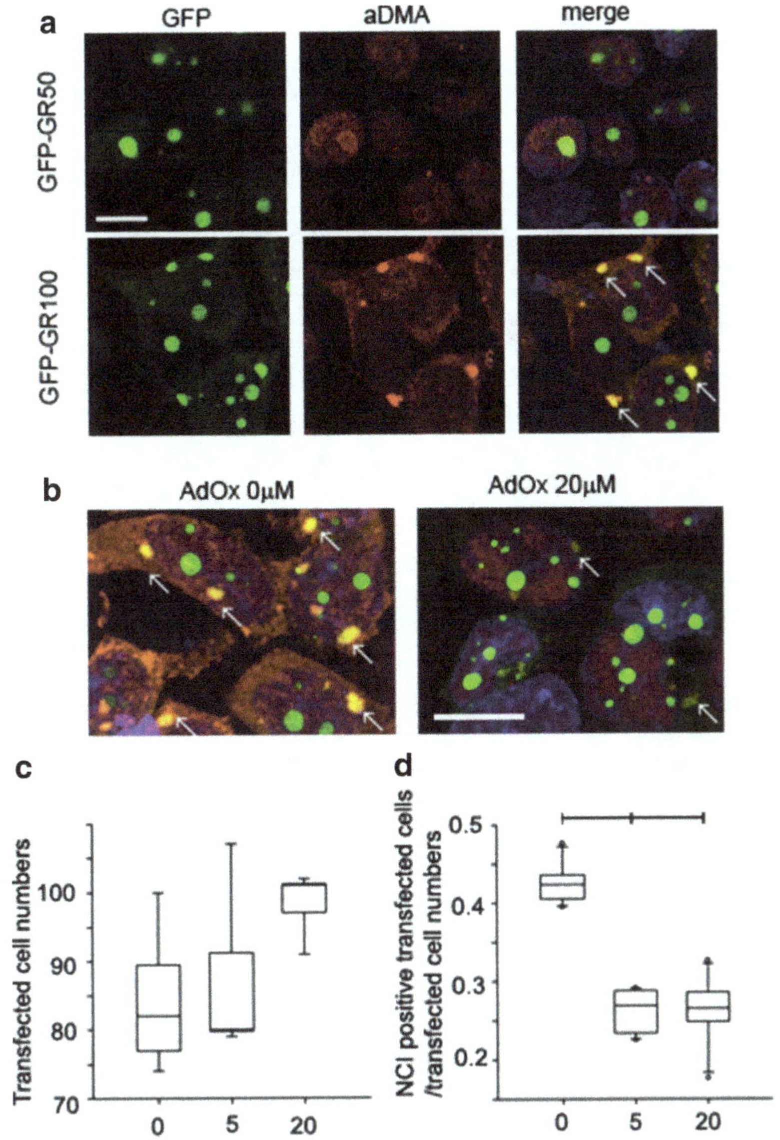

Fig. 5 Poly-GR proteins form cytoplasmic inclusions in HEK-293 T cultured cells. **a** Expression of GFP-$(GR)_{50}$ in HEK-293 T cells accumulate in nucleus. No cytoplasmic inclusions are detected. Expression of GFP-$(GR)_{100}$ in HEK-293 T cells show immunoreactivity in nucleus and cytoplasm, with formation of cytoplasmic inclusions. Double immunofluorescence of GFP-$(GR)_{100}$ and aDMA in HEK-293 T cells. **b** GFP-$(GR)_{100}$ and aDMA. GFP-$(GR)_{100}$ and no arginine methyltransferase inhibitor (AdOx) (left) versus AdOx 20 μM (right). Arrows indicate poly-GR and aDMA positive cytoplasmic aggregation (**c, d**) Effects of AdOx on poly-GR100 cytoplasmic inclusion formation. AdOx did not significantly decrease GFP positive, transfected cell numbers. **c** AdOx significantly decreased ratio of cytoplasmic inclusions in transfected cells – 43% at 0 mM, 27% at 5 mM and 25% at 20 mM. **d** Quantitative analysis and representative image showing cytoplasmic inclusions at different concentration of AdOx. Counts were made of over 500 transfected cells for each condition (with at least duplicate counts performed for each field analyzed). All variables analyzed with Kruskal-Wallis ANOVA on Ranks followed by Tukey's post hoc analysis and data are displayed as median (25th and 75th range). *Statistically significant *p*-value ($p < 0.05$); all *p*-values for ANOVA on Ranks comparison of all three groups. Scale bars in (**a**) and (**b**): 20 μm

FTLD than both FTLD-MND and MND cases, but neither poly-PR nor poly-GA correlated with neurodegeneration [26]. In contrast, we found correlations between poly-GR and neurodegeneration in a larger series of cases using quantitative digital microscopic methods. Another unique finding in our study was that patients with the most severe clinicopathologic phenotype, namely those with both FTLD and MND, had higher lesion burden that the other two clinicopathologic groups. Like Schludi and coworkers [26], we found the highest density of poly-GR in FTLD-MND. On the other hand, we were not able to detect any difference between FTD and MND. The FTD group had the oldest age at death and longest disease duration; therefore, greater neurodegeneration might be associated with clearance of poly-GR pathology. While the three largest neuropathologic studies

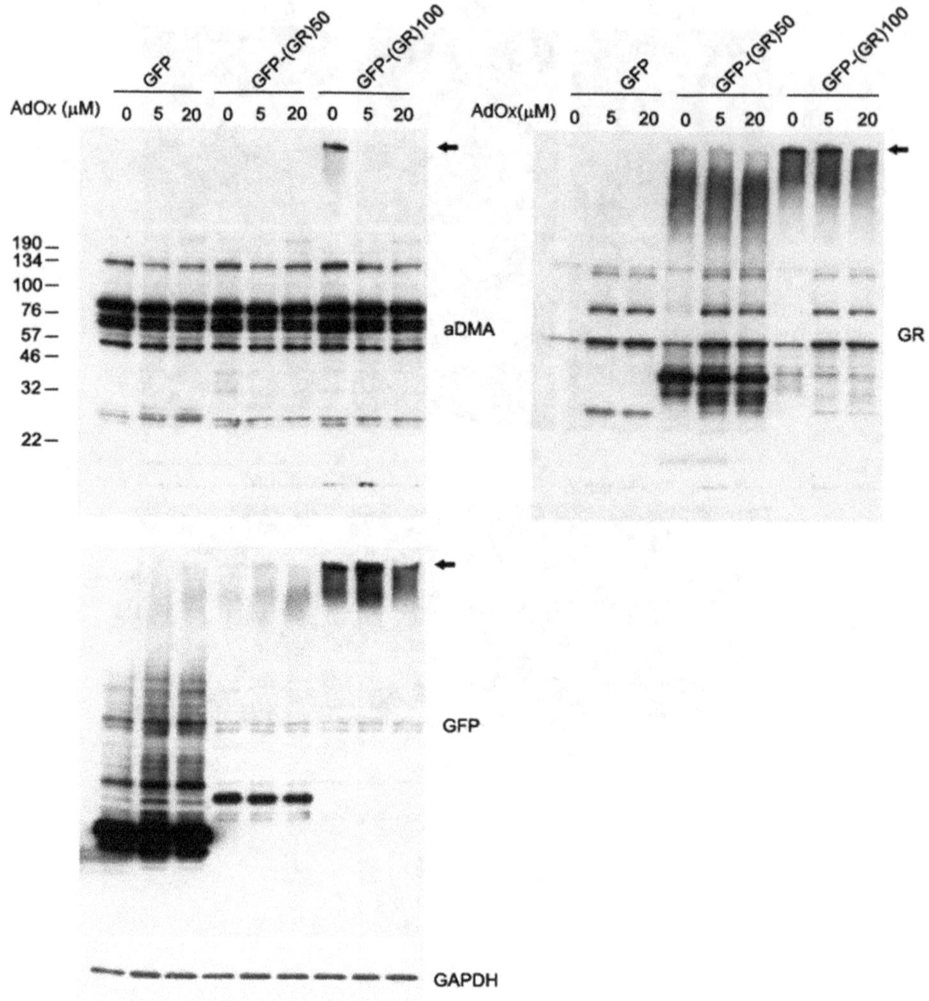

Fig. 6 Western blot analysis of soluble and insoluble cell lysates. Immunoblots show poly-GR in high molecular weight species. Arrows mark the top of the gel. Only GFP-$(GR)_{100}$ cells had dimethylarginine in high molecular species, which was lost after treatment with AdOx at 5- μM and 20-μM. $^*p < 0.05$. ANOVA All p-value for ANOVA on ranks comparison of all three groups. Mann-Whitney U test was employed for the statistical analysis

of DPR pathology in *C9ORF72*-related disease and a range of clinicopathologic subtypes, different quantitative methods and different antibodies for immunohistochemistry, there were several notable similarities. All found that poly-GR inclusions were less abundant than poly-GA (and poly-GP) inclusions and that certain brain regions had propensity for DPR inclusions, such as specific hippocampal subregions (DF, CA4 and CA2/3) and the cerebellar internal granular cell layer. The current study is the first to use digital pathology and quantitative methods, including color deconvolution image analysis, to objectively assess the burden of DPR pathology and histologic markers of neurodegeneration.

A recent study by Saberi and coworkers suggested poly-GR inclusions co-localize with TDP-43 in dendritic structures in a small series ($n = 5$) of MND compared with sporadic ALS ($n = 3$) [25]. These findings differ from our results and those of others [17, 26], who find little evidence for poly-GR immunoreactive dystrophic neurites.

Various pathomechanisms have been proposed for *C9ORF72*-related disease based on animal and cell culture models, including loss of function of *C9ORF72* leading to neuroinflammation [23], nuclear dysfunction due to alternative RNA splicing, perturbations in RNA metabolism, formation of DNA/RNA hybrids, RNA foci and defects in nucleocytoplasmic transport. The most characteristic pathologic hallmark of *C9ORF72*-related is widespread and regionally-specific neuronal DPR polymer inclusions and RNA foci. Given that two of the DPR contain arginine polymers, we hypothesized that post-translational modification of these DPR by methylarginine transferases might uniquely contribute to their greater toxicity. We found evidence to support methylation of poly-GR, while poly-PR was not amenable to study due to the paucity of these inclusions and the lack of reliable and sensitive reagents for their detection. Double immunostaining methods showed colocalization of aDMA immunoreactivity in poly-GR inclusions (Fig. 3). In contrast, there was very little colocalization of poly-GA and aDMA in neuronal inclusions (data not shown). Moreover, the distribution of poly-GR was highly correlated with the distribution of aDMA (Additional file 6: Table S2). We found that aDMA immunoreactivity was present in normal nuclei of various cell types, which is assumed to be physiologic methylation of nuclear proteins, such as histones and RNA-binding proteins [10]. Boeynaems and coworkers previously reported nuclear signal of aDMA in dentate fascia neurons of healthy controls [3]. We also detected nuclear aDMA in control cases (Additional file 7: Figure S5). Therefore, it is reasonable the aDMA nuclear labeling represents physiological methylation. In these proteins, DMA post-translational modification occurs at sites with a consensus glycine/arginine rich (GAR) motif, which may be mimicked by poly-GR. Recent studies show that in addition to GAR-domain class of proteins, other proteins can be targeted by arginine methyltransferases [10]. Based upon histologic features and morphology, the nuclear aDMA we detected was not only in intranuclear inclusions, but also in other nuclear structures. Unlike normal controls, in c9FTLD-MND aDMA was found in the neuronal cytoplasm and it co-localized with poly-GR, especially in the hippocampus.

Given the strong correlation between poly-GR and aDMA, their association with neurodegeneration, and their relative abundance in patients with the most severe clinicopathologic phenotype (FTLD-MND), we hypothesized that post-translational modification of poly-GR may be a novel mechanism of gain of toxicity of poly-GR. In support of this, poly-GR cytoplasmic inclusions in cultured cells expressing GFP-$(GR)_{100}$ were frequently co-labeled with a sensitive and specific antibody to aDMA. Treating the cells with an arginine methyltransferase inhibitor (AdOx), which has intrinsic cytotoxic properties, decreased the numbers of poly-GR cytoplasmic inclusions at times and concentrations not associated with significant cytotoxicity. These findings suggest that formation of poly-GR cytoplasmic inclusions might be influenced by aDMA modification.

Although post-translational modification of proteins with aDMA is often toxic in various tissues in human diseases, including the brain [5, 27, 29], the effects of post-translational aDMA modification is not well understood in the brain. Regarding clinical and experimental studies of CNS disease and aDMA, in hepatic encephalopathy, elevated aDMA levels could potentially contribute to cognitive dysfunction through oxidative stress, restriction of cerebral blood flow and inflammation [5]. In ischemic stroke, elevated levels of aDMA might contribute to brain injury through endothelial cell damage, and aDMA also might be involved in nitric oxide associated oxidative stress and excitotoxicity [4]. In neurodegenerative disorders, Suarez-Calved and coworkers reported that mono-methylated arginine is frequent in FTLD-FUS, but not in ALS-FUS. Unmethylated and mono-methylated methylarginine FUS had much higher binding affinities to the nuclear receptor of FUS, transportin-1, compared to aDMA FUS [28]. To complicate matters, DMA modification is also considered to both positively and negatively regulate protein-protein interactions [10].

A limitation of our study is the inability to detect specific methylated forms (e.g., mono-methylation, symmetrical di-methylation and asymmetrical di-methylation) of poly-GR (and poly-PR). There is also no direct way to know the effect of the DPR polymer repeat length on post-translational modification. Our in vitro cell culture studies used repeat lengths of 50- and 100-mers. These are much smaller repeats that seen in disease brain based upon their mobility on western blots. In this regard, it is interesting to note that Bennion Callister and co-workers pointed out that repeat length effects subcellular distribution of DPR, with smaller repeats producing inclusions in the nucleus (specifically in nucleoli) and larger repeats (> 1000) producing inclusions in the cytoplasm [2]. We were able to detect both nuclear and cytoplasmic inclusions in our cell culture models with much smaller repeats. It remains to be determined if repeat length affects methylation modification. Nevertheless, we suggest that current studies provide preliminary evidence from human neuropathology that post-translational modification of arginine residues may play a role in the toxicity of poly-GR. Clearly, there is need for further study.

Conclusions

In summary, we provide evidence that poly-GR is more closely associated with markers of neurodegeneration than poly-GA and poly-GP. Preliminary evidence suggests that methylation may contribute to this toxicity. Furthermore, in our small clinicopathologic series poly-GR seems to be more abundant in patients with FTLD-MND compared to FTLD or MND. Investigating the contribution of poly-GR to neuronal dysfunction, TDP-43 pathology and neurodegeneration may shed additional light on disease pathogenesis and lead to new therapeutic targets.

Additional files

Additional file 1: Figure S1. Semiquantitative assessment of neurodegeneration. Grading neurodegeneration in FCtx, hippocampal DF, CA4 and CA2/3 are shown. In FCtx, neurodegeneration was assessed by superficial microvacuolation and spongiosis. In DF, gaps in granular cell density were assessed as neurodegeneration. In CA4 and CA2/3, neuronal cell loss and gliosis were assessed as neurodegeneration. Neurodegeneration was graded as absent (G0), mild (G1), moderate (G2) or severe (G3). (TIF 1630 kb)

Additional file 2: Figure S2. Correlation between manual counts and positive pixel burden from color deconvolution in poly-GR staining. Plot shows the correlation of manual counts of neuronal cytoplasmic inclusions and positive pixel burden from color deconvolution in poly-GR staining. The line shows linear regression CD color deconvolution. Ctx frontal cortex, DF dentate fascia, CA - *cornu ammonis*, MCtx motor cortex. (TIF 2581 kb)

Additional file 3: Table S1. Quantitative assessment of DPR density by color deconvolution algorithm in clinicopathologic subgroups of C9ORF72-related disease. In frontal cortex, $p = 0.019$, FTLD vs. FTLD-MND. In CA4, $p = 0.055$, FTLD vs. FTLD-MND. In CA2/3, $p = 0.03$, FTLD vs. FTLD-MND. Significant *p*-values (< 0.05) are indicated in bold. All variables were analyzed with Kruskal-Wallis ANOVA on Ranks and data are displayed as median (25th and 75th range). *Statistically significant p-value ($p < 0.05$); all p-value for ANOVA on Ranks comparison of all three groups. FCtx = frontal cortex, MCtx = Motor cortex, DF dentate fascia, CA hippocampal subfields. (DOCX 15 kb)

Additional file 4: Figure S3. Dot plot graph of semiquantitative assessment of neurodegeneration and DPR. Note that X axis is neurodegeneration score (0 to 3), Y-axis is density of DPR. FCtx - frontal cortex, DF - dentate fascia, CA4 - *cornu ammonis* sector 4. (TIF 1325 kb)

Additional file 5: Figure S4. Western blot analysis of aDMA and sDMA in brains of C9FLTD-MND and sporadic FTLD-MND. The high molecular weight aDMA and sDMA signals are visible in c9FTD/ALS, but not in sporadic FTD/ALS cases. (TIF 2960 kb)

Additional file 6: Table S2. Correlation between DPR and aDMA inclusions. *P*-values are from Pearson's test of correlation. Significant *p*-values (< 0.05) are indicated in bold. FCtx frontal cortex, DF dentate fascia, CA - *cornu ammonis*, MCtx motor cortex. (DOCX 14 kb)

Additional file 7: Figure S5 Comparison of immunostaining with aDMA between C9ORF72 cases and non- neurodegeneration control in parahippocampal cortex. The nuclear signal of aDMA is variable in both cases and controls. Note sparse cytoplasmic inclusions labeled with aDMA in in C9ORF72 cases (arrows). Scale bar represents 50 μM. (TIF 2898 kb)

Acknowledgements
We thank the patients and their families who donated brains to help further our knowledge of c9FTLD-MND. We are grateful to Linda Rousseau and Virginia Phillips for histological support; and to Monica Castanedes-Casey for immunohistochemistry support.

Funding
This study is supported by NIH: P01 NS084974–04, R01 AG037491–08, P50 AG016574–19.

Authors' contributions
NS, KFB, Y-JZ, KR, TFG, MEM and RR contributed to data acquisition and analysis. LP and DWD provided support and scientific oversight for the studies. All authors contributed in writing the final manuscript. All authors have approved the final version of the manuscript.

Competing interests
The authors declare that they have no competing interests.

References

1. Ash PE, Bieniek KF, Gendron TF, Caulfield T, Lin WL, Dejesus-Hernandez M, van Blitterswijk MM, Jansen-West K, Paul JW 3rd, Rademakers R, Boylan KB, Dickson DW, Petrucelli L (2013) Unconventional translation of C9ORF72 GGGGCC expansion generates insoluble polypeptides specific to c9FTD/ALS. Neuron 77:639–646
2. Bennion Callister J, Ryan S, Sim J, Rollinson S, Pickering-Brown SM (2016) Modelling C9orf72 dipeptide repeat proteins of a physiologically relevant size. Hum Mol Genet 25:5069–5082
3. Boeynaems S, Bogaert E, Michiels E, Gijselinck I, Sieben A, Jovicic A, De Baets G, Scheveneels W, Steyaert J, Cuijt I, Verstrepen KJ, Callaerts P, Rousseau F, Schymkowitz J, Cruts M, Van Broeckhoven C, Van Damme P, Gitler AD, Robberecht W, Van Den Bosch L (2016) Drosophila screen connects nuclear transport genes to DPR pathology in c9ALS/FTD. Sci Rep 6:20877
4. Chen S, Li N, Deb-Chatterji M, Dong Q, Kielstein JT, Weissenborn K, Worthmann H (2012) Asymmetric dimethyarginine as marker and mediator in ischemic stroke. Int J Mol Sci 13:15983–16004
5. Czarnecka A, Milewski K, Zielinska M (2017) Asymmetric Dimethylarginine and hepatic encephalopathy: cause, effect or association? Neurochem Res 42:750–761
6. Davidson YS, Barker H, Robinson AC, Thompson JC, Harris J, Troakes C, Smith B, Al-Saraj S, Shaw C, Rollinson S, Masuda-Suzukake M, Hasegawa M, Pickering-Brown S, Snowden JS, Mann DM (2014) Brain distribution of dipeptide repeat proteins in frontotemporal lobar degeneration and motor neurone disease associated with expansions in C9ORF72. Acta Neuropathol Commun 2:70
7. DeJesus-Hernandez M, Mackenzie IR, Boeve BF, Boxer AL, Baker M, Rutherford NJ, Nicholson AM, Finch NA, Flynn H, Adamson J, Kouri N, Wojtas A, Sengdy P, Hsiung GY, Karydas A, Seeley WW, Josephs KA, Coppola G, Geschwind DH, Wszolek ZK, Feldman H, Knopman DS, Petersen RC, Miller BL, Dickson DW, Boylan KB, Graff-Radford NR, Rademakers R (2011) Expanded GGGGCC hexanucleotide repeat in noncoding region of C9ORF72 causes chromosome 9p-linked FTD and ALS. Neuron 72:245–256
8. Dickson DW, Josephs KA, Amador-Ortiz C (2007) TDP-43 in differential diagnosis of motor neuron disorders. Acta Neuropathol 114:71–79
9. Freibaum BD, Taylor JP (2017) The role of dipeptide repeats in C9ORF72-related ALS-FTD. Front Mol Neurosci 10:35
10. Gayatri S, Bedford MT (2014) Readers of histone methylarginine marks. Biochim Biophys Acta 1839:702–710
11. Gendron TF, Bieniek KF, Zhang YJ, Jansen-West K, Ash PE, Caulfield T, Daughrity L, Dunmore JH, Castanedes-Casey M, Chew J, Cosio DM, van Blitterswijk M, Lee WC, Rademakers R, Boylan KB, Dickson DW, Petrucelli L (2013) Antisense transcripts of the expanded C9ORF72 hexanucleotide repeat form nuclear RNA foci and undergo repeat-associated non-ATG translation in c9FTD/ALS. Acta Neuropathol 126:829–844
12. Geser F, Brandmeir NJ, Kwong LK, Martinez-Lage M, Elman L, McCluskey L, Xie SX, Lee VM, Trojanowski JQ (2008) Evidence of multisystem disorder in whole-brain map of pathological TDP-43 in amyotrophic lateral sclerosis. Arch Neurol 65:636–641
13. Geser F, Stein B, Partain M, Elman LB, McCluskey LF, Xie SX, Van Deerlin VM, Kwong LK, Lee VM, Trojanowski JQ (2011) Motor neuron disease clinically limited to the lower motor neuron is a diffuse TDP-43 proteinopathy. Acta Neuropathol 121:509–517
14. Josephs KA, Stroh A, Dugger B, Dickson DW (2009) Evaluation of subcortical pathology and clinical correlations in FTLD-U subtypes. Acta Neuropathol 118:349–358
15. Kwon I, Xiang S, Kato M, Wu L, Theodoropoulos P, Wang T, Kim J, Yun J, Xie Y, McKnight SL (2014) Poly-dipeptides encoded by the C9orf72 repeats bind nucleoli, impede RNA biogenesis, and kill cells. Science 345:1139–1145
16. Mackenzie IR, Arzberger T, Kremmer E, Troost D, Lorenzl S, Mori K, Weng SM, Haass C, Kretzschmar HA, Edbauer D, Neumann M (2013) Dipeptide repeat protein pathology in C9ORF72 mutation cases: clinico-pathological correlations. Acta Neuropathol 126:859–879
17. Mackenzie IR, Frick P, Grasser FA, Gendron TF, Petrucelli L, Cashman NR, Edbauer D, Kremmer E, Prudlo J, Troost D, Neumann M (2015) Quantitative analysis and clinico-pathological correlations of different dipeptide repeat protein pathologies in C9ORF72 mutation carriers. Acta Neuropathol 130:845–861
18. Mackenzie IR, Neumann M, Baborie A, Sampathu DM, Du Plessis D, Jaros E, Perry RH, Trojanowski JQ, Mann DM, Lee VM (2011) A harmonized classification system for FTLD-TDP pathology. Acta Neuropathol 122:111–113
19. Mann DM (2015) Dipeptide repeat protein toxicity in frontotemporal lobar degeneration and in motor neurone disease associated with expansions in C9ORF72-a cautionary note. Neurobiol Aging 36:1224–1226
20. Mizielinska S, Gronke S, Niccoli T, Ridler CE, Clayton EL, Devoy A, Moens T, Norona FE, Woollacott IOC, Pietrzyk J, Cleverley K, Nicoll AJ, Pickering-Brown S, Dols J, Cabecinha M, Hendrich O, Fratta P, Fisher EMC, Partridge L, Isaacs AM (2014) C9orf72 repeat expansions cause neurodegeneration in Drosophila through arginine-rich proteins. Science 345:1192–1194

21. Mori K, Arzberger T, Grasser FA, Gijselinck I, May S, Rentzsch K, Weng SM, Schludi MH, van der Zee J, Cruts M, Van Broeckhoven C, Kremmer E, Kretzschmar HA, Haass C, Edbauer D (2013) Bidirectional transcripts of the expanded C9orf72 hexanucleotide repeat are translated into aggregating dipeptide repeat proteins. Acta Neuropathol 126:881–893
22. Murray ME, Przybelski SA, Lesnick TG, Liesinger AM, Spychalla A, Zhang B, Gunter JL, Parisi JE, Boeve BF, Knopman DS, Petersen RC, Jack CR Jr, Dickson DW, Kantarci K (2014) Early Alzheimer's disease neuropathology detected by proton MR spectroscopy. J Neurosci 34:16247–16255
23. O'Rourke JG, Bogdanik L, Yanez A, Lall D, Wolf AJ, Muhammad AK, Ho R, Carmona S, Vit JP, Zarrow J, Kim KJ, Bell S, Harms MB, Miller TM, Dangler CA, Underhill DM, Goodridge HS, Lutz CM, Baloh RH (2016) C9orf72 is required for proper macrophage and microglial function in mice. Science 351:1324–1329
24. Renton AE, Majounie E, Waite A, Simon-Sanchez J, Rollinson S, Gibbs JR, Schymick JC, Laaksovirta H, van Swieten JC, Myllykangas L, Kalimo H, Paetau A, Abramzon Y, Remes AM, Kaganovich A, Scholz SW, Duckworth J, Ding J, Harmer DW, Hernandez DG, Johnson JO, Mok K, Ryten M, Trabzuni D, Guerreiro RJ, Orrell RW, Neal J, Murray A, Pearson J, Jansen IE, Sondervan D, Seelaar H, Blake D, Young K, Halliwell N, Callister JB, Toulson G, Richardson A, Gerhard A, Snowden J, Mann D, Neary D, Nalls MA, Peuralinna T, Jansson L, Isoviita VM, Kaivorinne AL, Holtta-Vuori M, Ikonen E, Sulkava R, Benatar M, Wuu J, Chio A, Restagno G, Borghero G, Sabatelli M, Heckerman D, Rogaeva E, Zinman L, Rothstein JD, Sendtner M, Drepper C, Eichler EE, Alkan C, Abdullaev Z, Pack SD, Dutra A, Pak E, Hardy J, Singleton A, Williams NM, Heutink P, Pickering-Brown S, Morris HR, Tienari PJ, Traynor BJ (2011) A hexanucleotide repeat expansion in C9ORF72 is the cause of chromosome 9p21-linked ALS-FTD. Neuron 72:257–268
25. Saberi S, Stauffer JE, Jiang J, Garcia SD, Taylor AE, Schulte D, Ohkubo T, Schloffman CL, Maldonado M, Baughn M, Rodriguez MJ, Pizzo D, Cleveland D, Ravits J (2017) Sense-encoded poly-GR dipeptide repeat proteins correlate to neurodegeneration and uniquely co-localize with TDP-43 in dendrites of repeat-expanded C9orf72 amyotrophic lateral sclerosis. Acta Neuropathol
26. Schludi MH, May S, Grasser FA, Rentzsch K, Kremmer E, Kupper C, Klopstock T, Arzberger T, Edbauer D (2015) Distribution of dipeptide repeat proteins in cellular models and C9orf72 mutation cases suggests link to transcriptional silencing. Acta Neuropathol 130:537–555
27. Schwedhelm E, Boger RH (2011) The role of asymmetric and symmetric dimethylarginines in renal disease. Nat Rev Nephrol 7:275–285
28. Suarez-Calvet M, Neumann M, Arzberger T, Abou-Ajram C, Funk E, Hartmann H, Edbauer D, Kremmer E, Gobl C, Resch M, Bourgeois B, Madl T, Reber S, Jutzi D, Ruepp MD, Mackenzie IR, Ansorge O, Dormann D, Haass C (2016) Monomethylated and unmethylated FUS exhibit increased binding to Transportin and distinguish FTLD-FUS from ALS-FUS. Acta Neuropathol 131:587–604
29. Tain YL, Hsu CN (2017) Toxic Dimethylarginines: asymmetric Dimethylarginine (ADMA) and symmetric Dimethylarginine (SDMA). Toxins (Basel) 9
30. Tao Z, Wang H, Xia Q, Li K, Li K, Jiang X, Xu G, Wang G, Ying Z (2015) Nucleolar stress and impaired stress granule formation contribute to C9orf72 RAN translation-induced cytotoxicity. Hum Mol Genet 24:2426–2441
31. Todd TW, Petrucelli L (2016) Insights into the pathogenic mechanisms of chromosome 9 open reading frame 72 (C9orf72) repeat expansions. J Neurochem 138(Suppl 1):145–162
32. Vatsavayai SC, Yoon SJ, Gardner RC, Gendron TF, Vargas JN, Trujillo A, Pribadi M, Phillips JJ, Gaus SE, Hixson JD, Garcia PA, Rabinovici GD, Coppola G, Geschwind DH, Petrucelli L, Miller BL, Seeley WW (2016) Timing and significance of pathological features in C9orf72 expansion-associated frontotemporal dementia. Brain 139:3202–3216
33. Wen X, Tan W, Westergard T, Krishnamurthy K, Markandaiah SS, Shi Y, Lin S, Shneider NA, Monaghan J, Pandey UB, Pasinelli P, Ichida JK, Trotti D (2014) Antisense proline-arginine RAN dipeptides linked to C9ORF72-ALS/FTD form toxic nuclear aggregates that initiate in vitro and in vivo neuronal death. Neuron 84:1213–1225
34. Yang D, Abdallah A, Li Z, Lu Y, Almeida S, Gao FB (2015) FTD/ALS-associated poly(GR) protein impairs the notch pathway and is recruited by poly(GA) into cytoplasmic inclusions. Acta Neuropathol 130:525–535

3

Alzheimer's associated amyloid and tau deposition co-localizes with a homeostatic myelin repair pathway in two mouse models of post-stroke mixed dementia

Thuy-Vi V. Nguyen[1,2], Megan Hayes[1], Jacob C. Zbesko[1], Jennifer B. Frye[1], Nicole R. Congrove[4], Nadia P. Belichenko[5], Brian S. McKay[4], Frank M. Longo[5] and Kristian P. Doyle[1,2,3*]

Abstract

The goal of this study was to determine the chronic impact of stroke on the manifestation of Alzheimer's disease (AD) related pathology and behavioral impairments in mice. To accomplish this goal, we used two distinct models. First, we experimentally induced ischemic stroke in aged wildtype (wt) C57BL/6 mice to determine if stroke leads to the manifestation of AD-associated pathological β-amyloid (Aβ) and tau in aged versus young adult wt mice. Second, we utilized a transgenic (Tg) mouse model of AD (hAPP-SL) to determine if stroke leads to the worsening of pre-existing AD pathology, as well as the development of pathology in brain regions not typically expressed in AD Tg mice. In the wt mice, there was delayed motor recovery and an accelerated development of cognitive deficits in aged mice compared to young adult mice following stroke. This corresponded with increased brain atrophy, increased cholinergic degeneration, and a focal increase of Aβ in areas of axonal degeneration in the ipsilateral hemisphere of the aged animals. By contrast, in the hAPP-SL mice, we found that ischemia induced aggravated behavioral deficits in conjunction with a global increase in Aβ, tau, and cholinergic pathology compared to hAPP-SL mice that underwent a sham stroke procedure. With regard to a potential mechanism, in both models, we found that the stroke-induced Aβ and tau deposits co-localized with increased levels of β-secretase 1 (BACE1), along with its substrate, neuregulin 1 (NGR1) type III, both of which are proteins integral for myelin repair. Based on these findings, we propose that the chronic sequelae of stroke may be ratcheting-up a myelin repair pathway, and that the consequent increase in BACE1 could be causing an inadvertent cleavage of its alternative substrate, AβPP, resulting in greater Aβ seeding and pathogenesis.

Keywords: Stroke, Alzheimer's disease, Mixed dementia, Amyloid, Tau, BACE1, Neuregulin, Myelin repair

Introduction

People over the age of 55 have a 1 in 6 lifetime risk of suffering a stroke, and 1 in 10 people aged 65 years or older are diagnosed with Alzheimer's disease (AD) [6, 17]. Currently, there are more than 6.5 million stroke survivors in the United States, a third of whom will develop post-stroke dementia, within 3-6 months of the ischemic event, and there are more than 5 million Americans living with AD [83]. In light of these facts, it is unsurprising that the most common form of mixed dementia is the co-morbidity of vascular pathology, such as the presence of chronic stroke infarcts, alongside AD-associated pathology. Indeed, post-mortem analyses from the National Institute of Health's Rush Memory and Aging Project suggest that nearly 50% of clinically diagnosed AD patients have a mixture of infarct and AD (amyloid plaques and neurofibrillary tangles) pathologies [27, 80, 82]. Yet despite this evidence for the co-existence of stroke and AD-like pathology, little is known about the role that ischemic infarcts play in the pathogenesis, distribution, and burden of toxic amyloid and tau species seen in AD.

* Correspondence: doylekr@email.arizona.edu
[1]Department of Immunobiology, University of Arizona, 1656 E. Mabel Street, Tucson, AZ 85719, USA
[2]Department of Neurology, University of Arizona, 1656 E. Mabel Street, Tucson, AZ 85719, USA
Full list of author information is available at the end of the article

With regard to prior animal research that has examined the impact of stroke on the pathology and cognitive decline related to the AD phenotype, Qui and colleagues have shown that 2 months of cerebral hypoperfusion enhances phosphorylated (p)-tau in adult Aβ precursor protein (AβPP) transgenic (Tg) mice [70]. In addition, Lee and colleagues have demonstrated that cerebral hypoperfusion worsens cognitive dysfunction in adult AβPP Tg mice [52]. Likewise, Pimentel-Coelho and colleagues found that 6 weeks of cerebral hypoperfusion induces cognitive dysfunction in young adult AβPP/presenilin 1 (PS1) Tg mice that is strongly correlated with Aβ plaque burden, but not in their wildtype (wt) littermates [68]. However, these cerebral hypoperfusion studies do not provide information with regard to how amyloid manifests in response to the chronic consequences of a distinct infarct.

This gap in knowledge is partly filled by work from the Simpkins research group, which has shown that a middle cerebral artery occlusion (MCAO) in young adult rats results in apoptosis and tau pathology at 2 and 24 hours post-stroke, respectively [101, 102]. Similarly, Garcia-Alloza and colleagues have reported that a MCAO or photothrombotic (PT) stroke in adult and mature AβPP/PS1dE9 mice correlates with significant accumulation of Aβ plaques at 7 days post-stroke [30]. Whitehead and colleagues found that giving a vasoconstrictor, endothelin-1 (ET-1), to adult AβPP Tg mice results in a stroke with increased AβPP and tau-2 expression by 8 days post-stroke [104]. However, these studies have only investigated the effect of ischemia on the development of AD-associated amyloid, tau, AβPP proteins in the post-stroke timeframe of hours and days.

With regard to the long-term impact of stroke on the development of pathology and other phenotypic markers associated with AD, Back and colleagues recently reported that chronic cerebral hypoperfusion following MCAO in rats results in synergistic impairment of spatial memory, enhanced neuroinflammation, and aggravated amyloid pathology after 12 weeks; however, they only found a significant increase in amyloid burden and inflammation in the ipsilateral hemisphere [7]. Likewise, in another rat model, after waiting 12 weeks post-stroke, Sharp and colleagues detected the presence of Aβ in the ipsilateral cortex surrounding the infarct, but only after administering lipopolysaccharide (LPS) as an inflammatory stimulus [109]. Recently, Ong and colleagues found toxic Aβ oligomers in the thalami of adult mice at 6 weeks following PT stroke. Using rats instead of mice, they also found exacerbation of pathology, but only when the rats were exposed to chronic behavior-induced stress in addition to a PT stroke [66]. These studies, however, have only utilized wt mice and rats rather than Tg mouse models of AD, which have proven useful for revealing disease-related mechanisms.

Taken together, these studies all support the hypothesis that the genesis of AD-associated pathology is a chronic sequela of ischemic stroke under certain circumstances, and they have introduced important models of mixed dementia (i.e., the co-existence of infarct and AD-related pathologies) that can be used to help untangle causality. However, to fill a gap that still remains in the field, the goal of this study was to evaluate the impact of stroke on the development of pathology, degeneration, and behavioral dysfunction associated with the AD phenotype over a chronic time period in aged and young wildtype mice, as well as a Tg AβPP mouse line (hAPP-SL).

To accomplish this goal, we employed a distal MCAO plus hypoxia stroke model, which our research group previously demonstrated causes delayed cognitive decline [21]. Considering that AD-related pathology has been reported in the brains of patients with post-stroke dementia, this is a pertinent model for investigating the pathophysiology of post-stroke mixed dementia. However as a caveat, and to be clear, this study is not modeling mixed AD vascular dementia, associated with the presence of white matter lesions, lacunar infarcts, microinfarcts, and microbleeds [39]. Rather, this study is using mice to specifically emulate how an ischemic stroke in a large to medium size artery impacts AD related pathology in humans.

Using our model of post-stroke mixed dementia, we found that multiple neuropathological abnormalities associated with AD develop over the course of 8 weeks in the white matter tracts (mainly in the internal capsule and thalamus regions, where axonal degeneration resulting from a stroke can be found) in the ipsilateral hemisphere of aged wt mice, but not young adult mice following stroke. Aged AβPP Tg mice, however, develop exacerbated archetypal London/Swedish mutation AD pathology in both hemispheres, as well as in the ipsilateral white matter tract regions apparent in wt mice at 12 weeks following stroke. In both of these models, Aβ and tau pathology overlapped with increased levels of BACE1 and its substrate NGR1 type III, both of which are critical components of a myelin repair pathway [10, 15]. Although this is not evidence of causality, these observations are in agreement with George Bartzokis' proposed myelin model of AD as a homeostatic response to myelin breakdown [11]. That is to say, a possible interpretation of the findings reported here is that the chronic sequelae of stroke may be ratcheting-up a neuregulin dependent myelin repair pathway, and the consequent increase in BACE1 may be causing inadvertent cleavage of AβPP, resulting in greater Aβ seeding and pathogenesis. The two mouse models of post-stroke mixed dementia introduced in this study now provide powerful tools to test this working hypothesis, as well as alternative hypotheses.

Materials and methods

C57BL/6 and hAPP-SL mice

For the purpose of investigating the chronic impact of a stroke infarct on pathogenesis related to AD in mice with no known predisposition for AD-like pathology (see Study design in Fig. 1a), we considered different ages and used both young adult and aged male C57BL/6 mice, which were purchased from The Jackson Laboratory (stock number: 000664). Each wt mouse was given a stroke or sham surgery starting at either 3 or 18 months old (mo). Behavioral testing was performed a week before surgery, and final testing completed during week 7, after which mice were sacrificed at week 8 post-surgery, when they were then 5 and 20 mo, respectively. A cohort of 17-18 mo wt mice were sacrificed at 12 weeks after surgery, when they were 20-21 mo, to extend the post-stroke time interval in order to determine the kinetics of deleterious processes that may still be progressing.

For the purpose of investigating the effects of a chronic stroke on existing AD pathology (see Study design in Fig. 2a), aged male hAPP-SL (Thy1-hAβPP$^{\text{Lond/Swe}}$) mice were used. This transgenic mouse line 41 over-expresses human AβPP751 containing the London

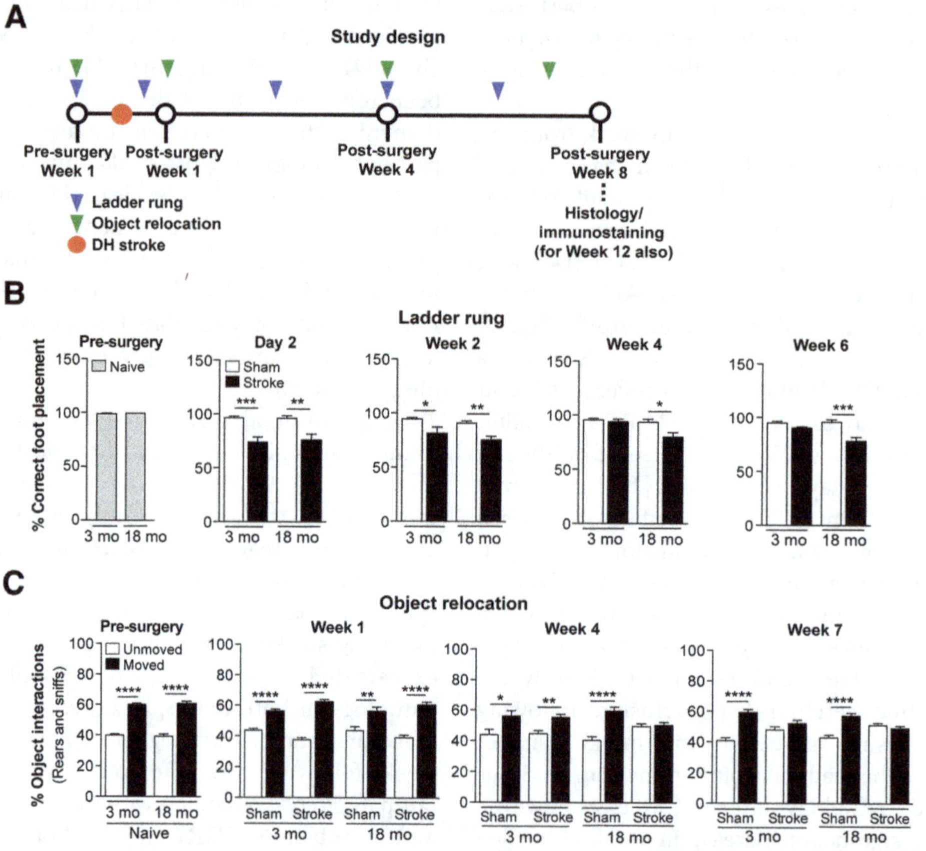

Fig. 1 Motor recovery is impaired and there is accelerated onset of cognitive impairment in aged versus young adult C57BL/6 mice following stroke. **a** Study design: 3 and 18 month-old (mo) C57BL/6 mice were assessed on the ladder rung and object relocation tests prior to a distal hypoxic (DH) stroke or sham surgery at the indicated timepoints. Following behavioral testing, mice were euthanized and brains were harvested for histology and immunostaining at either 8 or 12 weeks post-surgery. **b** Motor ability on the ladder rung test was assessed at 1 week pre-surgery, and at 2 days, 2 weeks, 4 weeks, and 6 weeks post-surgery. At 1 week prior to a stroke, there was no difference in motor performance between 3 and 18 mo mice, as both age groups displayed a similar number of correct (nearly 100%) foot placements on the rungs. At 2 days and 2 weeks post-surgery, 3 and 18 mo stroked mice exhibited a motor deficit, as both age groups displayed a significantly fewer number of correct foot placement relative to age-matched sham mice. However, at 4 and 6 weeks post-surgery, 3 mo stroked mice exhibited motor recovery, as they displayed an indistinguishable number of correct foot placements as age-matched sham mice, which was once again nearly 100% correct. 18 mo stroked mice, however, continued to exhibit a motor deficit relative to age-matched sham mice at 4 and 6 weeks post-surgery. **c** Cognitive function using the object relocation test was assessed at 1 week pre-surgery, and at 1 week, 4 weeks, and 7 weeks post-surgery. At 1 week prior to a stroke, there was no difference in cognitive function between 3 and 18 mo mice, as both age groups displayed significantly more interactions (sniffs and rears) with moved (novel location) verses unmoved objects relative to age-matched sham mice. However, at 4 weeks post-surgery, the 18 mo stroked mice exhibited cognitive dysfunction, as they were now interacting with the two sets of objects equally, indicating that they could no longer distinguish between the moved and unmoved objects. Not until 7 weeks post-surgery did the 3 mo stroked mice exhibit cognitive dysfunction. Data represent mean ± SEM. *p<0.05, **p<0.01, ***p<0.001, and ****p<0.0001

(V717I) and Swedish (K670M/N671L) mutations under the control of the Thy1 promoter [25, 33, 38, 47, 67, 75–77, 79], and is maintained on a C57BL/6 background. Because of a month age gap between the youngest and oldest hAPP-SL mice, they were randomized to either stroke or sham surgery groups such that there was no significant difference in age (reflective of extent of pathology) between experimental conditions. Each hAPP-SL mouse was given either a stroke or sham operation at 17-18 mo. Behavioral testing in these mice was performed a week before surgery, and final testing completed during week 11, after which mice were sacrificed 12 weeks after surgery at 20-21 mo to ensure that enough time passed to discern any enhancement in pathology due to a stroke.

All mice were housed under a 12-hour light/dark schedule with *ad libitum* access to food and water. In behavioral experiments, mice were handled by the experimenter in the procedure room for 5 days before testing, and habituated to the procedure room 2 hours prior to testing. Each behavioral testing arena and each object was thoroughly cleaned with 10% ethanol and allowed to dry between each trial. At study completion, mice were anesthetized with 5% isoflurane, followed by intracardial perfusion with 0.9% saline. Brains were extracted, and either the target regions dissected and snap frozen in liquid nitrogen for biochemical assays, or the whole brain was post-immersed in 4% paraformaldehyde and cyroprotected in 30% sucrose prior to sectioning. All behavioral testing and analyses, including biochemical and morphological analyses were performed with blinding to experimental condition, except in the case of tissue processing due to the visibility of the stroke lesion. Experiments were performed in accordance with protocols approved by the University of Arizona Institutional Animal Care and Use Committee, and were based on the National of Health Guide for the Care and Use of Laboratory Animals.

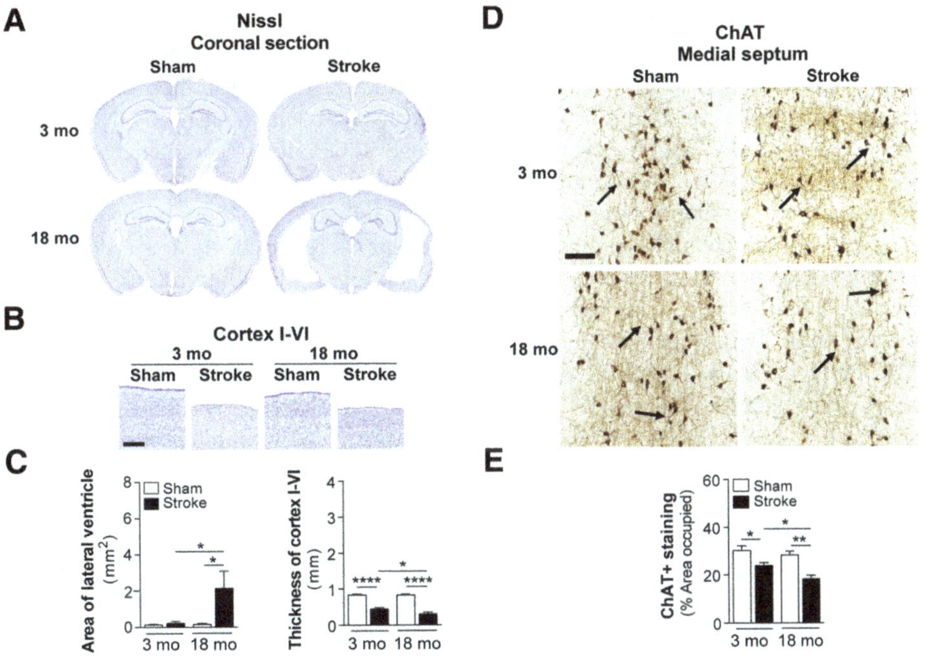

Fig. 2 Brain atrophy and cholinergic degeneration is more pronounced in aged versus young adult C57BL/6 mice following stroke. **a** Representative 4× images of Nissl-stained whole brain sections from 3 and 18 month-old (mo), sham- and stroke-operated C57BL/6 mice at 8 weeks post-surgery. **b** Representative 2× images of Nissl-stained cortical layers I-VI of the ipsilateral primary somatosensory cortex in 3 and 18 mo, sham- and stroke-operated mice at 8 weeks post-surgery. Scale bar, 250 μm. **c** Quantification of the lateral ventricle (left graph) in the ipsilateral hemisphere revealed significant ventricle enlargement in the 18 mo stroked mice relative to the age-matched sham-operated mice. Furthermore, the 18 mo stroked mice had a significantly larger ventricle area compared to the 3 mo stroked mice. Quantification of cortical thickness (right graph) in the ipsilateral hemisphere revealed significant tissue loss or shrinkage in both the 3 and 18 mo stroked mice relative to age-matched sham-operated mice. Furthermore, the 18 mo stroked mice had significantly more tissue loss compared to the 3 mo stroke mice. **d** Representative 5× images of choline acetyltransferase (ChAT)-immunolabeled neuronal cell bodies, their neurites, and innervating projection fibers in the medial septum of the basal forebrain in 3 and 18 mo, sham- and stroke-operated C57BL/6 mice at 8 weeks post-surgery. Many neurites (arrows) in the stroked mice displayed qualitative degenerative changes, including decreased length relative to sham mice. Scale bar, 100 μm. **e** Quantification of cholinergic somas, neurites, and fibers revealed a significant reduction of ChAT+ staining in both the 3 and 18 mo stroked mice relative to the age-matched sham mice. Furthermore, the 18 mo stroked mice exhibited significantly more loss of ChAT+ staining compared to the 3 mo stroked mice. Data represent mean ± SEM. *p<0.05, **p<0.01, and ****p<0.0001

Stroke and sham surgeries

Distal MCAO plus hypoxia (DH stroke) was performed in mice, as previously described [22, 63, 108]. Mice were anesthetized by isoflurane inhalation, and an incision was made to expose the temporalis muscle. A pocket was created in the muscle to expose the skull underneath, and the right MCA identified. A microdrill was used to expose the underlying MCA. The meninges were cut, and the vessel cauterized using a small vessel cauterizer. The wound was then closed using surgical glue. Immediately following surgery, mice were placed in a large chamber containing 9% oxygen and 91% nitrogen for 45 minutes. Sham mice underwent the same surgical steps, except for cauterization of the MCA, and were also given 9% oxygen and 91% nitrogen for 45 minutes immediately after surgery. Core body temperature was maintained at 37°C throughout surgery and hypoxia.

This stroke model creates a large infarct comprising approximately 25% of the ipsilateral hemisphere, and is adjacent to the hippocampus, but does not incorporate it to avoid an immediate memory deficit. This model has little variability, and excellent long-term survivability [22]. Hypoxia is necessary with this model because C57BL/6 mice that underdo distal MCAO without hypoxia have significantly smaller infarcts [22]. Although hypoxia is required for DH stroke, we found that other stroke paradigms such as PT stroke, which does not require hypoxia, or BALB/c mice that undergo distal MCAO without hypoxia, have similar infarct size and degree of morphological and biochemical outcomes in similar regions of the brain as C57BL/6 mice given DH stroke [22, 23, 63, 108]. Furthermore, we found that naïve mice do not differ from sham mice that undergo a sham procedure and hypoxia on behavioral, morphological, and biochemical parameters at 12 weeks post-surgery.

Ladder rung test

The ladder rung test [69] was adapted from the ladder rung walking task [26, 59]. The apparatus consisted of two plexiglass walls (0.64 cm width × 76.20 cm length × 15.24 cm height) spaced 3.18 cm apart, just wide enough for the animal to pass through. Plexiglass rungs (10.16 cm long with a 0.32 cm diameter) were inserted across the length of the walls and spaced at a constant distance of 0.64 cm apart. Both ends of the apparatus were placed atop standard mouse housing cages so that the rungs are 38 cm from the tabletop. A desk lamp illuminating the start zone incentivized the animals to traverse the ladder, and a small igloo leading to the home cage was placed at the end zone.

The test was performed at 1-week pre-surgery for all mice, at 1, 4, and 7 weeks post-surgery for C57BL/6 mice (n=8-10 per experimental group), and at 1, 6, and 11 weeks post-surgery for hAPP-SL mice (n=16-17 per experimental group). Prior to pre-surgery testing, training was necessary to ensure that the animals were able to spontaneously traverse the apparatus. Eight training trials were required for animals to make an acceptable minimum number of limb placing errors (<12% error). Traversing animals were recorded from below the ladder with a handheld video recorder. Each animal was tested once for a given day, and each trial was analyzed frame-by-frame using standard film play-back software (VLC media player for Mac OSX). Tallying began once the first visible full gait cycle had been completed (i.e., all four limbs had been placed). If a limb was placed on a rung and was not subsequently removed, a correct step was recorded. If a limb was placed and subsequently slipped off the rung, a missed step was recorded. If a limb was placed and subsequently replaced on the same rung, a correction step was recorded. Tallying was complete after the animal's final gait cycle. The percent correct foot placement was calculated as 100 × [correct step/(correct step + missed step + correction step)].

Object relocation (OR) test

C57BL/6 mice (n=10-16 per experimental group) were habituated for 5 minutes to an empty arena (50 cm width × 50 cm length × 50 cm height) composed of beige acrylonitrile butadiene styrene (ABS) plastic, and containing spatial cues on two of the walls. Mice were then returned to their home cage while four different objects were placed in the arena. The objects consisted of children's building blocks of different shapes and colors, and each was placed in a corner of the arena, 5 cm from the walls. Baseline studies showed no innate preference between objects (data not shown). Mice were allowed to explore the objects for 5 minutes and were then returned to their home cage. The positions of two of the objects were then switched. Rodents have a natural tendency to explore novelty, and in this test, spend more time exploring or interacting with objects that have been relocated. After 5 minutes, mice were then returned to the arena, and the number of interactions (rears and sniffs) for moved and unmoved objects was recorded for 5 minutes. Different sets of objects were used for each timepoint to control for biases from previously exposed objects.

Y-maze spontaneous alternation behavior (SAB) test

hAPP-SL mice (n=16-17 per experimental group) were tested in a Y-shaped maze composed of beige ABS plastic, and consisted of two symmetrical arms and one longer arm set at a 120° angle from each other (equal arms: 7.5 cm width × 37.0 cm length × 12.5 cm height; longer arm: 7.5 cm width × 42.0 cm length × 12.5 cm height). Mice were placed at the end of the longest arm of the maze, facing outward, and allowed to freely explore the three arms for 5 minutes. Over the course of multiple entries, mice normally exhibited a tendency to visit new arms of the maze rather than visiting a recently visited arm. An entry was recorded when all four limbs of the mouse were within an arm. The number of arm entries and the number of triads were recorded by an ANY-maze behavioral video tracking software (Stoelting), and the percentage of SAB was calculated by the software.

Novel object recognition (NOR) test

On day 1, hAPP-SL mice (n=14-16 per experimental group) were placed with cage mates for 15 minutes in the testing apparatus, a white opaque arena (38 cm width × 48 cm length × 20 cm height) made of ABS plastic. On day 2, each mouse was allowed to explore the arena alone for 15 minutes. On day 3 (object exposure and testing), each mouse was placed in the arena along with two identical objects located at different corners of the arena 5 cm from the walls. The objects consisted of children's building blocks of different shapes and colors. Baseline studies showed no innate preference between objects (data not shown). Mice were allowed to explore the objects until 5 minutes of exploration had accrued. Object exploration was defined as contact with the object by the mouse's nose within 2 cm of the object, which was recorded by ANY-maze behavioral video tracking software. An object recognition test lasting for 5 minutes was performed 4 hours later. For testing, mice were placed back in the box with a "familiar" object (FO), which they had previously explored earlier in the day, and a novel object (NO). The object role (novel versus familiar) and position (left versus right) were balanced within each experimental group. Different sets of objects were used for each timepoint to control for biases from previously exposed objects. The percentage of recognition index was calculated as 100 × [(NO Time)/(NO Time + FO Time)] using total time spent exploring each object computed by the software.

Light dark transition (LDT) test

The apparatus used for the LDT test consisted of an arena (40 cm width × 40 cm length × 35 cm height) divided into two equally sized chambers (each 20 cm width × 40 cm length × 35 cm height) with an opening (5 cm × 5 cm) between them. One chamber was made of Plexiglas that was transparent, opened on top, and brightly illuminated (390 lux) overhead. The other chamber was made of black ABS plastic, enclosed with a top lid, and kept dark (2 lux). hAPP-SL mice (n=17 per experimental group) were each placed in the enclosed, dark chamber of the arena at the beginning of the 10-minute trial, while being tracked by ANY-maze behavioral video tracking software once it entered the transparent, light chamber by placement of the center of its body in the doorway. The time spent in the light chamber was recorded and reported by the software.

Body weight, spleen weight, and frailty score

Physiological parameters of body and spleen weights were taken from each animal. For body weight, hAPP-SL mice (n=15-17 per experimental group) were each weighed at the pre-surgery (baseline timepoint), and at 1 week (early timepoint), 6 weeks (mid-timepoints), and 11 weeks (final timepoints) post-surgery. Spleen weights, however, were taken from mice (n=16 per experimental group) following tissue harvest at the end of the study, at 12 weeks post-surgery.

Frailty was assessed using a noninvasive scoring system developed by Whitehead and colleagues using aged C57BL/6 mice [103], in which an overall clinical frailty index was calculated for each animal based on scores across frailty parameters, age, and clinical comparisons to humans. Frailty in hAPP-SL mice (n=16-17 per experimental group) was assessed at the pre-surgery and post-surgery timepoints.

Nissl staining

Mounted, dehydrated brain sections were cleared in xylenes, rehydrated, immersed in 0.5% cresyl violet acetate (Millipore Sigma) solution for 1 minute, rinsed with distilled water, differentiated in 0.25% acetic alcohol, dehydrated though a graded ethanol series, cleared, and coverslipped with mounting media.

Immunostaining

Frozen coronal sections (40 μm) were taken through the entire brain using a freezing Microm HM 450 sliding microtome (ThermoFisher Scientific), and immunostained according to standard protocols [64]. The following antibodies were used: rabbit anti-Aβ_{42} (abcam; RRID: AB_443253), mouse anti-AT8 [recognizes tau phosphorylated at serine 202 and threonine 205 (p-tau$^{Ser202/Thr205}$, ThermoFisher Scientific; RRID: AB_223647)], rabbit anti-tau (abcam, Cat No: ab32057), goat anti-choline acetyl transferase (ChAT, Millipore Sigma; RRID: AB94647), rabbit anti-BACE1 (Cell Signaling; AB_1903900), and rabbit anti-NRG1 type III (abcam, Cat No: ab23248). Briefly, free floating sections were immunolabeled with antibodies (1:300 for Aβ_{42}, 1:1500 for AT8, 1:800 for ChAT, 1:400 for BACE1, and 1:200 for NRG1 type III) in conjunction with M.O.M (for AT8), ABC Vector Elite, and 3,3'-diaminobenzidine or Vector VIP kits (for AT8) (Vector Laboratories) for visualization. For immunofluorescence staining, rabbit anti-NRG1 type III (1:50), mouse anti-AT8 (1:100), chicken anti-glial fibrillary acidic protein (GFAP, 1:500, Millipore Sigma; RRID: AB_177521), and chicken anti-ionized calcium binding adaptor molecule 1 (Iba1, 1:100, abcam; RRID: AB_2728648) antibodies were used, followed by goat anti-rabbit and donkey anti-chicken Alexa Fluor secondary antibodies (Molecular Probes), or a DyLight Fluor fluorescent dye (ThermoFisher Scientific) was used following secondary antibody incubation using the M.O.M kit for AT8. Images of sections co-stained with immunofluorescence antibodies were captured with a Keyence BZ-X700 fluorescence microscope using 488 nm and 647 nm filters. Amyloid plaques were stained with 1% Thioflavin S (ThioS; Millipore Sigma), and viewed under a fluorescence microscope using the 488 filter.

Fluoro-Jade staining and analysis

To identify the area of axonal degeneration following DH stroke, brain sections were pre-mounted on slides, air-dried, and subjected to Fluoro-Jade staining. For consistency to the methodology of measuring white matter tracts labeled with $A\beta_{42}$, p-tau, BACE1, and NRG1 type III, one section per mouse (n=4 per experimental group) at bregma -1.70 was also analyzed for Fluoro-Jade staining. This section allows one 10× field per section (landmark: starting at the reticular thalamus nucleus) to be taken for each of the following white matter tracts in a hemisphere. Briefly, the sections were immersed in a 1% NaOH and 80% ethanol solution for 5 minutes, followed by 2 minutes each in 70% ethanol and distilled water. The sections were then transferred to a solution of 0.06% potassium permanganate (Sigma-Aldrich) for 10 minutes and rinsed in distilled water for 2 minutes. The sections were then immersed to a 0.0001% solution of Fluoro-Jade C (Biosensis) dissolved in 0.1% acetic acid (pH 3.5) for 10 minutes, washed with distilled water 3 times for 1 minute each, and then left to dry overnight at room temperature in darkness and coverslipped with Entellan (Electron Microscopy Sciences). Fluoro-Jade sections were viewed under a Keyence BZ-X700 fluorescence microscope using a 488 nm filter, and digital images captured. Fluoro-Jade fluorescent staining was measured from the digital images using histogram thresholding with NIH ImageJ analysis software and computed. The threshold was set manually to identify dense immunostaining that was distinct from the background. Values for each field within a given mouse were averaged to yield one value per mouse. The Fluoro-Jade+ staining area was expressed as a percentage of the total area analyzed.

Western blotting

To authenticate the specificity of BACE1 and NRG1 type III antibodies, white matter regions (thalamus/internal capsule) were dissected from stroked mouse brains and sonicated in ice-cold 0.1 M phosphate buffered saline (PBS) containing 1% triton X-100 and 0.1% sodium deoxycholate, Protease Inhibitor Cocktail (1:100; Millipore Sigma), and Phosphatase Inhibitor Cocktail 2 (1:100; Millipore Sigma). Following centrifugation, the total protein concentration of each supernatant was measured using a Direct Detect Infrared Spectrometer (Millipore Sigma). Samples were then resolved by electrophoresis, transferred to a nitrocellulose membrane, and probed with the same BACE1 or NRG1 type III antibodies used for immunostaining throughout the manuscript: rabbit anti-BACE1 (1:1000, Cell Signaling) and rabbit anti-NRG1 type III (1:1000, Abcam). Following incubation with the appropriate secondary antibodies, proteins were visualized using a chemiluminescence detection system (GE Healthcare Life Sciences).

Anti-$A\beta_{42}$ antisera affinity subtraction

Affinity chromatography was used to verify specificity of the anti-$A\beta_{42}$ antibody produced against the $A\beta_{1-42}$ peptide (rat/mouse form, abcam, Cat No: ab120959). Briefly, the immunizing peptide was immobilized on aldehyde-activated agarose beads (AminoLink Plus Coupling Resin, ThermoFisher Scientific), as per the manufacturer's directions. After coupling the peptide covalently to the immobilized support, the column was washed extensively in quenching buffer to block any remaining active sites. Subsequently, the column was flushed with 10 mL of 0.1 M PBS. To remove antibodies against $A\beta_{42}$ from the antisera, the sera was passed over the resin bed subtracting antibodies with affinity to the $A\beta_{1-42}$ peptide. We performed parallel immunostaining using the complete antisera and the $A\beta_{1-42}$ peptide subtracted antisera as a negative control. There was no staining detected using the peptide subtracted sera, indicating the specificity of staining achieved with the complete sera.

Quantitation of brain atrophy

Two coronal brain sections (containing the hippocampi) per mouse (n=4-5 per experimental group) at bregma -1.70 and -1.94 based on the mouse brain atlas of Franklin and Paxinos 3rd edition [28] were analyzed for anatomical abnormalities via Nissl staining. The area of the lateral ventricles, and the thickness of the primary somatosensory cortex (landmarks: from the corpus callosum through cortical layers I-VI) of each hemisphere per section were manually traced using ImageJ (National Institute of Health) analysis software. The area of the ventricles and the thickness of the cortex were then computed by ImageJ. For each mouse, the values from each section were averaged to yield one value for each measurement (area of the ventricle or thickness of the cortex) per mouse.

Quantitation of cholinergic degeneration

ChAT-immunolabeled cholinergic somas and their neurites in the medial septum of the basal forebrain, which innervate hippocampal and cortical areas, as well as innervating fibers into the medial septum, were assessed in two sections per mouse (n=4-8 mice per experimental group). To generate an image of the complete medial septal nucleus in each section, four 10× fields were taken throughout the medial septum between bregma +1.18 and +0.74 per section, and stitched together to generate the entire medial septum for quantification. ChAT+ staining was measured from the digital images using histogram thresholding with NIH ImageJ analysis software and computed. The threshold was set manually to identify dense immunostaining that was distinct from the background. Values for each section within a given mouse were averaged to yield one value per mouse. The immunostained area was expressed as a percentage of the total area analyzed.

For assessment of dystrophic cholinergic neurites in the cortex, 5-6 sections per mouse (n=7-9 per experimental group) were analyzed. Two non-overlapping, adjacent 10× fields of the cortex comprising the cingulate, motor, and primary somatosensory areas in each hemisphere between bregma +1.18 and -1.94 were analyzed, for a total of 10-12 fields per mouse. ChAT+ staining of dystrophic neurites was measured from the digital images using histogram thresholding with NIH ImageJ analysis software and computed. The threshold was set manually to identify dense immunostaining that was distinct from the background. Values for each field within a given mouse were averaged to yield one value per mouse. The immunostained area was expressed as a percentage of the total area analyzed.

Quantitation of $A\beta_{42}$ immunoreactivity

In C57BL/6 mice (n=4-8 per experimental group), one section per mouse containing regions of white matter tracts following DH stroke surgery at bregma -1.70 were analyzed. This section allows two to three non-overlapping, adjacent 10× fields to be taken for each of the following white matter tracts in each hemisphere: (i) 2 fields for the internal capsule region (landmarks: in the upper part bordered by the stria terminalis); (ii) 2 fields for the thalamus regions (landmarks: at the reticular thalamus nucleus to the ventrolateral thalamic nucleus); and (iii) 3 fields for the corpus callosum region (landmarks: bordered by the indusium griseum and the dorsal fornix). Aβ+ immunoreactivity was measured from the digital images using histogram thresholding with NIH ImageJ analysis software and computed. The threshold was set manually to identify dense immunostaining that was distinct from the background. Values for each field within a given mouse were averaged to yield one value per mouse. The immunostained area was expressed as a percentage of the total area analyzed.

For consistency, one section per mouse at bregma -1.70 was also analyzed for $A\beta_{42}$ immunoreactivity in the hAPP-SL mice (n=6-8 per experimental group). However, both white matter tracts as well as grey matter regions in these mice were quantified due to the much more widespread deposition of $A\beta_{42}$ following stroke or sham surgery. Therefore, two to three non-overlapping, adjacent 10× fields were taken from each hemisphere: (i) 3 fields of the cortex (landmarks: beginning at the retrosplenial granular/dysgranular to the primary/secondary somatosensory areas); (ii) 2 fields of the central part of the hippocampus (landmarks: comprising the oriens layer into the dentate gyrus to CA1 to CA2/3; (iii) 2 fields for the internal capsule region (landmarks: in the upper part bordered by the stria terminalis); and (iv) 2 fields for the thalamus (landmarks: at the reticular thalamus nucleus to the ventrolateral thalamic nucleus). Aβ+ immunoreactivity was measured from the digital images using histogram thresholding with NIH ImageJ analysis software and computed. The threshold was set manually to identify dense immunostaining that was distinct from the background. Values for each field within a given mouse were averaged to yield one value per mouse. The immunostained area was expressed as a percentage of the total area analyzed.

In the same hAPP-SL mice, 3 sections per mouse (n=7-8 per experimental group) between bregma -1.34 and -2.18 were also analyzed for ThioS-stained fibrillary Aβ. 4× fields were imaged from each brain section. The percentage occupied by ThioS+ staining was computed using NIH ImageJ software and computed. Values for each section per mouse were averaged to yield one value per mouse. The area of ThioS+ staining was expressed as a percentage of the total area analyzed.

Quantitation of tau immunoreactivity

For assessment of AT8 (p-tau) immunoreactivity, sections in regions encompassing areas of white matter tracts following DH stroke surgery between bregma -1.46 and -2.18 were analyzed (n=7-9 per experimental group). For each of the following regions, two to three non-overlapping, adjacent 10× fields were taken for each section from each hemisphere: (i) Cortex: 3 sections per mouse, 3 fields per section (landmark: at the retrosplenial granular/dysgranular to the primary/secondary somatosensory areas); (ii) Internal capsule: 3 sections per mouse, 1 field per section (landmark: starting at the upper part bordered by the stria terminalis); and (iii) Thalamus: 1 section per mouse, 1 field per section (landmark: starting at the reticular thalamus nucleus). p-tau+ staining was quantified from the digital images using histogram thresholding with NIH ImageJ analysis software and computed. The threshold was set manually to identify dense immunostaining that was distinct from the background. The immunostained area was expressed as the percentage of the total area analyzed.

Quantitation of BACE1 and NRG1 type III immunoreactivity

Similar to quantification of tau immunoreactivity, for assessment of BACE1-immunolabeled dystrophic neurites, sections in regions encompassing areas of white matter tracts following DH stroke surgery between bregma -1.46 and -2.18 were analyzed (n=6-11 per experimental group). Briefly, for each of the following regions, two to three non-overlapping, adjacent 10× fields were taken for each section from each hemisphere: (i) Cortex: 3 sections per mouse, 3 fields per section (landmark: at the retrosplenial granular/ dysgranular to the primary/secondary somatosensory areas); (ii) CA1 region of the hippocampus: 2-3 sections per mouse, 2-3 fields per section (landmark: from the oriens layer to the radiatum layer); and (iii) Thalamus: 3 sections per mouse, 1 field per section (landmark: at the reticular thalamus nucleus). BACE1 + and NRG1 type III+ staining was quantified from the digital images using histogram thresholding with NIH ImageJ analysis software and computed. The threshold was set manually to identify dense immunostaining that was distinct from the background. The immunostained area was expressed as the percentage of the total area analyzed.

Multiplex immunoassays

For mouse brains, the cortex (excluding the stroke lesion) and white matter regions (thalamus/internal capsule) were dissected. Following dissections, mouse brain samples were snap frozen in liquid nitrogen. Tissue samples were then sonicated in ice-cold 0.1 M PBS containing 1% triton X-100 and 0.1% sodium deoxycholate, Protease Inhibitor Cocktail, and Phosphatase Inhibitor Cocktail 2. Following centrifugation, the total protein concentration of each supernatant was measured using a Direct Detect Infrared Spectrometer. Total soluble $A\beta_{42}$ in mouse brain regions were then quantified using a customized mouse single-plex magnetic bead assay kit (Millipore Sigma), according to the manufacturer's recommendations and protocols. Each lysate sample, standard, and quality control were measured in duplicate. Plates were read using a MAGPIX instrument platform (Luminex), and results were analyzed using MILLIPLEX Analyst 5.1 software (Millipore Sigma).

Statistics

Data were presented as mean ± SEM. To determine normality, the Shapiro-Wilk and the Kolmogorov-Smirnov normality tests were performed. After the dataset passed the normality test, then when analyzing data consisting of the interaction of age (young adult versus aged) and experimental condition (stroke versus sham), a two-way ANOVA, followed by post-hoc Newman-Keuls testing (with the exception of brain atrophy analysis, which employed the Fisher's LSD as the post-hoc test) was performed. For planned comparisons with explicit predictions as to the direction of difference, an ANOVA, followed by a one-tailed t-test was used. All other analyses were evaluated using an ANOVA and a two-tailed t-test. In the case that the dataset did not pass the normality test, a Mann-Whitney test or an ANOVA, followed by a Dunnett's post-hoc test was used. Significance was set at $p<0.05$. For all figures, $^{*}p$ is <0.05, $^{**}p$ is <0.01, $^{***}p$ is <0.001, and $^{****}p$ is <0.0001.

Results

Motor recovery is impaired and there is accelerated onset of cognitive impairment in aged versus young adult C57BL/6 mice following stroke

Most stroke, AD, and mixed dementia patients are 65 years of age or older [4, 46]. Therefore, in the first part of this study, we examined the impact of age on the development of AD-associated pathological markers following a stroke in wt mice. To accomplish this goal, we induced a DH stroke or sham surgery in young adult (3 mo) and aged (18 mo) C57BL/6 mice and compared behavioral outcomes over the course of 8 weeks, and neuropathological outcomes at the end of 8 weeks (see Study design in Fig. 1a). To measure motor recovery, we performed an assessment of spontaneous gait using the horizontal ladder rung test. This test measures limb placement errors on a ladder [22], and previously, we showed that following DH stroke, C57BL/6 mice at 5 months of age display a significant motor impairment of the front limb contralateral to the stroke starting at day 1, which continues until week 2 post-surgery [22]. At baseline or pre-surgery testing, we found no difference in the ability of the 3 and 18 mo mice to traverse the ladder (Fig. 1b). However, as expected, on day 2 following a stroke, performance was significantly impaired on the ladder, which localized to the contralateral (left) front limb in both age groups.

This motor deficit persisted in both the 3 and 18 mo mice into the second week following a stroke. However, between 2 and 4 weeks post-surgery, there was a significant recovery of ladder traversing ability in the 3 mo mice, with the stroked mice performing at an equivalent level to their age-matched sham-operated counterparts at 4 and 6 weeks post-surgery. This recovery of limb function did not occur in the 18 mo stroked mice. The 18 mo stroked mice continued to perform significantly worse than their aged-matched sham-operated counterparts for the duration of the study. These data indicate that motor recovery following a stroke is impaired in aged compared to young adult C57BL/6 mice.

Next, we assessed cognitive status through the use of the OR test. We previously reported that DH stroke in 3-5 mo C57BL/6 mice results in impairment of hippocampal function at 7 weeks post-surgery, as assessed by both the Y-maze SAB and OR tests [23]. Here, we employed the OR test to determine how age in wt mice affects the chronic impact of a stroke on a task of short-term spatial memory [53, 111]. As seen in Fig. 1c, prior to surgery, the 3 and 18 mo mice were equally able to distinguish between a set of moved and unmoved objects by spending significantly more time interacting with the relocated objects. At 1 week post-surgery, stroke- and sham-operated mice from both age groups continued to be able to distinguish between the moved and unmoved objects. However, at 4 weeks post-surgery, though the 3 mo stroke- and sham-operated mice, and 18 mo sham-operated mice were able to distinguish between the moved and unmoved objects, suggesting intact short-term spatial memory, the 18 mo stroked mice were unable to recognize which objects were relocated. An equivalent, but delayed cognitive deficit subsequently appeared at 7 weeks post-surgery in the 3 mo stroked mice. These data indicate that stroke induces an accelerated onset of cognitive impairment in aged compared to young adult wt mice.

Brain atrophy is more pronounced in the ipsilateral hemisphere of aged versus young adult C57BL/6 mice following stroke

Enlargement of the lateral ventricles and cortical shrinkage appear in both human [5, 58] and animal models [1, 34, 73, 112] of dementia. Atrophy of the brain likely results from progressive degeneration of neurons, and the loss of these neurons is a likely contributor to the manifestation of dementia. Previously, we demonstrated that DH stroke causes delayed ipsilateral cortical atrophy in 3-5 mo C57BL/6 mice at 8 weeks post-surgery, and that atrophy is correlated with a loss of neuronal specific nuclear protein (NeuN)+ cells in the peri-infarct cortex and external capsule [108]. Here, we investigated using Nissl-staining, whether the severe behavioral deficits present in aged wt stroked mice (Fig. 1b and c) were associated with more severe brain atrophy than occurs in 3 mo mice. This analysis revealed no significant difference in the area of the ipsilateral lateral ventricle of the 3 mo stroked mice compared to their aged-matched sham operated counterparts at 8 weeks post-surgery (Fig. 2a and c). However, there was a significant increase in the area of the ipsilateral lateral ventricle of the 18 mo stroked mice compared to their 18 mo sham operated counterparts (Fig. 2a and c). Furthermore, although there was a significant difference in cortical tissue loss, or thinning, of the ipsilateral hemisphere in stroke- compared to sham-operated mice of both age groups, the 18 mo stroked mice exhibited significantly more tissue loss than the 3 mo stroked mice (Fig. 2b and c). These data demonstrate that brain atrophy is more pronounced in the ipsilateral hemisphere of aged versus young adult C57BL/6 mice following stroke.

There is increased cholinergic degeneration in aged versus young adult C57BL/6 mice following stroke

The dysfunction and loss of cholinergic neurons and their projections are among the earliest pathological events in age-related dementias such as AD and vascular dementia. Cholinergic neurons primarily originate in the basal forebrain, though they are found in lower density in regions such as the cortex and striatum. They provide the main source of acetylcholine to the cortex and hippocampus through their projection fibers, and as a result, are critical for attention, cognition, and psychological well-being [18, 24, 65, 99, 105]. Previously, we observed loss of cholinergic neurons in the ipsilateral cortex of 3-5 mo C57BL/6 mice at 7 weeks post-stroke [108]. Here, we also found significant loss of ChAT+ cells in the medial septum of the basal forebrain of stroke- and sham-operated mice from both age groups at 8 weeks post-surgery (Fig. 2d and e). However, the 18 mo stroked mice had significantly more cholinergic loss than the 3 mo stroked mice.

Stroke induces accumulation of Aβ and tau in white matter tracts of the ipsilateral hemisphere in aged versus young adult C57BL/6 mice

As previously mentioned, approximately 50% of clinically diagnosed AD patients are verified at post-mortem to have mixed pathology, most commonly infarct and Aβ and tau accumulation [27, 80, 82]. Therefore, we next surveyed Aβ and tau levels in the 3 and 18 mo C57BL/6 mice that had undergone stroke or sham surgery.

As depicted in Fig. 3a-c, toxic $A\beta_{42}$ was not significantly detected in either the 3 mo mice that underwent stroke or sham surgery, or the 18 mo mice that underwent sham surgery. However, significant accumulation of $A\beta_{42}$ was detected in the 18 mo stroked mice at 8 weeks post-surgery. In these mice, $A\beta_{42}$ appeared in the white matter tracts of the ipsilateral hemisphere, including the internal capsule (Fig. 3a), thalamus (Fig. 3b), and corpus callosum (Fig. 3c). Notably, quantitation revealed that there was a non-significant trend towards more $A\beta_{42}$ deposits in the 3 mo stroked mice compared to their aged-matched sham counterparts, however, there was significantly more $A\beta_{42}$ accumulation in the 18 mo stroked mice compared to the 3 mo stroked mice for every brain region quantified (Fig. 3d). The specificity of the $A\beta_{42}$ antibody was confirmed by pre-absorbing the antibody with its target antigen, the $A\beta_{1\text{-}42}$ peptide.

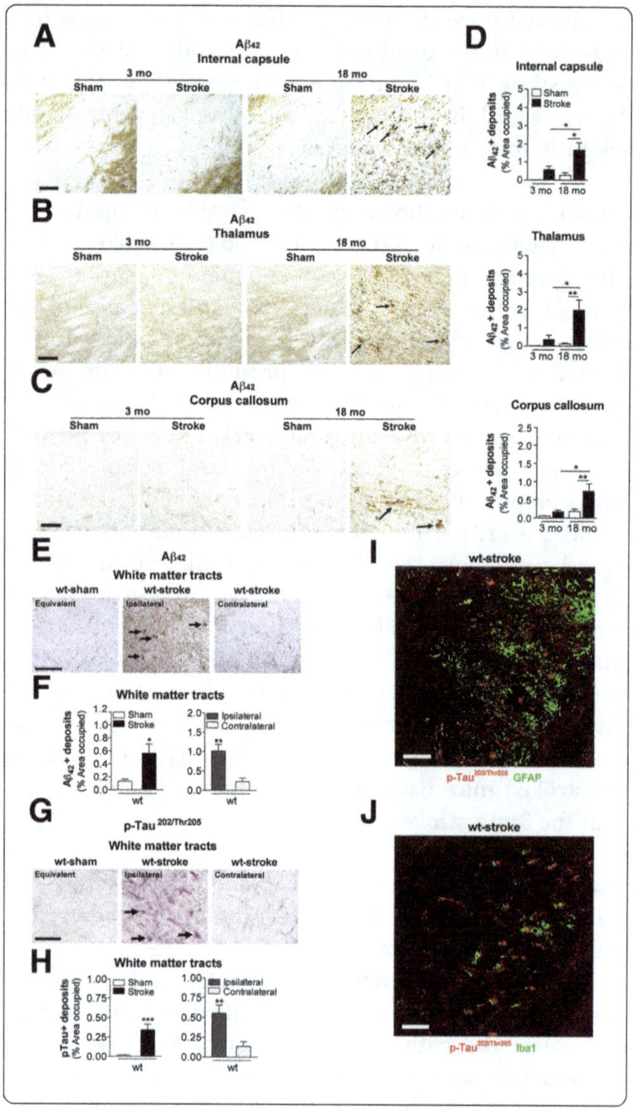

Fig. 3 Stroke causes β-amyloid (Aβ) and phosphorylated (p) tau deposition in the white matter tracts of aged wildtype (wt) mice compared to young adult mice. Representative 10× images of $A\beta_{42}$-immunolabeled deposits (arrows) in the white matter tracts of the (**a**) internal capsule, **b** thalamus, and (**c**) corpus callosum of the 3 and 18 mo, sham- and stroke-operated C57BL/6 mice at 8 weeks post-surgery. Scale bar, 100 μm (internal capsule and thalamus), 50 μm (corpus callosum). Nissl-stained sections to the left of each image delineate where representative images were taken. **d** Quantification of the ipsilateral hemisphere revealed a significant deposition of $A\beta_{42}$ in the internal capsule (top graph), thalamus (middle graph), and corpus callosum (bottom graph) of the 18 mo stroked mice relative to the age-matched sham-operated mice. Furthermore, the 18 mo stroked mice had significantly more $A\beta_{42}$ accumulation in three of the brain regions analyzed compared to the 3 mo stroked mice. **e-h** Representative 10× images of (**e**) $A\beta_{42}$- and (**g**) p-tau-immunolabeled deposits (arrows) in white matter tracts (thalamus-internal capsule) of the 18 mo mice at 12 weeks after sham or stroke surgery (Equivalent = area imaged in wt-sham mice that is equivalent to the ipsilateral hemisphere imaged in wt-stroke mice; Contralateral = area imaged in the contralateral hemisphere of wt-stroke mice that is equivalent to the ipsilateral hemisphere of wt-stroke mice). Scale bar, 125 μm ($A\beta_{42}$ and p-tau). Quantification of the ipsilateral and contralateral hemispheres revealed significantly more deposits of (**f**) $A\beta_{42}$ and (**h**) p-tau in the white matter tracts of the 18 mo stroked mice compared to the age-matched sham-operated mice. Furthermore, there was also significantly more $A\beta_{42}$ and p-tau accumulation in the white matter tracts of the ipsilateral versus the contralateral hemisphere. No $A\beta_{42}$ signal was detected in (**i**) astrocytes (GFAP, green; n=3 mice/experimental group) or (**j**) microglia (Iba1, green; n=3 mice/experimental group). Scale bar, 125 μm. Data represent mean ± SEM. *$p<0.05$, **$p<0.01$, and ***$p<0.001$

There was no $A\beta_{42}$+ staining detected in the pre-absorbed immunostaining sections of 18 mo stroked mice. These findings suggest that stroke alone can cause some of the abnormalities associated with AD, and that age exacerbates the manifestation of post-stroke AD-related pathological markers, such as $A\beta_{42}$ in wt mice.

Next, to understand the kinetics of deleterious processes that may still be occurring, and to capture more advanced pathology or degeneration, we extended the post-stroke time interval to 12 weeks post-surgery in the aged mice. Similar to 8 weeks post-stroke, we saw an abundant amount of $A\beta_{42}$ deposits in the white matter tracts of the 18 mo stroked mice compared to age-matched sham operated mice (Fig. 3e). Quantitation revealed that there was significantly more $A\beta_{42}$ deposition in the ipsilateral hemisphere than in the contralateral hemisphere (Fig. 3f). This finding demonstrates that $A\beta_{42}$ accumulation in response to stroke in aged wt mice is focal, rather than global, and based on its anatomical localization, it appears to localize to the area of axonal degeneration.

It is well established that $A\beta_{42}$ promotes signal transduction mechanisms such as the activation of calpain and stress kinases, and increases p-tau, and that these events can lead to neurite and synapse degeneration, and eventual neuronal death [49, 92, 100]. Ser202 and Thr205, the epitopes on tau that is recognized by the antibody AT8 when they are phosphorylated, are among the tau residues that contribute to the pathological conformation of p-tau [41]. Therefore, we next sought to determine whether $A\beta_{42}$ coincides with the presence of p-tau at these epitopes in the weeks following stroke. As seen in Fig. 3g, the expression of p-tau was significantly higher in the white matter tracts of the 18 mo stroked mice compared to their age-matched sham counterparts, and quantitation revealed that the ipsilateral hemisphere contained significantly more p-tau deposits than the contralateral hemisphere of the stroked mice (Fig. 3h).

Based on morphological assessment, the p-tau staining appeared to be in a linear arrangement consistent with axons. However, to gather more information with regard to the localization of p-tau in our tissue, we performed fluorescent co-staining with GFAP for astrocytes and Iba1 for microglia. We did not detect that p-tau colocalized with the GFAP-labeled astrocytes (Fig. 3i) or with the Iba1-labeled microglia (Fig. 3j).

Stroke-induced accumulation of Aβ in C57BL/6 mice is associated with expression of BACE1 and NRG1 type III

Axonal degeneration and myelin damage distal to stroke injury sites takes months, if not years to resolve [93], and the dysregulation of myelin repair mechanisms has been proposed to contribute to the genesis of AD pathology [11]. A critical myelin homeostasis repair pathway in the CNS involves the upregulation of BACE1 and the cleavage of NRG1 type III [10, 15]. Soluble NRG1 type III β-subunit or transmembrane-bound NRG1 type III then binds to ErbB (epidermal growth factor, EGF) receptors on oligodendrocytes, initiating their myelinating function through the activation of intracellular signaling cascades [19, 39, 87, 89]. However, BACE1 also cleaves AβPP, and causes the release of the pathogenic Aβ peptide [110]. Therefore, because the chronic sequalae of stroke, such as axonal degeneration and chronic inflammation, may place stress on myelin homeostasis, we determined whether BACE1 expression co-localized with the areas of $A\beta_{42}$ deposition following stroke. First, we authenticated the specificity of the BACE1 antibody though Western blotting, and detected a single band at the appropriate molecular weight for mature glycosylated BACE1 of ~70 kDa (Fig. 4a). Then we discovered, as seen in Fig. 4a, that BACE1 was indeed present in the ipsilateral white matter tracts of 18 mo stroked C57BL/6 mice compared to their age-matched sham counterparts at 12 weeks post-surgery. BACE1 was not detected in the contralateral hemisphere of these stroked mice.

To support the hypothesis that BACE1 and NRG1 type III are part of a chronically activated myelin repair mechanism following stroke, we then tested if NRG1 type III expression is chronically increased in stroked wt mice, and if it colocalizes with areas of BACE1 expression and $A\beta_{42}$ deposition. First, we authenticated the specificity of the NRG1 type III antibody though Western blotting, and detected a single band at the appropriate molecular weight of ~50 kDa (Fig. 4b). We then found, as depicted in Fig. 4b, that NRG1 type III was present in the ipsilateral white matter tracts of the 18 mo stroked C57BL/6 mice compared to their age-matched sham counterparts at 12 weeks post-surgery. NRG1 type III was not detected in the contralateral hemisphere of these stroked mice. Taken together, these findings lend support to the possibility that deposition of $A\beta_{42}$ following stroke is a by-product of a chronically activated myelin repair process in areas of axonal degeneration in aged C57BL/6 mice.

To confirm that the expression of BACE1 and NRG1 type III in the white matter tracts of the wt stroked mice was correlating with the area of axonal degeneration, we performed immunostaining for total tau and Fluoro-Jade staining. The total tau immunostaining revealed a chronic loss of total tau immunoreactivity in the ipsilateral white matter tracts compared to the contralateral white matter tracts of the aged wt stroked mice (Fig. 4c), and the Fluoro-Jade staining revealed a delayed and sustained area of degenerating axons in the ipsilateral white matter tracts (Fig. 4d).

Stroke exacerbates motor, cognitive, and psychological behavioral deficits in aged hAPP-SL mice

In the first part of this study, we used aged C57BL/6 mice as one model of post-stroke mixed dementia. To complement this model, in the second part of the study, we used a combination of age, stroke, and Tg AβPP mice, which are an *in vivo* chronic Aβ deposition and degeneration model of AD (see Study design in Fig. 5a). Evidence in humans suggest that vascular risk factors such as stroke increase the risk of developing AD [91], with a synergistic effect in some cases [32]. Furthermore, in human mixed dementia, most patients have more varied pathology with respect to Aβ accumulation, brain atrophy, and neurodegeneration than typical "pure" AD patients [43]. Therefore, this second model of post-stroke mixed dementia is useful for determining how a typical AD phenotype evolves into an atypical subtype over time, or vice versa, when interacting with the chronic sequelae of stroke.

First, we assessed the motor ability of aged hAPP-SL mice, using the ladder rung test following an ischemic stroke with a chronic post-surgery timeframe of 12 weeks. Baseline data showed no impairment in ladder performance before surgery in the 18 mo hAPP-SL mice (Fig. 5b). The naïve mice were then allocated into

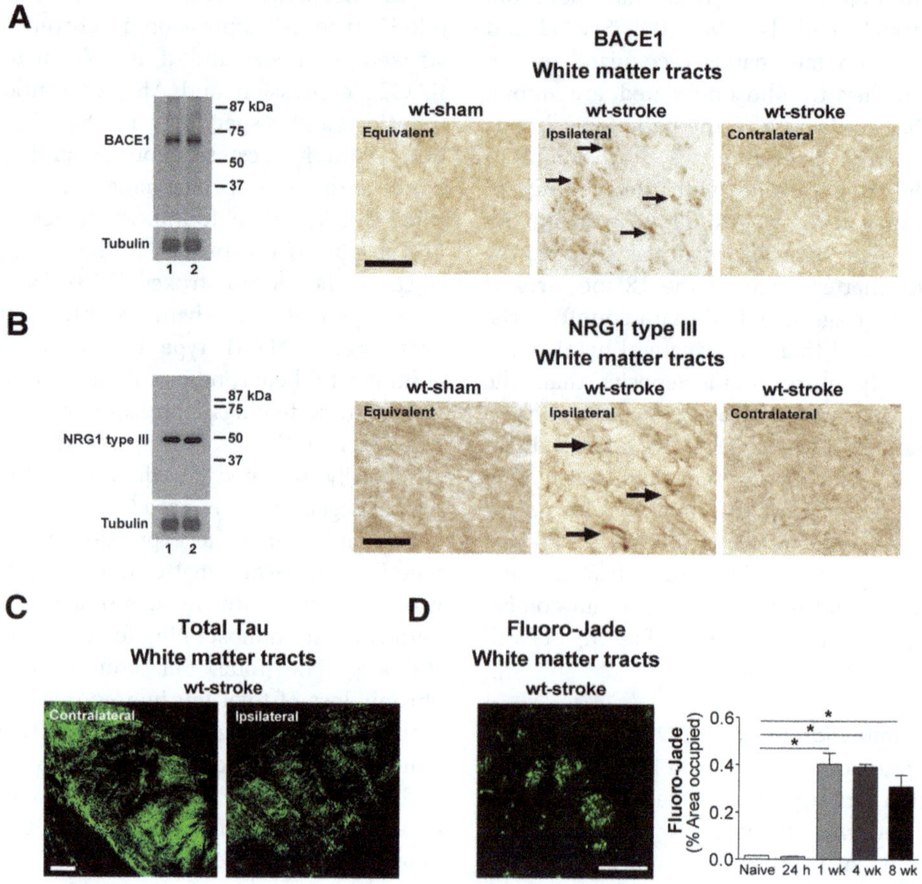

Fig. 4 Stroke induces β-secretase (BACE) 1 and neuregulin (NRG) 1 type III expression in the white matter tracts of aged wildtype (wt) mice compared to young adult mice. **a-c** Western blotting with a BACE1 (~70 kDa) or NRG type III (~50 kDa) antibody detected a single band at the appropriate molecular weight in mouse brain lysates for each protein. Representative 20× images (n=3 mice/experimental group) of (**a**) BACE1+ and (**b**) NRG1 type III+ immunostaining (arrows) in the white matter tracts (thalamus-internal capsule) of 18 mo mice at 12 weeks after sham or stroke surgery (Equivalent = area imaged in wt-sham mice that is equivalent to the ipsilateral hemisphere imaged in wt-stroke mice; Contralateral = area imaged in the contralateral hemisphere of wt-stroke mice that is equivalent to the ipsilateral hemisphere of wt-stroke mice). Scale bar, 50 μm (BACE1 and NRG1 type III). Images revealed BACE1 and NRG1 type III expression in the ipsilateral white matter tracts of stroked, but not in sham-operated mice. **c** Representative 10× immunofluorescence images (n=3 mice/experimental group) of total tau+ immunostaining in the ipsilateral and contralateral white matter tracts of wt mice after stroke surgery. Scale bar, 125 μm. **d** Image: Representative 40× Fluoro-Jade staining in the ipsilateral white matter tracts of wt mice after stroke confirms that this is an area of axonal degeneration following DH stroke. Scale bar, 100 μm. Graph: Relative to naïve mice, there is significant Fluoro-Jade staining starting at 1 week (wk) post-stroke, continuing into at least 8 wk post-stroke. Data represent mean ± SEM from n=5 mice/experimental group. *$p<0.05$

experimental groups and given either a stroke or sham surgery. At 1-week post-surgery, there was a significant difference in motor function between experimental groups, as the stroked hAPP-SL mice performed significantly worse compared to their age-matched sham counterparts. This difference in motor function was still present when mice were tested at 6 weeks post-surgery and at 11 weeks post-surgery.

We have previously demonstrated that AβPP mice exhibit a host of behavioral deficits (contextual fear conditioning, delayed-matching-to-place in a modified Barnes maze and Morris water maze, Y-maze SAB, T-maze, NOR, and social novelty compared to their age-matched wt littermates on a C57BL/6 background [25, 33, 48, 64, 74, 76, 77, 79]). Therefore, we proceeded to examine the effect of stroke on the cognitive status of aged hAPP-SL mice by using the Y-maze SAB to assess spatial working memory. As seen in Fig. 5c, spontaneous alternation of Y-maze arm choices between naïve hAPP-SL mice, which were later allocated into stroke or sham experimental groups, were indistinguishable from each other pre-surgery, and continued to be indistinguishable during weeks 1-6 post-surgery. However, at week 11 post-surgery, significantly poorer spontaneous alternation performance was detected in the stroke- compared to the sham-operated hAPP-SL mice.

To corroborate these findings, NOR testing was also performed. In NOR testing, mice tend to spend more

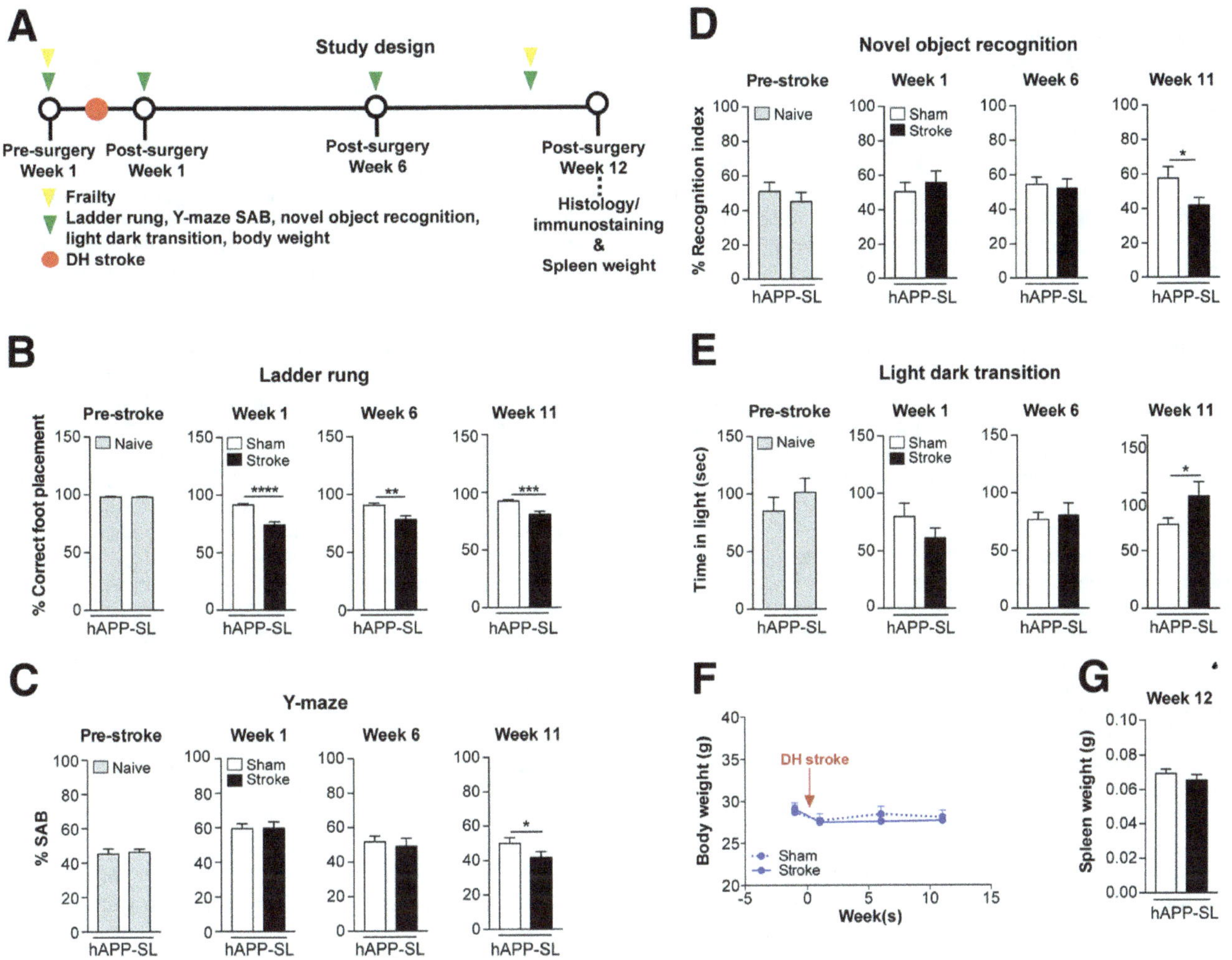

H

Frailty parameter score	Pre-stroke				Post-stroke Week 11			
	Sham		Stroke		Sham		Stroke	
	Mean	SEM	Mean	SEM	Mean	SEM	Mean	SEM
Overall frailty	2.324	±0.39	1.813	±0.18	2.500	±0.50	2.469	±0.19
Alopecia	0.118	±0.05	0.063	±0.06	0.088	±0.05	0.063	±0.04
Kyphosis	0.206	±0.06	0.125	±0.06	0.235	±0.09	0.531*	±0.07
Piloerection	0.412	±0.06	0.406	±0.05	0.265	±0.09	0.406	±0.05
Hearing loss	0.324	±0.10	0.250	±0.10	0.706	±0.11	0.625	±0.12
Body condition	0.294	±0.75	0.013	±0.03	0.147	±0.08	0.094	±0.05
Cataracts/cloudy eyes	0.058	±0.06	0.000	±0.00	0.118	±0.07	0.059	±0.04
Fur color	0.323	±0.07	0.313	±0.06	0.353	±0.08	0.281	±0.06
Coat condition	0.147	±0.07	0.063	±0.04	0.147	±0.08	0.156	±0.06
Forelimb grip strength	0.000	±0.00	0.000	±0.00	0.059	±0.04	0.031	±0.03
Microphthalmia	0.000	±0.00	0.059	±0.06	0.029	±0.03	0.088	±0.06
Weight	0.309	±0.07	0.297	±0.07	0.235	±0.07	0.133	±0.08
Temperature	0.132	±0.04	0.141	±0.05	0.000	±0.00	0.000	±0.00

Fig. 5 (See legend on next page.)

(See figure on previous page.)
Fig. 5 Stroke exacerbates behavioral deficits in aged hAPP-SL mice on tests of motor, cognition, and anxiety. **a** Study design: 18 month-old (mo) hAPP-SL mice were assessed on the ladder rung, Y-maze spontaneous alternation behavior (SAB), novel object recognition, and light dark transition tests prior to a distal hypoxic (DH) stroke or sham surgery at the indicated timepoints. Mice were also weighed at each indicated timepoint. Mice were euthanized and brains were harvested for histology and immunostaining at 12 weeks post-surgery, along with spleen for organ weight. **b** Motor ability on the ladder rung test was assessed at 1-week pre-surgery, and at 1 week, 6 weeks, and 11 weeks post-surgery. At 1 week prior to a stroke, there was no difference in motor performance in the naïve hAPP-SL mice, as mice displayed a similar number of acceptable (<12% error) baseline foot placements on the rungs. These naïve mice would later be assigned into the sham or stroke experimental groups. At 1 week post-surgery, stroked hAPP-SL mice exhibited an enhanced motor deficit, as they displayed a significantly fewer number of correct foot placements relative to sham-operated hAPP-SL mice. Significant motor deficits continued to manifest in stroked hAPP-SL mice at 6 and 11 weeks post-surgery compared to sham-operated hAPP-SL mice at those timepoints. **c** Cognitive function using the Y-maze SAB test was assessed at 1 week pre-stroke, and at 1 week, 6 weeks, and 11 weeks post-surgery. At 1 week prior to surgery, there was no difference in cognitive function in naïve hAPP-SL mice, as mice displayed similar levels of spontaneous alternations. At 1 and 6 weeks post-surgery, there was no difference in the cognitive status of sham- and stroke-operated hAPP-SL mice. However, at 11 weeks post-surgery, stroked hAPP-SL mice exhibited aggrevated short-term spatial memory impairment, as they displayed significantly less spontaneous alternations compared to sham-operated hAPP-SL mice. **d** Cognitive function using the novel object recognition test was assessed at 1 week pre-stroke, and at 1 week, 6 weeks, and 11 weeks post-surgery. At 1 week prior to surgery, there was no difference in cognitive function in naïve hAPP-SL mice, as mice displayed similar recognition indexes, which corresponds to similar exploration time for an unfamiliar (novel) and a familiar object. At 1 and 6 weeks post-surgery, there was no difference in the cognitive status of the sham- and stroke-operated hAPP-SL mice. However, at 11 weeks post-surgery, the stroked hAPP-SL mice exhibited worsened intermediate recognition memory impairment, as they displayed significantly lower recognition indexes calculated from less time spent distinguishing and exploring an unfamiliar/novel object compared to the sham-operated hAPP-SL mice. **e** Using the light dark transition test, we assessed mice on the anxiety-impulsivity spectrum of behavior at 1 week pre-surgery, and at 1 week, 6 weeks, and 11 weeks post-surgery. At 1 week prior to surgery, there was no difference in the amount of time spent in the light, open (intimidating space) versus the dark, enclosed (safe space) arenas of the chamber in the naïve hAPP-SL mice. At 1 week prior to surgery, the amount of time spent in each arena remained similar between sham- and stroke-operated hAPP-SL mice, and this pattern was seen at 6 weeks post-surgery. However, at 11 weeks post-surgery, stroked hAPP-SL mice spent significantly more time in the light arena than sham-operated hAPP-SL mice, suggesting that stroke initiated behavioral impulsivity or a lack of inhibition in the hAPP-SL mice by reducing their anxiety of open spaces. **f** No significant weight changes were seen in the sham- and stroke-operated experimental hAPP-SL mouse groups at pre- and post-surgery timepoints. **g** There was no spleen weight difference between experimental groups at 12 weeks post-surgery. **h** There was no significant difference in any of the selected frailty outcomes depicted, with the exception of kyphosis, in the 18 mo sham- versus stroke-operated hAPP-SL mice at pre- and post-surgery timepoints. Data represent mean ± SEM. *$p<0.05$, **$p<0.01$, ***$p<0.001$, and ****$p<0.0001$

time exploring a novel object relative to a familiar object. Because the inter-trial-interval (ITI) here was 4 hours, this ITI timeframe has been reported to test intermediate memory retention [9] as opposed to spatial working memory from the SAB test. Also, the NOR test is a test of recognition memory. Naïve hAPP-SL mice, which were later allocated into stroke or sham experimental groups, had similar recognition indexes (RI) to each object at the pre-surgery timepoint (Fig. 5d). Recognition indexes between stroke- and sham-operated mice were also equivalent during week 1-6 post-surgery. However, a loss of object recognition ability became apparent in the stroked hAPP-SL mice at 11 weeks post-surgery, as they had a significantly lower RI compared to the sham-operated hAPP-SL mice.

Psychological disturbances, including depression, anxiety-impulsivity, aggression-submission, and psychosis are increasingly recognized as a manifestation of the pathological features present in AD and other age-related neurodegenerative diseases [12, 45, 71, 95]. Adult hAPP-SL mice display significant psychological disturbances such as anxiety- and submissive-like behaviors, and sensorimotor gating deficits compared to their wt littermates (Nguyen TV et al., unpublished data). Here, we determined the chronic impact of stroke on a psychological measurement of anxiety-impulsivity in aged hAPP-SL mice. The LDT test measures the spontaneous exploratory behavior of mice in response to mild stressors, such as a novel environment and brighter lighting after some habituation [50]. As seen in Fig. 5e, naïve hAPP-SL mice, which were later allocated into stroke or sham experimental groups, experienced comparable levels of exploration in the light chamber pre-surgery. The amount of exploration time in the light chamber was also comparable between the stroke- and sham-operated hAPP-SL mice during weeks 1-6 post-surgery. However, at 11 weeks post-surgery, the stroked hAPP-SL mice spent significantly more time in the light chamber compared to the sham-operated hAPP-SL mice. This increased time spent in the open, light, and what should be an intimidating arena, by the stroked hAPP-SL mice, supports a display of behaviors resembling the impulsive, uninhibited, or risk-taking behaviors exhibited by patients with dementia, including frontotemporal dementia and AD [54].

Because of reports suggesting changes in body and spleen weights (correlated with inflammatory signals), and the development of frailty in age-related dementias, such as AD [35, 78, 81, 96, 106], we evaluated the impact of stroke on these physiological parameters in aged hAPP-SL mice. However, we did not detect a significant difference in the body weights of both the stroke- and sham-operated hAPP-SL mice at pre- and post-surgery timepoints (Fig. 5f). Likewise, there was no significant difference in the spleen weights of both the stroke- and sham-operated hAPP-SL mice at 12 weeks post-surgery (Fig. 5g). Furthermore, there was no significant difference in any of the selected frailty outcomes indicated, with the exception of kyphosis, in the stroke- versus sham-operated hAPP-SL mice at pre- and post-surgery timepoints (Fig. 5h). Overall, the hAPP-SL mice appeared physiologically similar at the end of the study regardless of having undergone a stroke or sham procedure.

Stroke exacerbates global cholinergic degeneration in aged hAPP-SL mice

Given that chronic stroke exacerbates behavioral deficits in aged hAPP-SL mice, we evaluated whether these manifestations are correlated with neurodegeneration. Adult hAPP-SL mice exhibit cholinergic neurite degeneration in the basal forebrain, as well as a loss of projection fibers and prominent dystrophic neurites in the cortex [48, 64, 85]. Accumulation of Aβ in AD is associated with the appearance of dystrophic neurites [57], which likely impair neuronal and synaptic function. Dystrophic neurites are swollen, bulbous, and tortuous processes that cluster together [13], are intrinsic to degenerative changes that result from cytoskeletal derangement [36], manifest early in AD [14], and precede neuronal death [31]. Here, we assessed whether stroke impacts cholinergic dystrophic neurites in aged hAPP-SL mice. As seen in Fig. 6a, clusters of cholinergic dystrophic neurites appeared more abundant, as indicated by significantly more ChAT-labeled dystrophic neurites occupied in the cortex of the 18 mo stroked mice compared to the sham-operated hAPP-SL mice (Fig. 6b). There was no difference in the percentage occupied by dystrophic neurite clusters in the ipsilateral versus the contralateral hemisphere of the stroked hAPP-SL mice, suggesting not only an exacerbated effect of a stroke on cholinergic pathology in hAPP-SL mice, but also a global effect.

Stroke exacerbates global tau pathology in aged hAPP-SL mice

Previous studies report that cholinergic dystrophic neurites are found in the vicinity of tau and amyloid deposits in the cortex of adult hAPP-SL mice [48, 64]. Dystrophic neurites have been shown to contain abnormal filaments of hyperphosphorylated tau proteins [8, 97]. Here, we assessed whether stroke impacts p-tau+ dystrophic neurites in aged hAPP-SL mice up to 12 weeks post-stroke. As seen in Fig. 6c, clusters of p-tau+ containing dystrophic neurites were more abundant in the 18 mo stroked hAPP-SL mice compared to the sham-operated hAPP-SL mice, as indicated by significantly more p-tau+ dystrophic neurites in the cortex and white matter tracts of the internal capsule of these mice (Fig. 6d). There was also significantly more p-tau+ staining in both the white matter tracts of the thalamus and the internal capsule of the stroked hAPP-SL mice versus the sham-operated hAPP-SL mice. Furthermore, for each brain region, there was no difference in the area occupied by p-tau+ dystrophic neurite clusters in the ipsilateral compared to the contralateral hemisphere of the stroked hAPP-SL mice, suggesting once more not only an exacerbated effect of a stroke on AD-related pathology in hAPP-SL mice, but also a global effect.

Stroke exacerbates global Aβ burden in aged hAPP-SL mice

Previous work has shown that increased p-tau expression in hAPP-SL mice results from Aβ-induced signal transduction mechanisms, including activation of calpain and stress kinases (cdk5, GSK3β, c-Jun, and p38) [64, 107]. Because there was significantly more p-tau expression in the stroke- versus sham-operated hAPP-SL mice, we wanted to determine whether abnormally high p-tau expression correlated with stroke-induced exacerbation of Aβ pathology at 12 weeks post-surgery. Therefore, we examined amyloid plaque distribution in ThioS-stained brain sections from 18 mo hAPP-SL mice given stroke or sham surgery. ThioS primarily stains fibrillary forms of Aβ, and notably, ThioS pathology was not detected in the young adult or aged wt C57BL/6 mice that underwent stroke surgery. However, as seen in Fig. 7a, we found more abundant amyloid plaques, as detected by ThioS's intrinsic fluorescence, in the brains of the stroked hAPP-SL mice compared to the sham-operated hAPP-SL mice. Quantitation revealed a significantly higher percentage of cortical and hippocampal areas occupied by ThioS-stained deposits in the stroke- versus sham-operated hAPP-SL mice (Fig. 7b). Also, there were significantly more ThioS-stained deposits in both the white matter tracts of the thalamus of the stroked versus sham hAPP-SL mice. For each brain region, there was no significant difference in the area occupied by ThioS-stained deposits in the ipsilateral versus the contralateral hemisphere of the stroked hAPP-SL mice. This again suggests not only an exacerbated effect of stroke on amyloid pathology, as revealed by ThioS staining, in hAPP-SL mice, but also a global effect.

Though ThioS stains primarily fibrillary forms of Aβ, it may also stain some dystrophic neurites [61]. Therefore, to more accurately determine the effect of stroke on Aβ pathology, we next probed for the pathological $A\beta_{1\text{-}42}$ peptide using a DAB-linked secondary antibody to a specific $A\beta_{42}$ antibody. We detected abundant $A\beta_{42}$-immunolabeled deposits in the cortex of the 18 mo stroke- compared to sham-operated hAPP-SL mice at 12 weeks post-surgery (Fig. 7c). Quantitation showed significantly more $A\beta_{42}$+ deposits in the cortex, thalamus, and

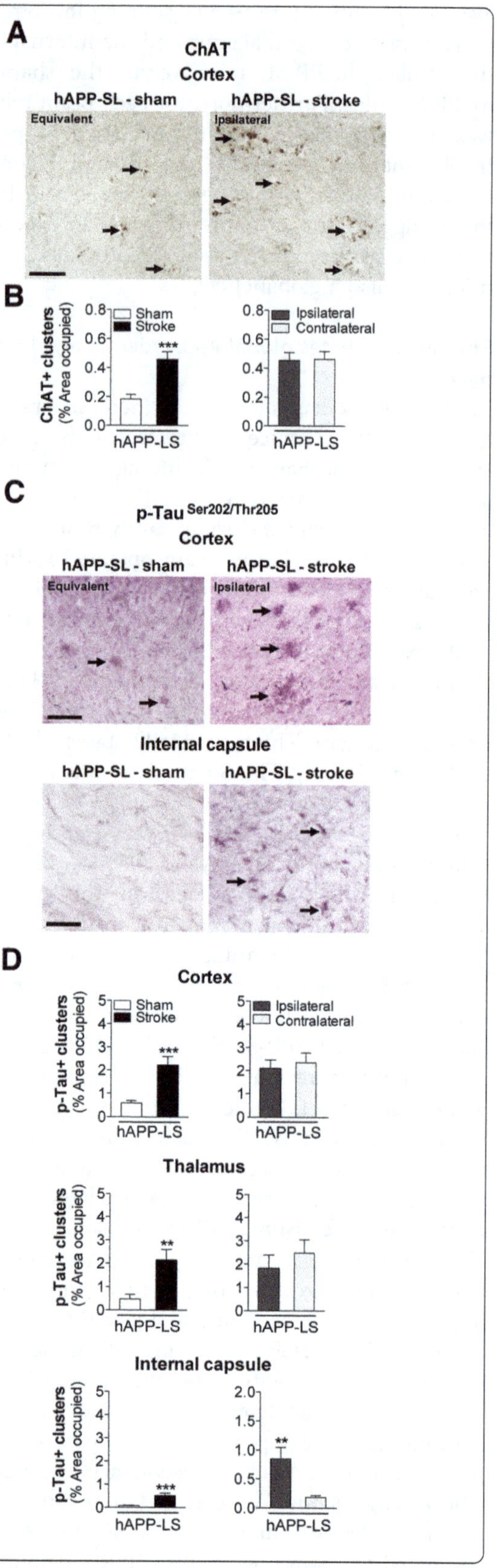

Fig. 6 Stroke increases cholinergic neurodegeneration and levels of tau phosphorylation (p) in aged hAPP-SL mice. **a** Representative 10× images of choline acetyltransferase (ChAT)-immunolabeled dystrophic neurites (arrows) in the primary somatosensory cortex of 18 mo sham- or stroke-operated hAPP-SL mice (Equivalent = area imaged in wt-sham mice that is equivalent to the ipsilateral hemisphere imaged in wt-stroke mice). Scale bar, 125 μm. **b** Quantification revealed that relative to sham-operated hAPP-SL mice, the area occupied by cholinergic dystrophic neurites in the cortex was significantly higher in the stroked hAPP-SL mice; no significant difference in the amount of cholinergic dystrophic neurites was found between the ipsilateral versus contralateral cortex. **c** Representative 10× images of AT8 (p-tau$^{Ser202/Thr205}$)-immunolabeled dystrophic neurites (arrows) in the primary somatosensory cortex of 18 mo sham- or stroke-operated hAPP-SL mice (Equivalent = area imaged in wt-sham mice that is equivalent to the ipsilateral hemisphere imaged in wt-stroke mice). Scale bar, 125 μm. **d** Quantification revealed that relative to sham-operated hAPP-SL mice, the area occupied by p-tau+ dystrophic neurites was significantly higher in the cortex (top graph), thalamus (middle graph), and internal capsule (bottom graph) of the stroked hAPP-SL mice; no significant difference in the amount of p-tau+ dystrophic neurites was found between the ipsilateral versus contralateral cortex and thalamus, although the ipsilateral internal capsule showed significantly more p-tau+ dystrophic neurites than the contralateral region. $^{**}p<0.01$ and $^{***}p<0.001$

internal capsule (p value of 0.0751 in the hippocampus) of the stroke- versus sham-operated hAPP-SL mice (Fig. 7d). There was no significant difference in the area occupied by $A\beta_{42}$+ deposits in the ipsilateral versus the contralateral hemisphere of the stroked hAPP-SL mice in the cortex, hippocampus, or thalamus, but there was a non-significant trend (*p* value of 0.0606) of an increase in the internal capsule. These data again suggest not only an exacerbated effect of stroke on $A\beta_{42}$ pathology in hAPP-SL mice, but also a global effect.

To more precisely measure the concentration of $A\beta_{42}$ in hAPP-SL mice after stroke and sham surgery, we quantified $A\beta_{42}$ in dissected ipsilateral brain region homogenates 12 weeks after surgery. Using a single-plex immunoassay kit and the Luminex technology platform, we found significantly higher levels of soluble $A\beta_{42}$ in the ipsilateral cortex and the ipsilateral white matter (which included the thalamus and internal capsule) of the stroke- compared to sham-operated hAPP-SL mice (Fig. 7e). Taken together, the data so far suggest that stroke chronically exacerbates neurodegeneration in hAPP-SL mice, possibly through enhanced p-tau and $A\beta_{42}$ pathology.

BACE1 expression is chronically increased in aged hAPP-SL mice following stroke

In aged wt mice, we detected significant BACE1 accumulation in the white matter tracts of the ipsilateral hemisphere of the stroked compared to the sham-operated C57BL/6 mice (Fig. 4a). Our findings

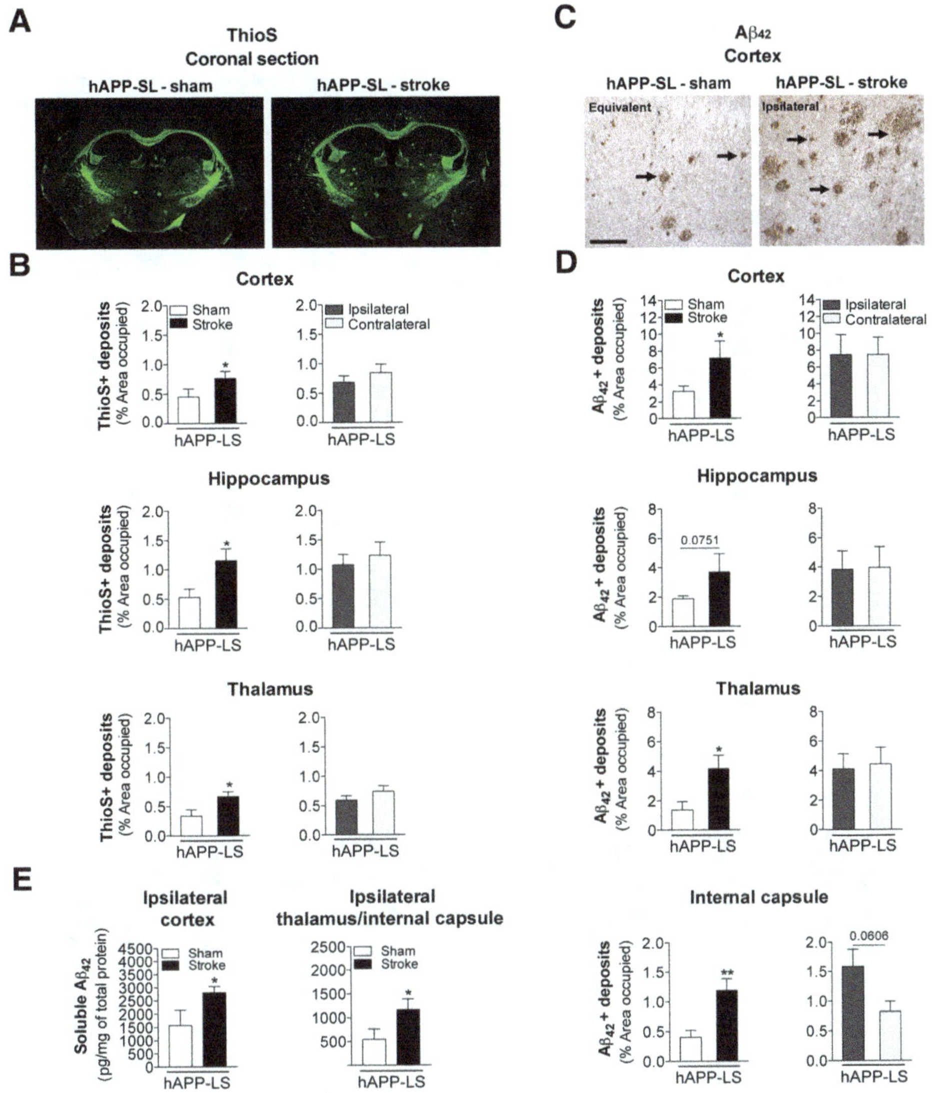

Fig. 7 Stroke exacerbates amyloid plaque burden and soluble $A\beta_{42}$ levels in aged stroke hAPP-SL mice. **a** Representative 4× stitched images of Thioflavin S (ThioS)-stained coronal brain sections of 18 mo sham- or stroke-operated hAPP-SL mice. **b** Quantification revealed that relative to sham-operated hAPP-SL mice, the area occupied by ThioS-labeled amyloid plaques was significantly greater in the cortex (top graph), hippocampus (middle graph), and thalamus (bottom graph) of the stroked hAPP-SL mice; no significant difference in the amount of amyloid plaques was found between the ipsilateral versus contralateral hemisphere. **c** Representative 10× images of $A\beta_{42}$-immunolabeled deposits (arrows) in the primary somatosensory cortex of the 18 mo sham- or stroke-operated hAPP-SL mice (Equivalent = area imaged in wt-sham mice that is equivalent to the ipsilateral hemisphere imaged in wt-stroke mice). Scale bar, 125 μm. **d** Quantification revealed that relative to sham-operated hAPP-SL mice, the area occupied by $A\beta_{42}$+ deposits was significantly higher in the cortex (top graph), thalamus (bottom middle graph), and internal capsule (bottom graph) of the stroked hAPP-SL mice (p value for the hippocampus shown in the top middle graph was 0.0751); no significant difference in the amount of $A\beta_{42}$+ deposits was found between the ipsilateral versus contralateral hemisphere. **e** A single-plex immunoassay of tissue samples from the ipsilateral cortex or thalamus/internal capsule regions showed that in hAPP-SL mice, significantly higher levels of soluble $A\beta_{42}$ are found in stroked mice compared to sham-operated mice. Data represent mean ± SEM. *$p<0.05$ and **$p<0.01$

parallel those of Hilunen and colleagues who reported a similar result after focal cerebral ischemia in adult rats [37]. Here, we determined whether a chronic sequela of stroke in hAPP-SL mice is a global increase in BACE1, thereby resulting in a global increase in production of $A\beta_{42}$. As seen in Fig. 8a, there was more BACE1 accumulation in the cortex of the 18 mo stroked-hAPP-SL mice compared to the sham-operated hAPP-SL mice at 12 weeks post-surgery. Quantitation showed significantly more BACE1+ deposits in the cortex, hippocampus, and thalamus of stroked versus sham-operated hAPP-SL mice (Fig. 8b). There was no significant difference, however, in the percentage area occupied by BACE1 staining in the ipsilateral versus the contralateral hemisphere of

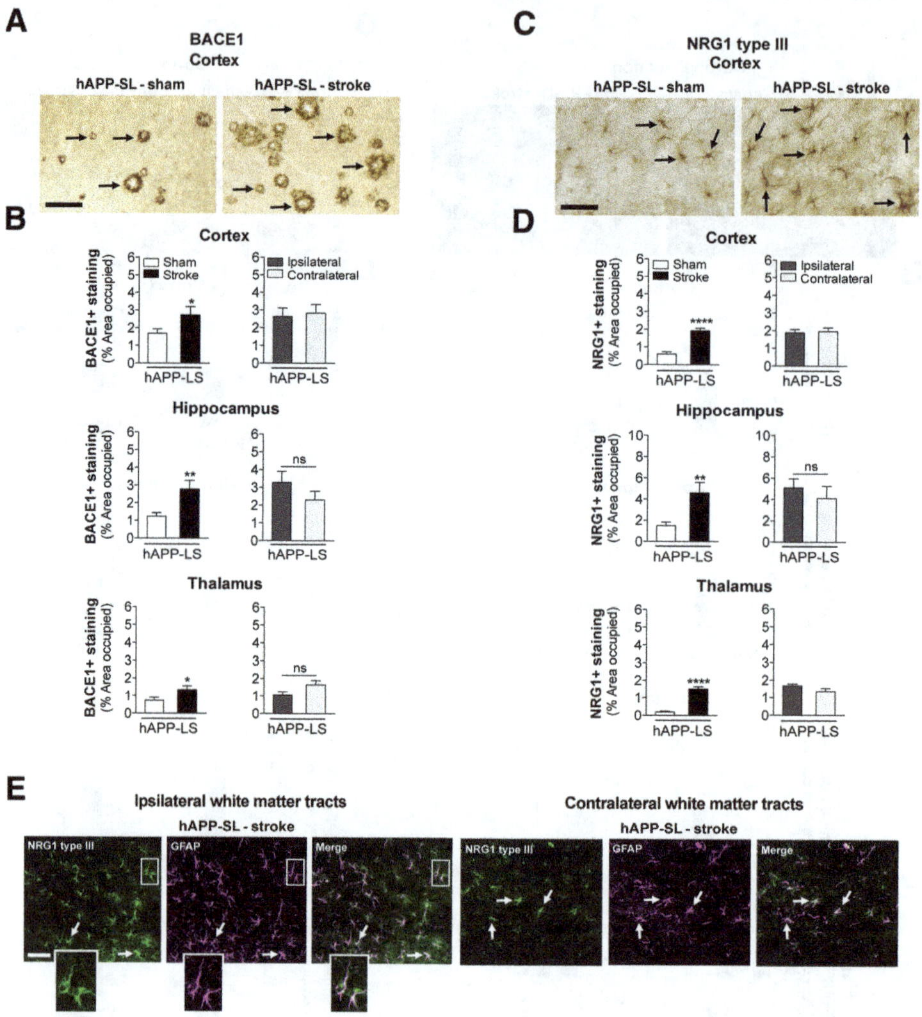

Fig. 8 Stroke increases β-secretase (BACE) 1 and neuregulin (NRG) 1 type III immunostaining in aged hAPP-SL mice. **a** Representative 10× images of BACE1+ immunostaining (arrows) in the primary somatosensory cortex of 18 mo sham- or stroke-operated hAPP-SL mice. Scale bar, 125 μm. **b** Quantification revealed that relative to sham-operated hAPP-SL mice, the area occupied by BACE1+ staining was significantly higher in the cortex (top graph), hippocampus (middle graph), and thalamus (bottom graph) of the stroked hAPP-SL mice; no significant difference in the amount of BACE1+ staining was found between the ipsilateral versus contralateral hemisphere. **c** Representative 20× images of NRG1 type III+ immunostaining (arrows) in the primary somatosensory cortex of 18 mo sham- or stroke-operated hAPP-SL mice. Scale bar, 125 μm. **d** Quantification revealed that relative to sham-operated hAPP-SL mice, the area occupied by NRG1 type III+ staining was significantly higher in the cortex (top graph), hippocampus (middle graph), and thalamus (bottom graph) of the stroked hAPP-SL mice; no significant difference in the amount of NRG1 type III+ staining was found between the ipsilateral versus contralateral hemisphere. Data represent mean ± SEM. *$p<0.05$, **$p<0.01$, and ****$p<0.0001$. **e** Representative 40× fluorescence images (n=3 mice/experimental group) from the 18 mo stroked hAPP-SL mouse sections showing NRG1 type III staining (green) within cells staining for the astrocytic marker, glial fibrillary acidic protein (GFAP, magenta), in the ipsilateral and contralateral white matter tracts (thalamus-internal capsule). Magnified outsets show GFAP+ astrocytes colocalized with NRG1 type III. Scale bar, 50 μm

the stroked hAPP-SL mice, indicating that there is indeed a global increase in BACE1 expression in hAPP-SL mice that lasts for weeks following stroke.

NRG1 type III expression is chronically increased in aged hAPP-SL mice following stroke

As previously discussed, soluble or transmembrane-bound NRG1 type III binds to ErbB receptors on oligodendrocytes as part of an endogenous myelin homeostasis mechanism. This induces oligodendrocyte myelination through receptor-mediated signaling, and it requires the cleavage of NRG1 type III by BACE1. Increased levels of NRG1 have been detected in Schwann cells of the PNS in response to spinal cord injury [2, 3], however, the impact of chronic stroke on NRG1 type III expression was previously unknown. Data in Fig. 4b show that NRG1 type III expression is present in the white matter tracts of the ipsilateral hemisphere of aged wt mice at 12 weeks post-stroke, and here, we determined the chronic impact of stroke on NRG1 type III expression in aged hAPP-SL mice. As seen in Fig. 8c, expression of NRG1 type III was more abundant in the cortex of the 18 mo stroked hAPP-SL mice compared to the sham-operated hAPP-SL mice at 12 weeks post-surgery. Quantitation showed significantly more NRG1 type III expression in the cortex, hippocampus, and thalamus of the stroked versus sham hAPP-SL mice (Fig. 8d). Similar to BACE1 expression, there was no significant difference in the percent area of each brain region occupied by NRG1 type III staining in the ipsilateral versus the contralateral hemisphere of the stroked hAPP-SL mice, indicating that there is a global rather than a focal increase in NRG1 type III expression in hAPP-SL mice.

NRG1 type III, either in its soluble or transmembrane-bound form, has been reported to be produced by astrocytes, [20, 29, 86, 88, 90]. Therefore, we next performed NRG1 type III and astrocyte (GFAP) co-staining. Assessment of GFAP-immunolabeled astrocytes in the white matter tracts (thalamus/internal capsule) from tissue samples of the 18 mo stroked hAPP-SL mice revealed medium to high levels of co-staining of NRG1 type III with GFAP in both the ipsilateral and contralateral hemispheres (Fig. 8e).

Discussion

In this study, we provide evidence that AD-related pathology is a chronic sequela of ischemic stroke in two mouse models of post-stroke mixed dementia. To our knowledge, this is one of the most comprehensive studies investigating the long-term impact of ischemia on the development of the pathology related to AD to date, and the first study to compare differences in stroke-induced pathology in wt and hAPP-SL mice. Importantly, our post-stroke mixed dementia models are able to track the development of pathology related to AD over the period of weeks and months following stroke in mice. This is because the stroke model employed has low mortality and variability, even though it causes a sizeable infarct that encompasses approximately 25% of the ipsilateral hemisphere.

In wt mice, we found that ischemic stroke impairs motor recovery and accelerates the onset of cognitive impairment in aged compared to young adult C57BL/6 mice. This finding correlated with more extensive brain atrophy, cholinergic neurodegeneration, and deposition of p-tau and $A\beta_{42}$ in the ipsilateral white matter tracts of the 18 mo stroked C57BL/6 mice compared to their 3 mo counterparts. Furthermore, increased levels of p-tau and $A\beta_{42}$ were still present at 12 weeks post-stroke in a separate cohort of 18 mo C57BL/6 mice that underwent stroke surgery. ThioS pathology, which labels fibrillary forms of Aβ, was not detected in the adult or aged wt C57BL/6 mice that underwent stroke surgery. These findings demonstrate that in aged animals, stroke by itself can cause a subset of the brain abnormalities associated with AD.

In the hAPP-SL mice, however, we found that stroke worsened a broader array of the stereotypical hallmarks of AD-like pathology, and that worsened pathology was evident throughout both hemispheres of the brain. In both of these models, the stroke-induced amyloid and tau deposition co-localized with AβPP cleavage enzyme, BACE1, and myelin-associated protein, NRG1 type III (Fig. 9a), both of which are critical for myelin repair. Based on these findings, we propose that a myelin homeostasis mechanism is focally malfunctioning or overwhelmed in response to stroke in aged wt mice, and is globally malfunctioning or overwhelmed in hAPP-SL mice. Due to a consequence of advanced age or having the hAPP-SL transgene, this is leading to the inadvertent cleavage of AβPP, Aβ deposition, and subsequent exacerbated neurodegeneration.

This possibility is in agreement with the hypothesis put forth by Bartzokis and colleagues that AD pathology may be the result of a defective homeostatic response to age-related myelin breakdown [11, 55]. This hypothesis suggests that because in addition to NRG1 type III, BACE1 has high cleavage affinity for AβPP, over activation of the NRG1/BACE1 myelin repair mechanism may result in the inadvertent cleavage of AβPP in aged animals (Fig. 9b). It is not fully understood which cell type or types produce NRG1 type III following stroke, however, recent data, as well as the data presented here, support reactive astrocytes as one source [20, 29, 86, 88, 90].

An important observation from our findings is that there was a difference in the development of AD-like pathology following stroke in the 3 mo and 18 mo wt mice. Unlike their aged counterparts, the 3 mo stroked C57BL/6 mice did not exhibit Aβ or p-tau pathology following stroke. Why the chronic consequences of stroke impacted AD-related pathology differently in the young adult versus the aged C57BL/6 mice could be due to myelin repair processes becoming less efficient or malfunctioning with increased age [62]. Alternatively, with advanced age comes an attenuated inflammatory response following stroke [84]. As a consequence, there may be diminished clearance of myelin debris in the repair process in the area of axonal degeneration by microglia/macrophages in the 18 mo stroked mice, thereby leading to a hyperactive or prolonged myelin repair process.

Another important observation from our findings is the difference in the regional distribution of Aβ and p-tau in the brains of the aged wt mice and the aged hAPP-SL mice. In the wt mice, AD-like pathology was primarily confined to the ipsilateral white matter tract areas, mainly including the thalamus and internal

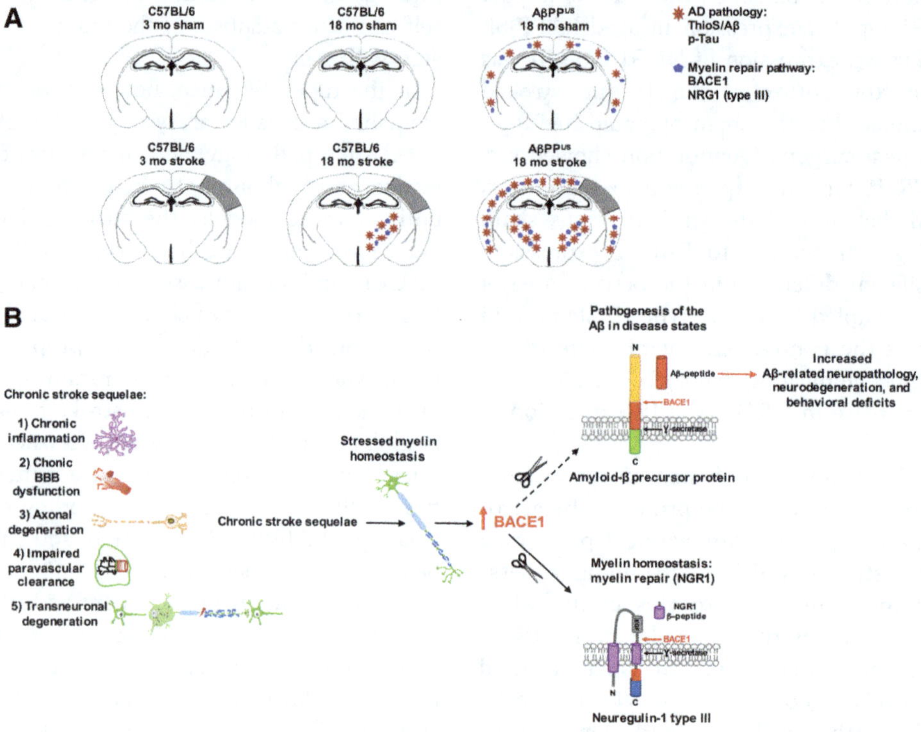

Fig. 9 Schematic representations summarizing key findings of our study. **a** In this study, we provide evidence that there is overlap of pathology (amyloid plaques, and Aβ_{42} and p-tau deposition) associated with AD following stroke with key components (BACE1 and NRG1 type III) of a myelin repair pathway in aged stroked wt and stroked hAPP-SL mice. **b** Working model proposing AD-associated pathology as a chronic sequela of ischemic stroke: chronic inflammation, chronic BBB dysfunction, axonal degeneration, impaired paravascular clearance, and transneuronal degeneration are all chronic sequalae of stroke that may result in stressed myelin homeostasis. BACE1's role as a protease that cleaves NRG1 type III at its β-site is critical in the formation of myelin sheaths by oligodendrocytes, and is a key regulator of myelination of axons in the central nervous system [10]. BACE1's cleavage of NRG1 type III initiates γ-secretase cleavage of NRG1 type III at its γ-site. However, in addition to NRG1 type III, BACE1 has high cleavage affinity for the Aβ precursor protein (AβPP). Therefore, the chronic sequelae of stroke may be causing myelin repair mechanisms involving NRG1 type III and BACE1 to be racheted up, resulting in the inadvertent cleavage of AβPP by BACE1 and γ-secretase, and the abnormal generation of amyloidogenic Aβ peptides

capsule, whereas in the hAPP-SL mice there was exacerbated distribution in grey and white matter areas of both hemispheres. We propose that this could be due to myelin repair being less effective in aged C57BL/6 mice than in younger mice, but not severely so. Therefore, perhaps in aged wt mice, AD-associated pathological amyloid and tau species only develop in an area of maximal myelin repair, such as the area of axonal degeneration. On the other hand, myelin homeostasis may be closer to a tipping point that leads to the deposition of Aβ throughout the brain in aged hAPP-SL mice. Following a stroke, the combined impact of multiple chronic sequelae of stroke may send myelin homeostasis over this tipping point in more brain regions in hAPP-SL mice.

Examples of chronic consequences of stroke, separate from axonal degeneration, that could be leading to the more widespread overload of this tipping point in hAPP-SL mice, include chronic inflammation, prolonged blood brain barrier (BBB) impairment, and impaired paravascular clearance. For instance, recently published data from our research group demonstrate that CNS infarcts in both humans and mice are sites of sustained expression of proinflammatory cytokines/chemokines, sustained foamy macrophage responses, and the sustained presence of T- and B-lymphocytes for at least 7 weeks following stroke [23, 63]. These responses are imperfectly sequestered from the rest of the brain by glial scars [108]. Another chronic consequence of stroke is prolonged BBB impairment, for instance our previously published data from adult C57BL/6 mice demonstrate that neovascularization following stroke results in the formation of a network of new blood vessels within the infarct that do not mature into vessels with full BBB competency [108]. Finally, studies by Wang and colleagues using micro-infarcts, recently demonstrated that paravascular clearance is perturbed in the vicinity of the infarct following stroke [98]. A consequence of this impairment may be the accumulation of potentially toxic molecules that could promote protein aggregation and inflammation. These "trapped" molecules may be proinflammatory cytokines and cytotoxic extracellular Aβ, or extracellular tau released into the brain interstitial fluid as a result of axonal damage [40] [56, 60]). Needless to say, each of these processes could also be contributing to AD pathogenesis following stroke via a mechanism independent of their impact on myelin homeostasis. However, they may have a pervasive impact on myelin homeostasis if they are sending toxic factors widespread and indiscriminately throughout the brain.

As a final caveat, a potential limitation of the models of post-stroke mixed dementia presented here is that the accumulation of amyloid and tau in the white matter is not a typical characteristic of AD, either with or without vascular brain injury. However, using sensitive imaging techniques several independent groups have recently reported elevated Aβ burden in the white matter of AD patients independent of cortical plaque severity [16], as well as in preclinical AD [72].

Conclusions

In conclusion, despite evidence of significant overlap in the incidence of stroke and AD, the impact of the chronic sequelae of stroke on the development and progression of AD-associated pathology is largely unknown. Here, we have developed two novel post-stroke mixed dementia models, which enable the long-term consequences of stroke injury on the development of AD-related pathological markers, such as amyloid and tau to be tracked. Because of the heterogeneity and complexity of human post-stroke mixed dementia [51, 94], each of our models are important for reflecting the varied clinical symptoms and pathological diversity exhibited in mixed dementia patients [42, 44], in which age and a predisposition for, or existing diagnosed or undiagnosed AD symptoms, may affect long-term outcome after a stroke. These models enable hypotheses, such as the myelin repair hypothesis highlighted here to be tested, and provide a platform for future preclinical drug studies.

Abbreviations

AD: Alzheimer's disease; wt: Wildtype; Tg: Transgenic; BACE1: β-secretase 1; NGR1: Neuregulin 1; Aβ: β-amyloid; AβPP: Aβ precursor protein; p: Phosphorylated; PS1: Presenilin 1; MCAO: Middle cerebral artery occlusion; PT: Photothrombotic; ET-1: Endothelin-1; LPS: Lipopolysaccharide; mo: Months old; Thy1-hAβPP$^{Lond/Swe}$ (hAPP-SL): Transgenic mouse line 41 over-expresses human AβPP751 containing the London (V717I) and Swedish (K670M/N671L) mutations under the control of the Thy1 promoter; DH stroke: Distal MCAO plus hypoxia; OR: Object relocation; SAB: Spontaneous alternation behavior; NOR: Novel object recognition; FO: Familiar object; LDT: Light dark transition; ChAT: Choline acetyl transferase; GFAP: Glial fibrillary acidic protein; Iba1: Ionized calcium binding adaptor molecule 1; ThioS: Thioflavin S; NeuN: Neuronal specific nuclear protein; epidermal growth factor, EGF: ErbB; ITI: Inter-trial-interval; BBB: Blood brain barrier

Funding

This research project was supported by funds from National Institute of Health (K99NR013593 and R01NS096091), and start-up funds provided by the University of Arizona, Tucson to KPD, the Jean Perkins Foundation to FML, and from National Institute of Health (R01EY026544) to BSM.

Authors' contributions

TN supervised and participated in the behavioral testing, tissue harvesting, immunostaining. TN and KD drafted the manuscript. KD and JF performed the mouse surgeries. MH performed the behavioral testing and immunostaining. MH and JZ performed the immunoassays. TN, MH, and KD participated in the statistical analyses. NC and BM performed the Western blotting for the authentication of the BACE1 and NRG1 type III antibodies used in immunostaining, and also performed anti-$A\beta_{42}$ antisera affinity subtraction experiment to pre-absorption the $A\beta_{42}$ antibody to confirm its specificity in immunostaining. NB and FL bred and provided the Alzheimer's disease model mice. TN and KD conceived of the study and oversaw its design and coordination. All authors read and approved the final manuscript.

Competing interests

The authors declare that they have no competing interests.

Author details

[1]Department of Immunobiology, University of Arizona, 1656 E. Mabel Street, Tucson, AZ 85719, USA. [2]Department of Neurology, University of Arizona, 1656 E. Mabel Street, Tucson, AZ 85719, USA. [3]Arizona Center on Aging, University of Arizona, 1656 E. Mabel Street, Tucson, AZ 85719, USA. [4]Department of Ophthalmology and Vision Science, University of Arizona, Tucson, AZ, USA. [5]Department of Neurology and Neurological Sciences, Stanford University, Stanford, CA, USA.

References

1. Akiguchi I, Pallas M, Budka H, Akiyama H, Ueno M, Han J, Yagi H, Nishikawa T, Chiba Y, Sugiyama H et al (2017) SAMP8 mice as a neuropathological model of accelerated brain aging and dementia: Toshio Takeda's legacy and future directions. Neuropathology 37:293–305. https://doi.org/10.1111/neup.12373.
2. Alizadeh A, Dyck SM, Kataria H, Shahriary GM, Nguyen DH, Santhosh KT, Karimi-Abdolrezaee S (2017) Neuregulin-1 positively modulates glial response and improves neurological recovery following traumatic spinal cord injury. Glia 65:1152–1175.
3. Alizadeh A, Santhosh KT, Kataria H, Gounni AS, Karimi-Abdolrezaee S (2018) Neuregulin-1 elicits a regulatory immune response following traumatic spinal cord injury. J Neuroinflammation 15:53.
4. Alzheimer's A (2016) 2016 Alzheimer's disease facts and figures. Alzheimers Dement 12:459–509.
5. Amtul Z, Nikolova S, Gao L, Keeley RJ, Bechberger JF, Fisher AL, Bartha R, Munoz DG, McDonald RJ, Naus CC et al (2014) Comorbid Abeta toxicity and stroke: hippocampal atrophy, pathology, and cognitive deficit. Neurobiol Aging 35:1605–1614. https://doi.org/10.1016/j.neurobiolaging.2014.01.005.
6. Alzheimer's Association (2018) https://www.alz.org/alzheimers-dementia/facts-figures.
7. Back DB, Kwon KJ, Choi DH, Shin CY, Lee J, Han SH, Kim HY (2017) Chronic cerebral hypoperfusion induces post-stroke dementia following acute ischemic stroke in rats. J Neuroinflammation 14:216. https://doi.org/10.1186/s12974-017-0992-5.
8. Ballatore C, Lee VM, Trojanowski JQ (2007) Tau-mediated neurodegeneration in Alzheimer's disease and related disorders. Nat Rev Neurosci 8:663–672. https://doi.org/10.1038/nrn2194.
9. Balogh SA, Kwon YT, Danenberg VH (2000) Varying intertrial interval reveals temporally defined memory deficits and enhancements in NTAN1-deficient mice. Learn Mem 7:279–286.
10. Bartus K, Galino J, James ND, Hernandez-Miranda LR, Dawes JM, Fricker FR, Garratt AN, SB MM, Ramer MS, Birchmeier C et al (2016) Neuregulin-1 controls an endogenous repair mechanism after spinal cord injury. Brain 139:1394–1416. https://doi.org/10.1093/brain/aww039.
11. Bartzokis G (2011) Alzheimer's disease as homeostatic response to age-related myelin breakdown. Neurobiol Aging 32:1341–1371.

12. Bemelmans SA, Tromp K, Bunnik EM, Milne RJ, Badger S, Brayne C, Schermer MH, Richard E (2016) Psychological, behavioral and social effects of disclosing Alzheimer's disease biomarkers to research participants: a systematic review. Alzheimers Res Ther 8:46. https://doi.org/10.1186/s13195-016-0212-z.
13. Benzing WC, Mufson EJ, Armstrong DM (1993) Alzheimer's disease-like dystrophic neurites characteristically associated with senile plaques are not found within other neurodegenerative diseases unless amyloid beta-protein deposition is present. Brain Res 606:10–18.
14. Braak H, Alafuzoff I, Arzberger T, Kretzschmar H, Del Tredici K (2006) Staging of Alzheimer disease-associated neurofibrillary pathology using paraffin sections and immunocytochemistry. Acta Neuropathol 112:389–404. https://doi.org/10.1007/s00401-006-0127-z.
15. Carroll SL, Miller ML, Frohnert PW, Kim SS, Corbett JA (1997) Expression of neuregulins and their putative receptors, ErbB2 and ErbB3, is induced during Wallerian degeneration. J Neurosci 17:1642–1659.
16. Collins-Praino LE, Francis YI, Griffith EY, Wiegman AF, Urbach J, Lawton A, Honig LS, Cortes E, Vonsattel JP, al CPD (2014) Soluble amyloid beta levels are elevated in the white matter of Alzheimer's patients, independent of cortical plaque severity. Acta Neuropathol Commun 2:1–10.
17. Centers for Disease Control and Prevention (2017) https://www.cdc.gov/stroke/facts.htm.
18. Davies P, Maloney AJ (1976) Selective loss of central cholinergic neurons in Alzheimer's disease. Lancet 2:1403.
19. Domingues HS, Portugal CC, Socodato R, Relvas JB (2016a) Oligodendrocyte, Astrocyte, and Microglia Crosstalk in Myelin Development, Damage, and Repair. Front Cell Dev Biol 4:71. https://doi.org/10.3389/fcell.2016.00071.
20. Domingues HS, Portugal CC, Socodato R, Relvas JB (2016b) Oligodendrocytes, astrocytes, and microglia crosstalk in myelin development, damage, and repair. Front Cell Dev Biol 4:1–16.
21. Doyle KP, Buckwalter MS (2016) Does B lymphocyte-mediated autoimmunity contribute to post-stroke dementia? Brain Behav Immun. https://doi.org/10.1016/j.bbi.2016.08.009.
22. Doyle KP, Fathali N, Siddiqui MR, Buckwalter MS (2012) Distal hypoxic stroke: a new mouse model of stroke with high throughput, low variability and a quantifiable functional deficit. J Neurosci Methods 207:31–40. https://doi.org/10.1016/j.jneumeth.2012.03.003.
23. Doyle KP, Quach LN, Sole M, Axtell RC, Nguyen TV, Soler-Llavina GJ, Jurado S, Han J, Steinman L, Longo FM,et al (2015) B-lymphocyte-mediated delayed cognitive impairment following stroke. J Neurosci 35:2133–2145. https://doi.org/10.1523/JNEUROSCI.4098-14.2015.
24. Erkinjuntti T. (2002) Diagnosis and management of vascular cognitive impairment and dementia. J Neural Transm Suppl. 63:91-109. Review.
25. Faizi M, Bader PL, Saw N, Nguyen TV, Beraki S, Wyss-Coray T, Longo FM, Shamloo M (2012) Thy1-hAPP(Lond/Swe+) mouse model of Alzheimer's disease displays broad behavioral deficits in sensorimotor, cognitive and social function. Brain Behav 2:142–154. https://doi.org/10.1002/brb3.41.
26. Farr TD, Liu L, Colwell KL, Whishaw IQ, Metz GA (2006) Bilateral alteration in stepping pattern after unilateral motor cortex injury: a new test strategy for analysis of skilled limb movements in neurological mouse models. J Neurosci Methods 153:104–113. https://doi.org/10.1016/j.jneumeth.2005.10.011.
27. Fernando MS, Ince PG, Function MRCC, Ageing Neuropathology Study G (2004) Vascular pathologies and cognition in a population-based cohort of elderly people. J Neurol Sci 226:13–17. https://doi.org/10.1016/j.jns.2004.09.004.
28. Fernando MS, Ince PG; MRC Cognitive Function and Ageing Neuropathology Study Group. (2004) Vascular pathologies and cognition in a population-based cohort of elderly people. J Neurol Sci. 226(1-2):13-17.
29. Frost GR, Li Y-M (2017) The role of astrocytes in amyloid production and Alzheimer's disease. Open Biol 7:1–14.
30. Garcia-Alloza M, Gregory J, Kuchibhotla KV, Fine S, Wei Y, Ayata C, Frosch MP, Greenberg SM, Bacskai BJ (2011) Cerebrovascular lesions induce transient beta-amyloid deposition. Brain 134:3697–3707. https://doi.org/10.1093/brain/awr300.
31. Grace EA, Rabiner CA, Busciglio J (2002) Characterization of neuronal dystrophy induced by fibrillar amyloid beta: implications for Alzheimer's disease. Neuroscience 114:265–273.
32. Hachinski V (2011) Stroke and Alzheimer disease: fellow travelers or partners in crime? Arch Neurol 68:797–798. https://doi.org/10.1001/archneurol.2011.118.
33. Havas D, Hutter-Paier B, Ubhi K, Rockenstein E, Crailsheim K, Masliah E, Windisch M (2011) A longitudinal study of behavioral deficits in an AbetaPP transgenic mouse model of Alzheimer's disease. J Alzheimers Dis 25:231–243. https://doi.org/10.3233/JAD-2011-101866.
34. Hebert F, Grand'maison M, Ho MK, Lerch JP, Hamel E, Bedell BJ (2013) Cortical atrophy and hypoperfusion in a transgenic mouse model of Alzheimer's disease. Neurobiol Aging 34:1644–1652. https://doi.org/10.1016/j.neurobiolaging.2012.11.022.
35. Hendriksz CJ, Anheim M, Bauer P, Bonnot O, Chakrapani A, Corvol JC, de Koning TJ, Degtyareva A, Dionisi-Vici C, Doss S et al (2017) The hidden Niemann-Pick type C patient: clinical niches for a rare inherited metabolic disease. Curr Med Res Opin 33:877–890. https://doi.org/10.1080/03007995.2017.1294054.
36. Heredia L, Helguera P, de Olmos S, Kedikian G, Sola Vigo F, LaFerla F, Staufenbiel M, de Olmos J, Busciglio J, Caceres A et al (2006) Phosphorylation of actin-depolymerizing factor/cofilin by LIM-kinase mediates amyloid beta-induced degeneration: a potential mechanism of neuronal dystrophy in Alzheimer's disease. J Neurosci 26:6533–6542. https://doi.org/10.1523/JNEUROSCI.5567-05.2006.
37. Hiltunen M, Makinen P, Peraniemi S, Sivenius J, van Groen T, Soininen H, Jolkkonen J (2009) Focal cerebral ischemia in rats alters APP processing and expression of Abeta peptide degrading enzymes in the thalamus. Neurobiol Dis 35:103–113. https://doi.org/10.1016/j.nbd.2009.04.009.
38. Huttunen HJ, Havas D, Peach C, Barren C, Duller S, Xia W, Frosch MP, Hutter-Paier B, Windisch M, Kovacs DM (2010) The acyl-coenzyme A: cholesterol acyltransferase inhibitor CI-1011 reverses diffuse brain amyloid pathology in aged amyloid precursor protein transgenic mice. J Neuropathol Exp Neurol 69:777–788. https://doi.org/10.1097/NEN.0b013e3181e77ed9.
39. Iadecola C (2013) The pathobiology of vascular dementia. Neuron 80: 844–866. https://doi.org/10.1016/j.neuron.2013.10.008.
40. Iliff JJ, Chen MJ, Plog BA, Zeppenfeld DM, Soltero M, Yang L, Singh I, Deane R, Nedergaard M (2014) Impairment of glymphatic pathway function promotes tau pathology after traumatic brain injury. J Neurosci 34:16180–16193. https://doi.org/10.1523/JNEUROSCI.3020-14.2014.
41. Jeganathan S, Hascher A, Chinnathambi S, Biernat J, Mandelkow EM, Mandelkow E (2008) Proline-directed pseudo-phosphorylation at AT8 and PHF1 epitopes induces a compaction of the paperclip folding of Tau and generates a pathological (MC-1) conformation. J Biol Chem 283:32066–32076. https://doi.org/10.1074/jbc.M805300200.
42. Jellinger KA (2007) The enigma of mixed dementia. Alzheimers Dement 3: 40–53. https://doi.org/10.1016/j.jalz.2006.09.002.
43. Kalaria RN (2016) Neuropathological diagnosis of vascular cognitive impairment and vascular dementia with implications for Alzheimer's disease. Acta Neuropathol 131:659–685. https://doi.org/10.1007/s00401-016-1571-z.
44. Kalaria RN, Akinyemi R, Ihara M (2016) Stroke injury, cognitive impairment and vascular dementia. Biochim Biophys Acta 1862:915–925. https://doi.org/10.1016/j.bbadis.2016.01.015.
45. Kim JS (2017) Management of post-stroke mood and emotional disturbances. Expert Rev Neurother 17:1179–1188. https://doi.org/10.1080/14737175.2017.1395281.
46. Kissela BM, Khoury JC, Alwell K, Moomaw CJ, Woo D, Adeoye O, Flaherty ML, Khatri P, Ferioli S, De Los Rios La Rosa F et al (2012) Age at stroke: temporal trends in stroke incidence in a large, biracial population. Neurology 79:1781–1787. https://doi.org/10.1212/WNL.0b013e318270401d.
47. Knowles JK, Rajadas J, Nguyen TV, Yang T, LeMieux MC, Vander Griend L, Ishikawa C, Massa SM, Wyss-Coray T, Longo FM (2009) The p75 neurotrophin receptor promotes amyloid-beta(1-42)-induced neuritic dystrophy in vitro and in vivo. J Neurosci 29:10627–10637. https://doi.org/10.1523/JNEUROSCI.0620-09.2009.
48. Knowles JK, Simmons DA, Nguyen TV, Vander Griend L, Xie Y, Zhang H, Yang T, Pollak J, Chang T, Arancio O et al (2013) Small molecule p75NTR ligand prevents cognitive deficits and neurite degeneration in an Alzheimer's mouse model. Neurobiol Aging 34:2052–2063. https://doi.org/10.1016/j.neurobiolaging.2013.02.015.
49. Krstic D, Knuesel I (2013) Deciphering the mechanism underlying late-onset Alzheimer disease. Nat Rev Neurol 9:25–34. https://doi.org/10.1038/nrneurol.2012.236.
50. Kulesskaya N, Voikar V (2014) Assessment of mouse anxiety-like behavior in the light-dark box and open-field arena: role of equipment and procedure. Physiol Behav 133:30–38. https://doi.org/10.1016/j.physbeh.2014.05.006.
51. Ladecola C (2013) The pathobiology of vascular dementia. Neuron 80:844–866.
52. Lee JS, Im DS, An YS, Hong JM, Gwag BJ, Joo IS (2011) Chronic cerebral hypoperfusion in a mouse model of Alzheimer's disease: an additional contributing factor of cognitive impairment. Neurosci Lett 489:84–88.

https://doi.org/10.1016/j.neulet.2010.11.071.
53. Lesburgueres E, Tsokas P, Sacktor TC, Fenton AA (2017) The Object Context-place-location Paradigm for Testing Spatial Memory in Mice. Bio Protoc 7. https://doi.org/10.21769/BioProtoc.2231.
54. Liscic RM, Storandt M, Cairns NJ, Morris JC (2007) Clinical and psychometric distinction of frontotemporal and Alzheimer dementias. Arch Neurol 64: 535–540. https://doi.org/10.1001/archneur.64.4.535.
55. Lu PH, Lee GJ, Shapira J, Jimenez E, Mather MJ, Thompson PM, Bartzokis G, Mendez MF (2014) Regional differences in white matter breakdown between frontotemporal dementia and early-onset Alzheimer's disease. J Alzheimers Dis 39:261–269.
56. Magnoni S, Esparza TJ, Conte V, Carbonara M, Carrabba G, Holtzman DM, Zipfel GJ, Stocchetti N, Brody DL (2012) Tau elevations in the brain extracellular space correlate with reduced amyloid-beta levels and predict adverse clinical outcomes after severe traumatic brain injury. Brain 135: 1268–1280. https://doi.org/10.1093/brain/awr286.
57. Masliah E, Alford M, Adame A, Rockenstein E, Galasko D, Salmon D, Hansen LA, Thal LJ (2003) Abeta1-42 promotes cholinergic sprouting in patients with AD and Lewy body variant of AD. Neurology 61:206–211.
58. Meier-Ruge W, Hunziker O, Iwangoff P (1991) Senile dementia: a threshold phenomenon of normal aging? A contribution to the functional reserve hypothesis of the brain. Ann N Y Acad Sci 621:104–118.
59. Metz GA, Whishaw IQ (2002) Cortical and subcortical lesions impair skilled walking in the ladder rung walking test: a new task to evaluate fore- and hindlimb stepping, placing, and co-ordination. J Neurosci Methods 115:169–179.
60. Morris M, Maeda S, Vossel K, Mucke L (2011) The many faces of tau. Neuron 70:410–426. https://doi.org/10.1016/j.neuron.2011.04.009.
61. Murray ME, Graff-Radford NR, Ross OA, Petersen RC, Duara R, Dickson DW (2011) Neuropathologically defined subtypes of Alzheimer's disease with distinct clinical characteristics: a retrospective study. Lancet Neurol 10:785–796. https://doi.org/10.1016/S1474-4422(11)70156-9.
62. Nave KA (2008) Neuroscience: An ageing view of myelin repair. Nature 455: 478–479. https://doi.org/10.1038/455478a.
63. Nguyen TV, Frye JB, Zbesko JC, Stepanovic K, Hayes M, Urzua A, Serrano G, Beach TG, Doyle KP (2016) Multiplex immunoassay characterization and species comparison of inflammation in acute and non-acute ischemic infarcts in human and mouse brain tissue. Acta Neuropathol Commun 4: 100. https://doi.org/10.1186/s40478-016-0371-y.
64. Nguyen TV, Shen L, Vander Griend L, Quach LN, Belichenko NP, Saw N, Yang T, Shamloo M, Wyss-Coray T, Massa SM et al (2014) Small molecule p75NTR ligands reduce pathological phosphorylation and misfolding of tau, inflammatory changes, cholinergic degeneration, and cognitive deficits in AbetaPP(L/S) transgenic mice. J Alzheimers Dis 42:459–483. https://doi.org/10.3233/JAD-140036.
65. Ofek K, Soreq H (2013) Cholinergic involvement and manipulation approaches in multiple system disorders. Chem Biol Interact 203:113–119. https://doi.org/10.1016/j.cbi.2012.07.007.
66. Ong LK, Zhao Z, Kluge M, Walker FR, Nilsson M (2017) Chronic stress exposure following photothrombotic stroke is associated with increased levels of Amyloid beta accumulation and altered oligomerisation at sites of thalamic secondary neurodegeneration in mice. J Cereb Blood Flow Metab 37:1338–1348. https://doi.org/10.1177/0271678X16654920.
67. Pickford F, Masliah E, Britschgi M, Lucin K, Narasimhan R, Jaeger PA, Small S, Spencer B, Rockenstein E, Levine B et al (2008) The autophagy-related protein beclin 1 shows reduced expression in early Alzheimer disease and regulates amyloid beta accumulation in mice. J Clin Invest 118:2190–2199. https://doi.org/10.1172/JCI33585.
68. Pimentel-Coelho PM, Michaud JP, Rivest S (2013) Effects of mild chronic cerebral hypoperfusion and early amyloid pathology on spatial learning and the cellular innate immune response in mice. Neurobiol Aging 34:679–693. https://doi.org/10.1016/j.neurobiolaging.2012.06.025.
69. Pollak J, Doyle KP, Mamer L, Shamloo M, Buckwalter MS (2012) Stratification substantially reduces behavioral variability in the hypoxic-ischemic stroke model. Brain Behav 2:698–706. https://doi.org/10.1002/brb3.77.
70. Qiu L, Ng G, Tan EK, Liao P, Kandiah N, Zeng L (2016) Chronic cerebral hypoperfusion enhances Tau hyperphosphorylation and reduces autophagy in Alzheimer's disease mice. Sci Rep 6:23964. https://doi.org/10.1038/srep23964.
71. Quinn TJ, Elliott E, Langhorne P (2017) Cognitive and Mood Assessment Tools for Use in Stroke. Stroke. https://doi.org/10.1161/STROKEAHA.117.016994.
72. Racine AM, Adluru N, Alexander AL, Christian BT, Okonkwo OC, Oh J, Cleary CA, Birdsill A, Hillmer AT, al MD (2014) Associations between white matter microstructure and amyloid burden in preclinical Alzheimer's disease: A multimodal imaging investigation. Neuroimage Clin 4:604–614.
73. Rattray I, Smith EJ, Crum WR, Walker TA, Gale R, Bates GP, Modo M (2017) Correlations of Behavioral Deficits with Brain Pathology Assessed through Longitudinal MRI and Histopathology in the HdhQ150/Q150 Mouse Model of Huntington's Disease. PLoS One 12:e0168556. https://doi.org/10.1371/journal.pone.0168556.
74. Rockenstein E, Adame A, Mante M, Moessler H, Windisch M, Masliah E (2003a) The neuroprotective effects of Cerebrolysin in a transgenic model of Alzheimer's disease are associated with improved behavioral performance. J Neural Transm (Vienna) 110:1313–1327. https://doi.org/10.1007/s00702-003-0025-7.
75. Rockenstein E, Adame A, Mante M, Moessler H, Windisch M, Masliah E (2003b) The neuroprotective effects of Cerebrolysin in a transgenic model of Alzheimer's disease are associated with improved behavioral performance. J Neural Transm 110:1313–1327.
76. Rockenstein E, Mallory M, Mante M, Sisk A, Masliaha E (2001) Early formation of mature amyloid-beta protein deposits in a mutant APP transgenic model depends on levels of Abeta(1-42). J Neurosci Res 66:573–582. https://doi.org/10.1002/jnr.1247.
77. Rockenstein E, Torrance M, Adame A, Mante M, Bar-on P, Rose JB, Crews L, Masliah E (2007) Neuroprotective effects of regulators of the glycogen synthase kinase-3beta signaling pathway in a transgenic model of Alzheimer's disease are associated with reduced amyloid precursor protein phosphorylation. J Neurosci 27:1981–1991. https://doi.org/10.1523/JNEUROSCI.4321-06.2007.
78. Rogers NT, Steptoe A, Cadar D (2017) Frailty is an independent predictor of incident dementia: Evidence from the English Longitudinal Study of Ageing. Sci Rep 7:15746. https://doi.org/10.1038/s41598-017-16104-y.
79. Schilling S, Zeitschel U, Hoffmann T, Heiser U, Francke M, Kehlen A, Holzer M, Hutter-Paier B, Prokesch M, Windisch M et al (2008) Glutaminyl cyclase inhibition attenuates pyroglutamate Abeta and Alzheimer's disease-like pathology. Nat Med 14:1106–1111. https://doi.org/10.1038/nm.1872.
80. Schneider JA, Bennett DA (2010) Where vascular meets neurodegenerative disease. Stroke 41:S144–S146. https://doi.org/10.1161/STROKEAHA.110.598326.
81. Searle SD, Rockwood K (2015) Frailty and the risk of cognitive impairment. Alzheimers Res Ther 7:54. https://doi.org/10.1186/s13195-015-0140-3.
82. Seshadri S, Beiser A, Kelly-Hayes M, Kase CS, Au R, Kannel WB, Wolf PA (2006) The lifetime risk of stroke: estimates from the Framingham Study. Stroke 37:345–350. https://doi.org/10.1161/01.STR.0000199613.38911.b2.
83. Seshadri S, Wolf PA (2007) Lifetime risk of stroke and dementia: current concepts, and estimates from the Framingham Study. Lancet Neurol 6: 1106–1114. https://doi.org/10.1016/S1474-4422(07)70291-0.
84. Sieber MW, Claus RA, Witte OW, Frahm C (2011) Attenuated inflammatory response in aged mice brains following stroke. PLoS One 6:e26288. https://doi.org/10.1371/journal.pone.0026288.
85. Simmons DA, Knowles JK, Belichenko NP, Banerjee G, Finkle C, Massa SM, Longo FM (2014) A small molecule p75NTR ligand, LM11A-31, reverses cholinergic neurite dystrophy in Alzheimer's disease mouse models with mid- to late-stage disease progression. PLoS One 9:e102136. https://doi.org/10.1371/journal.pone.0102136.
86. Simmons M, Trajkovic K (2006) Neuron-glia communication in the control of oligodendrocyte function and myelin biogenesis. J Cell Sci 119:4381–4389.
87. Simons M, Trajkovic K (2006) Neuron-glia communication in the control of oligodendrocyte function and myelin biogenesis. J Cell Sci 119:4381–4389. https://doi.org/10.1242/jcs.03242.
88. Sinha S, Anderson JP, Barbour R, Basi GS, Caccavello R, Davis D, Doan M, Dovey HF, Frigon N, al HJ (1999) Purification and cloning of amyloid precursor protein beta-secretase from human brain. Nature 402:537–540.
89. Tokita Y, Keino H, Matsui F, Aono S, Ishiguro H, Higashiyama S, Oohira A (2001a) Regulation of neuregulin expression in the injured rat brain and cultured astrocytes. J Neurosci 21:1257–1264.
90. Tokita Y, Keino H, Matsui F, Aono S, Ishiguro H, Higashiyama S, Oohira A (2001b) Regulation of neuregulin expression in the injured rat brain and cultured astrocytes. J Neurosci 21:1257–1264.
91. Tolppanen AM, Solomon A, Soininen H, Kivipelto M (2012) Midlife vascular risk factors and Alzheimer's disease: evidence from epidemiological studies. J Alzheimers Dis 32:531–540. https://doi.org/10.3233/JAD-2012-120802.
92. Ubhi K, Masliah E (2013) Alzheimer's disease: recent advances and future perspectives. J Alzheimers Dis 33(1):S185–S194. https://doi.org/10.3233/JAD-2012-129028.
93. Vargas ME, Barres BA (2007) Why is Wallerian degeneration in the CNS so

slow? Annu Rev Neurosci 30:153–179. https://doi.org/10.1146/annurev.neuro.30.051606.094354.
94. Vijayan M, Reddy PH (2016) Stroke, Vascular Dementia, and Alzheimer's Disease: Molecular Links. J Alzheimers Dis 54:427–443.
95. Villa RF, Ferrari F, Moretti A (2017) Post-stroke depression: Mechanisms and pharmacological treatment. Pharmacol Ther. https://doi.org/10.1016/j.pharmthera.2017.11.005.
96. Wang C, Ji X, Wu X, Tang Z, Zhang X, Guan S, Liu H, Fang X (2017a) Frailty in Relation to the Risk of Alzheimer's Disease, Dementia, and Death in Older Chinese Adults: A Seven-Year Prospective Study. J Nutr Health Aging 21: 648–654. https://doi.org/10.1007/s12603-016-0798-7.
97. Wang JZ, Xia YY, Grundke-Iqbal I, Iqbal K (2013a) Abnormal hyperphosphorylation of tau: sites, regulation, and molecular mechanism of neurofibrillary degeneration. J Alzheimers Dis 33(1):S123–S139. https://doi.org/10.3233/JAD-2012-129031.
98. Wang M, Ding F, Deng S, Guo X, Wang W, Iliff JJ, Nedergaard M (2017b) Focal Solute Trapping and Global Glymphatic Pathway Impairment in a Murine Model of Multiple Microinfarcts. J Neurosci 37:2870–2877. https://doi.org/10.1523/JNEUROSCI.2112-16.2017.
99. Wang X, Li J, Qian L, Zang XF, Zhang SY, Wang XY, Jin JL, Zhu XL, Zhang XB, Wang ZY et al (2013b) Icariin promotes histone acetylation and attenuates post-stroke cognitive impairment in the central cholinergic circuits of mice. Neuroscience 236:281–288. https://doi.org/10.1016/j.neuroscience.2012.12.074.
100. Weiner MW (2013) Dementia in 2012: Further insights into Alzheimer disease pathogenesis. Nat Rev Neurol 9:65–66. https://doi.org/10.1038/nrneurol.2012.275.
101. Wen Y, Yang S, Liu R, Simpkins JW (2004) Transient cerebral ischemia induces site-specific hyperphosphorylation of tau protein. Brain Res 1022: 30–38. https://doi.org/10.1016/j.brainres.2004.05.106.
102. Wen Y, Yang SH, Liu R, Perez EJ, Brun-Zinkernagel AM, Koulen P, Simpkins JW (2007) Cdk5 is involved in NFT-like tauopathy induced by transient cerebral ischemia in female rats. Biochim Biophys Acta 1772:473–483. https://doi.org/10.1016/j.bbadis.2006.10.011.
103. Whitehead JC, Hildebrand BA, Sun M, Rockwood MR, Rose RA, Rockwood K, Howlett SE (2014) A clinical frailty index in aging mice: comparisons with frailty index data in humans. J Gerontol A Biol Sci Med Sci 69:621–632. https://doi.org/10.1093/gerona/glt136.
104. Whitehead SN, Massoni E, Cheng G, Hachinski VC, Cimino M, Balduini W, Cechetto DF (2010) Triflusal reduces cerebral ischemia induced inflammation in a combined mouse model of Alzheimer's disease and stroke. Brain Res 1366:246–256. https://doi.org/10.1016/j.brainres.2010.10.008.
105. Whitehouse PJ, Price DL, Struble RG, Clark AW, Coyle JT, Delon MR (1982) Alzheimer's disease and senile dementia: loss of neurons in the basal forebrain. Science 215:1237–1239.
106. Yang SH, Kim J, Lee MJ, Kim Y (2015) Abnormalities of plasma cytokines and spleen in senile APP/PS1/Tau transgenic mouse model. Sci Rep 5:15703. https://doi.org/10.1038/srep15703.
107. Yang T, Knowles JK, Lu Q, Zhang H, Arancio O, Moore LA, Chang T, Wang Q, Andreasson K, Rajadas J et al (2008) Small molecule, non-peptide p75 ligands inhibit Abeta-induced neurodegeneration and synaptic impairment. PLoS One 3:e3604. https://doi.org/10.1371/journal.pone.0003604.
108. Zbesko JC, Nguyen TV, Yang T, Frye JB, Hussain O, Hayes M, Chung A, Day WA, Stepanovic K, Krumberger M et al (2018) Glial scars are permeable to the neurotoxic environment of chronic stroke infarcts. Neurobiol Dis 112: 63–78. https://doi.org/10.1016/j.nbd.2018.01.007.
109. Zhan X, Cox C, Ander BP, Liu D, Stamova B, Jin LW, Jickling GC, Sharp FR (2015) Inflammation Combined with Ischemia Produces Myelin Injury and Plaque-Like Aggregates of Myelin, Amyloid-beta and AbetaPP in Adult Rat Brain. J Alzheimers Dis 46:507–523. https://doi.org/10.3233/JAD-143072.
110. Zhang X, Song W (2013) The role of APP and BACE1 trafficking in APP processing and amyloid-β generation. Alzheimers Res Ther 5:1–8.
111. Zimmer HD, Speiser HR, Seidler B (2003) Spatio-temporal working-memory and short-term object-location tasks use different memory mechanisms. Acta Psychol (Amst) 114:41–65.
112. Zuloaga KL, Zhang W, Yeiser LA, Stewart B, Kukino A, Nie X, Roese NE, Grafe MR, Pike MM, Raber J et al (2015) Neurobehavioral and imaging correlates of hippocampal atrophy in a mouse model of vascular cognitive impairment. Transl Stroke Res 6:390–398. https://doi.org/10.1007/s12975-015-0412-z.

4

GJA1 (connexin43) is a key regulator of Alzheimer's disease pathogenesis

Yuji Kajiwara[1,7†], Erming Wang[2,3†], Minghui Wang[2,3], Wun Chey Sin[4], Kristen J. Brennand[1,2,5,6], Eric Schadt[2,3], Christian C. Naus[4], Joseph Buxbaum[1,3,5,6] and Bin Zhang[2,3*]

Abstract

GJA1 (connexin43) has been predicted as the top key driver of an astrocyte enriched subnetwork associated with Alzheimer's disease (AD). In this study, we comprehensively examined *GJA1* expression across 29 transcriptomic and proteomic datasets from post-mortem AD and normal control brains. We demonstrated that *GJA1* was strongly associated with AD amyloid and tau pathologies and cognitive functions. RNA sequencing analysis of *Gja1−/−* astrocytes validated that *Gja1* regulated the subnetwork identified in AD, and many genes involved in Aβ metabolism. Astrocytes lacking *Gja1* showed reduced Apoe protein levels as well as impaired Aβ phagocytosis. Consistent with this, wildtype neurons co-cultured with *Gja1−/−* astrocytes contained higher levels of Aβ species than those with wildtype astrocytes. Moreover, *Gja1−/−* astrocytes was more neuroprotective under Aβ stress. Our results underscore the importance of *GJA1* in AD pathogenesis and its potential for further investigation as a promising pharmacological target in AD.

Keywords: Alzheimer's disease, GJA1, Cx43, connexin43, Gene networks, amyloidβ, Astrocyte

Introduction

Alzheimer's disease (AD) reflects multifactorial genetic and environmental perturbations that, in turn, cause pleiotropic changes in molecular networks linking a host of biological processes. By employing an integrative network biology approach to analyze a large-scale genetic and gene expression dataset in late onset Alzheimer's disease (LOAD), we previously conducted an unbiased identification and prioritization of gene networks associated with clinical and pathological progression of the disease [98]. In addition to a prominent driver of LOAD, an immune response subnetwork (module) governed by *TYROBP*, we identified other network modules within which gene coexpression patterns were significantly changed in LOAD subjects compared to controls. In the current study, we focused on the identification and characterization of causal regulators of a module that shows a dramatic loss of coordination in AD and that includes *APOE*, a well-known risk factor of AD [18, 82]. This module was highly enriched in astrocyte specific genes, with *GJA1* predicted as its top regulator.

GJA1, also known as connexin43 (Cx43), is a member of the connexin family of proteins that is highly conserved among vertebrates. Members of the connexin family exist at the plasma membrane as hexameric complexes known as connexons, and function as connexin hemichannels allowing permeability to small molecules and ions [28]. Two connexons at the apposed cell surface of adjacent cells form a trans-dimer called a gap junction channel (GJC). Gap junctions are clusters of gap junction channels, and mediate efficient and rapid bidirectional inter-cellular transmission and transport of electrical and chemical signals [55, 80]. Cx43 also functions as a unitary channel (hemichannel) to participate in paracrine communication [17], but this activity is often associated with pathological conditions [21]. *GJA1* and *GJB6* (connexin30) are predominantly expressed in mature astrocytes [27, 93, 99], forming astrocytic networks facilitating propagation of calcium waves, potassium and glutamate buffering, and metabolic coupling [66, 70, 77, 78, 83, 89]. Astrocytic gap junctions are critical for neuronal function, as evidenced by the profound

* Correspondence: bin.zhang@mssm.edu; zhangb@hotmail.com
†Yuji Kajiwara and Erming Wang contributed equally to this work.
[2]Department of Genetics and Genomic Sciences, Icahn School of Medicine at Mount Sinai, New York, NY 10029, USA
[3]Mount Sinai Center for Transformative Disease Modeling, Icahn Institute of Genomics and Multiscale Biology, Icahn School of Medicine at Mount Sinai, New York, NY 10029, USA
Full list of author information is available at the end of the article

neurological phenotypes in *Gja1/Gjb6* double knockout mice [56].

Numerous autosomal dominant *GJA1* mutations have been reported to cause oculodentodigital dysplasia (ODDD), which is characterized by craniofacial and limb dysmorphisms [42]. Patients with ODDD frequently manifest neurological symptoms including paraparesis, white matter abnormalities, hearing and vision loss, and low IQ [29, 54]. *GJA1* mutations associated with ODDD are mostly loss-of-function, although a few gain-of-function cases have also been identified, indicating that diverse functional perturbations of *GJA1* can lead to ODDD [42].

Although mice deficient in astrocytic *Gja1* are grossly normal, they show reduced synaptic plasticity [30], increased propagation of synaptic depolarization and neuronal inactivation ("spreading depression") [84] and impaired in rotarod performance [26]. Mice deficient in both *Gja1* and *Gjb6* spontaneously develop pathological myelin degeneration without overt neuronal atrophy [56]. Loss or reduced expression of *Gja1* leads to enlarged infarct size upon induced-ischemia, and the loss of only the C-terminal tail of Cx43 appeared to mediate the damaging effects [41, 44, 51, 64, 65, 85]. These studies indicated that *Gja1* plays a neuroprotective function and restricts neuronal damage under oxidative and metabolic stress.

GJA1 has been previously investigated in the context of Alzheimer's disease. GJA1 (Cx43) immunoreactivity was found to be enriched in astrocytes surrounding amyloid plaques in post-mortem AD brain [63] and a APP/PS1 mouse model [59] and Cx43 hemichannel activity was increased in the APP/PS1 mouse model [96]. Cx43 deficiency or pharmacological blockade of connexins in APP/PS1 mice appeared to reduce dystrophic neurites, mitochondrial oxidative stress, and cognitive impairment without altering amyloid pathology [73, 96, 97].

Here we corroborated the evidence of *GJA1* dysregulation in AD by analyzing *GJA1* expression in a large number of transcriptomic and proteomic datasets from pathologically and clinically characterized LOAD brain samples. We showed that a number of known AD risk factor genes were significantly correlated with *Gja1* in multiple brain regions in AD. We constructed and validated *GJA1* regulated gene networks in AD. We revealed that *Gja1* regulated the expression of more than half of the known AD risk factor genes. We further demonstrated the effect of *Gja1*-deficiency on astrocyte function and the subsequent impact on co-cultured neurons.

Materials and methods

Data preprocessing

Three clinical cohorts of post-mortem brain samples from patients with Alzheimer's disease (AD) symptoms of various severity, and normal controls were subject to RNA microarray and/or RNA-seq analysis to detect changes in mRNA expression caused by AD pathology. As summarized in (64), RNA microarray assays were performed on RNAs extracted from prefrontal cortex (PFC), visual cortex (VC), and cerebellum (CB) of post-mortem brain cortex tissues in the Harvard Brain Tissue Bank (HBTRC) [98]. Details of the research such as neuropathological phenotypic traits of AD subjects and normal controls, RNA microarray assays, data preprocessing and covariate adjustment were described in [98]. Both RNA microarray and RNA-seq assays were conducted using RNAs collected from post-mortem brains in the Mount Sinai Brain Bank (MSBB) cohort [31, 91]. Experimental design and data analysis of RNA microarrays on 19 distinct brain regions of post-mortem brain tissues in the MSBB cohort were presented by Wang et al. [91]. Single-end RNA-seq assays were performed on RNAs extracted from four selected regions (BM10, frontal pole (FP); BM22, superior temporal gyrus (STG); BM36, parahippocampal gyrus (PHG); BM44, inferior frontal gyrus (IFG)) of post-mortem brain tissues in the MSBB cohort. The raw sequence reads were aligned to human genome hg19 with the star aligner (v2.3.0e) [22]. Then the gene level expression was quantified by featureCounts (v1.4.4) [49] based on Ensemble gene model GRCh37.70. The gene level read counts data was normalized using the trimmed mean of M-values normalization (TMM) [76] method to adjust for sequencing library size difference. The normalized data was further adjusted for the covariates postmortem interval (PMI), race, RNA integrity number (RIN), gender, rate of exonic reads, and batch using a linear mixed model [33], where batch was treated as a random effect. The residuals from the regression model were used for downstream analysis. In addition, proteomics assays were performed on proteins extracted from the BM10 region of post-mortem brains in the MSBB cohort, and raw counts summarized at the gene/protein level were provided by the Genomics Core at the Icahn School of Medicine at Mount Sinai. These raw counts were further corrected by covariates (PMI + AOD + batch + gender) using a linear model described by Wang et al. [91], and the residuals after correction were used for further downstream analysis.

The Religious Orders Study and Memory and Aging Project (ROSMAP) cohort consists of ROS and MAP studies [7]. The detailed information regarding ROSMAP study was described in previous studies [8, 9]. Normalized RNA-seq expression data were downloaded from the AMP-AD Knowledge Portal at Synapse upon authentication by the AMP-AD Consortium (doi:https://doi.org/10.7303/syn3388564). Genes with at least 1 FPKM in at least 10% of the samples were selected and then the data was corrected for confounding factors including batch, PMI, gender and RIN via a linear model.

The residuals after correction were used for further downstream analysis.

Bayesian causal network analysis

Bayesian causal network was constructed by integrating genome-wide gene expression, SNP genotype, and known transcription factor (TF)-target relationships. Briefly, we first computed expression quantitative trait loci (eQTLs) and then employed a formal statistical causal inference test (CIT) [62] to infer the causal probability between gene pairs associated with the same eQTL. The causal relationships inferred were used, together with TF-target relationships from the ENCODE project, as structural priors for building a causal gene regulatory network from the gene expression data through a Monte Carlo Markov Chain (MCMC) simulation based procedure [100]. We followed a network averaging strategy in which 1000 networks were generated from the MCMC procedure starting with different random structure, and links that shared by more than 30% of the networks were used to define a final consensus network structure. To ensure the consensus network is a directed acyclic graph, an iterative de-loop procedure was conducted, removing the most-weakly supported link of all links involved in any loop. Following Zhang et al. [98], we performed Key Driver Analysis (KDA) on the consensus Bayesian network to identify key hub genes which regulated many downstream nodes.

RNA sequencing and data processing

Total RNAs were sequenced via the Illumina HiSeq 2500 system with 100 nt paired-end read. Sequencing reads were aligned to mouse reference genome mm10 (GRCm38.75) STAR aligner [22] guided by UCSC gene model. Accepted mapped reads were summarized to gene levels using the featureCounts [49] program. Raw count data were normalized by the voom function in the R limma package [75], and then differential expression was called by the moderated t-test implemented in limma. Differentially expressed genes (DEGs) were defined to have at least 1.2-fold change in expression and BH-adjusted $p < 0.05$ for two comparisons including *Gja1−/−* astrocytes versus wildtype astrocytes and coculture of *Gja1−/−* astrocytes and neurons versus co-culture of wildtype astrocytes and neurons.

Construction of *GJA1* centric co-expression networks

We constructed *GJA1* centric consensus co-expression networks from 8 cohort datasets from three cohorts including MSBB (4 brain regions), ROSMAP (1 brain region) and HBTRC (3 brain regions). In each dataset, the genes significantly correlated with *GJA1* were identified based on BH-corrected p value < 0.05. From those significant correlations, a directional voting method was utilized to calculate the frequency of positive correlation as well as the frequency of negative correlations between *GJA1* and each other gene. *Gja1* centric networks were then defined as a function of frequency threshold n (=1, 2, ..., 8}.

Construction of *GJA1* signaling map

Starting from *GJA1* as the root, we searched through the khaki module based Bayesian network for further three layers of genetic neighborhood, and trimmed away those single leaf nodes while keeping the remaining nodes. Then, we used the individual nodes or its first neighborhood in the remaining network to query the reactome (https://reactome.org/) and MSigDB database for gene ontology enrichment. A *GJA1* signal map was constructed by replacing each individual nodes in the network plot with a relevant gene ontology entry acquired from the query.

Quantitative PCR

Quantitative PCR was performed as previously described [38]. Briefly, total RNA was isolated using Qiagen RNeasy kit, and 1–2 µg of total RNA was used to synthesize cDNA using Ecodry (Clontech, 639,543, Mountain view, CA). Universal probe library in combination with the primers listed (Additional file 1: Table S10) was used to perform qPCR with KAPA PROBE FAST qPCR master mix (KAPA Biosystems, KK4703, Wilmington, MA). Acquired Ct values were loaded onto qbase Plus software package (Biogazelle, Belgium) for data quality control and normalization. *Actb*, *Rpl13a*, and *Rplp0* were used as normalizer genes.

Cell culture and reagents

Generation of *Gja1−/−* astrocytes were previously described [66]. WT and *Gja1−/−* primary astrocytes were prepared by dissecting and dissociating forebrains of P1–3 pups and culturing for 2 weeks in DMEM containing 10% fetal bovine serum and penicillin/streptomycin in T75 flask. Contaminating microglia were reduced by vigorous shaking flasks at 500 rpm for 20 min and replacement of medium containing floating cells. Mouse TNFα (14–8321-62) and IL-1β (14–8012-62) were purchased from eBiosciences and used at concentration of 10 ng/ml. Carbenoxolone (C4790), lanthanum (575275), quinine (Q1125) were purchased from Sigma-Aldrich (St. Louis, MO, USA).

Neuron astrocyte cocultures

For RNA-seq in astrocytes and neuron/astrocyte cocultures, cortical neuron cultures were prepared from E15.5 wildtype C57BL6/J embryos as previously described [14]. 1×10^5 neurons were seeded in poly-D-lysine coated 6 well plates with or without 1×10^5 wildtype or *Gja1−/−*

astrocytes in neurobasal medium (Life Technologies, 21,103–049, Grand Island, NY, USA) supplemented with B27 (Life Technologies, 17,504–044), and cultured for 10 days. At div10, half of medium was replaced with neurobasal containing 20 μM $A\beta_{1-42}$ oligomer for four days, and total RNA was harvested using RNA-Bee (AMSBIO, Cambridge, MA, USA) following the manufacturer's instruction. Four replicate wells were used for each condition.

For MEA assays, E15.5 cortical neuron cultures were prepared from wildtype C57BL6/J as above. MEA wells were coated with poly-D-lysine and one day prior to plating 1×10^5 neurons, 5×10^4 wildtype or *Gja1−/−* astrocytes were plated in neurobasal medium supplemented with B27. At days in vitro (div) 16, neuron/astrocyte co-cultures were treated with 10 μM $A\beta_{1-42}$ oligomers until div 20.

For neuronal death and viability assays, 2×10^5 cortical neurons were plated onto PDL coated 12 well plate and 1×10^5 wildtype or *Gja1−/−* astrocytes are plated in Transwells (Costar, 3460, Kennebunk, ME USA). At div7, Transwells with astrocytes were inserted to neuronal cultures and incubated with the indicated $A\beta_{1-42}$ for 4 or 7 days. LDH assay was performed as in (Kajiwara, 2014) using LDH Cytotoxicity Detection Kit (Clontech, Mountain View, CA, USA). MTT assay was performed as described in (Bruban 2015).

Apoe and Aβ ELISA

Astrocytes were seeded in 6 well plates at the density of 100,000 cells per well in serum free DMEM medium for 48 h with vehicle, 2 or 20 μM $A\beta_{1-42}$ oligomers. Mouse Apoe secreted in conditioned medium was quantitated using mouse Apoe ELISA kit (Mybiosource, MBS705227, San Diego, CA, USA) following manufacture's instruction. Astrocytes attached to the plate were used to prepare cell lysates as described below. Mouse amyloidβ 40 and 42 species were quantitatively determined using Human/Rat Amyloid ELISA kits (294–64,701 and 294–64,501, Wako Chemicals, Richmond, VA, USA).

Immunoblotting

Lysates were prepared from astrocytes underwent above procedure in buffer containing phosphate buffered saline, protease inhibitor cocktail (Roche, Indianapolis, IN, USA), and 1x loading buffer. Lysates were resolved by denaturing SDS-PAGE gel and transferred to PVDF membrane. The membranes were blotted with following primary antibody: Cx43 (1:500, 3512, Cell Signaling Technology); Apoe (1:1000, sc-6384, Santa Cruz Biotechnology); Actin (1:1000, A5060, Sigma-Aldrich), and specific signals were detected with HRP-conjugated secondary antibodies followed by SuperSignal West Dura (34,075, Thermo-Fisher Scientific).

Multielectrode array recordings

Recordings of neuronal activity was performed on Axion 768 channel system (The Maestro, Axion Biosystems, Atlanta, GA, USA) using 48-well plate, which records or stimulates neuronal activity from up to 16 electrodes per well. Manufacture's recommended settings were used for detection of spikes, bursts and network bursts. Briefly, spikes were detected using Adaptive Threshold Crossing with 6x Standard Deviation; bursts were defined as minimum of 5 spikes with 100 ms of maximum inter-spike interval; and network bursts were defined as minimum of 10 spikes with 100 ms of maximum inter-spike interval and 20 ms of synchrony window. Spontaneous activities were recorded at days in vitro (div) 10, 14, 18, and 20 as follow. A MEA plate was set on heated stage at 37C for at least 5 min prior to initiation of recordings, which lasted for 10 min. All the recordings and analysis were performed on Axion Integrated Studio (Axion Biosystems). Stimulation was performed div 14 and 20 using the same spike and burst settings as in spontaneous recordings. A stimulation given was comprised of 3 repeated cycles of voltage-controlled (500 mV/− 500 mV), biphasic (500 μs each), and positive-first stimulus followed by 3 ms of floating duration [88], and was given to all electrodes. Stimulation was given 5 times with 5 s interval and stimulation data were analyzed using NeuralMetricTool (Axion Biosystems). Results are given as means of 5 stimulations.

Statistics

All of the statistical significance levels reported in this study were corrected for multiple testing unless otherwise specified. Statistical analysis was performed using either R programming language or SPSS version 20 or higher (IBM corporation, Somers, NY, USA). Amyloid uptake assays were analyzed by Student's t-test. Spontaneous neural recordings were analyzed by Man-Whitney, or Kruskal-Wallis non-parametric analysis.

Results

Figure 1 shows the workflow of the integrative network analysis and functional validation experiments performed in this study. We first examined the relationships between *GJA1* mRNA expression and clinical and pathological traits in 29 AD transcriptomic datasets. We also investigated the role of *GJA1* in gene networks underlying AD. We then performed in vitro experiments to study the role of *GJA1* in regulating AD gene networks and AD related phenotypes using primary astrocytes purified and cultured from wildtype and astrocyte specific *Gja1−/−* mice. *Gja1*'s target gene signatures identified from the RNA-seq data from the in vitro experiments were then projected onto the *GJA1* centric networks to validate these networks' structures.

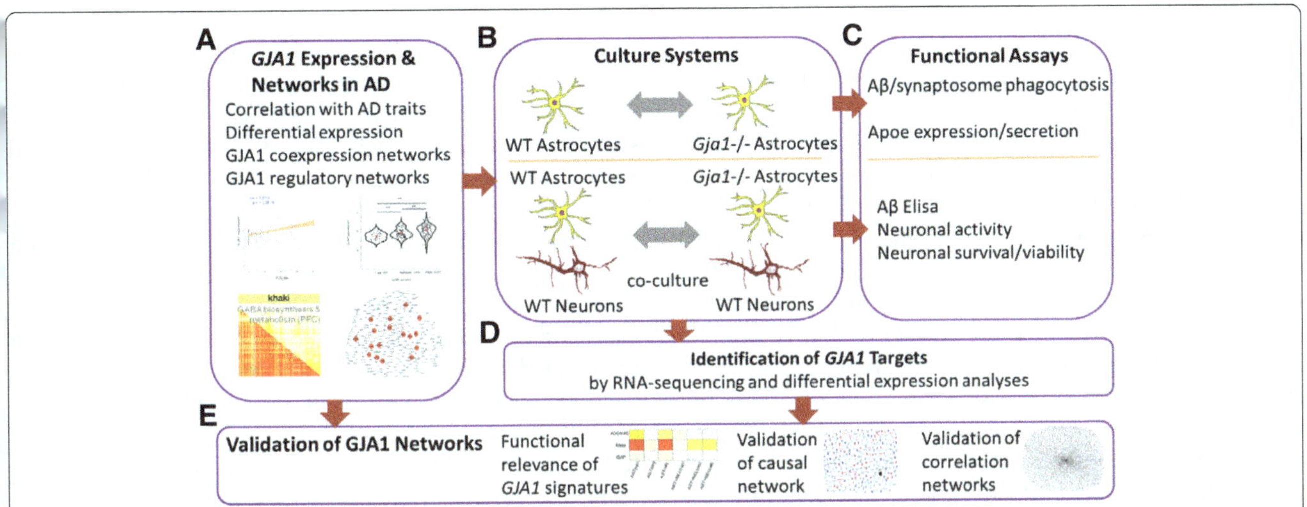

Fig. 1 Overview of the integrative network analyses and validation experiments performed in the study. **a**. *GJA1* mRNA expression changes and its correlations with clinical and pathological traits were systematically investigated in 29 datasets. *GJA1*-centric coexpression and regulatory networks. **b**. Workflow of in vitro functional validation study. Wildtype and *Gja1*−/− astrocytes with or without wildtype neurons were used to prepare RNA for sequencing and to perform various functional validations (**c**). **d**. *GJA1*'s gene signatures between wildtype and *Gja1*−/− astrocytes and between coculture of wildtype astrocytes and wildtype neurons and coculture of *Gja1*−/− astrocytes and wildtype neurons were identified from RNA-sequencing data from the experiments in **b**. **e**. *GJA1*'s gene signatures were used to validate the network structures predicted from the transcriptomic datasets in human AD brains. Functional relevance of *GJA1*'s gene signatures was also investigated

GJA1 is a key regulator of an astrocyte specific gene subnetwork dysregulated in LOAD

Several studies have used co-expression network analysis to find modules of co-regulated genes in AD [36, 60, 61]. Our previous study developed a novel network approach capable of integrating clinical and neuropathological data with large-scale genetic and gene expression [98]. This network biology approach led to a novel multiscale network model of LOAD, which identified a number of coexpressed gene modules that were strongly associated with AD pathological traits or underwent dramatic disruption of high-order gene-gene interactions [98]. One such module, referred to as the khaki module in the original construction of this network, was of particular interest since it included *APOE*, the top AD risk factor gene. Moreover, the average interaction strength among its member genes in LOAD was reduced by 71% compared to that in normal control at a false discovery rate (FDR) < 2%, suggesting a huge loss of coordination among this group of genes in AD. The khaki module was enriched for the genes in Gamma-aminobutyrate (GABA) biosynthesis and metabolism (24 fold enrichment (FE), Fisher's exact test (FET) $p = 0.046$) and harbored 12 (*ALDOC, APOE, AQP4, ATP1A2, CSPG3, CST3, EDG1, EMX2, GJA1, PPAP2B, PRDX6* and *SPARCL1*) of 46 known astrocyte marker genes, a 15-fold enrichment over what would be expected by chance (FET $p = 6.55\text{E-}9$). The module was also enriched for the expression of the common variants identified as genome-wide significant by AD genome wide association studies (GWAS) (3-FE, FET $p = 1.92\text{E-}11$). Bayesian causal network analysis showed that *GJA1* was the top driver of the module followed by *FXYD1*, *STON2* and *CST3* [98]. The key drivers of the corresponding causal network of the module were the nodes that had a large number of downstream nodes [90, 98]. These results indicate that *GJA1* is a potential regulator of molecular networks in AD. In the next subsection, we will investigate the association between *Gja1* mRNA expression and AD. All of the statistical significance levels reported were corrected for multiple testing unless otherwise specified.

GJA1 expression is associated with AD clinical and pathophysiological traits

To gain insight into the role of *GJA1* in cognitive functions and AD pathogenesis, we first extensively investigated how *GJA1* expression at the mRNA level was correlated with AD neuropathological traits in 29 gene expression datasets from three AD cohort studies of aging and dementia that included organ donation at death: the Mount Sinai/JJ Peters VA Medical Center Brain Bank (MSBB; Additional file 1: Table S1) [91], the Religious Orders Study and the Rush Memory and Aging Project (ROSMAP) [8, 9] and in the Harvard Brain Tissue Resource Center Alzheimer's Disease study (HBTRC) [98]. We chose six different clinical and pathological criteria to evaluate the clinical relevance of *GJA1* on AD pathology and cognitive functions: the Mini-Mental State Examination (MMSE) score [25, 32], the sum of NFT density estimates for all cortical regions examined (NTrSum), Mean Plaque density (PLQ_Mn) for the estimation of average plaque density, Braak stage score for quantitative assessment of neurofibrillary tangles

[11], the Consortium to Establish a Registry for Alzheimer's disease (CERAD: 1 for definite AD, 2 for probable AD, 3 possible AD, 4 for normal control) score for quantitative measure of neuritic plaques, and clinical dementia rating score (CDR ranging between 0 and 5 with 0 for normal control and 5 for severe dementia).

In the microarray data in the ROSMAP cohort, *GJA1* expression was significantly correlated with CERAD score ($r = -0.15$, $p = 3.3E\text{-}3$) and the MiniMental State Examination (MMSE) score ($r = -0.14$, $p = 6.4E\text{-}3$). Similar results were observed in the ROSMAP RNA-seq dataset (Fig. 2a, and Additional file 1: Table S2), suggesting that the mRNA expression of *GJA1* is associated with AD pathogenesis and dementia. The MSBB AD cohort includes microarray and RNA-seq data from a battery of distinct brain cortical regions and thus provides an excellent opportunity to investigate regional differences in the correlation between *GJA1* expression and AD neuropathological traits [91]. Among the 19 brain cortex regions investigated in the MSBB AD microarray data, *GJA1* expression in six cortex regions including BM10 (frontal pole), BM20 (inferior temporal gyrus), BM21 (middle temporal gyrus), BM32 (anterior cingulate), BM36 (parahippocampal gyrus) and BM46 (dorsolateral prefrontal cortex) was significantly correlated with at least three AD neuropathological traits (Fig. 2b, and Additional file 1: Table S2). Overall, *GJA1* expression in these six cortex regions displayed a significant positive correlation with Braak stage score, PLQ_Mn, NTrSum and CDR. The MSBB AD RNA-seq data revealed a consistent pattern of correlation between *GJA1* expression and AD clinic traits across the cortical regions studied (Fig. 2c-e; Additional file 1: Table S2). Notably, in BM10, BM36 and BM44 cortex regions, the microarray and RNA-seq data converged to show a consistent correlation between *GJA1* expression and AD neuropathological traits (Additional file 1: Table S2). Thus, in the MSBB cohort, the association between *GJA1* expression and AD neuropathological traits was cortex-specific. At the protein level, GJA1 in the brain cortex BM10 region was significantly correlated with CERAD ($r = -0.32$, $p = 1.26E\text{-}07$), PLQ_Mn ($r = 0.37$, $p = 4.08E\text{-}10$) (Fig. 2f) and CDR ($r = 0.35$, $p = 5.69E\text{-}9$) (Additional file 1: Table S2). Also the total soluble amyloidβ (Aβ) levels had a significant positive correlation with GJA1 protein levels in the BM10 region ($r = 0.18$, $p = 0.0036$).

We showed previously in the HBTRC cohort that *Gja1* had a significant correlation with Braak score ($r = 0.61$ and 0.52 for dorsolateral prefrontal cortex and cerebellum cortex regions, respectively) [98].

We further checked how *GJA1* mRNA expression was correlated with 30 known AD risk factor genes. As shown in Fig. 2g, a majority of those AD genes were significantly correlated to *GJA1* in the five RNA-seq datasets.

We also examined *GJA1* differential expression between various subgroups of AD severity with respect to each individual AD neuropathological or functional cognitive trait using pairwise Student's t-test. Consistent with the correlation analysis, *Gja1* expression increased significantly as the disease deteriorated (Additional file 1: Table S3).

Because *APOE* is one of the major AD risk factors, and age and sex are critical clinic covariables in AD neuropathology, we investigated whether age, sex and APOE genotypes had any impact on the association of *GJA1* expression with AD clinical and pathological traits. We stratified this cohort by age of death (AOD) (AOD > 85 versus AOD < 85), sex (female versus male), and *APOE* genotypes (E23, E34 and E33). As demonstrated in Additional file 1: Table S4 and Additional file 2: Figure S1, *GJA1* expression is more significantly associated with clinical dementia rating (CDR) in the group with AOD > 85 than that with AOD < 85, in females than males, and in the group with *APOE* E33 than that with E34 or E23, across four brain regions in the MSBB cohort, suggesting that age, sex and *APOE* genotypes impact the association of *GJA1* expression with clinical and pathological traits.

We further assessed if *GJA1* mRNA expression was correlated with the variants of the known AD risk genes using the RNA-seq data from the brain region BM36 in the MSBB cohort. Among the 28 ADGWAS genes that had identifiable variants in the present study, 18 had at least one variant that possessed a significant correlation with *GJA1* (Additional file 2: Figure S2). For example, the transcript/isoform ENST00000532146 of the risk factor *CELF1* is significantly correlated with *GJA1* expression in BM10 and BM44, but not BM22 and BM36 while ENST00000534614 and ENST00000539254 are correlated with *GJA1* expression only in BM36 and BM22, respectively (Additional file 2: Figure S2). These results suggested that variation in transcripts' abundance might be an important factor for determining the co-regulation between *GJA1* and AD risk factors.

In summary, both correlation and differential expression analyses revealed that *GJA1* was associated with amyloid and tau pathologies of AD as well as cognitive functions suggesting that *GJA1* may play an important role in AD.

Transcriptomic changes caused by *Gja1* deficiency in mouse astrocytes

To validate the role for *GJA1* in orchestrating the astrocytic transcriptome, we purified and cultured primary astrocytes from wildtype and astrocyte specific *Gja1−/−* mice, and identified differentially expressed genes (DEGs) by RNA-seq in *Gja1−/−* vs wildtype primary astrocytic cultures in the absence or presence of wildtype primary cortical neurons. Each group had four replicates. All

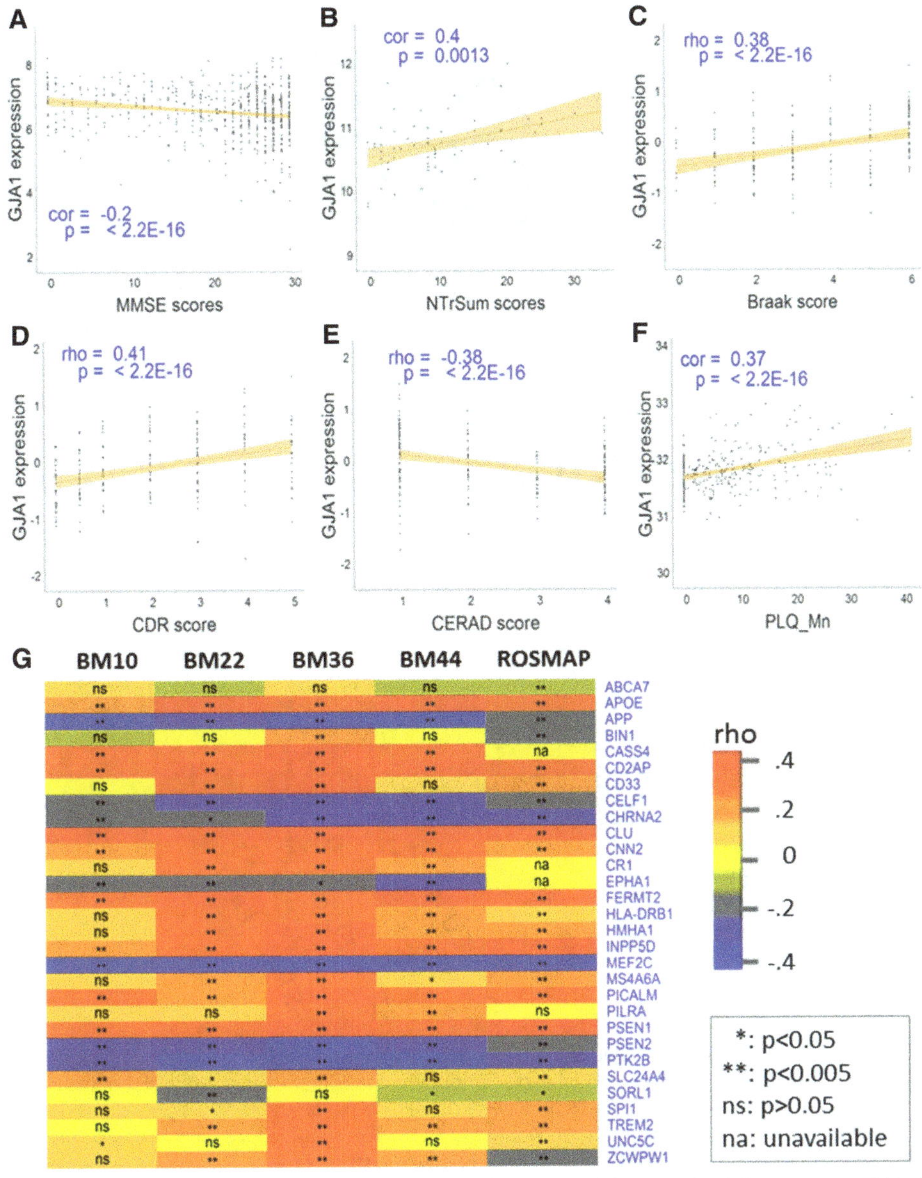

Fig. 2 *GJA1* mRNA/protein expression is correlated with AD pathogenesis, dementia and known AD risk factor genes. *GJA1* mRNA expression is correlated with the MMSE score in the prefrontal cortex region in the ROSMAP cohort (**a**), the NTrSum score in the cortex region frontal pole (BM10) the MSBB cohort (**b**), the Braak score in the parahippocampal gyrus (BM36) in the MSBB cohort (**c**), and the CDR score in BM36 in the MSBB cohort (**d**), and CERAD in BM36 in the MSBB cohort (**e**). The GJA1 protein level is also correlated with the plaque mean density (PLQ_Mn) in the frontal pole (BM10) in the MSBB cohort (**f**). Inset was the correlation coefficient along its *p* value between individual clinical traits and *GJA1* mRNA/protein level. Severity of AD symptoms was classified based on each individual AD neuropathological and cognitive traits according to the criteria established in the ROSMAP clinic codebook [91, 92]. **g**. *Gja1* mRNA expression is correlated with a vast majority of the ADGWAS genes in the MSBB (BM10, BM22, BM36 and BM44) and ROSMAP RNA-seq datasets. Colors represent Correlation coefficients: red, high; blue, low; yellow, in between. * and ** stand for significance at 5 and 0.5% level, respectively while ns indicates insignificant correlation and na stands for "not applicable". Shown in the heatmap are only the ADGWAS genes that passed RNA-seq data preprocessing, normalization and annotation

cultures were treated with 10 μM $A\beta_{1-42}$ oligomer from div 10 through 14, when total RNAs were harvested. We identified 2891 upregulated (termed AST(up)) and 2605 downregulated (termed AST(dn)) DEGs upon the ablation of the *Gja1* gene as compared to wildtype primary astrocytes (Fig. 3a). We identified 573 upregulated genes (termed AST + NEU(up)) and 1391 downregulated genes (termed AST + NEU(dn)) in *Gja1−/−* vs. wildtype primary astrocytes co-cultured with primary neurons (Fig. 3a). AST(up) shared 328 genes (11.3%) with AST + NEU(up) and 208 genes with AST + NEU(dn) while AST(dn) shared 672 and 60 genes with AST-NEU(dn) and AST-NEU(up), respectively (Fig. 3a). These DEG signatures were enriched for a variety of biological pathways including translational

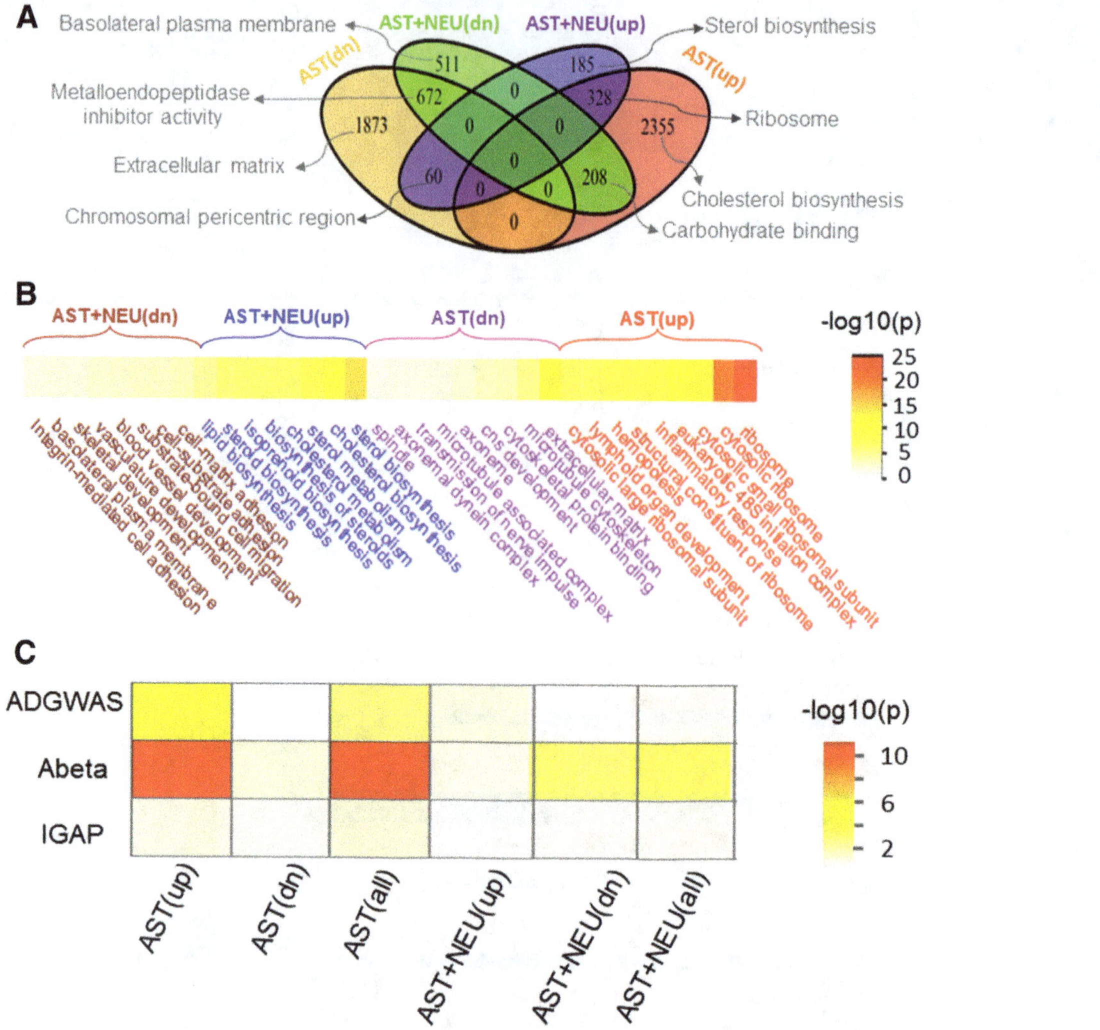

Fig. 3 The impact of GJA1 deficiency on AD relevant gene ontologies and AD risk networks. **a.** Venn diagram for genes overlapping among various differentially expressed genes (DEG) signatures. AST(dn) and AST(up) were down- and up- regulated DEG signatures in Gja1−/− vs. wildtype astrocyte cultures, while AST + NEU(dn) and AST + NEU(up) were down- and up- regulated DEG signatures in Gja1−/− vs. wildtype astrocytes co-cultured with neurons. Top gene ontology for each individual DEGs were shown above each cluster. **b.** Heatmap of Gene enrichment significance (−log10(p)) for the DEG signatures. Top 10 enriched gene ontologies were shown for each individual DEGs. **c.** *GJA1−/−* signatures including AST(all), AST(up), AST(dn), AST + NEU(all), AST + NEU(up) and AST + NEU(dn) are enriched for three AD genetic gene sets including the one identified by the International Genomics of Alzheimer's Project (IGAP) [1], the Abeta (Aβ) genetic network [16], the AD risk gene list (ADGWAS) [43]

processes, immune response, cell-cell communication, extracellular matrix, microtubule cytoskeleton, synaptic transmission, lipid biosynthesis, steroid biosynthesis, cholesterol biosynthesis and cell-matrix adhesion (Fig. 3a-b, Additional file 1: Table S5).

AST(up) was significantly enriched for the genes in an Aβ network signature [16] (2.03 FE, FET $p = 1.08$ E-10), the AD genome-wide significant risk factor gene signature (ADGWAS) (3.47 FE, FET $p = 6.58$E-6) (Fig. 2c) while AST + NEU(dn) was enriched for the genes in the Aβ network signature (1.68 FE, FET $p = 1.1$E-3) (Fig. 3c and Additional file 1: Table S6). These results suggested that *Gja1* is a critical regulator of the AD GWAS genes and may play an important role in Aβ metabolism.

We further intersected the *GJA1* KO DEG signatures with the signatures from other inflammatory diseases to better understand of the immune response component in *GJA1* regulated gene expression. We considered 2 well-established inflammatory gene signatures, an inflammatome signature of 2461 genes from eleven rodent inflammatory disease models [90] and the human macrophage and immune response enriched module of 2483 genes causally linked to obesity and diabetes [23]. These two inflammatory signatures share 758 genes [termed the core disease-related inflammatory gene (CDIG)]. About half of the CDIGs fall into AST(up) (accounting for about 12.6% of AST(up), 6.57 FE, FET $p = 1.85E\text{-}208$) and the intersection includes well known inflammatory markers (e.g., *CD44, CD53, FCER1G, HCK, TYROBP* and *TREM2*), inflammation complement component members (*C1QA, C1QB,* and *C1QC*), CXC chemokines (*CXCL10, CXCL3* and *CXCL6*) and TNF Receptors (*TNFRSF11B* and *TNFRSF13B*). The CDIGs are also significantly enriched in AST + NEU(up) (accounting for about 15% of AST + NEU(up), 7.84 FE, FET $p = 1.06E\text{-}49$). These results suggest that inflammation is a critical component in *GJA1*-regulated gene expression.

We then investigated expression changes of astrocyte- and neuron-specific genes in various gene signatures using the recently identified brain cell type specific signatures [57]. Astrocyte- and neuron-specific marker gene signatures are enriched in the down- and up-regulated gene signatures in the neuron and *Gja1−/−* astrocyte co-cultures versus the neuron and wildtype astrocyte co-cultures, respectively (Additional file 1: Table S9A). The co-culture systems with and without *Gja1−/−* upregulated a significant portion of the neuron-specific marker genes when compared with the respective astrocyte alone models (with or without *Gja1−/−*) while down-regulating many astrocyte marker genes (Additional file 1: Table S9B). The gene lists from the abovementioned intersection analyses can be found in (Additional file 1: Tables S9C and S9D).

Gja1 deficiency induced transcriptomic changes highly overlap the *GJA1* centric gene networks in AD

We further examined the molecular mechanisms of *GJA1* in AD pathogenesis and cognitive function. We first examined if these *Gja1−/−* DEG signatures were enriched in the Khaki module where *GJA1* resided based on our previous study [98]. As shown in Additional file 1: Table S7, AST + NEU(dn), AST(dn) and AST(up) were all significantly enriched in the khaki module with FET $p = 3.74E\text{-}54$ (9.0 FE), 3.64E-28 (4.4 FE), 1.28E-5 (2.1 FE), respectively. On the other hand, the overall signatures AST(all) and AST + NEU(all) also significantly overlapped the module with FET $p = 3.03E\text{-}32$ (3.2FE) and 1.9E-47 (6.7 FE), respectively .

To gain more insights into the signaling circuit of the *GJA1* regulation in AD, we constructed the Bayesian causal network for the khaki module and projected the *Gja1−/−* DEG signatures onto this network in order to delineate the underlying causal relationship among the molecular constituents of this module. As shown in Fig. 4a and Additional file 1: Table S7, 13 of the 19 predicted key drivers except for *GJA1* in the khaki module were regulated by *GJA1* (4.94 FE, FET $p = 4.70E\text{-}05$). Strikingly, 11 out of the 13 *GJA1* regulated key driver genes were within the *GJA1's* downstream network neighborhood (Additional file 2: Figure S3A). To better gain insights into the functions of the Bayesian causal network in Fig. 4a, we built up a *GIA1* signaling pathway map. As shown in Additional file 2: Figure S3B, *GIA1* regulates a diversity of pathways such as regulation of gap junction activity, innate immune system, TGFβ signaling, DNA repair and lipid metabolism. These results suggested that *Gja1* deficiency significantly impacted the khaki module and thus strongly validated our previous prediction of *GJA1* as a driver of this important AD related subnetwork.

To more comprehensively determine *GJA1*'s target genes in AD, we further systematically identified the genes correlated with *GJA1* in a number of human AD cohorts. Genes significantly correlated with *GJA1* (Benjamini-Hochberg (BH)-corrected *p*-value < 0.05) were first identified in each of eight datasets including four from the MSBB RNA-seq cohort, one from the ROSMAP RNA-seq data and three from the HBTRC cohort. Note that only the data from the AD subjects were used for the correlation analysis. A majority voting method was utilized to calculate the frequency of each correlation across the eight datasets (Additional file 1: Table S8). We defined consensus *GJA1*-centered correlation signature (CGCCS) as a function of frequency threshold n, i.e., $\text{CGCCS}(n) = \{g \mid \text{frequency}(r(g, GJA1)) \geq n\}$, where r(g, *GJA1*) represents a significant correlation between a gene g and *GJA1* at FDR < 0.05, and $n = 1, 2, \ldots, 8$. This process led to *GJA1* centered correlation networks, also denoted as CGCCS(n).

Additional file 2: Figure S4 shows the enrichment of the *GJA1* centered correlation networks for the previously identified DEGs in AST and AST + NEU. CGCCS (4) was most significantly enriched for the AST(all) and AST + NEU(all) DEG signatures with FET $p = 1.0E\text{-}330$ (3.2 FE) and 7.5E-311 (3.9 FE), respectively (Black lines, Additional file 2: Figure S4). CGCCS (6) is enriched for the DEG signature in AST with FET $p = 6.2E\text{-}309$ (3.8 FE). Figure 4b shows the network CGCCS (6) which includes 201 up-regulated (red nodes, termed GJA1_centered_AST(up)) and 307 down-regulated (blue nodes, termed GJA1_centered_AST(dn)) genes upon the knockout of *Gja1* in astrocytes. About 30% of the genes in each of the two *GJA1_centered_*signatures belonged to the khaki module (FET $p = 1.52E\text{-}90$, 32.37 FE). This *GJA1*-centered correlation network included eight driver genes (*AGT, BMPR1B, CST3, FXYD1, NTSR2, SLC15A2, SPON1, and STON2)* in the khaki module [98]. Similar results were derived for the AST + NEU(up) and AST + NEU(down) signatures. Therefore, *GJA1* impacts the expression of many key network drivers in the astrocytic subnetwork, suggesting its central role in this AD-related gene network. Furthermore, the analysis of the genes specific to the A1/A2 astrocytic activation in our DEG from *Gja1−/−* astrocytes [50] revealed that most of pan-, A1-, and A2-specific genes were generally upregulated (Additional file 2: Figure S5).

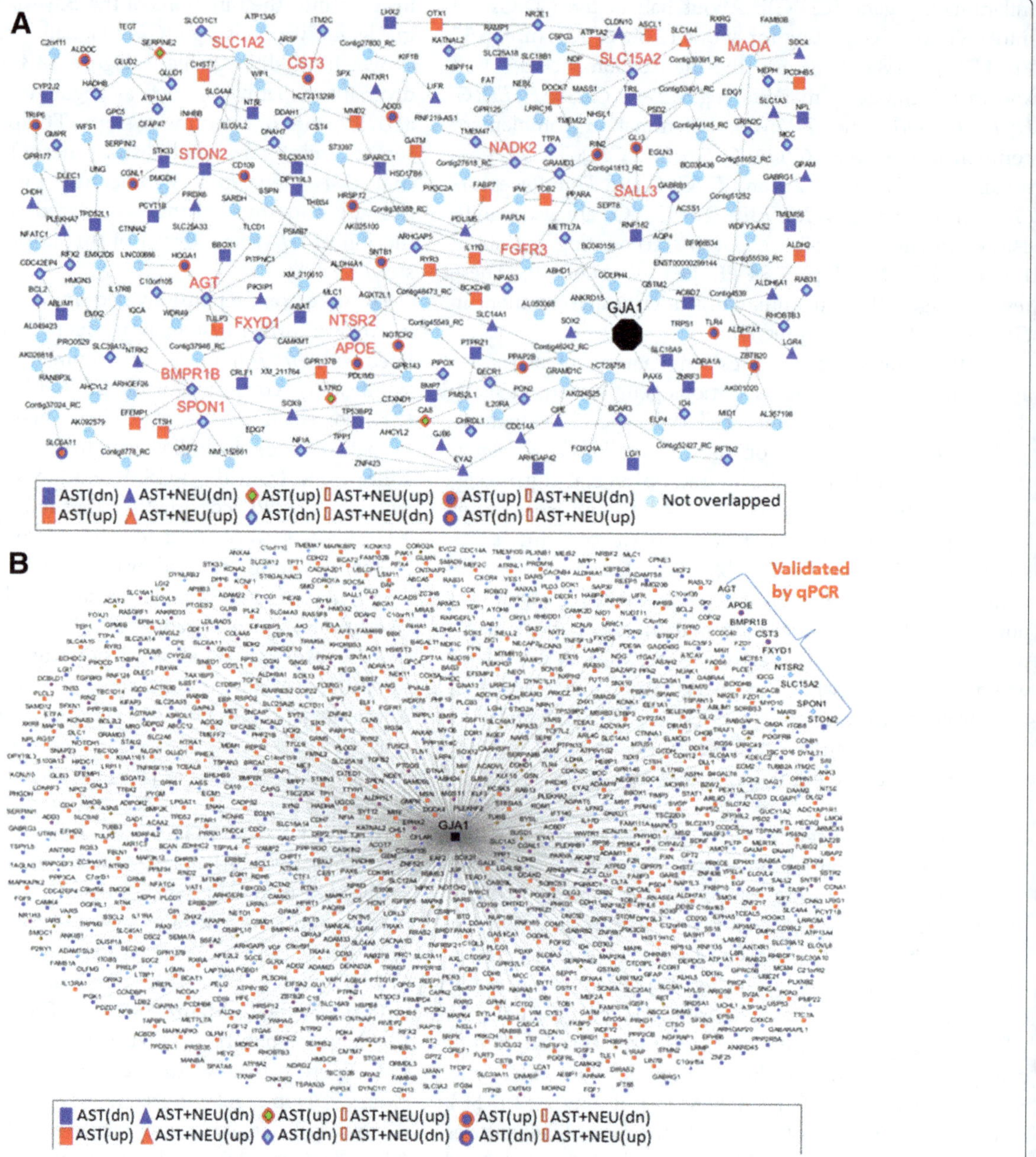

Fig. 4 Network analysis on GJA1 genetic networks. **a**. BN (Bayesian Network) based on astrocyte (khiki) module. *Gja1−/−* DEG signatures were projected onto BN to detect overlapped gene signatures, which were classified into eight categories: up-regulated only in AST (in red upright triangle), down-regulated only in AST (in blue downside triangle), only up-regulated in AST + NEU (red square), only down-regulated in AST + NEU (blue square), up-regulated in both AST and AST + NEU (in pink diamond), up-regulated in AST but down-regulated in AST + NEU (in pink hexagon), down-regulated in both AST and AST + NEU (in gray diamond), and down-regulated in AST but up-regulated in AST + NEU (in gray hexagon)). In enlarged label were genes that were validated experimentally. *Gja1* was in black. In turquoise circle were genes non-overlapped. AST, *Gja1−/−* astrocyte culture while AST + NEU, *Gja1−/−* astrocyte culture in the presence of co-cultured neurons. **b**. GJA1 centered genetic networks inferred by projecting *Gja1−/−* DEG signatures onto Gja1 correlation concensus network (CGCCS(6)). Overlapped gene nodes were denoted as in A

Inflammatory cytokines downregulate expression of *Gja1* and the astrocytic subnetwork module

Previously it has been shown that LOAD-relevant inflammatory cytokines such as TNFα and IL-1β downregulated expression of *Gja1* in astrocytes [19, 74]. Wildtype astrocytes were treated with TNFα, or IL-1β, or both for 7 days, confirming that Cx43 (Gja1 protein) was profoundly and synergistically reduced by both cytokines (Fig. 5a-b). Paradoxically, IL-1β significantly increased, but TNFα significantly decreased, Apoe protein

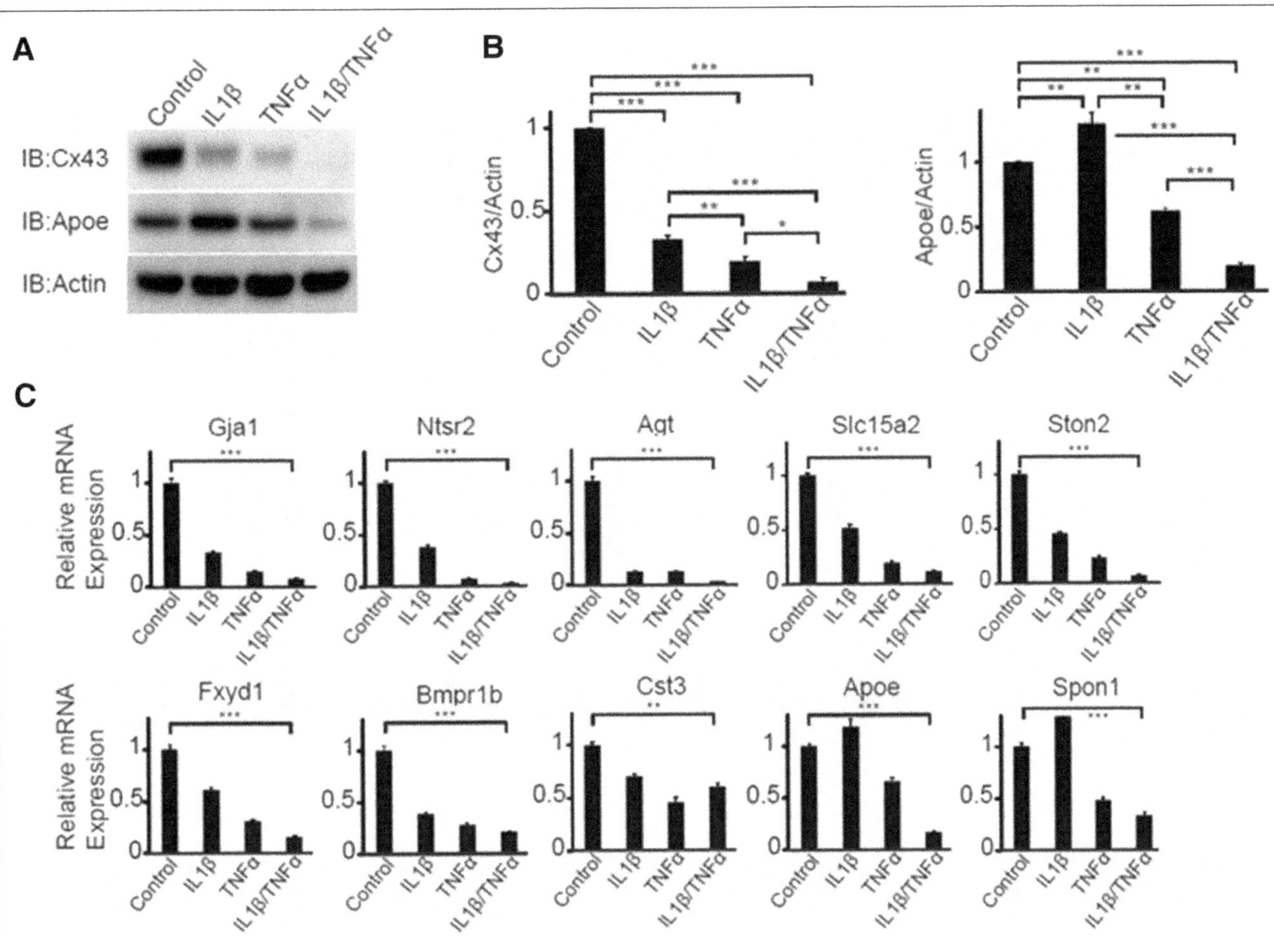

Fig. 5 Inflammatory cytokines downregulates Gja1, Apoe, and other network genes. **a**. Wildtype primary mouse astrocytes were treated with either IL-1β (10 ng/ml) or TNFα (10 ng/ml) or in combination for 7 days and levels of Cx43, Apoe expression were analyzed by immunoblot. Representative results from 4 (*Gja1*) and 3 (Apoe) independent experiments are shown. **b**. Protein levels of Cx43 (left) and Apoe (right) were quantitatively analyzed for these technical replicates after normalization to Actin. ANOVA followed by Bonferroni post-hoc tests are indicated by asterisks. * $p < 0.05$, ** $p < 0.01$, *** $p < 0.001$. **c**. Quantitative gene expression analysis in wildtype astrocytes with treatments similar to **a**) was performed to analyze the other key drivers of the *GJA1*-centered network. Results representative of two independent experiments are shown. Statistical analysis was performed as in B, and only the comparison between control and IL-1β/TNFα is shown

levels (Fig. 5b). Following cytokine treatment, we tested *Gja1, Apoe* and eight key network driver genes found to be differentially expressed in *Gja1−/−* astrocytes by RNA-seq analysis, as a proxy to capture the network changes. qPCR analysis revealed that *Gja1, Apoe* and the other astrocytic subnetwork drivers were similarly downregulated by these cytokines (Fig. 5c).

Gja1 channel activity increases the expression of the astrocytic subnetwork module

Since these cytokines inhibit GJC and potentiate hemichannel activities [74], we asked whether inhibition of GJC and hemichannel activities regulates *Gja1* and other astrocytic subnetwork drivers. Treatment of wildtype astrocytes with carbenoxolone (CBX, inhibitor of GJC and hemichannel [2, 95]) or lanthanum (La3+, inhibitor of hemichannel [2]) led to significant reduction of *Gja1* and Apoe protein levels (Fig. 6a-b). Interestingly, the CBX treatment had broader effects on the reduction of the driver genes (Fig. 6c), while La3+ had generally milder and more selective effects, suggesting that GJC and hemichannel activities contribute to the regulation of distinct sets of the genes.

We next tested whether *Gja1* channel activation can alter the astrocytic subnetwork. *Gja1* hemichannel activity can be increased by quinine [81]. Treatment of wildtype astrocytes with quinine significantly upregulated Gja1 and Apoe protein and mRNA levels, along with transcriptional upregulation of a subset of the driver genes (Additional file 2: Figure S6). These data collectively supports *Gja1*, and specifically its channel activity, as an important regulator of astrocytic gene coexpression network including *Apoe*.

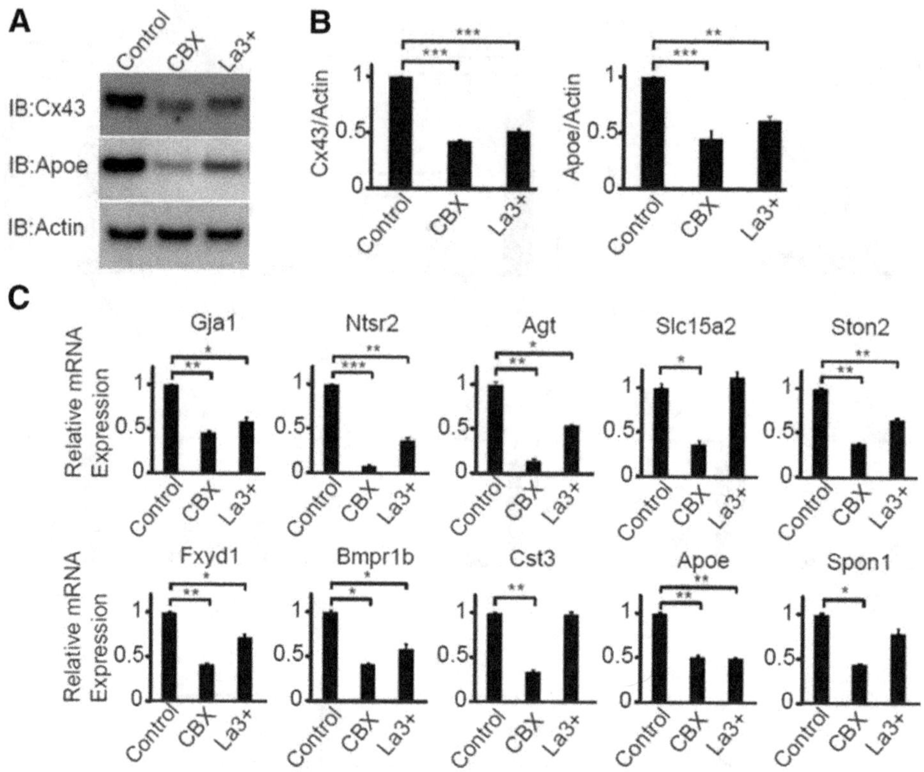

Fig. 6 *GJA1* inhibitors downregulate *Gja1* and Apoe, and other network genes. **a**. Wildtype primary mouse astrocytes were treated with 200 μM carbenoxolone (CBX, gap junction inhibitor) or Lanthanum (La3+, hemichannel inhibitor) for 3 days and levels of Cx43, Apoe were analyzed by immunoblot. **b**. Quantitative analysis of Cx43 and Apoe protein levels were normalized to Actin. ANOVA followed by Bonferroni post-hoc tests are indicated by asterisks. ** $p < 0.01$, *** $p < 0.001$. **c**. Quantitative gene expression analysis in wildtype astrocytes treated similar to A was performed to analyze GJA1 network drivers. Statistical analysis was performed as in **b**, and only the comparisons to control are shown. Results representative of two independent experiments are shown for all experiments

Increased neuronal survival following Aβ treatment when co-cultured with *Gja1−/−* astrocytes

We assessed the role for *Gja1* in neuronal death and viability in a transwell co-culture system, in which cortical neurons were grown on the bottom of the plate, while astrocytes were cultured on the transwell insert. This allowed physical separation of the two cell types, while maintaining chemical continuity. Incubation of wildtype neurons and wildtype astrocytes with the indicated concentration of $A\beta_{1-42}$ oligomers resulted in increased neuronal death [t (4) = − 2.941, $p = 0.030$ at 2 μM; t (4) = − 5.857, $p = 0.004$ at 20 μM] and decreased viability [t (6) = − 5.395, $p = 0.002$ at 2 μM; t (6) = 4.671, $p = 0.003$ at 20 μM] at day 7 (but not at day 4 (Fig. 7a)), in a dose dependent manner (Fig. 7b). Wildtype neurons cultured with *Gja1−/−* astrocytes were significantly resistant to death and loss of viability (Fig. 7b), consistent with a previous study showing that *Gja1−/−* deficient astrocytes conferred neuroprotection [69].

Reduced Apoe secretion and synthesis in *Gja1−/−* astrocytes

APOE is a well-known risk gene for LOAD and primarily produced by human and mouse astrocytes as well as microglia and neurons [52]. In addition, *APOE* was in the coexpression network module governed by *GJA1*. Therefore, we tested how Apoe levels were affected in the absence of *Gja1* in mouse primary astrocytes. Quantitative PCR revealed significantly reduced *Apoe* expression in *Gja1−/−* astrocytes (t (6) = − 5.330, $p = 0.002$) (Fig. 8a). Consistently, we found lower Apoe protein levels in *Gja1 −/−* astrocytes by immunoblot analysis of the lysates, with or without $A\beta_{1-42}$ oligomer treatment (Fig. 8b). We analyzed Apoe in the conditioned medium from these astrocytes and found that secreted Apoe in the conditioned medium was consistently reduced in Gja1−/− astrocytes compared to wildtype, with or without $A\beta_{1-42}$ oligomer treatment (Fig. 8c). Two way ANOVA revealed that there were significant main effects by genotype and treatment ($F(1, 18)=121.618$, $p < 0.0005$, $F(2, 18)=9.364$, $p = 0.0016$, respectively) but there was no interaction of genotype and treatment ($F(2, 18) = 0.305$, $p = 0.741$].

Neurons cocultured with Gja1−/− astrocytes produce higher levels of Aβ species

Since our RNA-seq analysis revealed that Gja1 regulated genes were highly enriched in Aβ network, we therefore

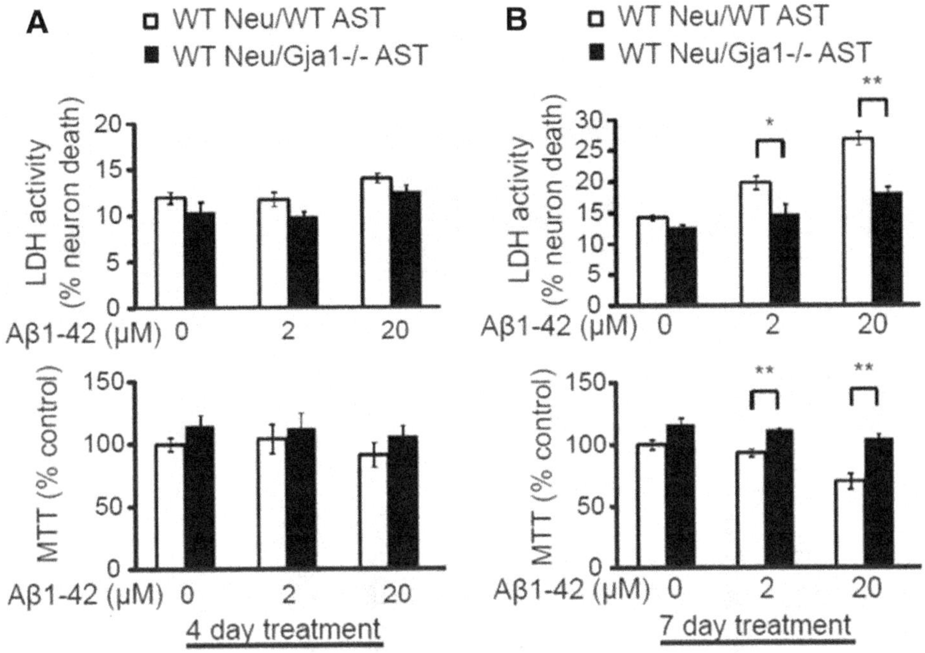

Fig. 7 *Gja1* contributes to neuronal death and reduces viability by $A\beta_{1-42}$ treatment. Cortical neurons were plated onto 12 well plate and wildtype or *Gja1−/−* astrocytes grown on transwells were inserted to the neuron cultures. Indicated concentration of $A\beta_{1-42}$ oligomers are applied for 4 days (**a**) or 7 days (**b**) and neuronal death and viability was determined by LDH and MTT assays, respectively. Student's t-tests were used for all the statistical analysis. * $p < 0.05$, ** $p < 0.01$, *** $p < 0.001$. For all experiments, representative of at least two independent experiments is shown

analyzed Aβ production in neuron/astrocyte cocultures. Indeed, we observed higher levels of both $A\beta_{40}$ and $A\beta_{42}$ species in the conditioned medium from neurons co-cultured with *Gja1−/−* astrocytes at all time points examined [$A\beta_{40}$; $t(4) = 17.684$, $p < 0.0005$ (div6), $t(4) = 3.447$, $p = 0.026$ (div13), $t(4) = 11.112$, $p < 0.0005$ (div16), $t(4) = 11.112$, $p < 0.0005$ (div20): $A\beta_{42}$; $t(4) = 8.422$, $p < 0.0005$ (div6), $t(4) = 2.047$, $p = 0.110$ (div13), $t(4) = 11.245$, $p < 0.0005$ (div16), $t(4) = 8.016$, $p < 0.001$ (div20)] (Fig. 8d-e). Because astrocytes have been shown to take up *Aβ*, preferentially oligomers [67], we investigated the role for *Gja1* in controlling Aβ clearance. When we tested whether wildtype and *Gja1−/−* astrocytes were proficient in taking up exogenously applied fluorescently labeled $A\beta_{1-42}$ oligomers, we found that the number of *Gja1−/−* astrocytes with cell-associated $A\beta_{1-42}$ oligomers was significantly reduced compared to wildtype astrocytes [$t(20) = -6.670$, $p < 0.0005$] (Additional file 2: Figure S7).

Reduced neuronal activity in response to Aβ treatment when co-cultured with *Gja1−/−* astrocytes

In order to understand the impact of the network perturbation by loss of astrocytic *Gja1−/−* on neuronal functions, we co-cultured wildtype cortical neurons with either wildtype or *Gja1−/−* astrocytes on multielectrode arrays and compared spontaneous and stimulated neuronal activities before and after $A\beta_{1-42}$ oligomer treatment (Fig. 9a). Although few significant differences were detected prior to Aβ treatment at 16 days in vitro (div), at 18 and/or 20 div (2 and 4 days after 10 μM $A\beta_{1-42}$ treatment) most metrics of spontaneous activity (i.e. number of spikes, bursts, network bursts, and spikes per network burst) were significantly reduced in *Gja1−/−* astrocyte-cocultured neurons (Fig. 9b). The reduced spontaneous neuronal activity at div 20 suggested that co-culture with *Gja1−/−* astrocytes made neurons less responsive to Aβ-induced changes. While stimulated neuronal activity at div 14 was not affected by co-culture with *Gja1−/−* astrocytes (Fig. 10a), it was reduced at 20 div (number of spikes, spikes per burst, mean firing rate, and burst duration) (Fig. 10b-c).

Discussion

Functional interaction between neurons and astrocytes is an appealing research area that has expanded vigorously in recent years. The involvement of astrocytes in the pathogenesis of neurodegenerative diseases such as AD is just beginning to be appreciated. Astrocyte-specific *GJA1* expression has been shown to be upregulated in the post-mortem AD brains [6, 34]. Consistent with but beyond these studies, we predicted and validated not only upregualtion of *GJA1* expression in AD but also its regulatory role in driving a large astrocyte-specific molecular network underlying AD. Indeed, our functional analysis using *Gja1 −/−* astrocytes revealed that the *Gja1* network contributed

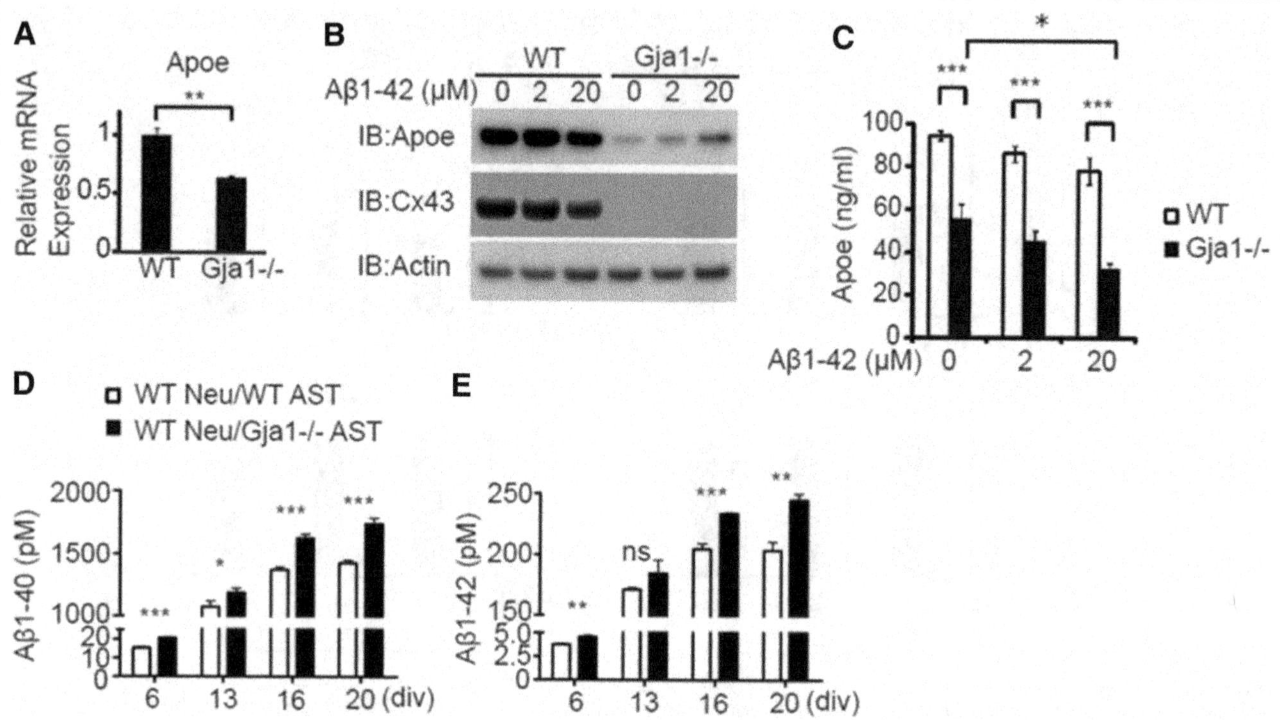

Fig. 8 *Gja1* deficiency causes reduction of Apoe production and promotes Aβ production in neuron/astrocyte cocultures. **a**. Quantitative PCR analysis of Apoe in wildtype (WT) and *Gja1−/−* astrocytes. **b**. Apoe, Cx43, and actin levels in wildtype and *Gja1−/−* astrocytes treated with the indicated concentration of $A\beta_{1-42}$ oligomers for 48 h were determined by immunoblot analysis of cell lysates. **c**. Apoe secreted into the conditioned medium of astrocytes in B was quantitatively determined by specific ELISA in quadruplicate wells. **d** and **e**. Amyloidβ secreted to the conditioned medium of wildtype cortical neurons cocultured with either wildtype or *Gja1−/−* astrocytes was quantitatively determined by $A\beta_{40}$ and $A\beta_{42}$ specific ELISA

to neuronal death and decreased their viability under $A\beta_{1-42}$ treatment and, which may explain synapse and neuron loss in the Alzheimer brains [20]. This is consistent with recent studies showing that *GJA1* play critical roles in AD-relevant phenotypes in AD mouse models [40, 73, 96, 97]. On the other hand, a number of other studies indicate that *Gja1* isneuroprotective [41, 44, 51, 64, 65, 85]. Indeed, our data showed that the *Gja1* network appeared to be involved in phagocytosis of Aβ, and maintenance of neuronal activities under Aβ stress. Taken together with the previous findings of the increase of Cx43 protein and its channel activity specifically in astrocytes surrounding plaques [59, 63, 96], we suggest that the upregulation of *GJA1* in AD brains may start as a neuroprotective response to amyloid plaques. It is interesting to note that previous clinical studies have consistently demonstrated an increased neuronal activity in the hippocampus and cortex in non-demented individuals at high risk for AD including *APOE4* carriers, minor cognitive impairment (MCI) or at presymptomatic stage of familial Alzheimer's disease [10, 72], and individuals with early Alzheimer's disease are prone to developing seizures [87]. Furthermore, the hippocampal hyperactivation is a viable therapeutic target for AD [4]. We speculate that the role of *GJA1* in supporting neuronal activity in the AD brain might explain partly the observation of elevated brain activity in the prodromal stage of AD.

In the present study, we demonstrated *GJA1* as a master regulator, which regulates not an AD-related astrocyte-specific gene subnetwork [98] but also an array of AD risk genes including the most important AD gene *APOE* (Fig. 4a-b). More broadly speaking, in in vitro cultured astrocytes, *Gja1* deficiency caused significant change in expression of 5496 genes involved a diverse of biological pathways and processes (Fig. 3b). Similarly, in in vitro astrocyte and neuron cocultures, thousands of genes were regulated by Gja1 (−/−). Of note, more than half of the known AD risk factor genes (Fig. 2g) and hundreds of inflammatome genes in chronic inflammation diseases [23] were the targets of *GJA1*. Upregulation of *GJA1* expression in AD brains of human subjects and in vitro or in vivo perturbation of *Gja1* (e.g., *Gja1* deficiency in primary cultured astrocytes in the present study) lead to a cascade of biological and pathological reactions and processes including subsequent alteration in cells' biological functions and responses to their environments, which are manifested as a complex and intertwined *GJA1* centered molecular network. Interestingly, our data pointed to the key role of Cx43 gap junction channel

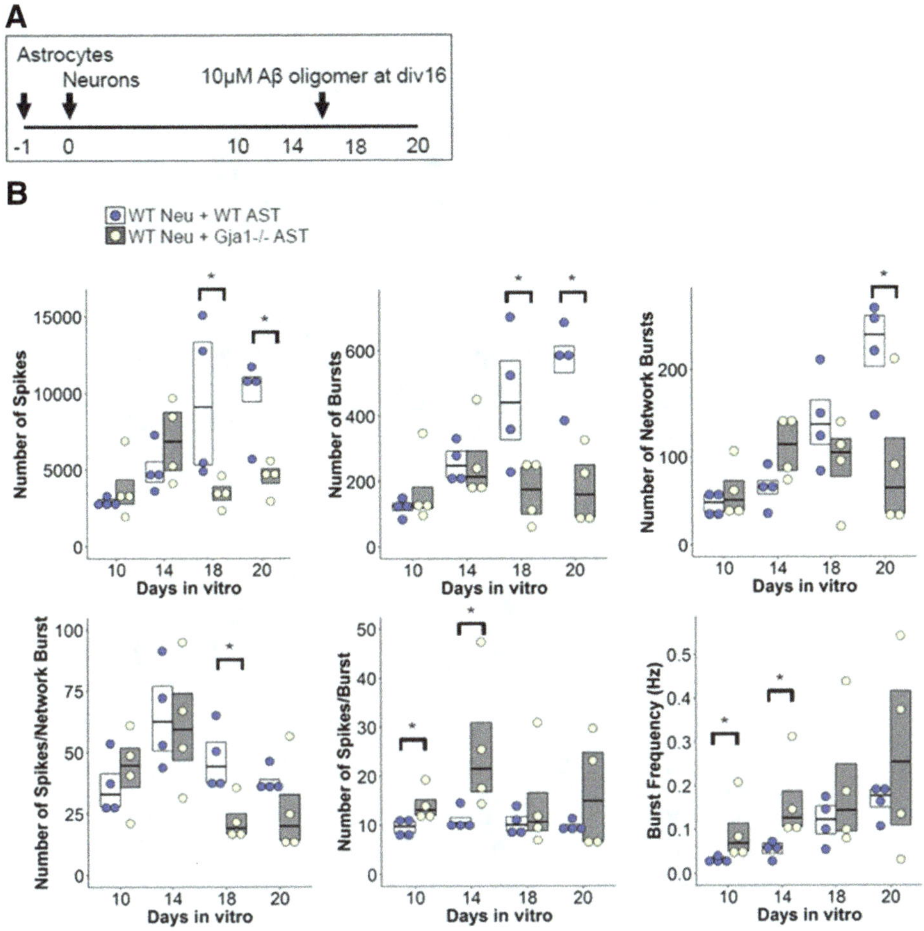

Fig. 9 *Gja1* deficiency reduces spontaneous neuronal activity in cortical neuron/astrocyte cocultures as determined by multielectrode array. **a**. Experimental scheme is indicated. One day prior to cortical neuron preparation and plating, wildtype or *Gja1−/−* astrocytes were plated onto 48-well MEA array plate in quadruplicate wells. Spontaneous activities of the cocultures were recorded at day 10, 14, 18 and 20 on Axion Maestro. At day 16, cocultures were treated with 10 μM $A\beta_{1-42}$ oligomers. **b**. Boxplots of the indicated metrics from the MEA recordings are shown. Each circles represent mean values of individual well, and the horizontal bars within the box indicates means of quadruplicates. Mann-Whitney U tests were used for statistical analysis. * $p < 0.05$

and hemichannel activities in regulating gene networks, and indicated that the network can be fine-tuned by pharmacologically modulating Cx43 channel activity (Fig. 6 and Additional file 2: Figures S5 and S8). Cx43 could be a useful therapeutic target in diseases such as LOAD, ODDD, and other neuropsychiatric disorders [71]. In support for such a hypothesis, recent studies showed that *Gja1*-deficiency or a connexin inhibitor (Boldine) treatment in APP/PS1 mice had beneficial effects [73, 96, 97], underscoring that Cx43 is a critical mediator of AD pathophysiology and an important therapeutic target for LOAD.

One of the important novel discoveries in the present study was the *Gja1* mediated production of ApoE in astrocytes. APOE is mainly produced in astrocytes, but also in neurons and microglia when under stress [35]. APOE is the major LOAD risk factor, critical to AD neuropathology and neurocognitions [15, 39]. We therefore focused on characterizing Apoe in *Gja1−/−* astrocytes. Manipulation of *Gja1* by genetic disruption, cytokines, CBX, and quinine in astrocytes as well as neuron/astrocyte/microglia culture system consistently resulted in the regulation of Apoe in the same direction as *Gja1*. Abnormal production of APOE, in particular, the risk-associated isoform APOE4, caused either gain of toxic functions, when over-expressed, such as neuronal toxicity, Aβ aggregation and tangle formation or loss of physiological functions, when under-expressed, such as Aβ clearance, synaptic function and neurogenesis. Consistent with this notion, we observed drastic reduction in uptake and retention of Aβ oligomers by Gja1(−/−) astrocytes (Additional file 2: Figure S7 A-B), with concomitant increase in concentration of both Aβ1−40 and Aβ1−42 species in in vitro culture medium (Fig. 8d-e). Since *APOE* is known to be regulated by transcription factors such as *LXR* and *RXR*

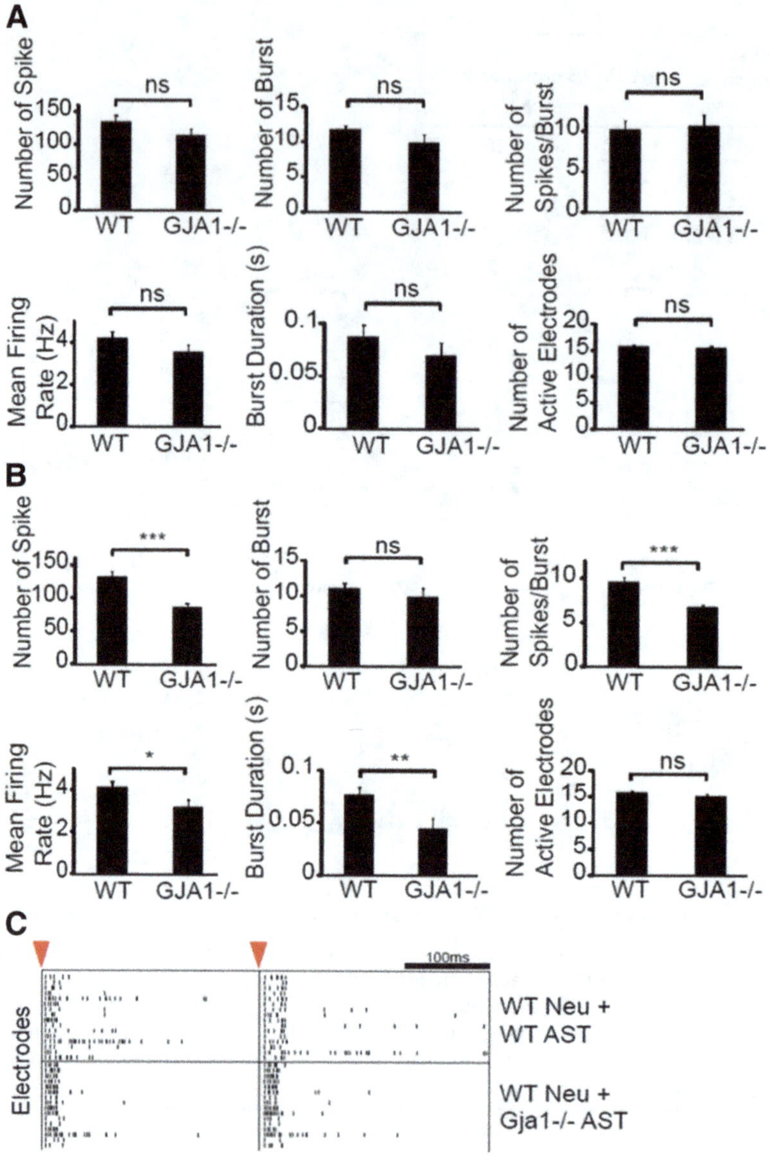

Fig. 10 *Gja1* deficiency reduces stimulated neuronal activity in cortical neuron/astrocyte cocultures as determined by multielectrode array. **a** and **b**. Cocultures were stimulated by 3 cycles of voltage-controlled biphasic stimulus from all electrodes within the wells at 14 days (**a**) and 20 days (**b**) in vitro. At least 5 times of repeated stimulations were recorded and analyzed. **c**. Two representative raster plots as recorded on day 20 are shown for wildtype neurons cocultured with wildtype astrocytes (upper panel) or with *Gja1−/−* astrocytes (lower panel). Y-axis represents 16 electrodes and X-axis represents time after stimulation indicated by red arrowhead. Black horizontal scale bar indicates 100 milliseconds (ms). Each vertical bar represents a detected spike

[48], and taken together with downregulation of *NR1H3* (LXRA) expression in our RNA-seq data, we speculate that *NR1H3* regulation by *GJA1* might have mediated the *APOE* expression. Further investigation is required to dissect the mechanism underlying GJA1-mediated expression of APOE and its biological significance, which would lead to the development of novel therapeutic strategies.

A recent study identified the transcriptomic basis of the two distinct polarization states of A1 neurotoxic and A2 neuroprotective astrocytes [50]. Interestingly, our RNA-seq analysis revealed that most of pan-reactive, A1 and A2 specific transcripts were significantly upregulated in *Gja1−/−* astrocytes (Additional file 2: Figure S5). This pattern of expression is most similar to those induced by combination of IL-1β and TNFα or C1q (Fig. 1a in [50]), and consistent with this, our data showed that IL-1β and TNFα caused downregulation of Cx43 and other key drivers, mimicking the loss of *Gja1*. This pattern of expression may indicate that *Gja1* deficiency induces non-specific activation of either A1 or A2 polarized-astrocytes, or A1/A2 overlapping polarization. Although these two possibilities need to be clarified by transcriptomic analysis at a single cell level, these mixed transcriptomic signatures suggest how *Gja1* may contribute to opposing neuroprotective (Figs. 8, 9 and 10) and neurotoxic (Fig. 7) phenotypes, as demonstrated here as well as in previous studies [41, 44, 51, 64, 65, 69, 85, 96, 97].

Based upon the results from this study and the discussion above, we developed a working hypothesis of *GJA1* dysregulation in AD (Fig. 11), in which upregulation of *GJA1*, a master regulator of astrocytic gene expression, concomitant with amyloid accumulation during Alzheimer pathogenesis ultimately drives AD clinical and pathological traits as evidenced by highly significant correlation with AD progression and AD GWAS genes (Fig. 2a-g). According to our model, *GJA1* induction initially serves to support neuronal functions by elevating gene expression signatures for the glial neurosupportive functions such as Abeta network (Fig. 3c), Apoe (Fig. 8a-c), vascular and neurodevelopment, extracellular matrix, and cytoskeletal and cell adhesion (Fig. 3a-b) as well as suppressing inflammatory response (Fig. 3b). These findings were supported by amyloid phagocytosis (Fig. 8d-e, Additional file 2: Figure S5) and multielectrode array (Figs. 9 and 10) assays showing that the amyloid uptake, Apoe expression, and neuronal activity are attenuated with Gja1−/− astrocytes. This is consistent with several key clinical and pathological observations in LOAD. For example, neuronal activity is found to be enhanced at the early stage of Alzheimer's disease subjects [4, 10, 72, 87] and evidence of cell cycle activation in AD neurons [3, 53, 58, 79, 86, 94], changes in extracellular matrix [12, 46], and neuronal cytoskeletal components [5, 13, 45, 91] have been reported. However, we speculate that chronic *GJA1* gain of function could lead to detrimental effects on neurons in a long run, as evidenced by our observation, in which prolonged neuron/astrocyte cocultures were better protected in the absence of *Gja1* in astrocytes (Fig. 7a-b) possibly due to excessive neuronal activity and glutamate-induced excitotoxicity [24, 37, 47, 68].

In summary, this study elucidated the previously unrecognized role for *GJA1* and its channel activity in regulating a key AD-related gene regulatory network comprised of *APOE* and other astrocyte-specific genes. We demonstrated that the disruption of this astrocytic gene coexpression network by knocking out *Gja1* can

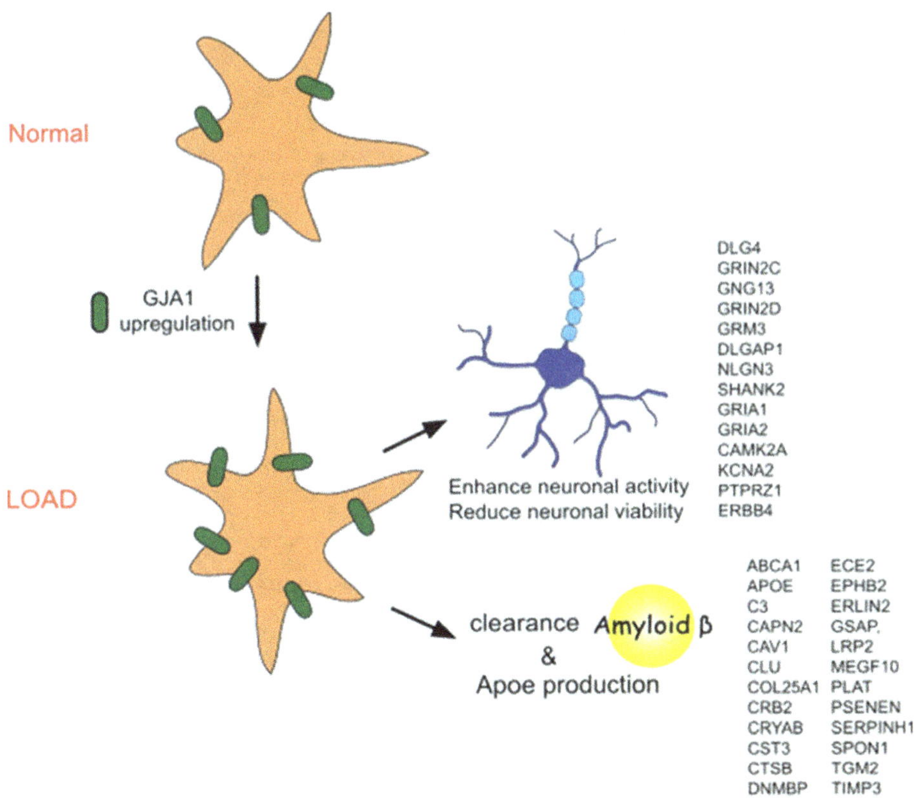

Fig. 11 A working hypothesis of *GJA1* dysregulation in AD. Progressive upregulation of *GJA1* in the brains during LOAD pathogenesis (in response to amyloid accumulation) serves to enhance the coordinated gene network function to orchestrate neuroprotective response by astrocytes including Aβ production and clearance (*CST3, CLU, CTSB, ECE2, MEGF10, PSENEN* and *GSAP*), APOE production (*APOE, ABCA1, CAV1* and *SPON1*), and supporting neuronal activity (*DLG4, NLGN3, GRINA* and *GRIN2D*). However, the enhanced neuronal activity due to chronic and prolonged *GJA1* upregulation triggers neuronal wear and eventual death

contribute to LOAD-related pathology. This study represents the first step towards a comprehensive functional characterization of one of the most significantly dysregulated modules in our previous integrative network analysis of LOAD brains. The strong validation of the predictive power of our multiscale gene network approach paves a way to dissect the complex pathogenic mechanisms of LOAD.

Additional files

Additional file 1: Tables S1. Clinical and pathological traits, brain regions analyzed by transcriptome profiling, and sample classification with respect to the severity stage of each trait. **Table S2.** Correlations between GJA1 expression and individual phenotypical traits. **Table S3.** Differential expression analysis. **TableS4.** Covariables' impacts on GJA1 association with AD traits. **Table S5.** Gene ontology analysis. **Table S6.** Intersection of GJA1 gene signatures and AD gene signatures. **Table S7.** Intersection of GJA1 gene signatures and the khiki module. **Table S8.** GJA1_centered genetic network analysis. **Table S9A.** GJA1 DEG signatures (AST+NEU) overlapped with brain cell type specific gene signatures. **Table S9B.** AST+NEU vs AST in Gja1 (-/-) or (+/+) DEG signatures overlapped with brain cell type specific gene signatures. **Table S9C.** differentially expressed genes in neurons upon GJA1 KO or not in astrocyte and neuron coculture. **Table S9D.** Difference of change degree in AST+NEU_vs_AST_Gja1(-/-) vs AST+NEU_vs_AST_Gja1(+/+). **Table S10.** List of primer sets and Universal Probe Library (UPL) probe for qRT-PCR. (XLSX 234 kb)

Additional file 2: Figure S1. Correlations between GIA1 and individual clinic traits stratified by AOD (age of death), gender and APOE genotypes in BM36 region. **Figure S2.** Correlation between Gja1 and individual transcripts of ADGWAS genes. **Figure S3.** GJA1-centric Bayesian causal network and GJA1 signaling pathway map. **Figure S4.** Enrichment of Gia1-/- gene signatures in GJA1 centric correlation networks. **Figure S5.** Regulation of A1/A2 astrocyte marker genes in Gja1-/- astrocytes. **Figure S6.** Quinine (GJA1 channel agonist) upregulates Gja1 and Apoe, and other network genes. **Figure S7.** A. Wildtype and Gja1-/- astrocytes were treated with fluorescently labeled Aβ1-42 oligomers for 24 hours and the number of astrocytes in association with Aβ1-42 oligomers were quantitatively estimated by counting total cells (DAPI+) and Aβ positive cells. B. Representative images of phase contrast, Hilyte Fluor488-labeled Aβ, and DAPI staining from wildtype (upper panels) and Gja1-/- (lower panels) astrocytes were shown. These images were taken by bright field microscope and the representatives of 2 independent experiments with similar results are shown. **Figure S8.** Complex regulation of Gja1 key drivers in neuron/astrocyte/microglia cocultures by carbenoxolone and quinine. (DOCX 1.4 kb)

Acknowledgments
This study was supported in parts by grants from the National Institutes of Health/National Institute on Aging (R01AG046170, RF1AG054014, RF1AG057440, R01AG057907). This study has been made possible through the support of Brain Canada and the financial support of Health Canada, Michael Smith Foundation for Health Research, Genome BC and the Pacific Alzheimer's Research Foundation to CCN and WCS. CCN holds a Canada Research Chair.

Competing interests
The authors declare that they have no competing interests.

Author details
[1]Department of Psychiatry, Icahn School of Medicine at Mount Sinai, New York, NY 10029, USA. [2]Department of Genetics and Genomic Sciences, Icahn School of Medicine at Mount Sinai, New York, NY 10029, USA. [3]Mount Sinai Center for Transformative Disease Modeling, Icahn Institute of Genomics and Multiscale Biology, Icahn School of Medicine at Mount Sinai, New York, NY 10029, USA. [4]Department of Cellular and Physiological Sciences, University of British Columbia, Vancouver, British Columbia V6T 1Z3, Canada. [5]Department of Neuroscience, Icahn School of Medicine at Mount Sinai, New York, NY 10029, USA. [6]Friedman Brain Institute, Icahn School of Medicine at Mount Sinai, New York, NY 10029, USA. [7]Current address: Denali Therapeutics,, South San Francisco,, CA 94080, USA.

References

1. (2015) Convergent genetic and expression data implicate immunity in Alzheimer's disease. Alzheimers Dement 11:658–671. https://doi.org/10.1016/j.jalz.2014.05.1757
2. Anselmi F et al (2008) ATP release through connexin hemichannels and gap junction transfer of second messengers propagate Ca2+ signals across the inner ear. Proc Natl Acad Sci U S A 105:18770–18775. https://doi.org/10.1073/pnas.0800793105
3. Arendt T, Rodel L, Gartner U, Holzer M (1996) Expression of the cyclin-dependent kinase inhibitor p16 in Alzheimer's disease. Neuroreport 7:3047–3049
4. Bakker A et al (2012) Reduction of hippocampal hyperactivity improves cognition in amnestic mild cognitive impairment. Neuron 74:467–474. https://doi.org/10.1016/j.neuron.2012.03.023
5. Bamburg JR, Bloom GS (2009) Cytoskeletal pathologies of Alzheimer disease. Cell Motil Cytoskeleton 66:635–649. https://doi.org/10.1002/cm.20388
6. Begcevic I et al (2013) Semiquantitative proteomic analysis of human hippocampal tissues from Alzheimer's disease and age-matched control brains. Clin Proteomics 10:5. https://doi.org/10.1186/1559-0275-10-5
7. Bennett DA (2006) Postmortem indices linking risk factors to cognition: results from the Religious Order Study and the Memory and Aging Project. Alzheimer Dis Assoc Disord 20:S63–S68
8. Bennett DA, Schneider JA, Arvanitakis Z, Wilson RS (2012) Overview and findings from the religious orders study. Current Alzheimer Research 9:628–645
9. Bennett DA et al (2005) The rush memory and aging project: study design and baseline characteristics of the study cohort. Neuroepidemiology 25: 163–175
10. Bookheimer SY et al (2000) Patterns of brain activation in people at risk for Alzheimer's disease. N Engl J Med 343:450–456. https://doi.org/10.1056/NEJM200008173430701
11. Braak H, Braak E (1991) Neuropathological stageing of Alzheimer-related changes. Acta Neuropathol 82:239–259
12. Brandan E, Inestrosa NC (1993) Extracellular matrix components and amyloid in neuritic plaques of Alzheimer's disease. Gen Pharmacol 24:1063–1068
13. Brion JP (1992) The pathology of the neuronal cytoskeleton in Alzheimer's disease. Biochim Biophys Acta 1160:134–142
14. Bruban J et al (2015) Presenilin 1 is necessary for neuronal, but not glial, EGFR expression and neuroprotection via gamma-secretase-independent transcriptional mechanisms. FASEB J 29:3702–3712. https://doi.org/10.1096/fj.15-270645
15. Bu G (2009) Apolipoprotein E and its receptors in Alzheimer's disease: pathways, pathogenesis and therapy. Nat Rev Neurosci 10:333–344. https://doi.org/10.1038/nrn2620
16. Campion D, Pottier C, Nicolas G, Le Guennec K, Rovelet-Lecrux A (2016) Alzheimer disease: modeling an Abeta-centered biological network. Mol Psychiatry 21:861–871. https://doi.org/10.1038/mp.2016.38
17. Chever O, Lee CY, Rouach N (2014) Astroglial connexin43 hemichannels tune basal excitatory synaptic transmission. J Neurosci 34:11228–11232. https://doi.org/10.1523/JNEUROSCI.0015-14.2014
18. Corder EH et al (1993) Gene dose of apolipoprotein E type 4 allele and the risk of Alzheimer's disease in late onset families. Science 261:921–923
19. De Vuyst E et al (2007) Connexin hemichannels and gap junction channels are differentially influenced by lipopolysaccharide and basic fibroblast growth factor. Mol Biol Cell 18:34–46. https://doi.org/10.1091/mbc.E06-03-0182
20. DeKosky ST, Scheff SW (1990) Synapse loss in frontal cortex biopsies in Alzheimer's disease: correlation with cognitive severity. Ann Neurol 27:457–

464. https://doi.org/10.1002/ana.410270502
21. D'Hondt C, Iyyathurai J, Himpens B, Leybaert L, Bultynck G (2014) Cx43-hemichannel function and regulation in physiology and pathophysiology: insights from the bovine corneal endothelial cell system and beyond. Front Physiol 5:348. https://doi.org/10.3389/fphys.2014.00348
22. Dobin A et al (2013) STAR: ultrafast universal RNA-seq aligner. Bioinformatics 29:15–21. https://doi.org/10.1093/bioinformatics/bts635
23. Emilsson V et al (2008) Genetics of gene expression and its effect on disease. Nature 452:423–428
24. Esposito Z et al (2013) Amyloid beta, glutamate, excitotoxicity in Alzheimer's disease: are we on the right track? CNS Neurosci Ther 19: 549–555. https://doi.org/10.1111/cns.12095
25. Folstein MF, Folstein SE, McHugh PR (1975) "Mini-mental state". A practical method for grading the cognitive state of patients for the clinician. J Psychiatr Res 12:189–198
26. Frisch C et al (2003) Mice with astrocyte-directed inactivation of connexin43 exhibit increased exploratory behaviour, impaired motor capacities, and changes in brain acetylcholine levels. Eur J Neurosci 18:2313–2318
27. Giaume C et al (1991) Gap junctions in cultured astrocytes: single-channel currents and characterization of channel-forming protein. Neuron 6:133–143
28. Goodenough DA, Paul DL (2003) Beyond the gap: functions of unpaired connexon channels. Nat Rev Mol Cell Biol 4:285–294. https://doi.org/10.1038/nrm1072
29. Gutmann DH, Zackai EH, McDonald-McGinn DM, Fischbeck KH, Kamholz J (1991) Oculodentodigital dysplasia syndrome associated with abnormal cerebral white matter. Am J Med Genet 41:18–20. https://doi.org/10.1002/ajmg.1320410106
30. Han Y et al (2014) Astrocyte-restricted disruption of connexin-43 impairs neuronal plasticity in mouse barrel cortex. Eur J Neurosci 39:35–45. https://doi.org/10.1111/ejn.12394
31. Haroutunian V, Katsel P, Schmeidler J (2009) Transcriptional vulnerability of brain regions in Alzheimer's disease and dementia. Neurobiol Aging 30: 561–573. https://doi.org/10.1016/j.neurobiolaging.2007.07.021
32. Harrell LE, Marson D, Chatterjee A, Parrish JA (2000) The severe mini-mental state examination: a new neuropsychologic instrument for the bedside assessment of severely impaired patients with Alzheimer disease. Alzheimer Dis Assoc Disord 14:168–175
33. Hoffman GE, Schadt EE (2016) variancePartition: interpreting drivers of variation in complex gene expression studies. BMC Bioinformatics 17:483. https://doi.org/10.1186/s12859-016-1323-z
34. Hokama M et al (2014) Altered expression of diabetes-related genes in Alzheimer's disease brains: the Hisayama study. Cereb Cortex 24:2476–2488. https://doi.org/10.1093/cercor/bht101
35. Huang Y, Mucke L (2012) Alzheimer mechanisms and therapeutic strategies. Cell 148:1204–1222. https://doi.org/10.1016/j.cell.2012.02.040
36. Humphries CE et al (2015) Integrated whole transcriptome and DNA methylation analysis identifies gene networks specific to late-onset Alzheimer's disease. J Alzheimers Dis 44:977–987. https://doi.org/10.3233/JAD-141989
37. Hynd MR, Scott HL, Dodd PR (2004) Glutamate-mediated excitotoxicity and neurodegeneration in Alzheimer's disease. Neurochem Int 45:583–595. https://doi.org/10.1016/j.neuint.2004.03.007
38. Kajiwara Y et al (2016) The human-specific CASP4 gene contributes to Alzheimer-related synaptic and behavioral deficits. Hum Mol Genet. https://doi.org/10.1093/hmg/ddw265
39. Kim J, Basak JM, Holtzman DM (2009) The role of apolipoprotein E in Alzheimer's disease. Neuron 63:287–303. https://doi.org/10.1016/j.neuron.2009.06.026
40. Koulakoff A, Mei X, Orellana JA, Saez JC, Giaume C (2012) Glial connexin expression and function in the context of Alzheimer's disease. Biochim Biophys Acta 1818:2048–2057. https://doi.org/10.1016/j.bbamem.2011.10.001
41. Kozoriz MG et al (2010) The connexin43 C-terminal region mediates neuroprotection during stroke. J Neuropathol Exp Neurol 69:196–206. https://doi.org/10.1097/NEN.0b013e3181cd44df
42. Laird DW (2014) Syndromic and non-syndromic disease-linked Cx43 mutations. FEBS Lett 588:1339–1348. https://doi.org/10.1016/j.febslet.2013.12.022
43. Lambert JC et al (2013) Meta-analysis of 74,046 individuals identifies 11 new susceptibility loci for Alzheimer's disease. Nat Genet 45:1452–1458. https://doi.org/10.1038/ng.2802
44. Le HT et al (2014) Gap junction intercellular communication mediated by connexin43 in astrocytes is essential for their resistance to oxidative stress. J Biol Chem 289:1345–1354. https://doi.org/10.1074/jbc.M113.508390
45. Lee VM (1995) Disruption of the cytoskeleton in Alzheimer's disease. Curr Opin Neurobiol 5:663
46. Lepelletier FX, Mann DM, Robinson AC, Pinteaux E, Boutin H (2017) Early changes in extracellular matrix in Alzheimer's disease. Neuropathol Appl Neurobiol 43:167–182. https://doi.org/10.1111/nan.12295
47. Lewerenz J, Maher P (2015) Chronic glutamate toxicity in neurodegenerative diseases-what is the evidence? Front Neurosci 9:469. https://doi.org/10.3389/fnins.2015.00469
48. Liang Y et al (2004) A liver X receptor and retinoid X receptor heterodimer mediates apolipoprotein E expression, secretion and cholesterol homeostasis in astrocytes. J Neurochem 88:623–634
49. Liao Y, Smyth GK, Shi W (2014) featureCounts: an efficient general purpose program for assigning sequence reads to genomic features. Bioinformatics 30:923–930. https://doi.org/10.1093/bioinformatics/btt656
50. Liddelow SA et al (2017) Neurotoxic reactive astrocytes are induced by activated microglia. Nature 541:481–487. https://doi.org/10.1038/nature21029
51. Lin JH et al (2008) A central role of connexin 43 in hypoxic preconditioning. J Neurosci 28:681–695. https://doi.org/10.1523/JNEUROSCI.3827-07.2008
52. Liu CC, Liu CC, Kanekiyo T, Xu H, Bu G (2013) Apolipoprotein E and Alzheimer disease: risk, mechanisms and therapy. Nat Rev Neurol 9:106–118. https://doi.org/10.1038/nrneurol.2012.263
53. Liu WK, Williams RT, Hall FL, Dickson DW, Yen SH (1995) Detection of a Cdc2-related kinase associated with Alzheimer paired helical filaments. Am J Pathol 146:228–238
54. Loddenkemper T, Grote K, Evers S, Oelerich M, Stogbauer F (2002) Neurological manifestations of the oculodentodigital dysplasia syndrome. J Neurol 249:584–595. https://doi.org/10.1007/s004150200068
55. Lohman AW, Isakson BE (2014) Differentiating connexin hemichannels and pannexin channels in cellular ATP release. FEBS Lett 588:1379–1388. https://doi.org/10.1016/j.febslet.2014.02.004
56. Lutz SE et al (2009) Deletion of astrocyte connexins 43 and 30 leads to a dysmyelinating phenotype and hippocampal CA1 vacuolation. J Neurosci 29:7743–7752. https://doi.org/10.1523/JNEUROSCI.0341-09.2009
57. McKenzie AT et al (2018) Brain cell type specific gene expression and co-expression network architectures. Sci Rep 8:8868. https://doi.org/10.1038/s41598-018-27293-5
58. McShea A, Harris PL, Webster KR, Wahl AF, Smith MA (1997) Abnormal expression of the cell cycle regulators P16 and CDK4 in Alzheimer's disease. Am J Pathol 150:1933–1939
59. Mei X, Ezan P, Giaume C, Koulakoff A (2010) Astroglial connexin immunoreactivity is specifically altered at beta-amyloid plaques in beta-amyloid precursor protein/presenilin1 mice. Neuroscience 171:92–105. https://doi.org/10.1016/j.neuroscience.2010.08.001
60. Miller JA, Oldham MC, Geschwind DH (2008) A systems level analysis of transcriptional changes in Alzheimer's disease and Normal aging. J Neurosci 28:1410–1420
61. Miller JA, Woltjer RL, Goodenbour JM, Horvath S, Geschwind DH (2013) Genes and pathways underlying regional and cell type changes in Alzheimer's disease. Genome Medicine 5:48
62. Millstein J, Zhang B, Zhu J, Schadt EE (2009) Disentangling molecular relationships with a causal inference test. BMC Genet 10:23. https://doi.org/10.1186/1471-2156-10-23
63. Nagy JI, Li W, Hertzberg EL, Marotta CA (1996) Elevated connexin43 immunoreactivity at sites of amyloid plaques in Alzheimer's disease. Brain Res 717:173–178
64. Nakase T, Fushiki S, Naus CC (2003) Astrocytic gap junctions composed of connexin 43 reduce apoptotic neuronal damage in cerebral ischemia. Stroke 34:1987–1993. https://doi.org/10.1161/01.STR.0000079814.72027.34
65. Nakase T, Sohl G, Theis M, Willecke K, Naus CC (2004) Increased apoptosis and inflammation after focal brain ischemia in mice lacking connexin43 in astrocytes. Am J Pathol 164:2067–2075. https://doi.org/10.1016/S0002-9440(10)63765-0
66. Naus CC et al (1997) Altered gap junctional communication, intercellular signaling, and growth in cultured astrocytes deficient in connexin43. J Neurosci Res 49:528–540

67. Nielsen HM et al (2010) Astrocytic a beta 1-42 uptake is determined by a beta-aggregation state and the presence of amyloid-associated proteins. Glia 58:1235–1246. https://doi.org/10.1002/glia.21004
68. Ong WY, Tanaka K, Dawe GS, Ittner LM, Farooqui AA (2013) Slow excitotoxicity in Alzheimer's disease. J Alzheimers Dis 35:643–668. https://doi.org/10.3233/JAD-121990
69. Orellana JA et al (2011) Amyloid beta-induced death in neurons involves glial and neuronal hemichannels. J Neurosci 31:4962–4977. https://doi.org/10.1523/JNEUROSCI.6417-10.2011
70. Pannasch U et al (2011) Astroglial networks scale synaptic activity and plasticity. Proc Natl Acad Sci U S A 108:8467–8472. https://doi.org/10.1073/pnas.1016650108
71. Parikshak NN, Gandal MJ, Geschwind DH (2015) Systems biology and gene networks in neurodevelopmental and neurodegenerative disorders. Nat Rev Genet 16:441–458. https://doi.org/10.1038/nrg3934
72. Quiroz YT et al (2010) Hippocampal hyperactivation in presymptomatic familial Alzheimer's disease. Ann Neurol 68:865–875. https://doi.org/10.1002/ana.22105
73. Ren R, Zhang L, Wang M (2018) Specific deletion connexin43 in astrocyte ameliorates cognitive dysfunction in APP/PS1 mice. Life Sci 208:175–191. https://doi.org/10.1016/j.lfs.2018.07.033
74. Retamal MA et al (2007) Cx43 hemichannels and gap junction channels in astrocytes are regulated oppositely by proinflammatory cytokines released from activated microglia. J Neurosci 27. https://doi.org/10.1523/JNEUROSCI.2042-07.2007
75. Ritchie, M. E. et al. limma powers differential expression analyses for RNA-sequencing and microarray studies. Nucleic Acids Res 43, e47, doi:https://doi.org/10.1093/nar/gkv007 (2015)
76. Robinson MD, McCarthy DJ, Smyth GK (2010) edgeR: a Bioconductor package for differential expression analysis of digital gene expression data. Bioinformatics 26:139–140. https://doi.org/10.1093/bioinformatics/btp616
77. Rouach N, Koulakoff A, Abudara V, Willecke K, Giaume C (2008) Astroglial metabolic networks sustain hippocampal synaptic transmission. Science 322:1551–1555. https://doi.org/10.1126/science.1164022
78. Scemes E, Giaume C (2006) Astrocyte calcium waves: what they are and what they do. Glia 54:716–725. https://doi.org/10.1002/glia.20374
79. Smith TW, Lippa CF (1995) Ki-67 immunoreactivity in Alzheimer's disease and other neurodegenerative disorders. J Neuropathol Exp Neurol 54:297–303
80. Sohl G, Maxeiner S, Willecke K (2005) Expression and functions of neuronal gap junctions. Nat Rev Neurosci 6:191–200. https://doi.org/10.1038/nrn1627
81. Stout CE, Costantin JL, Naus CC, Charles AC (2002) Intercellular calcium signaling in astrocytes via ATP release through connexin hemichannels. 277:10482–10488. https://doi.org/10.1074/jbc.M109902200
82. Strittmatter WJ et al (1993) Apolipoprotein E: high-avidity binding to beta-amyloid and increased frequency of type 4 allele in late-onset familial Alzheimer disease. Proc Natl Acad Sci U S A 90:1977–1981
83. Tabernero, A., Giaume, C. & Medina, J. M. Endothelin-1 regulates glucose utilization in cultured astrocytes by controlling intercellular communication through gap junctions. Glia 16, 187–195, doi:https://doi.org/10.1002/(SICI)1098-1136(199603)16:3<187::AID-GLIA1>3.0.CO;2-# [pii]. https://doi.org/10.1002/(SICI)1098-1136(199603)16:3<187::AID-GLIA1>3.0.CO;2-# (1996)
84. Theis M et al (2003) Accelerated hippocampal spreading depression and enhanced locomotory activity in mice with astrocyte-directed inactivation of connexin43. J Neurosci 23:766–776
85. Theodoric N, Bechberger JF, Naus CC, Sin WC (2012) Role of gap junction protein connexin43 in astrogliosis induced by brain injury. PLoS One **7**: e47311. https://doi.org/10.1371/journal.pone.0047311
86. Vincent I, Rosado M, Davies P (1996) Mitotic mechanisms in Alzheimer's disease? J Cell Biol 132:413–425
87. Vossel KA et al (2013) Seizures and epileptiform activity in the early stages of Alzheimer disease. JAMA Neurol 70:1158–1166. https://doi.org/10.1001/jamaneurol.2013.136
88. Wagenaar DA, Pine J, Potter SM (2004) Effective parameters for stimulation of dissociated cultures using multi-electrode arrays. J Neurosci Methods 138:27–37. https://doi.org/10.1016/j.jneumeth.2004.03.005
89. Wallraff A et al (2006) The impact of astrocytic gap junctional coupling on potassium buffering in the hippocampus. J Neurosci 26:5438–5447. https://doi.org/10.1523/JNEUROSCI.0037-06.2006
90. Wang IM et al (2012) Systems analysis of eleven rodent disease models reveals an inflammatome signature and key drivers. Mol Syst Biol 8:594. https://doi.org/10.1038/msb.2012.24
91. Wang M et al (2016) Integrative network analysis of nineteen brain regions identifies molecular signatures and networks underlying selective regional vulnerability to Alzheimer's disease. Genome Med 8:104. https://doi.org/10.1186/s13073-016-0355-3
92. Wilson RS, Arnold SE, Schneider JA, Li Y, Bennett DA (2007) Chronic distress, age-related neuropathology, and late-life dementia. Psychosom Med 69:47–53. https://doi.org/10.1097/01.psy.0000250264.25017.21
93. Yamamoto T, Ochalski A, Hertzberg EL, Nagy JI (1990) On the organization of astrocytic gap junctions in rat brain as suggested by LM and EM immunohistochemistry of connexin43 expression. J Comp Neurol 302:853–883. https://doi.org/10.1002/cne.903020414
94. Yang Y, Mufson EJ, Herrup K (2003) Neuronal cell death is preceded by cell cycle events at all stages of Alzheimer's disease. J Neurosci 23:2557–2563
95. Ye ZC, Oberheim N, Kettenmann H, Ransom BR (2009) Pharmacological "cross-inhibition" of connexin hemichannels and swelling activated anion channels. Glia 57:258–269. https://doi.org/10.1002/glia.20754
96. Yi C et al (2016) Astroglial connexin43 contributes to neuronal suffering in a mouse model of Alzheimer's disease. Cell Death Differ 23:1691–1701. https://doi.org/10.1038/cdd.2016.63
97. Yi C et al (2017) Inhibition of glial hemichannels by boldine treatment reduces neuronal suffering in a murine model of Alzheimer's disease. Glia 65:1607–1625. https://doi.org/10.1002/glia.23182
98. Zhang B et al (2013) Integrated systems approach identifies genetic nodes and networks in late-onset Alzheimer's disease. Cell 153:707–720. https://doi.org/10.1016/j.cell.2013.03.030
99. Zhang Y et al (2016) Purification and characterization of progenitor and mature human astrocytes reveals transcriptional and functional differences with mouse. Neuron 89:37–53. https://doi.org/10.1016/j.neuron.2015.11.013
100. Zhu J et al (2007) Increasing the power to detect causal associations by combining genotypic and expression data in segregating populations. PLoS Comput Biol 3:e69. https://doi.org/10.1371/journal.pcbi.0030069

5

Enhancement of therapeutic potential of a naturally occurring human antibody targeting a phosphorylated Ser^{422} containing epitope on pathological tau

Jeroen van Ameijde[1†], Rosa Crespo[1†], Roosmarijn Janson[1†], Jarek Juraszek[1†], Berdien Siregar[1], Hanneke Verveen[1], Imke Sprengers[1], Tariq Nahar[1], Jeroen J. Hoozemans[2], Stefan Steinbacher[3], Roland Willems[4], Lore Delbroek[4], Marianne Borgers[4], Koen Dockx[5], Kristof Van Kolen[4], Marc Mercken[4], Gabriel Pascual[6], Wouter Koudstaal[1] and Adrian Apetri[1*]

Abstract

Aggregation of tau protein and spreading of tau aggregates are pivotal pathological processes in a range of neurological disorders. Accumulating evidence suggests that immunotherapy targeting tau may be a viable therapeutic strategy. We have previously described the isolation of antibody CBTAU-22.1 from the memory B-cell repertoire of healthy human donors. CBTAU-22.1 was shown to specifically bind a disease-associated phosphorylated epitope in the C-terminus of tau (Ser^{422}) and to be able to inhibit the spreading of pathological tau aggregates from P301S spinal cord lysates in vitro, albeit with limited potency. Using a combination of rational design and random mutagenesis we have derived a variant antibody with improved affinity while maintaining the specificity of the parental antibody. This affinity improved antibody showed greatly enhanced potency in a cell-based immunodepletion assay using paired helical filaments (PHFs) derived from human Alzheimer's disease (AD) brain tissue. Moreover, the affinity improved antibody limits the in vitro aggregation propensity of full length tau species specifically phosphorylated at position 422 produced by employing a native chemical ligation approach. Together, these results indicate that in addition to being able to inhibit the spreading of pathological tau aggregates, the matured antibody can potentially also interfere with the nucleation of tau which is believed to be the first step of the pathogenic process. Finally, the functionality in a P301L transgenic mice co-injection model highlights the therapeutic potential of human antibody dmCBTAU-22.1.

Keywords: Tau, Nucleation, Aggregation, Phosphorylation, Monoclonal antibody, Intervention

Introduction

Aggregated tau protein is associated with a range of neurological disorders, including Alzheimer's disease [31]. Tau is predominantly expressed in neurons where, in its native state, it facilitates axonal transport and cytoskeletal remodeling by interacting with tubulin [17, 19]. This interaction is thought to be modulated through regulated phosphorylation of some of the many potential phosphorylation sites present in tau [6, 39]. However, under pathogenic conditions tau becomes hyperphosphorylated and aggregates into paired helical filaments (PHFs) and insoluble neurofibrillary tangles (NFTs) which impair axonal transport and synaptic function and ultimately lead to cell death (reviewed in [26]). The aggregation of tau is believed to follow a nucleation dependent polymerization (NDP) process [2, 16, 22, 45], characterized by an initial nucleation step followed by an exponential growth. Accumulating evidence indicates that misfolded tau aggregates released from neurons can

* Correspondence: AApetri@its.jnj.com
†Jeroen van Ameijde, Rosa Crespo, Roosmarijn Janson and Jarek Juraszek contributed equally to this work.
1 Janssen Prevention Center, Janssen Pharmaceutical Companies of Johnson and Johnson, Archimedesweg 6, 2333 Leiden, CN, the Netherlands
Full list of author information is available at the end of the article

be taken up by synaptically connected neurons and cause normal tau in the recipient neurons to aggregate, resulting in spreading of tau pathology trough neuronal connectivity [13, 21, 24, 29, 40]. This propagation through extracellular transfer of tau between cells suggests tau immunotherapy may be a viable therapeutic strategy for tauopathies. Indeed, promising results have been reported for both active and passive immunization targeting tau in animal models [3, 5, 7, 43, 44, 47, 50, 51].

We have previously described the isolation of a panel of monoclonal antibodies directed against pathological tau structures from the memory B cell repertoire of apparently healthy individuals [35]. One of these antibodies, CBTAU-22.1, was shown to recognize the C-terminus domain of tau, its binding being dependent on phosphorylation of Ser^{422}. Phospho-Ser422 is not observed on tau under physiological conditions, but only on pathological tau and associated with numerous neurodegenerative disorders [4, 10, 12, 23, 41]. In line with this notion, CBTAU-22.1 detects pathological tau structures in AD, PART, PSP, FTDP-17 and Pick's disease, but does not stain healthy brain tissue [35]. Using a cell-based biosensor assay adapted from Yanamandra et al. [51], we previously showed that CBTAU-22.1 is able to inhibit seeding activity of PHFs from P301S spinal cord lysates, suggesting that this fully human antibody might be able to slow the propagation of tau pathology in vivo [35]. However, its in vitro inhibitory effect was low, i.e. compared to that of murine anti-PHF antibody AT8 [32], which would likely limit any therapeutic potential. We hypothesized that this relatively low potency was caused by a relatively low affinity for PHFs. Here we used a combination of rational and random approaches to derive a variant antibody with improved affinity and assessed its specificity as well as its functionality.

Materials and methods

Expression, purification and analysis of recombinant IgG and tau

Human IgG1, chimeric IgG2a antibodies, Fab fragment, as well as recombinant tau were constructed, produced and purified in the same manner as previously described [1]. After purification, the antibodies as well as 2N4R-tau were characterized by size exclusion chromatography coupled with multi angle light scattering (SEC-MALS) by in-line coupled detectors on a TSKgel G3000SWxl gel filtration column (Tosoh Bioscience) equilibrated with 150 mM sodium phosphate, 50 mM sodium chloride pH 7.0 at a flow rate of 1 mL/min. The following detectors were used: UV (Agilent 1260 Infinity MWD, Agilent Technologies), refractive index (Optilab T-rEX, Wyatt Technology) and 8-angle static light scattering (DAWN HELEOS 8+, Wyatt Technology). The molar mass as well as the monomeric status of the samples were assessed and if samples contained > 5% of aggregates or fragments they were gel filtrated using a Superdex HiLoad 26/60 Superdex 200 pg column (GE Healthcare). The antibodies were furthermore analyzed by SDS-Page and their functionality confirmed by binding to cognate tau peptide V1089–24 (Pepscan, The Netherlands), sequence SSTGSIDMVD(pS)PQLATLA corresponds to residues 412–429 of tau with phosphorylation at Ser^{422} (Additional file 1: Table S2), by Octet biolayer interferometry (Octet Red 384, ForteBio).

Qualitative association and dissociation measurements by octet biolayer interferometry

Biolayer interferometry (Octet Red 384, ForteBio). was used to screen CBTAU-22.1 affinity matured mutants for improved binding (Additional file 1: Table S2). Biotinylated tau peptides (Additional file 1: Table S2) were immobilized on Streptavidin (SA) Dip and Read biosensors for kinetics (ForteBio) at a concentration of 2.5 μg/ml. Real-time binding curves were measured by applying the sensor in ForteBio's kinetics buffer containing 100 nM CBTAU mAbs for 600 s. To induce dissociation, the biosensor containing the mAb-tau peptide complex was immersed in ForteBio's kinetic buffer without antibody for 600 s. The relative association and dissociation kinetic curves were compared to qualitatively assess the efficiency of CBTAU binding to peptides under different conditions. To assess the nature of interaction, binding profiles were determined using different ionic strengths buffers. To gauge specificity a set of phosphorylated tau peptides outside the epitope region were taken along (Additional file 1: Table S2).

Binding affinities by octet biolayer interferometry

An indication for the improvement of the dmCBTAU-22.1 was obtained by measuring the affinity (K_D) of both Fab-CBTAU-22.1 and Fab-dmCBTAU-22.1 using the Steady State Analysis. Fabs were used to get a 1:1 stoichiometry. Biotinylated tau peptide V1089–24 (Additional file 1: Table S2) at 1 μg/ml was immobilized on Streptavidin (SA) biosensors till a shift of ~ 1 nm is reached. Then it was dipped into ForteBio's kinetics buffer containing a range of 13 Fab concentrations for each construct. This association step had a duration of 600 s for each concentration to reach equilibrium, followed by a 600 s dissociation step. The value of the equilibrium dissociation constant (K_D) is obtained via steady state analysis by fitting a plot of response values, which is the average of the last 5 s of the association step, against the respective Fab concentrations.

Affinity maturation

The coding sequence for scFv directed against CBTAU-22.1 epitope was cloned into an inducible prokaryotic expression vector containing the phage M13 pIII gene. Random mutations were deliberately introduced in the scFv by error prone PCR (Genemorph II EZClone Domain Mutagenesis kit) after which the DNA was transformed into TG1 bacteria. The transformants were grown to mid-log phase and infected with helper phages which provide all the genes required for phage assembly. ScFv expressing phages were rescued by a CT helper phage genome which lacks the infectivity domains N1 and N2 of protein pIII, rendering phage particles which are only infective if they display the scFv linked to the full length pIII [27]. Phage libraries were screened using magnetic beads coated with CBTAU-22.1 cognate peptide V1089–24 (Additional file 1: Table S2) in immunotubes. After three rounds of panning, individual phage clones were isolated and screened in phage ELISA for binding to V1089–24. Based on ELISA, clones were selected and converted into an IgG1 format to assess affinity in solution.

Crystallization, data collection and structure determination of fab-CBTAU-22.1 in complex with peptide V1088–5 and fab-dmCBTAU-22.1 in complex with peptide V1088–23

For crystallization the Fab fragments (in 20 mM HEPES/NaOH pH 7.5, 7.55 mM NaCl) were incubated with 4 mM of the respective peptide on ice overnight and concentrated to a final concentration of about 50 mg/ml. The Fab:peptide complexes were subjected to a broad crystallization screening by mixing 0.1 μL protein solution and 0.1 μL reservoir with sitting drop vapor diffusion, varying also the protein concentration. Fab-CBTAU-22.1 with peptide V1088–5 (Additional file 1: Table S2) was crystallized from 0.20 M KCl, 0.10 M Hepes/NaOH pH = 7, 21.2% (*w*/*v*) PEG 5 K MME at a concentration of 25 mg/mL. Fab-dmCBTAU-22.1 with peptide V1088–23 (Additional file 1: Table S2) was crystallized from 10% (w/v) PEG8K, 0.10 M Tris/HCl pH = 7.0, 0.20 M $MgCl_2$ at a concentration of 30 mg/mL. For cryo-protection crystals were briefly immersed in a cryo-solution consisting of 75% reservoir and 25% glycerol. X-ray diffraction data were collected at temperature of 100 K at the Swiss Light Source. Data were integrated, scaled and merged using XDS [25]. The structure was solved with MOLREP [48] and refined with REFMAC5 [49]. Manual model completion was carried out using Coot [18]. The quality of the final model was verified PROCHECK [28] and the validation tools available through Coot [18]. Data collection and refinement statistics for Fab-CBTAU-22.1 in complex with peptide V1088–5 and Fab-dmCBTAU-22.1 in complex with peptide V1088–23 are listed in Additional file 1: Tables S3 and S4.

FRET based cellular immunodepletion assay

Homogenates were prepared from cryopreserved cortical grey matter of 17 sporadic AD patients acquired from the Newcastle Brain Tissue Resource biobank and post mortally assessed at Braak stages 5–6. Patients were all Caucasian between ages of 56 and 93 years old at time of death. Tissue was homogenized in homogenization buffer (10 mM Tris (Gibco), 150 mM NaCl (Gibco) containing protease inhibitors (cOmplete ULTRA tablets EDTA free, Roche) to obtain a 10% *w*/*v* pooled brain homogenate. The homogenate was centrifuged at 27.000×g, 10 min at 4 °C and supernatants of different patients were pooled and stored in aliquots at − 80 °C until used as seed in the immunodepletion assay. Individual antibody dilutions were prepared in PBS pH 7.4 (Sigma), mixed with brain extract in a 1:1 ratio in a 96 well PCR plate (Thermo Scientific), and incubated until the beads were washed. Protein-G DynaBeads (Life Technologies) were added in a 96-well PCR plate (Thermo Scientific) and washed twice with PBS, 0.01% Tween-20 (Sigma) by pulling down the beads with a magnet (Life Technologies). Wash buffer was removed completely and 10 μL of PBS, 0.1% Tween-20 were added to the beads together with 90 μL of the 1: 1 antibody-brain extract mixture. Samples were incubated over night at 4 °C, rotating at 5 rpm. The following day, the immunodepleted fractions were separated from the beads by pulling down the beads with the magnet, transferred to a new 96-well PCR plate and stored at − 80 °C until tested. Each condition was tested in duplicate. Immunodepleted fractions were incubated for 10 mins with Lipofectamine 2000 (Invitrogen) in Opti-MEM (Gibco) in a 96-well cell culture plate (Greiner Bio-one) before 5.5 × 103 HEK biosensor cells (provided by M. Diamond, Washington University School of Medicine) were added to each well. After a 2-day incubation at 37 °C, cells were washed twice with PBS, detached using Trypsin/EDTA (Gibco) and transferred to a polypropylene round bottom plate (Costar) containing FACS buffer (Hank's Balanced Salt Solution (Sigma), 1 mM EDTA (Invitrogen), 1% FBS (Biowest)). Cells were then analyzed for FRET positivity by flow cytometry using a FACS Canto II (BD Bioscience). Each plate contained a brain extract only condition (to assess baseline FRET response) and an antibody isotype control. Results are reported as normalized values, relative to condition without antibody.

Immunohistochemistry on post mortem human brain tissue

Post-mortem human brain tissues of asymptomatic (62–74 year old, Braak stage 1–2) and AD patients (62–81 years old, Braak stage 5) were obtained from the Netherlands Brain Bank (Amsterdam, The Netherlands). All donors, or their next of kin, had given informed consent for the use of brain tissue and clinical details for research purposes. Sections (5 µm-thick) from formalin-fixed paraffin embedded control and AD brain tissue (hippocampus) were mounted on coated glass slides (Menzel gläser superfrost plus, VWR international, Leuven, Belgium) and dried overnight at 37 °C. Slides were deparaffinized in xylene and rehydrated through descending alcohol concentrations. Endogenous peroxidase activity was blocked by incubating the slides 30 min in phosphate buffered saline (PBS; pH 7.4) containing 0.3% H_2O_2. Subsequently, sections were subjected to pre-treatment: slides were heated in 10 mM citrate buffer (pH 6.0) in the autoclave. After allowing the heated sections to re-equilibrate to room temperature (RT), sections were rinsed in PBS. CBTAU-22.1 and anti-phosphorylated Tau (Ser^{202}/Thr^{205}; clone AT8, Thermo Fisher) were diluted in antibody diluent (Immunologic, Duiven, The Netherlands) and incubated overnight at RT. After incubation, sections were thoroughly rinsed in PBS and incubated with ready-to-use goat-anti-mouse/rabbit EnVision+HRP (Dako, Glostrup, Denmark) for 30 min at RT, followed by rinsing in PBS. To visualise the staining 3,3′-diaminobenzidine (DAB; Dako) was used. Slides were counterstained with haematoxylin, dehydrated and mounted with Quick D mounting medium (Klinipath, Duiven, The Netherlands).

Production recombinant tau fragments (tau1–415-Mxe-CBD) for ligation

DNA inserts for tau fragments with suitable overlaps to the pTXB1 vector (New England Biolabs) were obtained commercially (IDT) and cloned into the expressed protein ligation vector using the IMPACT kit and associated protocols (New England Biolabs). After cloning, the plasmid was amplified in *E. coli* NEB5α cells (New England Biolabs). Transformation of *E. coli* BL11 cells (New England Biolabs) was performed by mixing 25 µL cell suspension and 2 µL plasmid and incubating on ice for 30 mins. The mixture was heated to 42 °C for 30 s after which 475 µL LB medium was added followed by incubation at 37 °C for 1 h. 100 µL was spread on LB-Ampicilin+ agar plates and incubated overnight at 37 °C. 4 colonies were picked and transferred to 4 mL LB-Ampicilin+ and incubated for 8 h at 37 °C after which the mixture was diluted to 50 mL and further incubated overnight. 8 × 500 mL LB-Ampicilin+ was inoculated with sufficient overnight culture to reach an OD500 of 0.2 and incubated at 37 °C for approximately 2 h until the OD280 had reached 0.6. IPTG (Sigma) was added to a final concentration of 1 mM followed by further incubation for 3 h. Cells were harvested by centrifugation and stored at − 80 °C as 8 pellets until further use.

Expressed protein ligation

A pellet containing tau (1–415)-Mxe-CBD was added to 20 mL of Bugbuster MasterMix (Millipore) supplemented with a Pierce cOmplete protease inhibitor tablet (Thermo Scientific) and incubated for 30 mins at RT. After centrifugation for 10 min, the 5 mL lysate was added in its entirety to 3 mL of chitin resin beads (New England Biolabs) and incubated for 2 h at RT. The resin was then added to 10 mL of PBS supplemented with 0.02% Tween-20 (Merck), 50 mM MESNa (Sigma) and 1 mM TCEP (Sigma) as well as 2 mg of phosphorylated tau peptide CL22D-P (CIDMVD(pS)PQLATLADEVSA-SLAKQGLEPEA, Pepscan, The Netherlands). The ligation mixture was incubated for 48 h at RT after which the resin was decanted, the supernatant concentrated on an Amicon 10 k filter (Sigma) and buffer exchanged to 3.5 mL PBS on a PD10 column (Thermo Scientific). The crude ligate was run by gravity assist over a bed of 2 mL CaptureSelect C-tag beads (Thermo Scientific), followed by washing with 20 mL PBST (PBS with 0.02% Tween-20) and elution with 10 mL 100 mM pH 3.5 citrate buffer. The eluate was concentrated and buffer exchanged on a PD10 column as above. The purified ligation product in PBS (typically 1 mg/mL) was stored at − 20 °C until use. SEC-MALS characterization was performed as described above for the other recombinant proteins. Western blot analysis was performed by running 2N4R-tau and pS422-tau on a 4–12% BisTris gel (Novex) at 200 Vc in MOPS buffer followed by transfer onto a PVDF membrane (Invitrogen) using iBlot equipment. Primary antibody concentrations was 5 µg/mL and a dilution of 1:20000 was employed for the HRP-goat-anti-human conjugate antibody (Jackson). The blot was stained with the FemtoWest kit (Pierce) and imaged on a Biorad ChemiDoc XRS.

In vitro tau aggregation assay

Stock solutions of 500 µM thioflavin T (ThT) (Sigma-Aldrich, St Louis, MO, USA) and 55 µM heparin (Mw = 17–19 kDa; Sigma-Aldrich, St Louis, MO, USA) were prepared by dissolving the dry powders in reaction buffer (0.5 mM TCEP in PBS, pH 6.7), and filtered through a sterile 0.22 µm pore size PES membrane filter (Corning, NY, USA) or a sterile 0.22 µm pore size PVDF membrane filter (Merck Millipore, Tullagreen, Cork, IRL) respectively. The concentration of the ThT solution was determined by measurement of the absorption at

411 nm (extinction coefficient 22,000 M^{-1} cm^{-1}). Concentration of pS422-tau was determined through its absorption at 280 nm (extinction coefficient 0.31 ml mg^{-1} cm^{-1}). For spontaneous conversions, mixtures of 6.5 μM pS422-Tau in 200 μl reaction buffer containing 7 μM heparin and 50 μM ThT were dispensed into 96-well plates (Thermo Scientific, Vantaa, Finland) that were subsequently sealed with plate sealers (R&D Systems, Minneapolis, MN). To assess the effect of IgG on the conversion, pS422-tau and IgG were mixed and incubated for 20 min in reaction buffer before the addition of heparin and ThT. Kinetic measurements were monitored at 37 °C in a Biotek Synergy Neo2 Multi-Mode Microplate Reader (Biotek, VT, USA) by measuring ThT fluorescence at 485 nm (20 nm bandwidth) upon excitation at 440 nm (20 nm bandwidth) under continuous shaking (425 cpm, 3 mm).

Atomic force microscopy

For each sample, 20 μl of pS422-tau was deposited onto freshly cleaved mica surface. After 3 min incubation, the surface was washed with double-distilled water and dried with air. Samples were imaged using the Scanasyst-air protocol using a MultiMode 8-HR and Scanasyst-air silicon cantilevers (Bruker Corporation, Santa Barbara, USA). Height images of 1024 × 1024 pixels in size and surface areas of 10 × 10 μm were acquired under ambient environmental conditions with peak force frequency of 2 KHz.

Preparation of post-mortem human AD brain-derived PHFs for co-injection in transgenic P301L mice

Post-mortem tissue from the parietal cortex obtained from 5 histologically confirmed Alzheimer patients was partially purified by a modified method from [20]. Briefly, 5 g of frontal cortex was homogenized in 10 volumes of cold buffer H (10 mM Tris, 800 mM NaCl, 1 mM EGTA and 10% sucrose, pH 7.4) using a glass/Teflon Potter tissue homogenizer (IKA Works, Inc.; Staufen, Germany) at 1000 rpm. The homogenized material was centrifuged at 27,000 x g for 20 min. The pellet was discarded and the supernatant was adjusted to a final concentration of 1% (*w*/*v*) *N*-lauroylsarcosine and incubated for 2 h at 37 °C. Subsequently the supernatant was centrifuged at 184,000 x g for 90 min at 20 °C. The pellet was carefully washed in PBS and resuspended in 750 μL PBS, aliquoted and frozen at − 80 °C. The quality of the PHF-tau preparations was evaluated by AT8/AT8 phospho-aggregate-selective MSD and by Western blotting (Additional file 1: Figure S4) using pan tau antibody hTau10 and anti phospho-tau antibody AT8 (pS^{202}/pT^{205}/pS^{208}) [30]. A range of 2.5–20 μl of 1: 10 diluted PHF were resolved on SDS-PAGE (4–12% Bis–Tris Novex NuPAGE gel; Invitrogen) and subsequently transferred onto a nitrocellulose membrane. The membrane was blocked overnight in 1X TBS-T with 5% non-fat dry milk (blocking buffer). In house HRPO-labelled AT8 and hTau10 were used at 1 μg/ml in 2.5% BSA in TBS-T and incubated for 2 h at room temperature. The membranes were then washed three times for 5 min each in TBS-T. The membrane was washed three times for 5 min and developed using the Supersignal West Pico kit (Pierce). Images were obtained on the ImageQuant LAS-4000 (GE Healthcare).

Animals and stereotactic injections

Transgenic Tau-P301L mice, expressing the longest human tau isoform with the P301L mutation (tau-4R/2 N-P301L) [46] were injected at the age of 3 months. Two groups of 15 mice received unilateral hippocampal injection of 1 pmol AD-derived PHFs (3 μl) in an equimolar mixture with dmCBTAU-22.1 or anti-rabies IgG2a isotype control antibody, respectively. The concentration of PHFs is expressed in mols of monomeric Tau and was determined by western blotting using recombinant tau protein as reference. Stereotactic injections in the right hippocampus (TILT-corrected point of injection; CA1, AP -2.0, ML + 1.6 (from bregma), DV 1.4 mm (from dura)) were performed with a semi-automatic stereodrive drill-injection robot (Neurostar) according to the following settings: Hamilton 10 μl syringe, 30G needle point type 4 (45° beveled, not curved), opening 30–45° angle outwards at an injection rate 0.20 μl/min). All experiments were performed in compliance with protocols approved by the local ethical committee and national institutions adhering to AAALAC guidelines.

PHF extraction from mouse brain

Two months after injection, tissue from the *ipsilateral* hemisphere was weighed and homogenized in 6 volumes of buffer H (10 mM Tris, 800 mM NaCl, 1 mM EGTA and 10% sucrose, pH 7.4) using a FastPrep-24 5G benchtop homogenizer (MP Biomedicals).

Biochemical analysis MesoScale Discovery (MSD).

Coating antibody (AT8) was diluted in PBS (1 μg/mL) and aliquoted into MSD plates (30 μL per well) (L15XA, MSD, Rockville, MD, USA), which were incubated overnight at 4 °C. After washing with 5 × 200 μL of PBS/0.5%Tween-20, the plates were blocked with 0.1% casein in PBS and washed again with 5 × 200 μl of PBS/0.5% Tween-20. After adding samples and standards (both diluted in 0.1% casein in PBS), the plates were incubated overnight at 4 °C. Subsequently, the plates were washed with 5 × 200 μL of PBS/0.5% Tween-20, and SULFO-TAG™ conjugated detection antibody (AT8) in 0.1% casein in PBS was added and incubated for 2 h at room temperature while shaking at 600 rpm. After a final wash (5 × 200 μL of PBS/0.5%Tween-20), 150 μL of

2 x buffer T (MSD) was added, and plates were read with an MSD imager. Raw signals were normalized against a standard curve consisting of 16 dilutions of a sarcosyl-insoluble prep from *post-mortem* AD brain (PHF) and were expressed as arbitrary unit (AU) PHFs. Statistical analysis (ANOVA with Bonferroni post test) was performed with the GraphPad prism software and with an 'in house' developed application for automated analysis.

Data deposition

The atomic coordinates and structure factors of the co-crystal structures of CBTAU-22.1 Fab in complex with tau peptide V1088–5 and dmCBTAU-22.1 Fab in complex with tau peptide V1088–23 are being deposited in the Protein Data Bank, www.rcsb.org (PDB ID codes 6H06 and 6H0E) and will be released immediately upon publication.

Results

To improve the affinity of CBTAU-22.1, we employed a combination of random mutagenesis and rational design approaches. The random error prone PCR approach led to the identification of several variants with improved affinity to peptides encompassing the epitope of CBTAU-22.1 (Additional file 1: Table S1), the best of which being a variant containing a $Ser^{52} \rightarrow Arg$ mutation in the CDR2 of the heavy chain. The rational design was based on a co-crystal structure of Fab CBTAU-22.1 with tau peptide (Fig. 1a), which revealed polar interaction with the Ser^{422} phosphate playing a pivotal role in the hotspot from the center of the complex. The phosphate, together with 4 water molecules, gets buried in the cavity formed in the groove between the heavy and the light chains (Fig. 1b). In addition to the bridging waters, it forms hydrogen bonds with the heavy side-chains His^{35}, His^{100}, Asn^{33} and the backbone amide nitrogen of Cys^{101}. Another charge buried upon binding of CBTAU-22.1 to tau is the guanidine group of Arg^{50} from the heavy chain (Fig. 1c). Looking for the opportunities to design mutants with better affinities, we focused on forming new hydrophobic interactions and identified Asn^{33} as one possible site for mutation (Fig. 1d). Asn^{33} forms a hydrogen bond with the phosphate, but does not efficiently interact with the rest of the tau peptide. Most interactions are mediated by waters filling the small cavity surrounding the sidechain of the residue. We have scanned through all possible mutations and hypothesized that the phenylalanine side chain would fill the entire pocket, expel the unstable water molecules and form hydrophobic contacts with Leu^{425}. Our assumption was that even though the hydrogen bond with the phosphate would be lost, a $Asn^{33} \rightarrow Phe$ mutation would result in net gain in binding free energy due to multiple unfavorable water molecules being expelled and additional interactions being formed. While the $Ser^{52} \rightarrow Arg$ and $Asn^{33} \rightarrow Phe$ mutations each enhanced binding, the combination of these two mutations led to a double mutant of CBTAU-22.1 (from here on referred to as dmCBTAU-22.1) with significantly improved binding affinity, emphasized especially by its strikingly slower dissociation profile (Fig. 1e). Affinity measurements showed that the binding of dmCBTAU-22.1 ($Kd = 240 \pm 35$ nM) to tau peptide is improved by a factor of ~25 relative to parental CBTAU-22.1 ($Kd = 5.6 \pm 0.6$ μM) (Additional file 1: Figure S1). In addition, the binding profiles of Fab fragments suggested that the much higher affinity of dmCBTAU-22.1 relative to the parental antibody is due to a much slower dissociation rate without significant effect on association kinetics. A co-crystal structure of the Fab of dmCBTAU-22.1 with tau peptide confirms the predicted phenylalanine conformation (Fig. 1f, left panel) and shows that the $Ser^{52} \rightarrow Arg$ mutation resulting from the random mutagenesis approach gives rise to a charge-charge interaction with Asp^{418}, explaining the improved binding affinity (Fig. 1f, right panel). Nevertheless, the double mutant reveals the same overall binding mode as the wild-type antibody (compare Fig. 1, panels a and g).

We have previously shown that the interaction between CBTAU-22.1 and tau is affected by ionic strength [35]. A similar dependency was observed for dmCBTAU-22.1 (Additional file 1: Figure S2) indicating that the maturation process did not alter the epitope binding mode. Furthermore, we observed that in addition to the intrinsic optimization of affinity, avidity plays an important role in binding of the antibodies to tau, resulting in a very slow dissociation of dmCBTAU-22.1. Further binding experiments employing a set of different phosphorylated tau peptides (Additional file 1: Table S2) confirmed also that the specificity of the parental antibody was retained (Additional file 1: Figure S3).

The ability of the affinity improved dmCBTAU-22.1 to specifically recognize pathogenic tau structures in AD brain was compared to that of parental antibody (Fig. 2). In post mortem AD brain tissue, CBTAU-22.1 (5 μg/mL) detects pathological tau structures, which include (pre)tangles, neurofibrillary threads, and neuritic plaques. No immunoreactivity was observed in nondemented control brain tissue. While AT8 shows strong immunoreactivity of pathological tau structures at a concentration of 0.25 μg/mL, parental CBTAU-22.1 showed weak immunoreactive staining of tangles at this concentration. The detection of pathological tau

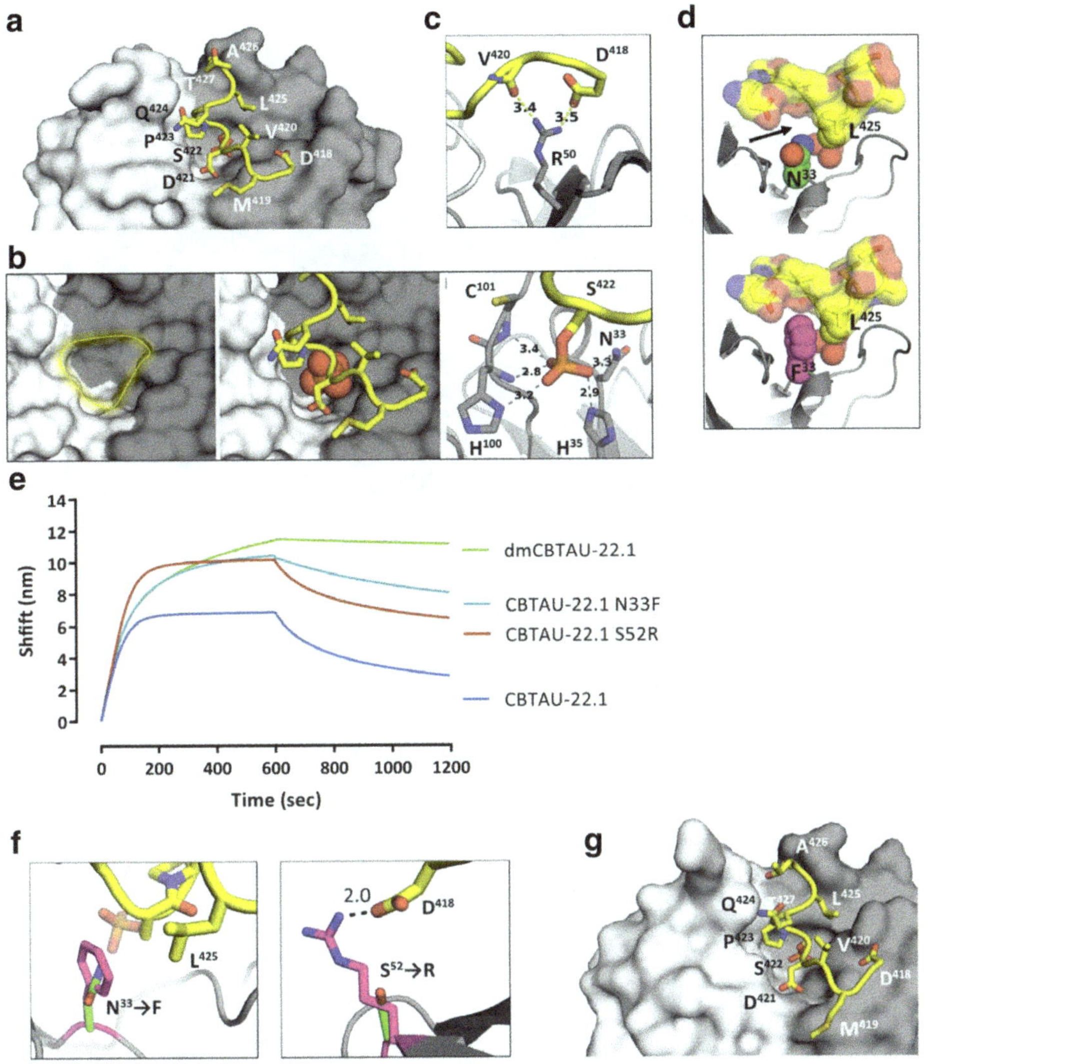

Fig. 1 Affinity maturation of CBTAU-22.1. **a** Co-crystal structure of Fab CBTAU-22.1 with tau peptide V1088-5. The Fab's molecular surface is plotted with heavy chain in grey and light chain in white. Tau peptide is plotted in yellow. **b** Peptide binding is driven by the Ser^{422} phosphate hotspot. Its binding pocket (left panel) is formed in the groove between light and heavy chains. The phosphate (plotted here as spheres) is buried deeply in the pocket and fully disolvated (central panel). Multiple hydrogen bonds are formed to bind the phosphate hotspot in the pocket (right panel). **c** Arg^{50} buried by peptide binding, second example of charge-charge interaction between CBTAU-22.1 and Tau. **d** Design of the Asn^{33} → Phe mutant based on the structure of the wild type CBTAU-22.1. Heavy chain Asn^{33} (green) interaction with tau is water mediated. Water cavity surrounding the residue in the co-crystal structure is indicated with black arrow in the upper panel. Phenylalanine (magenta, lower panel) has been identified as a mutation with high shape complementarity with the pocket, forming hydrophobic interactions with Leu^{425}. **e** Association and dissociation profiles for the parental antibody, variant antibodies with either the Ser^{52} → Arg mutation derived by random mutagenesis or the rationally-designed Asn^{33} → Phe, and a variant with both mutations combined (dmCBTAU-22.1) to peptide V1089-24 as determined by Octet biolayer interferometry. **f** Interactions introduced by the heavy chain mutations confirmed by the co-crystal structure of the double mutant. Wild type residues are plotted in green, and the mutations in magenta. Tau peptide amino-acids are plotted in yellow, and the antibody heavy chain in grey Left panel; Asn^{33} (green) mutated to Phenylalanine (magenta) resulted in formation of hydrophobic contacts with tau's Leu^{425}. Right panel: Ser^{52} (green) was mutated to Arginine (magenta) and resulted in addition of a charge-charge interaction with tau's Asp^{418}. **g** Co-crystal structure of Fab dmCBTAU-22.1 with tau peptide V1088-23. The Fabs' molecular surface is plotted with heavy chain in grey and light chain in white. Tau peptide is plotted in yellow. Tau peptide sequences are listed in Additional file 1: Table S2

was strongly improved with dmCBTAU-22.1 which showed intense staining of pathological tau at 0.25 μg/mL. These results further confirm the significant improvement in affinity and preservation of specificity of dmCBTAU-22.1.

We next assessed the effect of affinity improvement on the ability of the antibodies to bind PHFs and thus potentially block the propagation and spreading of tau pathology. To this end, the antibodies are incubated with AD brain homogenate in an immunodepletion

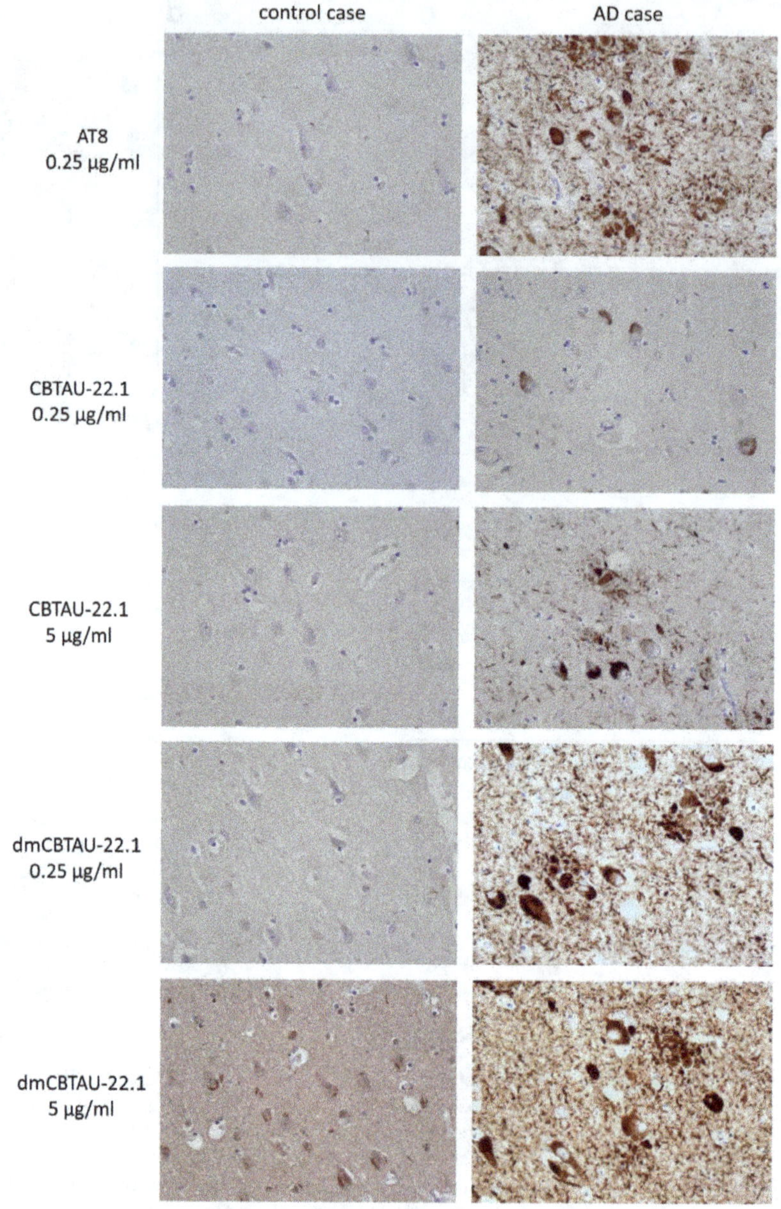

Fig. 2 Immunohistochemical detection of pathological tau in AD brain tissue. Immunohistochemistry with CBTAU-22.1 and dmCBTAU-22.1 on non-demented control and AD human brain tissue (hippocampus) was performed using two different concentrations of antibody: 0.25 µg/mL and 5 µg/mL. AT8 immunostaining (0.25 µg/mL) was applied on an adjacent section for comparison

step and subsequently residual seeding capacity is measured in a FRET-based assay [24]. As Fig. 3 shows, both CBTAU-22.1 and dmCBTAU-22.1 are capable of depleting PHFs from AD brain homogenate in a concentration dependent manner. As expected, dmCBTAU-22.1 was significantly more potent in this assay than parental CBTAU-22.1, with virtually complete seeding inhibition at he highest antibody concentration tested. Negative control antibody RSV-4.1 which does not bind tau was indeed unable to diminish PHF seeding efficiency even at the highest concentration.

Since the epitope recognized by CBTAU-22.1 is in the proximity of the MTBR which forms the core of PHF aggregates and is known to be crucial for the initial tau nucleation, we assessed the ability of the antibody to interfere with early stages in the tau aggregation process. We have previously reported on a highly reproducible rTau aggregation assay displaying all NDP features that can be used to assess the ability

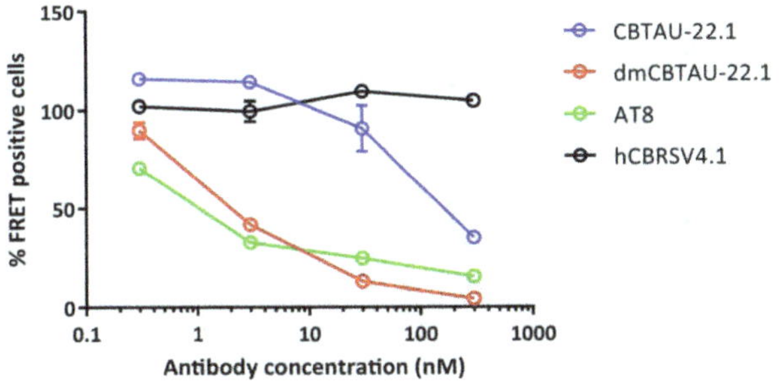

Fig. 3 Enhanced immunodepletion of AD seeds by affinity improved dmCBTAU-22.1. Residual seeding activity of human AD brain homogenates following immunodepletion with different concentrations of CBTAU-22.1 (blue) and dmCBTAU-22.1 (red) as measured by FRET signal in biosensor cells expressing the microtubule repeat domains of tau (aa 243–375) fused either to yellow or cyan fluorescent protein. Uptake of exogenous tau aggregates into the cells results in aggregation of the tau fusion proteins, which is detected by FRET. As positive and negative controls, a human IgG1 chimeric version of murine anti-PHF antibody AT8 (green) and anti-RSV-G antibody CBRSV-4.1 (black) were taken along, respectively. Error bars indicate the SD of two independent experiments

of antibodies to interfere with the aggregation of tau [1]. However, since CBTAU-22.1 recognizes an epitope phosphorylated at Ser^{422} which is not present on recombinantly produced tau we employed here a native protein ligation [33] strategy where a large recombinantly produced tau$^{1-415}$ protein fragment is coupled to a small, synthetic peptide encompassing tau$^{416-441}$ quantitatively phosphorylated at Ser^{422} (Fig. 4a). We employed a previously described ligation protocol for phosphorylated tau species [9, 37, 38], but modified it by selecting a different ligation site (as discussed in the Materials and Methods) and by adding an additional C-terminal purification tag. Progress of the ligation was monitored by capturing intermediates and visualizing on SDS-PAGE (Fig. 4b), and purification of the ligated product was performed by removal of the excess peptide and additives based on their low molecular weight followed by purification through the Ctag. Native size analysis of pS422-tau indicated that the ligated material was homogeneous, monomeric and had same molecular weight as 2N4R-tau (Fig. 4c). In addition, a Western Blot with dmCBTAU-22.1 confirmed that the phosphorylation at Ser^{422} is present in the pS422-tau ligation product (Fig. 4d).

Next, we investigated the behavior of pS422-tau in the in vitro aggregation assay. The aggregation kinetics profiles in Fig. 4e showed that, similar to 2N4R, the aggregation of pS422-tau shows the expected features of an NDP process with well-defined nucleation (nuclei formation) followed by an exponential fibril growth step [1]. AFM imaging further confirmed the formation of a homogeneous population of twisted fibrils similar in appearance to those observed for the aggregation of non-phosphorylated tau (Fig. 4f).

We have previously described an antibody, dmCBTAU-27.1, targeting the tau PHF motif located in the MTBR which is capable of completely blocking the aggregation process for non-phosphorylated recombinant tau [1]. Since the epitope of this antibody is distant from the C-terminus, its inhibiting ability should not be affected by phosphorylation introduced at Ser^{422}. Indeed, dmCBTAU-27.1 blocked the aggregation of pS422-tau at similar antibody concentrations as used before with non-phosphorylated tau (Fig. 4e, red traces). Upon incubation with dmCBTAU-22.1 at similar concentration we could clearly observe inhibition of the tau aggregation process (Fig. 4e, blue traces) even though the effect was not as strong as for dmCBTAU-27.1. This is most probably due to the epitope of CBTAU-22.1 being located outside of the key tau aggregation region as opposed to dmCBTAU-27.1 and is therefore arguably less well situated for blocking aggregation. Nonetheless, the observed behavior suggests that, in addition to a major inhibitory effect of PHF spreading, dmCBTAU-22.1 could also interfere with earlier stages of tau pathogenesis which broadens its scope both in prevention as well as therapeutic intervention.

To evaluate whether the in vitro functionality of dmCBTAU-22.1 translates to in vivo activity, we co-injected human AD-derived PHFs with equimolar amounts of dmCBTAU-22.1 expressed as mouse IgG2a in P301L mice following a protocol previously described for synthetic K18 seeds [36]. In this approach PHF-tau seeds derived from human AD brain are stereotactically injected in the hippocampal regions of P301L transgenic mice at the age of 3 months at which cell autonomous aggregation has not started. In the absence of antibody, PHF-tau seeds induce tauopathy in the injected hemisphere and to a lesser degree in the connected contralateral region. Biochemical analysis (AT8/AT8 MSD on total homogenates of the injected hemisphere) (Fig. 5) showed a 78% reduction in the amount of PHFs by the CBTAU-22.1 antibody ($P < 0.0001$) in comparison to the mouse anti-rabies IgG2a control group.

Discussion

Tau pathogenesis is a complex process characterized by a series of conformational changes, aggregation and a cascade of phosphorylation events. In the absence of reliable in vivo models there are numerous controversies regarding the most efficient strategies to interfere and prevent tau pathogenesis by passive immunotherapy. However, regardless of the targeted mechanism, both the

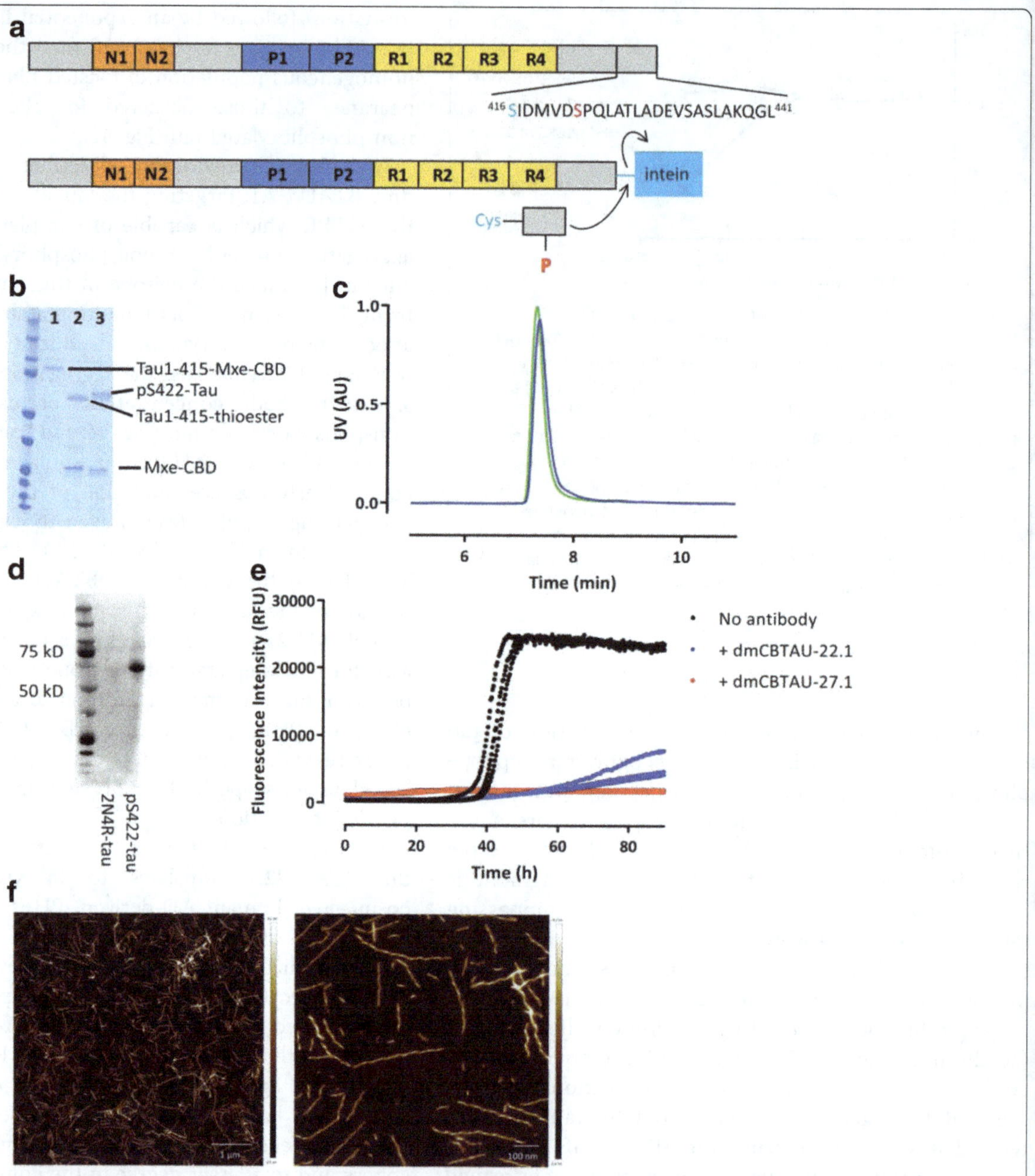

Fig. 4 Inhibition of in-vitro aggregation of pS422-tau by dmCBTAU-22.1. **a** Schematic representation of the chemical ligation process applied to preparation pS422-tau. Ser^{422} (red) is phosphorylated in the CBTAU-22.1 epitope and Ser^{416} (blue) is mutated into Cys as a result of the chemical ligation process. **b** SDS-PAGE analysis of the ligation reaction progress. Lane 1 corresponds to the full tau1–415-Mxe-CBD multidomain protein produced in *E. coli* after cloning into the pTXB1 vector. For the purposes of this analysis the protein was purified via His-tag affinity chromatography. Lane 2 corresponds to the thioester product obtained by treatment of the Lane 1 product with excess MESNa. Lane 3 represents the ligation product obtained by reaction of the Lane 2 product with tau peptide CL22D-P. **c** Size Exclusion Chromatography profiles of pS422-tau (green) and non-phosphorylated 2N4R-tau (blue). **d** Western blot of pS422-tau and non-phosphorylated 2N4R-tau with dmCBTAU-22.1. **e** Aggregation of pS422-tau in the absence (black) or presence of dmCBTAU-27.1 (red) or dmCBTAU-22.1 (blue) as monitored continuously by ThT fluorescence. The molar ratio between pS422-tau and IgG was 1: 0.6 in both cases. Each experimental condition was tested in three independent replicates, the red triplicates and two of the blue triplicates overlap and cannot be visually distinguished. **f** Atomic force microscopy of pS422-tau fibrils. The two panels correspond to AFM images with sizes of 6 × 6 μm and 1.5 × 1.5 μm, respectively

choice of tau epitope and the strength with which these are bound are expected to be pivotal. Antibody CBTAU-22.1 was, together with 51 other anti-tau antibodies, originally isolated from peripheral IgG^{+} memory B cells from asymptomatic donors [35]. We have previously reported that CBTAU-22.1 recognizes a Ser^{422} phosphorylated C-terminal epitope which has been associated with AD [4, 10, 12, 23, 41]. Furthermore,

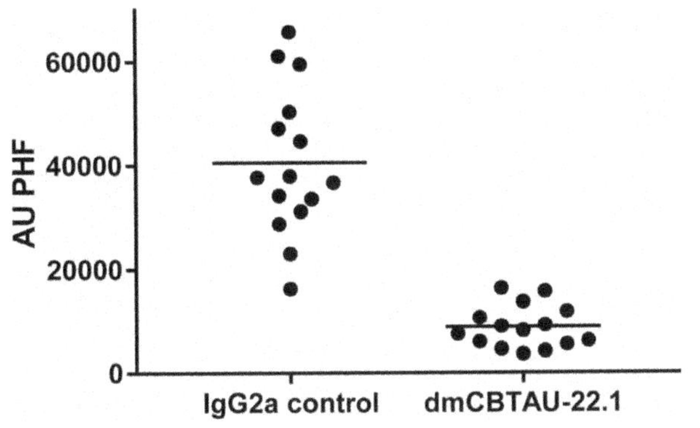

Fig. 5 Inhibition of PHF spreading by dmCBTAU-22.1 in a co-injection experiment using transgenic P301L mice. Two groups of 15 mice received unilateral (right hemisphere) hippocampal injection of 1 pmol AD-brain derived PHFs (concentration expressed in mols of monomeric tau) in an equimolar mixture with dmCBTAU-22.1 or an anti-rabies IgG2a isotype control antibody. Shown is the amount of PHF pathology, as determined by biochemical analysis (AT8/AT8 MSD) and displayed in arbitrary units (AU), in total P301L brain homogenates of the injected brain hemisphere two months after injection

CBTAU-22.1 was shown to specifically recognize pathological tau deposits in post-mortem brain tissue and to have inhibitory activity in an in vitro tau aggregation assay using PHFs derived from P301S mice, suggesting a therapeutic potential of this antibody. However, presumably due to its modest affinity for tau, this activity was low (e.g. compared to that of murine anti-PHF antibody AT8) which would likely limit its therapeutic application. We used a combination of random mutagenesis and structure-based design to generate a mutant antibody with increased affinity. Based on its apo structure (PDB 5V7U), we predicted that the Ser^{422} phosphate plays the major role in the hotspot interaction between the antibody and tau, with hydrogen bonds with heavy chain His^{35}, His^{100}, Asn^{33} and the backbone amide nitrogen of Cys^{101} as visible in the apo structure through the binding of a buffer phosphate molecule [35]. This hypothesis is confirmed here by the co-crystal structure of Fab CBTAU-22.1 with tau peptide which guided us in deriving the Asn33 → Phe mutation. By combining this mutation with a Ser^{52} → Arg that was identified by random mutagenesis, we generated a significantly improved antibody, dmCBTAU-22.1 that has the same binding mode as CBTAU-22.1 in all measured parameters.

In post mortem brain tissue, dmCBTAU-22.1 specifically stains pathological tau structures with similar intensities to well-known PHF antibody AT8. This affinity for pathological tau aggregates translates into a significantly increased ability to deplete and neutralize PHFs from AD brain lysates that again is comparable in efficiency to AT8. While CBTAU-22.1 reduced PHF seeding efficiency to 35% at its highest concentration tested, dmCBTAU-22.1 achieved a similar effect at a 100 times lower concentration and completely depleted the PHF seeding at the highest concentration tested. These results confirm that increased affinity leads to increased potency. This would translate into lower required drug dose and thus alleviate the difficulty of passing sufficient amounts of antibody across the blood brain barrier.

To assess the potential ability of dmCBTAU-22.1 to interfere with the aggregation of tau, we used chemical ligation to prepare homogeneous tau with phosphorylation at Ser^{422}. This strategy combines the advantage of peptide chemistry, the ability to introduce modified amino acids in a fully controlled way, with the advantage of recombinant expression, the ability to produce long sequences. In contrast to other conjugation methodologies, this approach is traceless: it requires no added linkers and affords a natural backbone. Selection of a suitable ligation site is key since the chemistry behind it demands the presence of a cysteine residue. One can: (1) take advantage of a cysteine residue already present, (2) employ the cysteine as a relatively close mimic of a serine residue or (3) chemically transform the cysteine into an alanine residue. Approach (1) was not available since there is no cysteine near the CBTAU-22.1 epitope. We decided on approach (2) since it leaves the possibility to maintain the two cysteine residues in tau, the oxidation state of which has an impact on aggregation; in contrast approach (3) would necessarily mutate these to alanines. We did not find in any of our studies any detrimental effect attributable to the resulting S416C mutation which we controlled for by preparing and testing ligated material from the corresponding non-phosphorylated peptide part. Using this tailor-made pS422-tau protein in the in vitro aggregation assay, we have shown that dmCBTAU-22.1 not only binds with high affinity to pathological tau, it also interferes with the tau aggregation process that underpins pathology formation. Interestingly, this represents the first time we observed such inhibition for an antibody binding outside the core aggregation domain. These two properties, neutralization of pathological tau species and ability to interfere with aggregation, translate into significant functionality in P301L transgenic mice. Immunotherapy against tau represents a promising strategy for treating AD and other tauopathies considering the direct link and strong association between tau pathology and loss of cognition [8, 34, 43]. Multiple studies in mice suggest that several anti-PHF antibodies of non-human origin may have therapeutic potential (reviewed in [42]). The only other antibody against pS422 that has been structurally characterized is rabbit antibody Rb86 (PDB 5DMG) [11]. While comparison of the structures reveals differences in the mode of binding of the two antibodies, i.e. binding of CBTAU-22.1 is centered around the buried phosphate pS422 while that of Rb86 is strongly driven by hydrophobic interactions, the demonstrated efficacy of a murine IgG1 version of Rb86 (MAb86) in reducing tau pathology in a mouse model of AD [14] provides further support for the potential of targeting the pS422 epitope. The data presented here in combination with the fact that dmCBTAU-22.1 is a fully human antibody, makes this antibody a particularly promising candidate for therapeutic intervention. As mentioned, the most efficient strategies to interfere and prevent tau pathogenesis by passive immunotherapy is subject of debate. For example, Congdon et al., [15] have shown that binding to soluble phospho tau, rather than to aggregated PHFs, correlated with both intro- and extracellular antibody-mediated clearance of phospho tau in primary neurons, and improvement in cognition in the htau mouse model. These findings suggest that, next to tau spreading and aggregation, prevention of neurotoxicity may be important for effective immunotherapy. Assessment of the ability of dmCBTAU-22.1 to prevent additional aspects of tau pathogenesis, like neurotoxicity and actual neurodegeneration, will be subject of future studies.

Additional file

Additional file 1: Table S1. Overview of mutations investigated during the maturation process. **Table S2.** Names and sequences of tau peptides used in this study. **Table S3**. Data collection for Fab-CBTAU-22.1 in complex with peptide V1088-5 and Fab-dmCBTAU-22.1 in complex with peptide V1088-23. **Table S4.** Refinement statistics for Fab-CBTAU-22.1 in complex with peptide V1088-5 and Fab-dmCBTAU-22.1 in complex with peptide V1088-23. **Figure S1.** Binding affinities of the antigen binding domains of CBTAU-22.1 (left) and dmCBTAU-22.1 (right) to biotinylated peptide V1089-24 as determined by Octet Biolayer Interferometry. **Figure S2.** Association and dissociation kinetics for the binding of CBTAU-22.1 (left) and dmCBTAU-22.1 (right) to peptide V1089-24 at different ionic strengths. **Figure S3.** Association and dissociation kinetics for the binding of CBTAU-22.1 (left) and dmCBTAU-22.1 (right) to a panel of phosphorylated tau-derived peptides. Neither of the antibodies shows unspecific binding to tau peptides that do not contain the $pSer^{422}$ epitope. **Figure S4.** Western blot detection of PHFs using anti-tau antibodies hTau10 (left) and AT8 (right). (DOCX 2093 kb)

Acknowledgements
Human brain tissue for the immunodepletion experiments performed in this study was provided by the Newcastle Brain Tissue Resource which is funded in part by a grant from the UK Medical Research Council (G0400074), by NIHR Newcastle Biomedical Research Centre and Unit awarded to the Newcastle upon Tyne NHS Foundation Trust and Newcastle University, and as part of the Brains for Dementia Research Programme jointly funded by Alzheimer's Research UK and Alzheimer's Society. We thank Frederique Bard and Jaap Goudsmit for fruitful discussions, David Zuijdgeest for expert support provided for the antibody affinity maturation process and Mohammed Drissi Saidi, Hector Quirante, Nasser Ouazrhari, Hanna Inganäs and Margot van Winsen for production, purification and analysis of proteins used in this study.

Authors' contributions
Project design by AA, JA, RC, RJ and JJ; native chemical ligation JA, TN and IS; aggregation assay and in vitro antibody screening by RC and AA; antibody discovery, optimization and protein expression and purification by JJ, GP, RJ, HV, BS and AA; FRET based cellular immunodepletion assay by MB, KD, KK, and MM; in vivo coinjection: RW, LD, KK and MM; biophysical characterization by RC, BS, JA and AA; atomic force microscopy by RC; immunohistochemical analysis by JJH, X-ray work and analysis by SS; and manuscript written by WK and AA. All authors read and approved the final manuscript.

Competing interest
This work was fully funded by Janssen. Patent applications relating to CBTAU-22.1 and dmCBTAU-22.1 have been filed.

Author details
[1]Janssen Prevention Center, Janssen Pharmaceutical Companies of Johnson and Johnson, Archimedesweg 6, 2333 Leiden, CN, the Netherlands. [2]Department of Pathology, Amsterdam Neuroscience, VU University Medical Center, De Boelelaan 1117, 1081, HV, Amsterdam, the Netherlands. [3]Proteros Biostructures GmbH, Bunsenstraße 7a, 82152 Planegg, Germany. [4]Janssen Neuroscience Discovery, Janssen Pharmaceutical Companies of Johnson and Johnson, Turnhoutseweg 30, 2340 Beerse, Belgium. [5]Molecular and Cellular Pharmacology, Discovery Sciences, Janssen Pharmaceutical Companies of Johnson and Johnson, Turnhoutseweg 30, 2340 Beerse, Belgium. [6]Janssen Prevention Center, Janssen Pharmaceutical Companies of Johnson and Johnson, 3210 Merryfield Row, San Diego, CA 92121, USA.

References

1. Apetri A, Crespo R, Juraszek J, Pascual G, Janson R, Zhu X, Zhang H, Keogh E, Holland T, Wadia J, Verveen H, Siregar B, Mrosek M, Taggenbrock R, Ameijde J, Inganas H, van Winsen M, Koldijk MH, Zuijdgeest D, Borgers M, Dockx K, Stoop EJM, Yu W, Brinkman-van der Linden EC, Ummenthum K, van Kolen K, Mercken M, Steinbacher S, de Marco D, Hoozemans JJ, Wilson IA, Koudstaal W, Goudsmit J (2018) A common antigenic motif recognized by naturally occurring human VH5-51/VL4-1 anti-tau antibodies with distinct functionalities. Acta Neuropathol Commun 6:43. https://doi.org/10.1186/s40478-018-0543-z
2. Apetri AC, Vanik DL, Surewicz WK (2005) Polymorphism at residue 129 modulates the conformational conversion of the D178N variant of human prion protein 90–231. Biochemistry 44:15880–15888. https://doi.org/10.1021/bi051455+
3. Asuni AA, Boutajangout A, Quartermain D, Sigurdsson EM (2007) Immunotherapy targeting pathological tau conformers in a tangle mouse model reduces brain pathology with associated functional improvements. J Neurosci 27:9115–9129. https://doi.org/10.1523/JNEUROSCI.2361-07.2007
4. Augustinack JC, Schneider A, Mandelkow EM, Hyman BT (2002) Specific tau phosphorylation sites correlate with severity of neuronal cytopathology in Alzheimer's disease. Acta Neuropathol 103:26–35
5. Bi M, Ittner A, Ke YD, Gotz J, Ittner LM (2011) Tau-targeted immunization impedes progression of neurofibrillary histopathology in aged P301L tau transgenic mice. PLoS One 6:e26860. https://doi.org/10.1371/journal.pone.0026860
6. Billingsley ML, Kincaid RL (1997) Regulated phosphorylation and dephosphorylation of tau protein: effects on microtubule interaction, intracellular trafficking and neurodegeneration. Biochem J 323(Pt 3):577–591
7. Boimel M, Grigoriadis N, Lourbopoulos A, Haber E, Abramsky O, Rosenmann H (2010) Efficacy and safety of immunization with phosphorylated tau against neurofibrillary tangles in mice. Exp Neurol 224:472–485. https://doi.org/10.1016/j.expneurol.2010.05.010
8. Braak H, Braak E, Bohl J (1993) Staging of Alzheimer-related cortical destruction. Eur Neurol 33:403–408. https://doi.org/10.1159/000116984
9. Broncel M, Krause E, Schwarzer D, Hackenberger CP (2012) The Alzheimer's disease related tau protein as a new target for chemical protein engineering. Chemistry 18:2488–2492. https://doi.org/10.1002/chem.201103032
10. Buee L, Bussiere T, Buee-Scherrer V, Delacourte A, Hof PR (2000) Tau protein isoforms, phosphorylation and role in neurodegenerative disorders. Brain Res Brain Res Rev 33:95–130
11. Bujotzek A, Lipsmeier F, Harris SF, Benz J, Kuglstatter A, Georges G (2016) VH-VL orientation prediction for antibody humanization candidate selection: a case study. MAbs 8:288–305. https://doi.org/10.1080/19420862.2015.1117720

12. Bussiere T, Hof PR, Mailliot C, Brown CD, Caillet-Boudin ML, Perl DP, Buee L, Delacourte A (1999) Phosphorylated serine422 on tau proteins is a pathological epitope found in several diseases with neurofibrillary degeneration. Acta Neuropathol 97:221–230
13. Clavaguera F, Akatsu H, Fraser G, Crowther RA, Frank S, Hench J, Probst A, Winkler DT, Reichwald J, Staufenbiel M, Ghetti B, Goedert M, Tolnay M (2013) Brain homogenates from human tauopathies induce tau inclusions in mouse brain. Proc Natl Acad Sci U S A 110:9535–9540. https://doi.org/10.1073/pnas.1301175110
14. Collin L, Bohrmann B, Gopfert U, Oroszlan-Szovik K, Ozmen L, Gruninger F (2014) Neuronal uptake of tau/pS422 antibody and reduced progression of tau pathology in a mouse model of Alzheimer's disease. Brain 137:2834–2846. https://doi.org/10.1093/brain/awu213
15. Congdon EE, Lin Y, Rajamohamedsait HB, Shamir DB, Krishnaswamy S, Rajamohamedsait WJ, Rasool S, Gonzalez V, Levenga J, Gu J, Hoeffer C, Sigurdsson EM (2016) Affinity of tau antibodies for solubilized pathological tau species but not their immunogen or insoluble tau aggregates predicts in vivo and ex vivo efficacy. Mol Neurodegener 11:62. https://doi.org/10.1186/s13024-016-0126-z
16. Crespo R, Rocha FA, Damas AM, Martins PM (2012) A generic crystallization-like model that describes the kinetics of amyloid fibril formation. J Biol Chem 287:30585–30594. https://doi.org/10.1074/jbc.M112.375345
17. Drechsel DN, Hyman AA, Cobb MH, Kirschner MW (1992) Modulation of the dynamic instability of tubulin assembly by the microtubule-associated protein tau. Mol Biol Cell 3:1141–1154
18. Emsley P, Lohkamp B, Scott WG, Cowtan K (2010) Features and development of coot. Acta Crystallogr Sect D Biol Crystallogr 66:486–501. https://doi.org/10.1107/S0907444910007493
19. Goedert M, Klug A, Crowther RA (2006) Tau protein, the paired helical filament and Alzheimer's disease. J Alzheimer's Dis 9:195–207
20. Greenberg SG, Davies P (1990) A preparation of Alzheimer paired helical filaments that displays distinct tau proteins by polyacrylamide gel electrophoresis. Proc Natl Acad Sci U S A 87:5827–5831
21. Guo JL, Narasimhan S, Changolkar L, He Z, Stieber A, Zhang B, Gathagan RJ, Iba M, McBride JD, Trojanowski JQ, Lee VM (2016) Unique pathological tau conformers from Alzheimer's brains transmit tau pathology in nontransgenic mice. J Exp Med 213:2635–2654. https://doi.org/10.1084/jem.20160833
22. Harper JD, Lansbury PT Jr (1997) Models of amyloid seeding in Alzheimer's disease and scrapie: mechanistic truths and physiological consequences of the time-dependent solubility of amyloid proteins. Annu Rev Biochem 66:385–407. https://doi.org/10.1146/annurev.biochem.66.1.385
23. Hasegawa M, Jakes R, Crowther RA, Lee VM, Ihara Y, Goedert M (1996) Characterization of mAb AP422, a novel phosphorylation-dependent monoclonal antibody against tau protein. FEBS Lett 384:25–30
24. Holmes BB, Furman JL, Mahan TE, Yamasaki TR, Mirbaha H, Eades WC, Belaygorod L, Cairns NJ, Holtzman DM, Diamond MI (2014) Proteopathic tau seeding predicts tauopathy in vivo. Proc Natl Acad Sci U S A 111:E4376–E4385. https://doi.org/10.1073/pnas.1411649111
25. Kabsch W (2010) Xds. Acta Crystallogr Sect D Biol Crystallogr 66:125–132. https://doi.org/10.1107/S0907444909047337
26. Kolarova M, Garcia-Sierra F, Bartos A, Ricny J, Ripova D (2012) Structure and pathology of tau protein in Alzheimer disease. Int J Alzheimers Dis 2012:731526. https://doi.org/10.1155/2012/731526
27. Kramer RA, Cox F, van der Horst M, van der Oudenrijn S, Res PC, Bia J, Logtenberg T, de Kruif J (2003) A novel helper phage that improves phage display selection efficiency by preventing the amplification of phages without recombinant protein. Nucleic Acids Res 31:e59
28. Laskowski RA, MacArthur MW, Moss DS, Thornton JM (1993) PROCHECK: a program to check the stereochemicai quality of protein structures. J Appl Crystallogr 26:283–291
29. Liu L, Drouet V, Wu JW, Witter MP, Small SA, Clelland C, Duff K (2012) Trans-synaptic spread of tau pathology in vivo. PLoS One 7:e31302. https://doi.org/10.1371/journal.pone.0031302
30. Malia TJ, Teplyakov A, Ernst R, Wu SJ, Lacy ER, Liu X, Vandermeeren M, Mercken M, Luo J, Sweet RW, Gilliland GL (2016) Epitope mapping and structural basis for the recognition of phosphorylated tau by the anti-tau antibody AT8. Proteins 84:427–434. https://doi.org/10.1002/prot.24988
31. Mandelkow EM, Mandelkow E (2012) Biochemistry and cell biology of tau protein in neurofibrillary degeneration. Cold Spring Harb Perspect Med 2:a006247. https://doi.org/10.1101/cshperspect.a006247
32. Mercken M, Vandermeeren M, Lubke U, Six J, Boons J, Van de Voorde A, Martin JJ, Gheuens J (1992) Monoclonal antibodies with selective specificity for Alzheimer tau are directed against phosphatase-sensitive epitopes. Acta Neuropathol 84:265–272
33. Muir TW, Sondhi D, Cole PA (1998) Expressed protein ligation: a general method for protein engineering. Proc Natl Acad Sci U S A 95:6705–6710
34. Oddo S, Caccamo A, Cheng D, LaFerla FM (2009) Genetically altering Abeta distribution from the brain to the vasculature ameliorates tau pathology. Brain Pathol 19:421–430. https://doi.org/10.1111/j.1750-3639.2008.00194.x
35. Pascual G, Wadia JS, Zhu X, Keogh E, Kukrer B, van Ameijde J, Inganas H, Siregar B, Perdok G, Diefenbach O, Nahar T, Sprengers I, Koldijk MH, der Linden EC, Peferoen LA, Zhang H, Yu W, Li X, Wagner M, Moreno V, Kim J, Costa M, West K, Fulton Z, Chammas L, Luckashenak N, Fletcher L, Holland T, Arnold C, Anthony Williamson R, Hoozemans JJ, Apetri A, Bard F, Wilson IA, Koudstaal W, Goudsmit J (2017) Immunological memory to hyperphosphorylated tau in asymptomatic individuals. Acta Neuropathol 133:767–783. https://doi.org/10.1007/s00401-017-1705-y
36. Peeraer E, Bottelbergs A, Van Kolen K, Stancu IC, Vasconcelos B, Mahieu M, Duytschaever H, Ver Donck L, Torremans A, Sluydts E, Van Acker N, Kemp JA, Mercken M, Brunden KR, Trojanowski JQ, Dewachter I, Lee VM, Moechars D (2015) Intracerebral injection of preformed synthetic tau fibrils initiates widespread tauopathy and neuronal loss in the brains of tau transgenic mice. Neurobiol Dis 73:83–95. https://doi.org/10.1016/j.nbd.2014.08.032
37. Reimann O, Glanz M, Hackenberger CP (2015) Native chemical ligation between asparagine and valine: application and limitations for the synthesis of tri-phosphorylated C-terminal tau. Bioorg Med Chem 23:2890–2894. https://doi.org/10.1016/j.bmc.2015.03.028
38. Reimann O, Smet-Nocca C, Hackenberger CP (2015) Traceless purification and desulfurization of tau protein ligation products. Angew Chem Int Ed Eng 54:306–310. https://doi.org/10.1002/anie.201408674
39. Sanchez C, Diaz-Nido J, Avila J (2000) Phosphorylation of microtubule-associated protein 2 (MAP2) and its relevance for the regulation of the neuronal cytoskeleton function. Prog Neurobiol 61:133–168
40. Sanders DW, Kaufman SK, DeVos SL, Sharma AM, Mirbaha H, Li A, Barker SJ, Foley AC, Thorpe JR, Serpell LC, Miller TM, Grinberg LT, Seeley WW, Diamond MI (2014) Distinct tau prion strains propagate in cells and mice and define different tauopathies. Neuron 82:1271–1288. https://doi.org/10.1016/j.neuron.2014.04.047
41. Schraen-Maschke S, Sergeant N, Dhaenens CM, Bombois S, Deramecourt V, Caillet-Boudin ML, Pasquier F, Maurage CA, Sablonniere B, Vanmechelen E, Buee L (2008) Tau as a biomarker of neurodegenerative diseases. Biomark Med 2:363–384. https://doi.org/10.2217/17520363.2.4.363
42. Schroeder SK, Joly-Amado A, Gordon MN, Morgan D (2016) Tau-directed immunotherapy: a promising strategy for treating Alzheimer's disease and other Tauopathies. J NeuroImmune Pharmacol 11:9–25. https://doi.org/10.1007/s11481-015-9637-6
43. Sigurdsson EM (2008) Immunotherapy targeting pathological tau protein in Alzheimer's disease and related tauopathies. J Alzheimers Dis 15:157–168
44. Sigurdsson EM (2009) Tau-focused immunotherapy for Alzheimer's disease and related tauopathies. Curr Alzheimer Res 6:446–450
45. Surewicz WK, Jones EM, Apetri AC (2006) The emerging principles of mammalian prion propagation and transmissibility barriers: insight from studies in vitro. Acc Chem Res 39:654–662. https://doi.org/10.1021/ar050226c
46. Terwel D, Lasrado R, Snauwaert J, Vandeweert E, Van Haesendonck C, Borghgraef P, Van Leuven F (2005) Changed conformation of mutant tau-P301L underlies the moribund tauopathy, absent in progressive, nonlethal axonopathy of tau-4R/2N transgenic mice. J Biol Chem 280:3963–3973. https://doi.org/10.1074/jbc.M409876200
47. Troquier L, Caillierez R, Burnouf S, Fernandez-Gomez FJ, Grosjean ME, Zommer N, Sergeant N, Schraen-Maschke S, Blum D, Buee L (2012) Targeting phospho-Ser422 by active tau immunotherapy in the THYTau22 mouse model: a suitable therapeutic approach. Curr Alzheimer Res 9:397–405
48. Vagin A, .Teplyakov, A. (1997) MOLREP: an automated program for molecular replacement J Appl Crystallogr 30:1022–1025
49. Vagin AA, Steiner RA, Lebedev AA, Potterton L, McNicholas S, Long F, Murshudov GN (2004) REFMAC5 dictionary: organization of prior chemical knowledge and guidelines for its use. Acta Crystallogr Sect D Biol Crystallogr 60:2184–2195. https://doi.org/10.1107/S0907444904023510

50. Yanamandra K, Jiang H, Mahan TE, Maloney SE, Wozniak DF, Diamond MI, Holtzman DM (2015) Anti-tau antibody reduces insoluble tau and decreases brain atrophy. Ann Clin Transl Neurol 2:278–288. https://doi.org/10.1002/acn3.176
51. Yanamandra K, Kfoury N, Jiang H, Mahan TE, Ma S, Maloney SE, Wozniak DF, Diamond MI, Holtzman DM (2013) Anti-tau antibodies that block tau aggregate seeding in vitro markedly decrease pathology and improve cognition in vivo. Neuron 80:402–414. https://doi.org/10.1016/j.neuron.2013.07.046

6

Environmental enrichment reverses Aβ pathology during pregnancy in a mouse model of Alzheimer's disease

Stephanie Ziegler-Waldkirch[1,2], Karin Marksteiner[1,2], Johannes Stoll[1,2], Paolo d´Errico[1,2], Marina Friesen[1,3,4], Denise Eiler[1,2], Lea Neudel[1,2], Verena Sturn[1,2], Isabel Opper[1,2], Moumita Datta[2,4], Marco Prinz[2,4,5] and Melanie Meyer-Luehmann[1,2,6*]

Abstract

Several studies suggest that women have a higher risk to develop Alzheimer's disease (AD) than men. In particular, the number of pregnancies was shown to be a risk factor for AD and women with several pregnancies on average had an earlier onset of the disease, thus making childbearing a risk factor. However, the impact of being pregnant on Aβ plaque pathology and adult neurogenesis still remains elusive. Postmortem analysis revealed that pregnant 5xFAD transgenic mice had significantly more Aβ plaques in the hippocampus from G10 onwards and that the number of Ki67 and DCX positive cells dramatically decreased during the postpartum period. Furthermore, 5 months old 5xFAD transgenic mice that also nursed their offsprings for 4 weeks had a similar Aβ plaque load than merely pregnant mice, indicating that pregnancy alone is sufficient to elevate Aβ plaque levels. Interestingly, housing in an enriched environment reduced the Aβ plaque load and vivified neurogenesis. Our results suggest that pregnancy alters Aβ plaque deposition in 5xFAD transgenic mice and diminishes the generation of newborn neurons. We conclude that pregnancy alone is sufficient to induce this phenotype that can be reversed upon environmental enrichment.

Keywords: Alzheimer's disease, Pregnancy, Amyloid-β plaques, Adult neurogenesis, Estrogens, Progesterone, Environmental enrichment

Introduction

Alzheimer's disease (AD) is the most common type of dementia that is characterized by a decline in memory. The majority of AD cases are sporadic [9] and the greatest non-genetic risk factors for the development of AD are age and gender. The incidence of the disease is higher in women than in men, which was previously attributed to the higher longevity of women versus men. Several epidemiological studies suggest however that there may be other factors contributing to the disease beyond longevity. In particular, women with multiple pregnancies had an earlier onset of AD [6, 7, 31] and nulliparous women had significantly less age related cognitive decline [25], while the number of children had no effect on the risk of developing AD [31]. Together, these studies indicate reproductive experience being a risk factor for AD, but the underlying mechanism for this higher risk of AD in women is still largely unknown.

In agreement with those aforementioned studies, gender-dependent elevated Aβ plaque formation has been observed in several APP transgenic mouse models. Female APP transgenic mice that exhibit massive cerebral amyloid deposition while aging developed more Aβ pathology with an earlier onset than their male siblings [1, 5, 14, 35, 39]. Additionally, fertility experience of those female APP transgenic mice altered Aβ plaque pathology, resulting in even higher Aβ plaque numbers and larger plaque sizes when compared to non-breeders [8]. Furthermore, these neuropathological changes were associated with spatial memory impairment and the down-regulation of synaptophysin levels in APP transgenic breeders.

* Correspondence: melanie.meyer-luehmann@uniklinik-freiburg.de
[1]Department of Neurology, Medical Center – University of Freiburg, Freiburg, Germany
[2]Faculty of Medicine, University of Freiburg, Freiburg, Germany
Full list of author information is available at the end of the article

Adult neurogenesis is a lifelong process in the healthy adult mammalian brain, where functional neurons are generated from adult neural stem cells and adult neural precursor cells. Emerging evidence has indicated that altered neurogenesis in the adult hippocampus represents a critical event in the course of AD and that cognitive deficits, learning difficulties and memory loss in AD patients may be due to impaired adult neurogenesis [10, 15, 20, 21]. Intriguingly, environmental enrichment and voluntary exercise were shown to increase the number of newborn granule cells in the dentate gyrus [18, 19, 26, 37, 38] and to reduce Aβ plaque formation in APP transgenic mice [16, 22]. Despite the immense interest in the therapeutic potential of environmental enrichment during pregnancy, the impact on the mother however still remains elusive since most studies focus on the offspring [3, 13].

Therefore, we aimed to investigate neuropathological changes such as Aβ plaque load and adult neurogenesis during the course of pregnancy at different gestation days. Our results demonstrate that pregnant 5xFAD transgenic mice had a significantly higher Aβ plaque load in different brain regions such as hippocampus, cortex and the olfactory bulb. Interestingly, 5 month old 5xFAD transgenic mice that also nursed their offspring for 4 weeks had an Aβ plaque load similar to merely pregnant mice, indicating that pregnancy alone is sufficient to elevate Aβ plaque levels. Furthermore, neurogenesis was dramatically decreased in both groups during the postpartum period compared to 5xFAD mice. Exposure of pregnant 5xFAD mice to an enriched environment reduced Aβ deposits and stimulated the generation of newborn neurons, thus underlining the beneficial effects of exercise and enrichment during pregnancy.

Material and methods

Animals

We used heterozygous 5xFAD transgenic mice co-expressing human APP $^{K670N/M671L\ (Sw) + I716V\ (Fl) + V717I(Lo)}$ and PS1$^{M146L + L286V}$ under the control of the neuron-specific Thy-1 promoter [27]. We backcrossed 5xFAD mice with C57BL/6 mice to generate heterozygous 5xFAD mice and non-transgenic littermates on the same genetic background. Only female mice were used in the present study. Animals were group-housed under specific pathogen-free conditions. Mice were kept under a 12-h light, 12-h dark cycle with food and water ad libitum. All animal experiments were carried out in accordance with the policies of the state of Baden-Württemberg under license number X14/02A and X17/01A.

Female mice were mated at the age of 12 weeks. The matings were initiated in the afternoon and the mice were separated after a positive plug check on the following morning. The day of vaginal plaque formation was estimated as gestation day 1 (G1). In order to analyze female mice at different stages of pregnancy, they were sacrificed on G5, G10 and G18. Non- pregnant 5xFAD female mice of the same age and from the same litters were used as control groups. To study the lactation period, female mice were mated at the age of 12 weeks and were divided into three groups. One group delivered and lactated the offspring for 4 weeks. One group was separated from their litter directly after the delivery and the third group was not pregnant and did not lactate. All mice were analyzed at postpartum day 20 (P20). To study how multiple pregnancies might affect Aβ pathology, 10 months old female mice were analyzed. Two groups of female mice, nulliparous and multiparous (4 times pregnant and lactating) were used.

Environmental enrichment

5xFAD female mice were mated at the age of 12 weeks. One group of mice was housed in standard cages and another group of mice in an enriched environment until G18 or P20. The environmental enrichment consisted of larger cages (40 × 60 cm) that contained 1 running wheel, tunnel systems, small plastic houses and extra nesting material. The animals had free access to the running wheel. Mice were housed in groups of 5. All mice were sacrificed at the end of the experiment at G18 or P20.

Histology

Mice were deeply anesthetized with a mixture of ketamine (300 mg per kg) and xylazine (20 mg per kg) before they were transcardially perfused with 20 ml of ice-cold PBS followed by 20 ml of ice-cold 4% paraformaldehyde in PBS. Brains were isolated and postfixed in 4% PFA for 24 h, followed by incubation in 30% sucrose (in PBS, pH 7.5) for a further 48 h. Frozen brains were cut into 25 μm thick coronal sections on a sliding microtome (SM2000R, Leica Biosystems, Wetzlar, Germany) and collected in PBS. Immunohistochemistry was performed on free floating sections using the following antibodies diluted in PBS containing 5% normal goat serum and 0.5% Triton X-100: anti-Aβ 3552 (rabbit polyclonal antibody specific for Aβ 1–40 [40] (kindly provided by E. Kremmer, Ludwig Maximilians University, Munich, Germany); diluted 1:3000), anti-doublecortin (rabbit, DCX; 1:5000, abcam, ab18723), anti-Ki67 (rabbit, 1:500, abcam, ab15580). Appropriate secondary antibodies conjugated to Alexa 488 or 555 (1:1500) were used. Dense-core plaques were stained with Thiazinred (Sigma, T3272). Staining was done according to standard protocols. In brief, sections were washed 3 times in PBS and incubated in Thiazinred (2 μM solution in PBS) for 5 min at RT followed by 3 × 5 min washes with PBS.

Assessment of Aβ and cell analysis

Fluorescence images of brain slices were taken using a Zeiss fluorescent microscope (Axio Imager M2M). For analysis every tenth brain section of one hemisphere was used. The total Aβ load was determined by counting the Aβ-positive stained plaques using the imaging software ImageJ (National Institutes of Health freeware). Ten sections per animal were analyzed for the hippocampus and cortex and 8 sections per animal for the olfactory bulb, in total 4–6 animals per group were investigated. Aβ plaque load is presented in % and normalized to the non-pregnant control group (set to 100%).

The cell number was quantified by counting the number of positively labeled cells in the animal's whole dentate gyrus. Four to six animals per group and 10 sections per animal were analyzed. Cell counting was done in the dentate gyrus and its area was measured with the ImageJ software. The area of the gyrus was defined according to the mouse brain atlas [29]. Cell numbers are presented as the quantity of positively labeled cells per mm^2. All analyses were conducted in a blinded manner.

Western blot analysis

Total protein from hippocampus was extracted in RIPA buffer (50 mM HEPES pH 7.5, 150 mM NaCl, 1 mM EDTA, 10% Glycerin, 1% Triton X-100, 10 mM $Na_4O_7P_2$, Protease Inhibitor). Protein concentration was determined by Pierce BCA Protein Assay Kit (ThermoFisher). Samples were separated by 4–12% NuPAGE Bis-tris mini gels using NuPAGE LDS sample buffer, NuPAGE sample reducing agent and NuPAGE MES SDS running buffer (Invitrogen). Proteins were transferred on PVDF membranes (Biorad) and visualized using Clarity Western ECL Substrate (Biorad). Antibodies against APP and CTFs (rabbit polyclonal antibody against the APP C-terminus, 6687, 1:1000) [34], anti-Aβ (mouse, 1:3000, Covance, 6E10), anti-insulin degrading enzyme (anti-IDE) (rabbit, 1:5000, abcam, ab109538), anti-neprilysin 1:2500 (rabbit, 1:2500, abcam, ab79423) and anti-β-actin-HRP (mouse, 1:5000, abcam, ab20272) were used.

ELISA

For the measurement of estrogen and progesterone levels, blood samples were taken from the ventricle before the perfusion of the mice at G5, G10 or G18. Blood was centrifuged immediately for 10 min at 1800 g. The supernatant was frozen at – 20 °C until analysis. Serum samples were prepared and analyzed by Mouse/Rat Estradiol ELISA kit (Calbiotech, catalog no. ES180S-100) or Progesterone ELISA Kit (Enzo, Enzo Life Science) according to the manufacturer's protocols. Samples were measured in duplicates and the ELISA was conducted in two to three independent experiments.

For the quantification of Aβ40 and 42 species in the soluble and insoluble hippocampal extracts, hippocampal tissue was homogenized (10% *w*/*v*) in PBS + protease inhibitor and sequentially extracted with PBS (soluble fraction), PBS + 0.1% TritonX100 (membrane bound fraction) and finally with 8 M guanidine hydrochloride solution. Protein concentration in each fraction was measured with Bradford reagent (Roth) and ELISA was performed using Human Aβ42 ultrasensitive ELISA kit (Life Technologies, catalog no. KHB3544) and Human Aβ40 ELISA kit (Life Technologies, catalog no. KHB3481), according to the manufacturer's protocol.

Statistical analysis

GraphPad Prism 6 (GraphPad Software, Inc) was used for statistical analysis. All data sets were tested for normality with the D'Agostino-Pearson omnibus K2 normality test with a significance level set to $P = 0.05$ before carrying out the appropriate parametric or nonparametric statistical comparison test. The Mann-Whitney test or Kruskal-Wallis test followed by Dunn's posthoc test were applied. Reported values are means ± S.D. Significance level α was set to 0.05. $^{*}P < 0.05$; $^{**}P < 0.01$; $^{***}P < 0.001$.

Results

Pregnancy-related alteration of Aβ plaque pathology in female 5xFAD mice

To investigate if pregnancy induces pathological alterations, we first determined the Aβ plaque load in 5xFAD transgenic female mice at different stages of pregnancy/gestation days and compared them to their age-machted non-pregnant littermates. 5xFAD transgenic mice were mated at the age of 12 weeks and were analyzed on gestation day 5, 10 and 18 (G5, 10, 18) (Fig. 1a). At G5, there was no difference between the Aβ plaque load of pregnant mice and non-pregnant littermates (Fig. 1b and c). While the total number of Aβ plaques was already increased in pregnant mice at G10, particularly in the subiculum, the number of thiazin red positive compact Aβ plaques did not differ (Fig. 1d and e). At G18, both, the number of total and of compact Aβ plaques significantly increased in pregnant 5xFAD mice when compared to controls (non-breeders) at the same age (Fig. 1f and g). In accordance with this higher plaque load in pregnant 5xFAD mice, we found that soluble and insoluble levels of Aβ40 and Aβ42 were increased but did not reach statistical significance in pregnant mice at G18 (Fig. 1h and i). To further determine if multiple pregnancies augment this effect, we next analyzed 40 weeks old female 5xFAD mice that had been pregnant 4 times (multiparous) and compared them with nulliparous mice of the same age (Fig. 2a). Although many plaques were detected in the hippocampi of nulliparous and multiparous 5xFAD transgenic mice

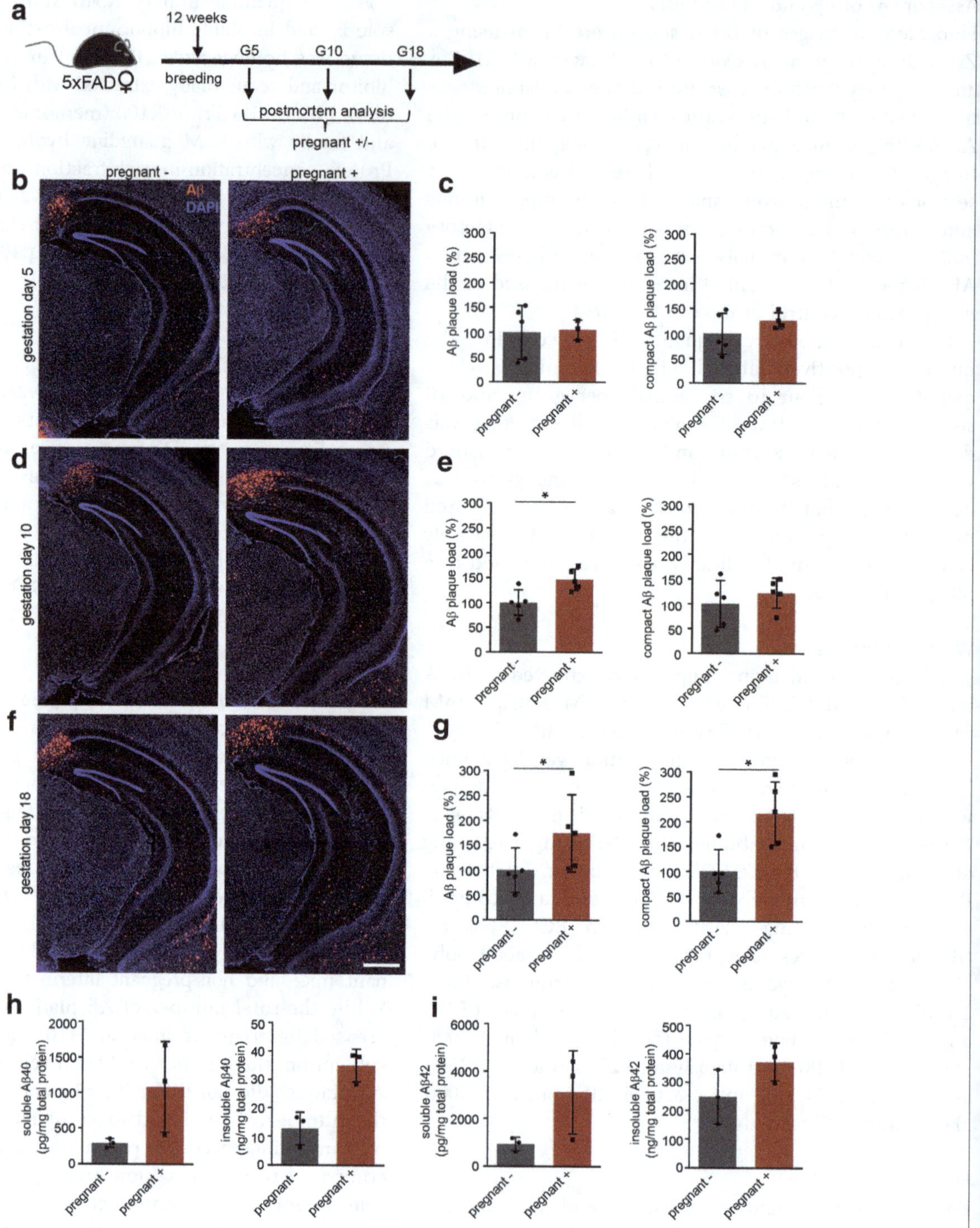

Fig. 1 (See legend on next page.)

(See figure on previous page.)

Fig. 1 Aβ plaque load increases during pregnancy from gestation day 5 to gestation day 18 in 5xFAD female mice. **a** Schematic overview of the experimental setup. Twelve weeks old 5xFAD female mice were breed and either sacrificed at gestation day 5 (G5), G10 or G18. **b** Fluorescence microscopy of Aβ (red) and DAPI (blue). Shown are representative images of hippocampi from female 5xFAD mice not pregnant or pregnant at G5. **c** Quantification of Aβ plaque load (left) and compact Aβ plaque load (right) of not pregnant and pregnant 5xFAD mice at G5 showed no differences between the groups. **d** Fluorescence microscopy of Aβ (red) and DAPI (blue). Shown are representative images of hippocampi from female 5xFAD mice not pregnant or pregnant at G10. **e** Aβ plaque load (left) is significantly increased in pregnant 5xFAD female mice compared to not pregnant mice at G10. Mann-Whitney test, $^*P = 0.03$. **f** Fluorescence microscopy of Aβ (red) and DAPI (blue). Shown are representative images of hippocampi from female 5xFAD mice not pregnant or pregnant at G18. **g** The number of Aβ plaques exhibited significant increase in pregnant 5xFAD mice compared to not pregnant 5xFAD mice at G18. Mann-Whitney test, $^*P = 0.03$. **h** Sandwich immunoassay for Aβ40 soluble and insoluble fractions of hippocampal brain extracts from non-pregnant and pregnant female 5xFAD mice at G18 ($n = 3$). **i** Sandwich immunoassay for Aβ42 soluble and insoluble fractions of hippocampal brain extracts from non-pregnant and pregnant female 5xFAD mice at G18 ($n = 3$). Data are presented as mean ± S.D. Each symbol represents data from one mouse, with four to five mice per group. Scale bar represents 500 μm. G = gestation day

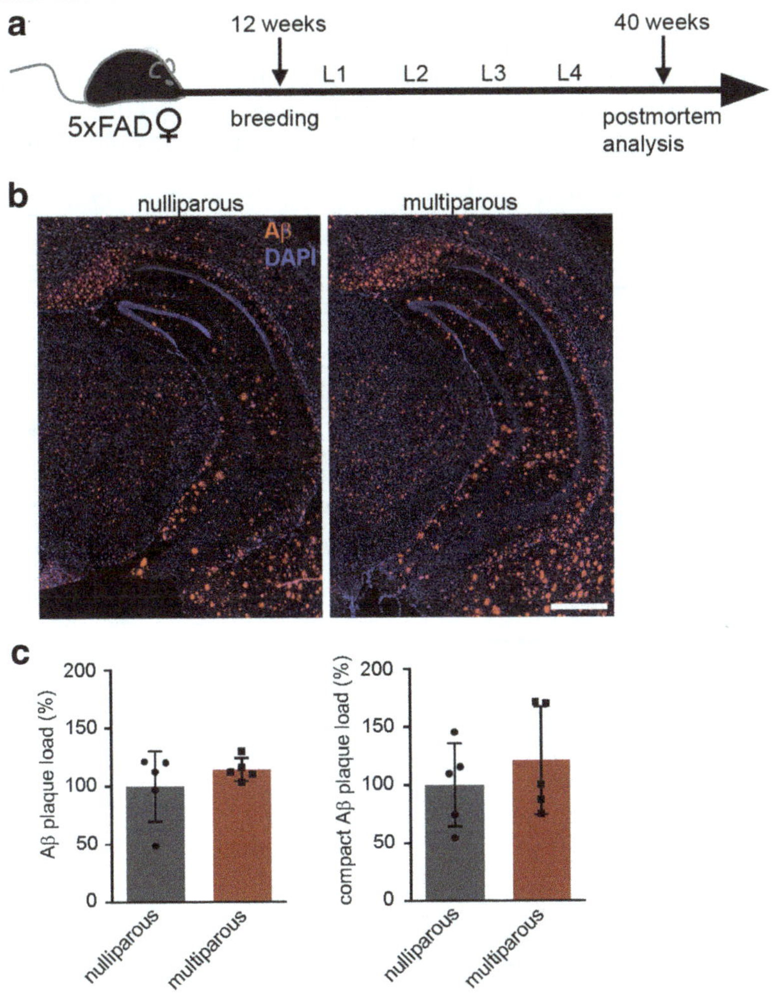

Fig. 2 Unaltered Aβ plaque load in 10 months old nulliparous and multiparous 5xFAD female mice. **a** Schematic overview of the experimental setup. Twelve weeks old 5xFAD female mice were bred and sacrificed at the age of 10 months. Females had either no litter or 4 litters. **b** Fluorescence microscopy of Aβ (red) and DAPI (blue). Shown are representative images of hippocampi from nulliparous and multiparous female 5xFAD mice. **c** Quantification of Aβ plaque load (left) and compact Aβ plaque load (right) of nulliparous and multiparous 5xFAD mice showed no differences between the groups. Data are presented as mean ± S.D. Each symbol represents data from one mouse, with five mice per group. Scale bar represents 500 μm. L = litter

(Fig. 2b), Aβ plaque load did not differ between both groups (Fig. 2c) most likely due to an Aβ overload.

In order to elucidate whether higher Aβ plaque load and Aβ levels in pregnant mice (G18) (Fig. 3a) result from either increased Aβ production or decreased Aβ degradation, we performed Western blot analyses. While full length APP levels were similar, there was a strong increase in monomeric Aβ and APP C-terminal fragments (in particular CTF-β) in pregnant mice, indicating that pregnancy affects the processing of APP and augments Aβ production (Fig. 3b).

Next, we collected blood samples to determine serum estrogen and progesterone levels of non-pregnant and pregnant 5xFAD female mice at G0, G5, G10 and G18. ELISA measurements revealed significant increases in estrogen levels both in pregnant WT and 5xFAD female mice from G5 onwards (Fig. 3c). Serum progesterone levels were enhanced at G10 in pregnant WT and 5xFAD mice. At G18, pregnant WT mice exhibited significantly higher progesterone levels when compared to non-pregnant littermates. Moreover, pregnant 5xFAD mice showed dramatically increased progesterone levels that even exceeded those of pregnant WT mice at G18 (Fig. 3d).

To rule out any effect of pregnancy on the clearance or degradation of Aβ, we determined the protein levels of the enzymes involved in Aβ degradation, neprilysin and IDE, which revealed mixed results. While neprilysin levels were not affected by pregnancy, we found increased IDE levels as measured by Western blotting in the hippocampus of pregnant mice (Fig. 3e), probably due to higher progesterone levels (Fig. 3d) that were shown to significantly increase IDE in vivo in rats [17].

Together, these data suggest that pregnancy modulates Aβ plaque load by increasing the generation of Aβ.

Pregnancy and lactation impair Aβ plaque load in several brain regions of 5xFAD mice

In search of a more detailed approach towards the relationship between pregnancy, motherhood and Aβ deposition, we tested the hypothesis that lactation itself might have an effect on Aβ pathology. Therefore, we mated 12 weeks old 5xFAD mice and subdivided

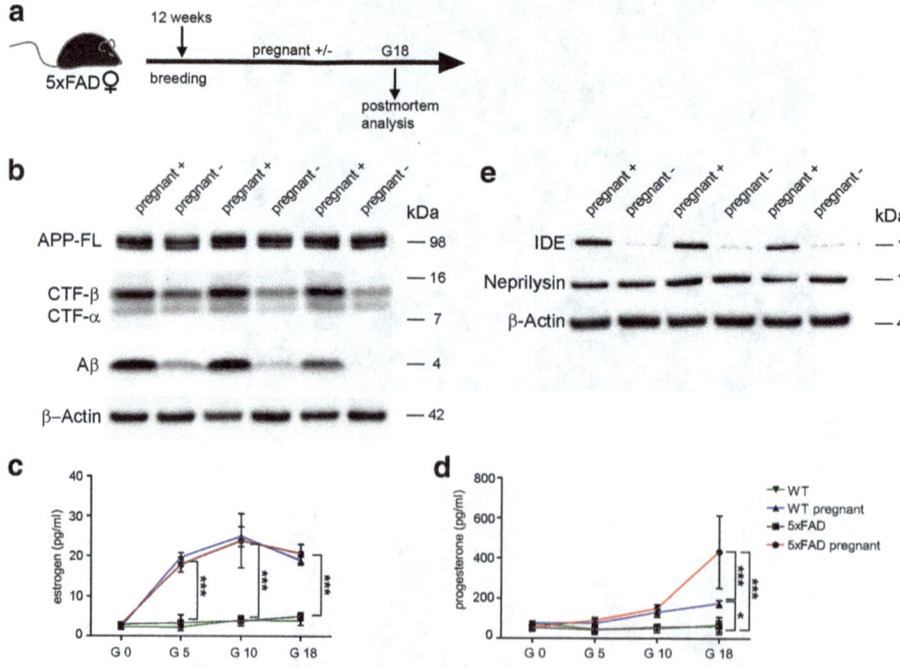

Fig. 3 APP processing is altered in pregnant 5xFAD mice during pregnancy. **a** Schematic overview of the experimental setup. Twelve weeks old 5xFAD female mice were bred and sacrificed at gestation day 18. **b** Immunoblot analysis of hippocampal brain homogenates from pregnant and non-pregnant 5xFAD mice at G18. Immunoblots were probed with antibodies that recognize human full length APP, CTF-β and CTFα (6687) and Aβ (6E10). β-Actin was used as loading control. Pregnant 5xFAD mice showed higher levels of CTF-β and Aβ while APP levels were unaltered. **c** Serum estrogen levels of 5xFAD and WT female mice were measured by ELISA at G0, G5, G10 and G18. Estrogen levels increased during pregnancy in 5xFAD and WT mice (***$P < 0.0001$, ***$P < 0.0001$; ***$P < 0.0001$). **d** Serum progesterone levels of female 5xFAD and WT mice were measured by ELISA at G0, G5, G10 and G18. Progesterone levels increased significantly during pregnancy in 5xFAD and WT mice (*$P = 0.03$; ***$P < 0.0001$; ***$P < 0.0001$). **e** Levels of IDE and neprilysin were detected by western blotting in pregnant and non-pregnant 5xFAD mice. β-Actin was used as loading control. Data are presented as mean ± S.D. Three mice per group were used.
G = gestation day, IDE = insulin-degrading-enzyme

the females after birth into the following 3 groups: a) non-pregnant, b) pregnant but non-lactating and c) pregnant and lactating. All mice were analyzed 4 weeks after delivery at postpartum day 20 (P20) (Fig. 4a). Aβ immunohistochemistry revealed a significantly higher Aβ plaque load in pregnant and lactating female mice compared to non-pregnant mice. Female mice that delivered but were separated from their litter directly after birth had enhanced hippocampal Aβ plaque numbers compared to non-pregnant ones but did not differ from the lactating group (Fig. 4b and c). To confirm these observations in other brain regions, Aβ plaques were analyzed in the cortex and olfactory bulb of the same 5xFAD mice by immunohistochemistry (Fig. 4d and f). In accordance with the results obtained in the hippocampus, the total and compact Aβ plaque load was significantly enhanced in pregnant and lactating female 5xFAD mice at P20 (Fig. 4e), albeit not reaching significance for the total Aβ plaque load in the olfactory bulb (Fig. 4g). In summary, we conclude from these results that pregnancy alone is sufficient to induce this phenotype as lactation has no influence on this pathology.

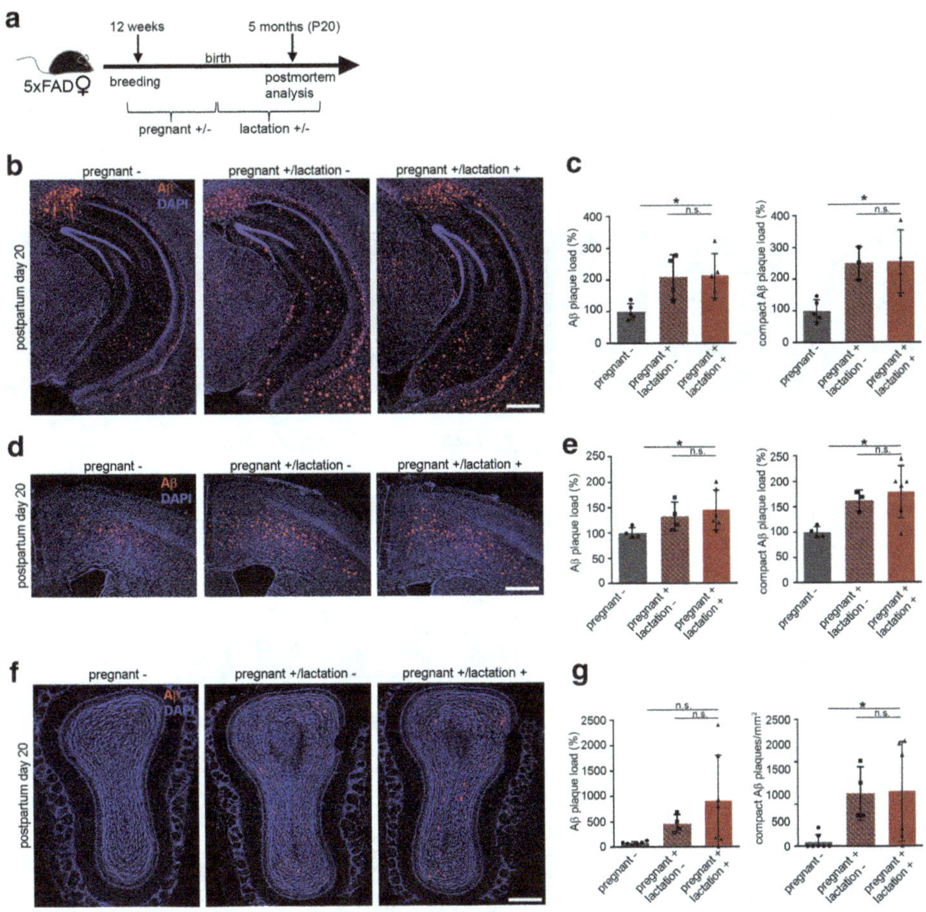

Fig. 4 Pregnancy and not lactation increases Aβ plaque pathology in different brain regions of 5xFAD female mice. **a** Schematic overview of the experimental setup. Twelve weeks old 5xFAD female mice were mated and sacrificed at the age of 5 months (postpartum day 20 (P20)) after the pregnancy and lactation period. One group of mice was separated from the litter directly after the delivery and analyzed 4 weeks later at P20. **b** Fluorescence microscopy of Aβ (red) and DAPI (blue). Shown are representative images of hippocampi from female 5xFAD mice either non-pregnant, pregnant but not lactating or pregnant and lactating at P20. **c** Quantification of Aβ plaque load exhibited significant increases in pregnant and lactating 5xFAD mice. Kruskal-Wallis test followed by Dunn's multiple comparison test, $^*P = 0.03$, $^*P = 0.03$. **d** Fluorescence microscopy of Aβ (red) and DAPI (blue). Shown are representative images of the cortex from female 5xFAD mice either non pregnant, pregnant but not lactating or pregnant and lactating at P20. **e** Quantification of Aβ plaque load in the cortex exhibited significant increases in pregnant and lactating 5xFAD mice compared to nulliparous 5xFAD female mice. Kruskal-Wallis test followed by Dunn's multiple comparison test, $^*p = 0.04$, $^*p = 0.03$. **f** Fluorescence microscopy of Aβ (red) and DAPI (blue). Shown are representative images of the olfactory bulb from female 5xFAD mice either non-pregnant, pregnant but not lactating or pregnant and lactating at P20. **g** Analysis of the number of compact Aβ plaques in the olfactory bulb exhibited significant increases in pregnant and lactating 5xFAD mice compared to nulliparous 5xFAD female mice. Kruskal-Wallis test followed by Dunn's multiple comparison test, $P = 0.056$, $^*P = 0.02$. Data are presented as mean ± S.D. Each symbol represents data from one mouse, with four to seven mice per group. Scale bar represents 500 μm. P = postpartum day

Adult hippocampal neurogenesis and cell proliferation are decreased during pregnancy and lactation period in 5xFAD mice

We determined proliferation and neurogenesis in 5xFAD transgenic and WT mice at P20 and compared them to their non-pregnant littermates to study the effect of pregnancy, lactation and Aβ plaque pathology on cells. While the number of doublecortin (DCX) positive cells dramatically declined during pregnancy in WT and 5xFAD mice, the number of DCX positive neuroblasts and immature neurons did not differ between pregnant/non-lactating and pregnant/lactating 5xFAD females at P20 (Fig. 5a and b), corroborating the aforementioned effect of pregnancy alone. Likewise, the number of Ki67 positive proliferating cells in pregnant WT and 5xFAD mice was significantly decreased (Fig. 5c and d).

Exposure to environmental enrichment and voluntary running during pregnancy circumvents Aβ plaque pathology and vivifies neurogenesis

Inspired by studies that report beneficial effects on the Aβ plaque burden in APP transgenic mice [22] upon exposure to an environmental enrichment (EE) and voluntary running, we exposed pregnant 5xFAD mice to EE during 18 days, based on a published protocol [3], and compared them with pregnant 5xFAD mice housed in standard cages (SH) (Fig. 6a). First, we focused on the question if exposure of the mice to an enriched environment influences their estrogen and progesterone levels. Indeed, progesterone levels of pregnant 5xFAD mice housed in EE dropped significantly to levels that were comparable to WT pregnant mice housed in SH, while estrogen levels remained unaffected (Fig. 6b). Intriguingly, hippocampal and cortical Aβ plaque pathology

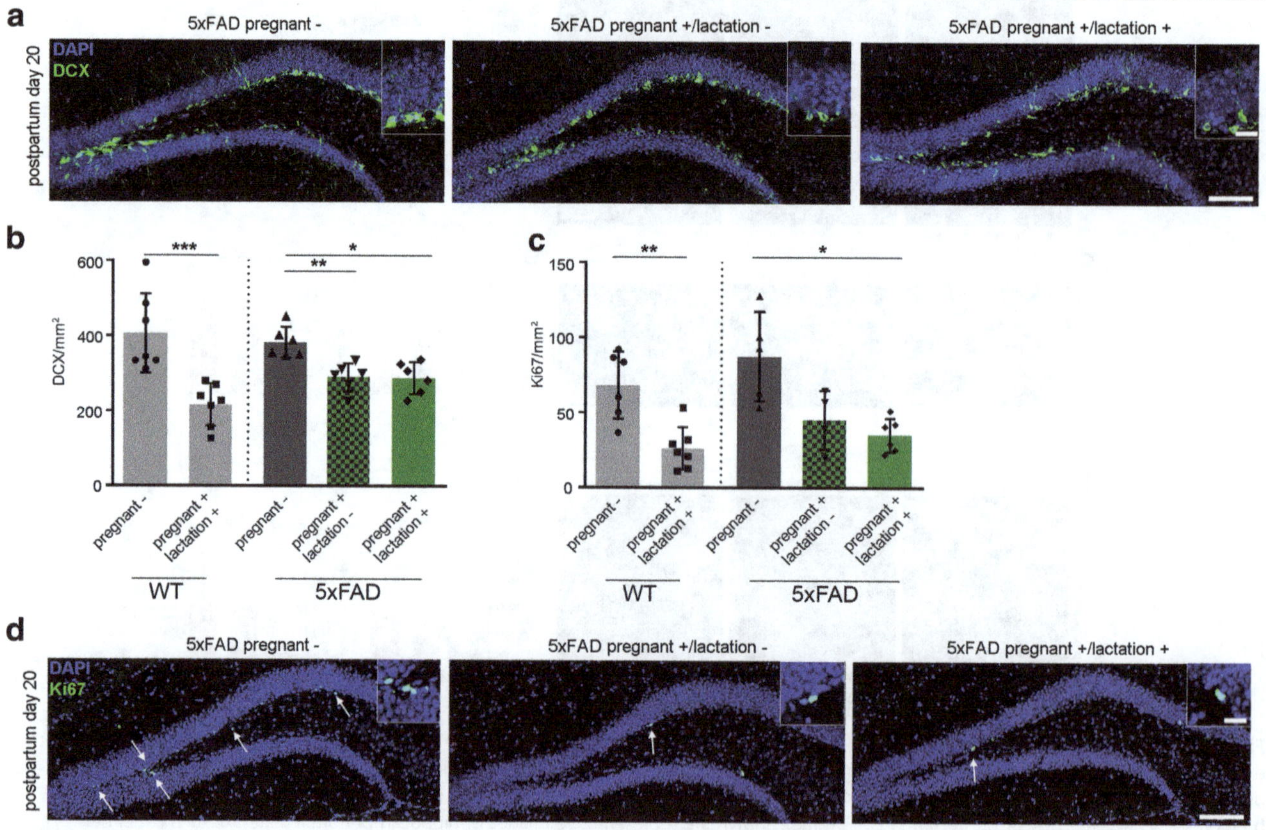

Fig. 5 Decreased adult neurogenesis in pregnant and lactating WT and 5xFAD female mice at P20. **a** Fluorescence microscopy of DCX (green) and DAPI (blue). Shown are representative images of the dentate gyrus from 5xFAD female mice sacrificed at the postpartum day 20 (P20). Inserts show higher magnifications. **b** Quantification of DCX positive cells displayed significant reductions in pregnant and lactating WT and 5xFAD female mice at P20. Mann-Whitney test, $^{**}P = 0.0015$, Kruskal-Wallis test followed by Dunn's multiple comparison test, $^{**}P = 0.0089$, $^{*}P = 0.012$. **c** Quantification of Ki67 positive cells exhibited significant reductions in pregnant and lactating WT and 5xFAD female mice at P20. Mann-Whitney test, $^{**}P = 0.0047$, Kruskal-Wallis test followed by Dunn's multiple comparison test, $^{*}P = 0.02$. **d** Fluorescence microscopy of Ki67 (green) and DAPI (blue). Shown are representative images of the dentate gyrus from 5xFAD female mice sacrificed at P20. White arrows indicate the presence of Ki67 positive cells. Inserts show higher magnifications. Scale bar represents 100 µm in the overview and 20 µm in the inserts. Data are presented as mean ± S.D. Each symbol represents data from one mouse, with five to seven mice per group. P = postpartum day, DCX = doublecortin

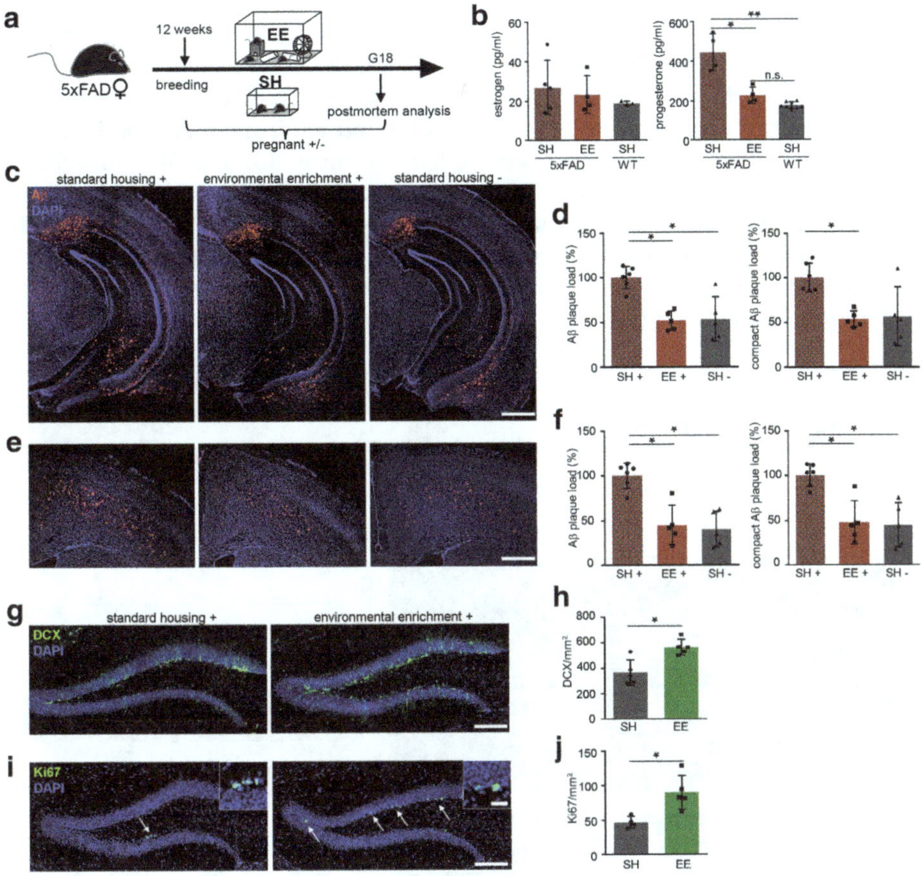

Fig. 6 Environmental enrichment prevents increase in Aβ plaque pathology during pregnancy in 5xFAD mice. **a** Schematic overview of the experimental setup. Twelve weeks old 5xFAD female mice were mated and either housed in standard housing (SH) or in environmental enrichment (EE) until they were sacrificed at gestation day 18 (G18). **b** Serum estrogen and progesterone levels of pregnant 5xFAD and WT female mice exposed to EE or SH were measured by ELISA at G18. Estrogen levels did not differ between EE and SH housed female mice. Progesterone levels decreased in 5xFAD mice housed in EE to the level of standard housed pregnant WT mice. Kruskal-Wallis test followed by Dunn's multiple comparison test, $^{*}P = 0.03$, $^{**}P = 0.0025$. **c** Fluorescence microscopy of Aβ (red) and DAPI (blue). Shown are representative images of hippocampi from pregnant female 5xFAD mice housed in SH or EE and non-pregnant housed in SH. **d** Quantification of Aβ plaque load (left) and compact Aβ plaque load (right) of pregnant 5xFAD mice housed in SH or EE displayed significant decreases in the number of Aβ plaques after housing in EE. Kruskal-Wallis test followed by Dunn's multiple comparison test, $^{*}P = 0.027$, $^{*}P = 0.0178$, $^{*}P = 0.0364$. **e** Fluorescence microscopy of Aβ (red) and DAPI (blue). Shown are representative images of the cortex from pregnant female 5xFAD mice housed in SH or EE and non-pregnant mice housed in SH. **f** Quantification of Aβ plaque load in the cortex of pregnant 5xFAD mice at G18 exhibited significant decreases in mice housed in EE. Kruskal-Wallis test followed by Dunn's multiple comparison test, $^{*}P = 0.040$, $^{*}P = 0.012$, $^{*}P = 0.033$, $^{*}P = 0.014$. **g** Fluorescence microscopy of DCX (green) and DAPI (blue). Shown are representative images of the dentate gyrus from pregnant 5xFAD female mice housed in SH or EE sacrificed at G18. **h** Quantification of DCX positive cells in pregnant 5xFAD mice showed significant increases in mice housed in EE. Mann-Whitney test, $^{*}P = 0.03$. **i** Fluorescence microscopy of Ki67 (green) and DAPI (blue). Shown are representative images of the dentate gyrus from pregnant female 5xFAD mice housed in SH or EE. **j** Analysis of Ki67 positive cells in pregnant 5xFAD mice revealed significant increases in mice housed in EE. Mann-Whitney test, $^{*}P = 0.02$. Inserts show higher magnifications. White arrows indicate Ki67 positive cells. Scale bar represents 500 μm in (**c** and **e**) and 100 μm in (g and i) and 20 μm in the insert. Data are presented as mean ± S.D. Each symbol represents data from one mouse, with four to six mice per group. SH = standard housing, EE = environmental enrichment, DCX = doublecortin, G = gestation day

was significantly decreased in pregnant 5xFAD mice housed in EE compared to pregnant mice housed in SH and even reached an Aβ plaque load similar to the non-pregnant control group housed in SH (Fig. 6c – f).

Since earlier studies reported beneficial effects on adult hippocampal neurogenesis upon exposure to an environmental enrichment (EE) [18, 19] and voluntary running [37, 38], we focused on the question whether EE could be beneficial for pregnant 5xFAD mice as well, by stimulating cell proliferation and adult neurogenesis. Consistent with the literature [18], pregnant 5xFAD mice housed under SH conditions had significantly less DCX labeled cells compared to mice housed in EE (Fig. 6g and h). Moreover, by quantifying Ki67 positive cells, it was clearly evident that pregnant mice housed in EE had significantly more proliferation compared to their counterparts in SH (Fig. 6i and j).

Given the positive effects of EE during pregnancy, we then tested whether the increased Aβ plaque burden during pregnancy and lactation could be reduced or even halted by exposure to an EE. Therefore, 5xFAD mice were mated at the age of 12 weeks and exposed directly to EE from G1 onwards until the end of the weaning period (P20) (Fig. 7a). Indeed, quantitative analysis of Aβ plaque numbers displayed a reduced hippocampal plaque burden in lactating mice housed in EE compared to mice housed in SH that even were comparable to those of the non-pregnant control group housed in SH (Fig. 7b and c). Similar results were obtained by examining Aβ plaques in the cortex (Fig. 7d and e), suggesting an overall beneficial effect of EE on Aβ plaque pathology.

Finally, we studied the influence of EE on cell proliferation and adult neurogenesis in pregnant and lactating 5xFAD mice. Consistent with our previous findings, housing 5xFAD female mice during pregnancy and the lactation period (P20) in EE resulted in a significantly enhanced number of DCX and Ki67 labeled cells compared to mice housed in SH (Fig. 7f – i), thus clearly indicating the beneficial effect of EE during pregnancy.

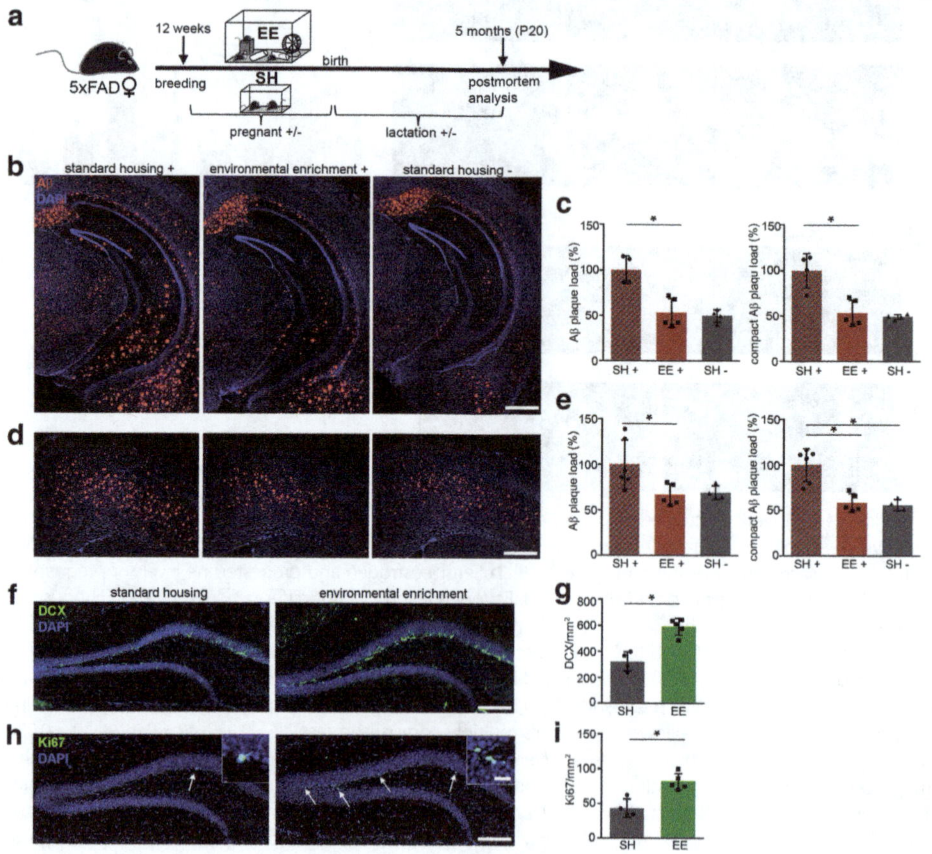

Fig. 7 Environmental enrichment during pregnancy and lactation rescues Aβ plaque pathology in 5xFAD mice. **a** Schematic overview of the experimental setup. Twelve weeks old 5xFAD female mice were mated and either housed in standard housing (SH) or in environmental enrichment (EE) until they were sacrificed at postpartum day 20 (P20). **b** Fluorescence microscopy of Aβ (red) and DAPI (blue). Shown are representative images of hippocampi from pregnant/lactating female 5xFAD mice housed in SH or EE and non-pregnant females housed in SH. **c** Quantification of Aβ plaque load (left) and compact Aβ plaque load (right) of pregnant/lactating 5xFAD mice housed in SH or EE displayed significant decreases in the number of Aβ plaques after housing in EE. Kruskal-Wallis test followed by Dunn's multiple comparison test, $^*P = 0.039$, $^*P = 0.03$. **d** Fluorescence microscopy of Aβ (red) and DAPI (blue). Shown are representative images of the cortex from pregnant/lactating female 5xFAD mice at P20 housed in SH or EE and non-pregnant females housed in SH. **e** Quantification of Aβ plaque load in the cortex of pregnant/lactating 5xFAD mice at P20 exhibited significant decreases in mice housed in EE. Kruskal-Wallis test followed by Dunn's multiple comparison test, $^*P = 0.024$, $^*P = 0.017$. **f** Fluorescence microscopy of DCX (green) and DAPI (blue). Shown are representative images of the dentate gyrus from pregnant 5xFAD female mice housed in SH or EE sacrificed at P20. **g** Quantification of DCX positive cells in pregnant/lactating 5xFAD mice showed significant increases in mice housed in EE. Mann-Whitney test, $^*P = 0.015$. **h** Fluorescence microscopy of Ki67 (green) and DAPI (blue). Shown are representative images of the dentate gyrus from pregnant female 5xFAD mice housed in SH or EE. **i** Analysis of Ki67 positive cells in pregnant/lactating 5xFAD mice revealed significant increases in mice housed in EE. Mann-Whitney test, $^*P = 0.015$. Inserts show higher magnifications. White arrows indicate Ki67 positive cells. Scale bar represents 500 μm in (**b** and **d**) and 100 μm in (**f** and **h**) and 20 μm in the insert. Data are presented as mean ± S.D. Each symbol represents data from one mouse, with four to six mice per group. SH = standard housing, EE = environmental enrichment, DCX = doublecortin, P = postpartum day

Discussion

Age and gender are the greatest non-genetic risk factors for developing sporadic AD. There are indications that reproductive experiences are the cause for an earlier onset of AD in women. However, only few studies have investigated the underlying mechanism for the higher risk of AD in women [6, 7, 31, 33]. Furthermore, the impact of pregnancy on Aβ plaque pathology and adult neurogenesis still remains elusive. To this end, we analyzed pregnant 5xFAD transgenic mice at different gestation days by immunohistochemical stainings and determined the Aβ plaque load as well as proliferation and neurogenesis. Indeed we found that pregnancy alters Aβ plaque pathology in female 5xFAD mice and reduces cell proliferation and the generation of newborn neurons in the hippocampus. Considering that female 5xFAD transgenic mice that also nursed their offspring for 4 weeks had a similar Aβ plaque load and Ki67- and DCX cell counts as merely pregnant mice, we conclude that pregnancy alone is sufficient to exacerbate this pathology.

Epidemiological studies reported that women with multiple pregnancies have an earlier onset of AD and that nulliparous women show less age-related cognitive decline [6, 7, 25, 31]. Our data do not support this view since we could not detect any difference in Aβ plaque load between nulliparous and multiparous 5xFAD female mice, suggesting no higher risk for multiparous female mice. However, we can't exclude the possibility that a significant difference would have been detectable in a slower Aβ aggregation mouse model such as APP23 or Tg2576 with an overall lower Aβ plaque burden at that age. Future studies will need to address this question. In further support of a mechanistic link between pregnancy, motherhood and an increased risk for the development of AD, it is observed that nulliparous women have higher estrogen levels later in life compared to women with reproductive experiences [2, 23]. Nevertheless, it is still under debate if estrogens could also have protective functions and eventually delay the onset of AD [11, 24, 28]. However, most findings in human studies should be taken cautiously because they contain insufficient information on the usage of birth control pills, especially in nulliparous women. While our results demonstrate a substantial increase in Aβ plaque formation during the course of pregnancy in 5xFAD transgenic mice compared to non-pregnant littermates, they also suggest that progesterone rather than estrogen levels might account for this result since estrogen levels were similar in pregnant WT and 5xFAD transgenic mice. The question whether estrogen levels change during aging in 5xFAD transgenic mice still remains open. This could give additional interesting hints specifically in comparison to the situation in humans. Recent work in rats has demonstrated that pregnancy-related hormones might also play a role in Aβ clearance by influencing Aβ clearance factors such as IDE [17]. In agreement with the proposed relationship between levels of pregnancy-related hormones and IDE [17], we indeed found higher IDE levels in pregnant than in non-pregnant 5xFAD mice that also had high progesterone levels. It still remains an open question why pregnant 5xFAD mice had increased Aβ levels despite elevated IDE levels that most likely were not able to execute its Aβ-degrading function. In contrast, neprilysin levels were not altered. Together, these experiments suggest that both, IDE and neprilysin did not affect the clearance of Aβ in a way that could account for the increased plaque density in pregnant mice. Instead, the high amount of CTF-β in pregnant mice might rather indicate that the observed increase in amyloid plaque density was primarily due to alterations in APP processing and Aβ production.

Given that lactation might also affect pathology, we further included non-lactating and lactating 5xFAD mice in our study, in order to determine if lactation could enlarge pathological changes during the postpartum period. In agreement with other studies we were able to confirm that breeders display higher numbers of Aβ plaques compared to non-breeders [8]. Importantly, this finding was applicable to other brain regions, such as the cortex and the olfactory bulb. Interestingly, there was no difference in Aβ plaque pathology between 5xFAD mice that nursed their offspring and those separated from the offspring directly after birth. Therefore we concluded that pregnancy alone is sufficient to induce this phenotype.

Reproductive experience, pregnancy and lactation influence physiological and endocrinological systems in women [4, 30, 32, 36]. Reproductive hormones that are produced during pregnancy and the postpartum period are known to alter neurogenesis and dendritic morphology [30, 32]. Cognitive deficits after reproductive experiences have been reported in human as well as in mouse studies [8, 12], although with inconclusive and contradictory results. While Cui et al [8] were able to show that WT breeders outperformed non-breeders in spatial working and memory they found the opposite in APP transgenic mice. Several studies provided evidence for the involvement of hippocampal neurogenesis in learning and memory and for its alteration under disease conditions such as AD and during reproductive experiences [10, 15, 20, 21]. To establish whether adult hippocampal neurogenesis is altered during the course of pregnancy and in the postpartum period, we carried out a detailed analysis and quantified Ki67 and DCX-positive cells. Indeed, adult hippocampal neurogenesis and cell proliferation were significantly diminished in 5 month old pregnant and lactating 5xFAD mice, suggesting that in the course of pregnancy the generation and maturation of newborn neurons is disturbed. Again, the lactation period alone had no influence on cell proliferation and adult neurogenesis. In summary, our data is in support of several human studies claiming that pregnancy is a risk factor for AD.

Previous work has demonstrated that voluntary running and EE can have beneficial effects on Aβ plaque formation and adult hippocampal neurogenesis [16, 18, 19, 22, 26, 37, 38, 41]. While there is no data published regarding the impact of voluntary running and EE on pregnant and lactating mothers, it has been reported that running during pregnancy reduces the Aβ plaque burden in transgenic offspring [13]. Inspired by a study that reports high running activity of pregnant mice until gestation day 10 [3], we exposed pregnant mice to an EE and investigated Aβ plaque pathology and adult neurogenesis during pregnancy and in the postpartum period. Intriguingly, maternal voluntary running and exercise prevented the pregnancy related increase in Aβ plaque pathology and stimulated cell proliferation as well as the generation of newborn neurons during the course of pregnancy. This beneficial effect of EE during the course of pregnancy was even more pronounced after the lactation period at P20, suggesting stronger effects with longterm EE. It remains to be seen if housing the pregnant mice in EE provides protection early on e.g. already at G10. Future experiments will have to test whether maternal voluntary running and exercise have long lasting effects on Aβ plaque pathology and adult neurogenesis as suggested by others [3] and whether maternal activity might lead to changes in hormone levels, such as estrogens or progesterone.

Conclusion

In conclusion, the present study demonstrates that Aβ plaque formation, cell proliferation and adult neurogenesis are dynamic processes, which can be influenced by reproductive activity on the one hand and physical exercise on the other hand. Together, our findings are unique and underscore the vulnerability of female brains during pregnancy and the effectiveness of EE as a non-pharmacological approach to counteract this happening.

Acknowledgements

We are grateful to J. Zbiegly for technical assistance and S. Kemna and M. Hüll for excellent comments on the manuscript. We also would like to thank E. Kremmer (Ludwig-Maximilians University, Munich) for the Aβ antibodies (3552 and 6687).

Funding

This work was supported by the Deutsche Forschungsgemeinschaft (DFG) ME 3542/2-1 (M.M-L.), the Hans and Ilse Breuer Foundation (M.M-L.) and the 'NeuroMac' Graduate School of the SFB/TRR 167 (M.F.).

Authors' contributions

SZ-W, KM, JS, PdE, MF, DE, LN, VS, IO and MD performed the experimental work. SZ-W and MM-L conceived and designed the experiments. SZ-W contributed to all aspects of the experimental work and data analysis. SZ-W, MP and MM-L discussed the results. SZ-W and MM-L wrote the manuscript; MM-L supervised the project. All authors edited the paper. All authors read and approved the final manuscript.

Competing interests

The authors declare that they have no competing interests.

Author details

[1]Department of Neurology, Medical Center – University of Freiburg, Freiburg, Germany. [2]Faculty of Medicine, University of Freiburg, Freiburg, Germany. [3]Faculty of Biology, University of Freiburg, Freiburg, Germany. [4]Institute of Neuropathology, Medical Center – University of Freiburg, Freiburg, Germany. [5]BIOSS Centre for Biological Signalling Studies, University of Freiburg, Freiburg, Germany. [6]Neurocenter, University of Freiburg, Breisacher Str.64, 79106 Freiburg, Germany.

References

1. Bayer TA, Schafer S, Simons A, Kemmling A, Kamer T, Tepest R, Eckert A, Schussel K, Eikenberg O, Sturchler-Pierrat C et al (2003) Dietary cu stabilizes brain superoxide dismutase 1 activity and reduces amyloid Abeta production in APP23 transgenic mice. Proc Natl Acad Sci U S A 100:14187–14192
2. Bernstein L, Pike MC, Ross RK, Judd HL, Brown JB, Henderson BE (1985) Estrogen and sex hormone-binding globulin levels in nulliparous and parous women. J Natl Cancer Inst 74:741–745
3. Bick-Sander A, Steiner B, Wolf SA, Babu H, Kempermann G (2006) Running in pregnancy transiently increases postnatal hippocampal neurogenesis in the offspring. Proc Natl Acad Sci U S A 103:3852–3857
4. Bridges RS (2016) Long-term alterations in neural and endocrine processes induced by motherhood in mammals. Horm Behav 77:193–203
5. Callahan MJ, Lipinski WJ, Bian F, Durham RA, Pack A, Walker LC (2001) Augmented senile plaque load in aged female beta-amyloid precursor protein-transgenic mice. Am J Pathol 158:1173–1177
6. Colucci M, Cammarata S, Assini A, Croce R, Clerici F, Novello C, Mazzella L, Dagnino N, Mariani C, Tanganelli P (2006) The number of pregnancies is a risk factor for Alzheimer's disease. Eur J Neurol 13:1374–1377
7. Corbo RM, Gambina G, Ulizzi L, Monini P, Broggio E, Rosano A, Scacchi R (2007) Combined effect of apolipoprotein e genotype and past fertility on age at onset of Alzheimer's disease in women. Dement Geriatr Cogn Disord 24:82–85
8. Cui J, Jothishankar B, He P, Staufenbiel M, Shen Y, Li R (2014) Amyloid precursor protein mutation disrupts reproductive experience-enhanced normal cognitive development in a mouse model of Alzheimer's disease. Mol Neurobiol 49:103–112
9. Cummings JL (2004) Alzheimer's disease. N Engl J Med 351:56–67
10. Ekonomou A, Savva GM, Brayne C, Forster G, Francis PT, Johnson M, Perry EK, Attems J, Somani A, Minger SL et al (2015) Stage-specific changes in neurogenic and glial markers in Alzheimer's disease. Biol Psychiatry 77:711–719
11. Henderson VW, Paganini-Hill A, Emanuel CK, Dunn ME, Buckwalter JG (1994) Estrogen replacement therapy in older women. Comparisons between Alzheimer's disease cases and nondemented control subjects. Arch Neurol 51:896–900
12. Henry JF, Sherwin BB (2012) Hormones and cognitive functioning during late pregnancy and postpartum: a longitudinal study. Behav Neurosci 126: 73–85
13. Herring A, Donath A, Yarmolenko M, Uslar E, Conzen C, Kanakis D, Bosma C, Worm K, Paulus W, Keyvani K (2012) Exercise during pregnancy mitigates Alzheimer-like pathology in mouse offspring. FASEB J 26:117–128
14. Hirata-Fukae C, Li HF, Hoe HS, Gray AJ, Minami SS, Hamada K, Niikura T, Hua F, Tsukagoshi-Nagai H, Horikoshi-Sakuraba Y et al (2008) Females exhibit more extensive amyloid, but not tau, pathology in an Alzheimer transgenic model. Brain Res 1216:92–103
15. Hollands C, Bartolotti N, Lazarov O (2016) Alzheimer's disease and hippocampal adult neurogenesis; exploring shared mechanisms. Front Neurosci 10:178

16. Hu YS, Xu P, Pigino G, Brady ST, Larson J, Lazarov O (2010) Complex environment experience rescues impaired neurogenesis, enhances synaptic plasticity, and attenuates neuropathology in familial Alzheimer's disease-linked APPswe/PS1DeltaE9 mice. FASEB J 24:1667–1681
17. Jayaraman A, Carroll JC, Morgan TE, Lin S, Zhao L, Arimoto JM, Murphy MP, Beckett TL, Finch CE, Brinton RD et al (2012) 17beta-estradiol and progesterone regulate expression of beta-amyloid clearance factors in primary neuron cultures and female rat brain. Endocrinology 153:5467–5479
18. Kempermann G, Kuhn HG, Gage FH (1997) More hippocampal neurons in adult mice living in an enriched environment. Nature 386:493–495
19. Kempermann G, Kuhn HG, Gage FH (1998) Experience-induced neurogenesis in the senescent dentate gyrus. J Neurosci 18:3206–3212
20. Lazarov O, Marr RA (2010) Neurogenesis and Alzheimer's disease: at the crossroads. Exp Neurol 223:267–281
21. Lazarov O, Mattson MP, Peterson DA, Pimplikar SW, van Praag H (2010) When neurogenesis encounters aging and disease. Trends Neurosci 33: 569–579
22. Lazarov O, Robinson J, Tang YP, Hairston IS, Korade-Mirnics Z, Lee VM, Hersh LB, Sapolsky RM, Mirnics K, Sisodia SS (2005) Environmental enrichment reduces Abeta levels and amyloid deposition in transgenic mice. Cell 120: 701–713
23. Lee JH, Jiang Y, Han DH, Shin SK, Choi WH, Lee MJ (2014) Targeting estrogen receptors for the treatment of Alzheimer's disease. Mol Neurobiol 49:39–49
24. Liang K, Yang L, Yin C, Xiao Z, Zhang J, Liu Y, Huang J (2010) Estrogen stimulates degradation of beta-amyloid peptide by up-regulating neprilysin. J Biol Chem 285:935–942
25. McLay RN, Maki PM, Lyketsos CG (2003) Nulliparity and late menopause are associated with decreased cognitive decline. J Neuropsychiatry Clin Neurosci 15:161–167
26. Nilsson M, Perfilieva E, Johansson U, Orwar O, Eriksson PS (1999) Enriched environment increases neurogenesis in the adult rat dentate gyrus and improves spatial memory. J Neurobiol 39:569–578
27. Oakley H, Cole SL, Logan S, Maus E, Shao P, Craft J, Guillozet-Bongaarts A, Ohno M, Disterhoft J, Van Eldik L et al (2006) Intraneuronal beta-amyloid aggregates, neurodegeneration, and neuron loss in transgenic mice with five familial Alzheimer's disease mutations: potential factors in amyloid plaque formation. J Neurosci 26:10129–10140
28. Paganini-Hill A, Henderson VW (1994) Estrogen deficiency and risk of Alzheimer's disease in women. Am J Epidemiol 140:256–261
29. Paxinos G, Franklin KBJ (2001) The mouse brain in stereotaxic coordinates 2n edn. San Diego, Academic Press
30. Prange-Kiel J, Rune GM (2006) Direct and indirect effects of estrogen on rat hippocampus. Neuroscience 138:765–772
31. Ptok U, Barkow K, Heun R (2002) Fertility and number of children in patients with Alzheimer's disease. Arch Womens Ment Health 5:83–86
32. Shingo T, Gregg C, Enwere E, Fujikawa H, Hassam R, Geary C, Cross JC, Weiss S (2003) Pregnancy-stimulated neurogenesis in the adult female forebrain mediated by prolactin. Science 299:117–120
33. Sobow T, Kloszewska I (2004) Parity, number of pregnancies, and the age of onset of Alzheimer's disease. J Neuropsychiatry Clin Neurosci. 16:120–121
34. Steiner H, Kostka M, Romig H, Basset G, Pesold B, Hardy J, Capell A, Meyn L, Grim ML, Baumeister R et al (2000) Glycine 384 is required for presenilin-1 function and is conserved in bacterial polytopic aspartyl proteases. Nat Cell Biol 2:848–851
35. Sturchler-Pierrat C, Staufenbiel M (2000) Pathogenic mechanisms of Alzheimer's disease analyzed in the APP23 transgenic mouse model. Ann N Y Acad Sci 920:134–139
36. Tomizawa K, Iga N, Lu YF, Moriwaki A, Matsushita M, Li ST, Miyamoto O, Itano T, Matsui H (2003) Oxytocin improves long-lasting spatial memory during motherhood through MAP kinase cascade. Nat Neurosci 6:384–390
37. van Praag H, Christie BR, Sejnowski TJ, Gage FH (1999a) Running enhances neurogenesis, learning, and long-term potentiation in mice. Proc Natl Acad Sci U S A 96:13427–13431
38. van Praag H, Kempermann G, Gage FH (1999b) Running increases cell proliferation and neurogenesis in the adult mouse dentate gyrus. Nat Neurosci 2:266–270
39. Wang J, Tanila H, Puolivali J, Kadish I, van Groen T (2003) Gender differences in the amount and deposition of amyloidbeta in APPswe and PS1 double transgenic mice. Neurobiol Dis 14:318–327
40. Yamasaki A, Eimer S, Okochi M, Smialowska A, Kaether C, Baumeister R, Haass C, Steiner H (2006) The GxGD motif of presenilin contributes to catalytic function and substrate identification of gamma-secretase. J Neurosci 26:3821–3828
41. Ziegler-Waldkirch S, d'Errico P, Sauer JF, Erny D, Savanthrapadian S, Loreth D, Katzmarski N, Blank T, Bartos M, Prinz M et al (2018) Seed-induced Abeta deposition is modulated by microglia under environmental enrichment in a mouse model of Alzheimer's disease. EMBO J 37:167–182

7

LRRK2 activity does not dramatically alter α-synuclein pathology in primary neurons

Michael X. Henderson, Chao Peng, John Q. Trojanowski and Virginia M. Y. Lee*

Abstract

Mutations in leucine-rich repeat kinase (LRRK2) are the most common cause of heritable Parkinson's disease (PD), and the most common mutations in LRRK2 lead to elevated kinase activity. For these reasons, inhibitors targeting LRRK2 have been the subject of intense research and development. However, it has been difficult to develop preclinical models that recapitulate PD-relevant LRRK2 phenotypes. The primary pathology in PD is the Lewy body (LB), which is a cytoplasmic aggregate of α-synuclein. The recent demonstration that LB-like aggregates of α-synuclein can be induced in primary neurons has provided a robust model for testing genetic modifiers of PD-relevant aggregation and neurodegeneration. In this study, we test the modulation of α-synuclein pathology by LRRK2 in primary neuron cultures using biochemistry and immunocytochemistry. We find that expression of familial mutant G2019S LRRK2 does not dramatically elevate the pathological burden of α-synuclein or neurodegeneration in neurons. We further test three LRRK2 inhibitors in two strains of wildtype neurons and find that even robust LRRK2 inhibition is insufficient to reduce α-synuclein pathology. LRRK2 inhibitors similarly had no effect in neurons with α-synuclein pathology seeded by human brain-derived pathological α-synuclein. Finally, we find that this lack of pathological modulation by LRRK2 was not confined to hippocampal neurons, but was also absent in midbrain dopaminergic neuron cultures. These data demonstrate that LRRK2 activity does not have more than minor effects on α-synuclein pathology in primary neurons, and more complex models may be needed to evaluate the ability of LRRK2 inhibitors to treat PD.

Keywords: LRRK2, Synuclein, pS129, Aggregates, Inhibitor, G2019S

Introduction

Parkinson's disease (PD) is the most common neurodegenerative movement disorder. Patients with this disease experience rigidity, resting tremors, and slowness of movement; 80% of patients will develop dementia throughout the disease course [15]. The clinical diagnosis of PD is confirmed post-mortem by the presence of intracytoplasmic inclusions termed Lewy bodies (LBs), which consist primarily of the synaptic protein α-synuclein [1, 29, 30]. While α-synuclein is thought to be pathogenic in this largely sporadic disease, mutations in several genes can increase the lifetime risk of developing disease. The most commonly mutated gene in hereditary PD is leucine-rich repeat kinase 2 (LRRK2, [11]).

LRRK2 is a widely expressed protein with unclear functions. It has kinase, GTPase and scaffolding domains and has been implicated in intracellular trafficking and cytoskeletal modeling [17]. LRRK2 mutations are found in 4% of hereditary and 1% of sporadic PD patients, and patients with LRRK2 mutations phenocopy sporadic PD patients, with similar onset of disease, α-synuclein pathology, and responsiveness to dopamine replacement [11]. The most common mutation (G2019S) in the kinase domain as well as mutations in the GTPase domain of LRRK2, elevate kinase activity of LRRK2 [8, 26, 31, 36], making LRRK2 an ideal candidate for small molecule inhibitor development. A large number of LRRK2 inhibitors have been developed and refined for increased potency and low off-target effects over the past decade. However, the lack of a reliable preclinical disease model for LRRK2 dysfunction has been a major challenge for validating the therapeutic potential of LRRK2 inhibitors.

To understand the relationship between LRRK2 and α-synuclein and develop a model of LRRK2-dependent PD phenotypes, early studies crossed mice expressing wildtype or G2019S LRRK2 mice with mice overexpressing α-synuclein with the familial A53T mutation. These

* Correspondence: vmylee@upenn.edu
Department of Pathology and Laboratory Medicine, Institute on Aging and Center for Neurodegenerative Disease Research, University of Pennsylvania School of Medicine, 3600 Spruce St, 3rd Floor Maloney, Philadelphia, PA 19104-4283, USA

studies all found little or no effect of LRRK2 expression on α-synuclein pathology [4, 14, 20]. However, later studies which injected adeno-associated virus into the substantia nigra of LRRK2 knockout or G2019S LRRK2 rats found that LRRK2 depletion rescued α-synuclein-induced neurodegeneration [5] and G2019S LRRK2 exacerbated degeneration [3]. Several cell culture studies have found that LRRK2 may directly interact with α-synuclein [9] or indirectly influence α-synuclein expression [23, 28], however none of these cell culture models recapitulate the phosphorylated, detergent-insoluble α-synuclein seen in PD patients. The recent finding that α-synuclein pathology can be induced in wildtype primary neurons by introduction of small amounts of recombinant α-synuclein pre-formed fibrils (PFFs) has allowed the study of α-synuclein pathology in neurons expressing wildtype or mutated LRRK2 [32]. A primary neuron model in which LRRK2 activity modulates α-synuclein pathology would be ideal for screening LRRK2 inhibitors and providing biological rationale for moving toward clinical intervention. We used robust immunocytochemical and biochemical assays for α-synuclein pathology in primary hippocampal and midbrain dopaminergic neurons derived from two strains of wildtype mice and mice expressing the LRRK2 with the familial G2019S mutation to test LRRK2 activity-dependent phenotypes. We induce α-synuclein pathology with addition of both recombinant and human-derived fibrillar α-synuclein. In order to manipulate LRRK2 activity, we used three validated LRRK2 inhibitors. In no system and by no measure did we observe more than very mild LRRK2-dependent changes in α-synuclein pathology.

Materials and methods

Animals

All housing, breeding, and procedures were performed according to the NIH Guide for the Care and Use of Experimental Animals and approved by the University of Pennsylvania Institutional Animal Care and Use Committee. C57BL/6 J (NTG, JAX 000664, RRID: IMSR_JAX:000664) and B6.Cg-Tg(Lrrk2*G2019S)2Yue/J (G2019S, JAX 012467, RRID: IMSR_JAX:012467) mice were obtained from Andrew West (University of Alabama, Birmingham). The G2019S mice have multiple inserts of the gene, but were heterozygous at these loci. Subsequently, mice were bred to homozygosity at loci as determined by quantitative PCR and outbreeding. The expression level of G2019S LRRK2 was thereby stabilized in this line of mice. All experiments shown use homozygous G2019S mice. CD1 (Strain 022, RRID: IMSR_CRL:22) mice were obtained from Charles River, Wilmington, MA.

α-Synuclein PFFs

Purification of recombinant α-synuclein and generation of α-synuclein PFFs was conducted as described elsewhere [21, 33, 34]. For treatment of neurons, α-synuclein PFFs, which were generated at a concentration of 5 mg/mL were vortexed and diluted with Dulbecco's phosphate-buffered saline (DPBS) to 100 μg/mL. They were then sonicated on high for 10 cycles of 30 s on, 30 s off (Diagenode Biorupter UCD-300 bath sonicator). α-Synuclein PFFs were then diluted in neuron media to 5 μg/mL and added to neuron cultures at a concentration of 1 μg/mL for immunocytochemistry experiments and 2.5 μg/mL for biochemistry experiments.

Primary hippocampal cultures

Primary hippocampal neuron cultures were prepared from postnatal day (P) 1 NTG and G2019S mice and embryonic day (E) 16–18 CD1 embryos. Dissociated hippocampal neurons were plated at 17,000 cells/well (96-well plate) or 1,000,000 cells/well (6-well plate) in neuron media (Neurobasal medium (ThermoFisher 21,103,049) (or Neurobasal A medium (Thermo Fisher 10,888–022) for postnatal cultures) supplemented with B27 (ThermoFisher 17,504,044), 2 mM GlutaMax (ThermoFisher 35,050,061), and 100 U/mL penicillin/streptomycin (ThermoFisher 15,140,122). LRRK2 inhibitors PF-475 and PF-360 were synthesized at Pfizer, Inc. MLi-2 was obtained from Tocris Bioscience (5756). All LRRK2 inhibitors were reconstituted at 10 mM in DMSO and stored at − 20 °C. There were further diluted to the final concentration indicated in neuron media with DMSO as a vehicle control. Neurons were either fixed with 4% paraformaldehyde, 4% sucrose in phosphate-buffered saline for immunocytochemistry or scraped for biochemistry.

Primary midbrain/striatum co-cultures

The ventral mesencephalon and striatum were dissected from P2 NTG and G2019S mice in Hibernate A medium (ThermoFisher A1247501) with B27 (ThermoFisher 17,504,044) and 0.5 mM GlutaMax (ThermoFisher 35,050,061). The tissue was then digested in papain (Worthington Biochemical LS003126) for ~ 20 min at 37 °C. Cells were mixed at a ratio of 1:1 and plated at a density of 34,000 cells/well in 96-well black-walled plates (Perkin Elmer 50–905-1605) in Neurobasal A medium (Thermo Fisher 10,888–022) supplemented with B27 and 0.4 mM GlutaMax, 50 ng/mL BDNF (PeproTech 450–02) and 30 ng/mL GDNF (Millipore Sigma GF030).

Neuron sequential detergent fractionation

Proteins from primary neuronal cultures treated with PBS or α-synuclein PFFs were sequentially extracted as described previously [21, 33, 34]. Briefly, neurons were scraped into 1 volume 1% TX-100 buffer, sonicated and spun at 100,000 x *g* for 30 min. The pellet was sonicated and again spun at 100,000 x *g* for 30 min in 1 volume 1% TX-100 solution to remove remaining TX-100-soluble proteins. This pellet was suspended in 0.5 volumes 2% SDS solution, sonicated and spun once more at 100,000 x *g* for 30 min. The first and final supernatant were kept for immunoblot analysis. Western Blot analysis was performed with primary antibodies targeting α-synuclein (SNL-4, CNDR, 1:10,000), pS129 α-synuclein (ab168381, Abcam, 1:1000), LRRK2 (3514–1, Epitomics, RRID: AB_10643781, 1:2000 or ab133474, Abcam, RRID: AB_2713963, 1:500), pS935 LRRK2 (ab133450, Abcam, 1:500), p62 (H00008878-M01, Abnova, RRID: AB_437085, 1:1000) or GAPDH (2-RGM2, Advanced Immunological, 1:5000). Primary antibodies were detected using IRDye 800 (Li-cor 925–32,210) or IRDye 680 (Li-cor 925–68,071) secondary antibodies, scanned on Li-cor Odyssey Imaging System and analyzed using Image Studio software. Values obtained from this program were normalized to average PFF alone values.

Human brain sequential detergent fractionation

Frozen postmortem human cingulate gyrus or frontal cortex brain tissue containing abundant α-synuclein-positive inclusions was selected for sequential extraction based on IHC examination of these samples as described [16] using previously established methods. These brains were sequentially extracted with increasing detergent strength as previously published [10]. After thawing, meninges were removed and gray matter was carefully separated from white matter. Gray matter was weighed and suspended in four volumes (*w*/*v*) high salt (HS) buffer (50 mM Tris-HCL (pH 7.4), 750 mM NaCl, 10 mM NaF, 5 mM EDTA, protease and phosphatase inhibitors), followed by homogenization with a dounce homogenizer and centrifugation at 100,000 x *g* for 30 min. The HS wash was repeated and the resulting pellet was then homogenized with 9 volumes HS buffer with 1% TX-100 and centrifuged at 100,000 x *g* for 30 min. The pellet fraction was then homogenized with 9 volumes HS buffer with 1% TX-100 and 30% sucrose and centrifuged at 100,000 x *g* for 30 min to float away the myelin, which was discarded. The pellet was then homogenized with 9 volumes HS buffer with 1% Sarkosyl, rotated for 1 h at room temperature and centrifuged at 100,000 x *g* for 30 min. The resulting pellets were washed once with Dulbecco's PBS and re-suspended in Dulbecco's PBS by brief sonication (QSonica Microson™ XL-2000; 20 pulses; setting 2; 0.5 s/pulse). This suspension was termed the "sarkosyl insoluble fraction" containing pathological α-synuclein and used for the cellular assays described here. The amounts of α-synuclein in the sarkosyl insoluble fractions were determined by sandwich ELISA as described previously [2] using Syn9027 (100 ng/well) as the capture antibody and MJF-R1 (1:1000 dilution) as the reporter antibody.

Immunocytochemistry

Immunostaining of neuronal cultures was carried out as described previously [12]. Briefly, cells were permeabilized in 3% BSA + 0.3% TX-100 in PBS for 15 min at room temperature. After a PBS wash, cells were blocked for 50 min with 3% BSA in PBS prior to incubation with primary antibodies for 2 h at room temperature. Primary antibodies used were targeting pS129 α-synuclein (81A, CNDR, 1:5000), MAP2 (17028, CNDR, 1:5000), NeuN (MAB377, Millipore, RRID: AB_2298772, 1:1500) or tyrosine hydroxylase (TH, T2928, Sigma-Aldrich, RRID: AB_477569, 1:1000). Cells were washed 5× with PBS and incubated with secondary antibodies for 1 h at room temperature. After 5× wash with PBS, cells were incubated in 1:10,000 DAPI in PBS. 96-well plates were imaged on In Cell Analyzer 2200 (GE Healthcare) and analyzed in the accompanying software. A standard intensity-based threshold was applied to MAP2 and pS129 α-synuclein channels and positive area was quantified. For NeuN quantification, an object-based analysis was applied to identify objects of specified size and intensity. TH+ cell analysis was based on intensity and size of objects (TH+ cells bodies are much more intense than associated processes). All quantification was optimized and applied equally across all conditions.

Statistical analysis

All statistical analyses were done in GraphPad Prism. The analysis used for each data set is described in the accompanying figure legend. More specifically, for experiments directly comparing only NTG and G2019S neurons (Fig. 1), unpaired t-tests with Welch's corrections were performed. For experiments in which various inhibitors were compared, one-way ANOVAs with Dunnett's multiple comparison test (Figs. 3 and 4b, d) or Kruskal-Wallis tests with Dunn's multiple comparisons tests (Figs. 4b, e, f and 5) were performed. Experiments which included both NTG and G2019S neurons and various treatment conditions (Figs. 2 and 6), we performed two-way ANOVAs with Dunnett's multiple comparison test to compare treatment type and Sidak's multiple comparison test to evaluate the difference between genotypes.

Results

G2019S LRRK2 expression does not affect soluble or insoluble α-synuclein in hippocampal neurons

To establish a model in which the effect of LRRK2 mutations on α-synuclein could be observed, we used a transgenic BAC mouse which expresses mouse LRRK2 with the familial G2019S mutation under the endogenous LRRK2 promoter (B6.Cg-Tg(Lrrk2*G2019S)2Yue/J, [19]). This allows overexpression of the mutated LRRK2 in a similar pattern to endogenous LRRK2 [35]. Upon

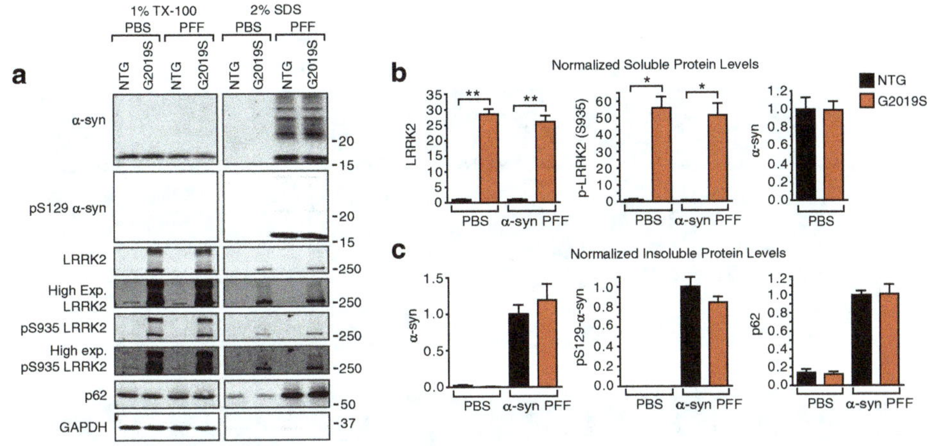

Fig. 1 G2019S LRRK2 hippocampal neurons do not have elevated α-synuclein pathology 14 days post-transduction. **a** Primary hippocampal neurons from NTG or G2019S pups were transduced with 2.5 μg/mL α-synuclein PFFs and allowed to age a further 14 days prior to sequential detergent fractionation. TX-100-insoluble α-synuclein and p62 are similar in both neuron types. **b** Quantification of soluble proteins shows ~ 25-fold elevation in the expression of LRRK2 and a commensurate ~ 50-fold elevation in pS395 LRRK2, indicative of the elevated LRRK2 kinase activity associated with the G2019S mutation. Soluble α-synuclein levels were equivalent between the cultures. **c** No significant differences were found between the genotypes in insoluble proteins by an unpaired t-test with Welch's correction. ($N = 3$ biological replicates for each protein). Means + s.e.m.; $**P < 0.01$; $*P < 0.05$ by an unpaired t-test with Welch's correction for unequal variances. All values are normalized to NTG neurons treated with α-synuclein PFFs and DMSO

initiation of breeding, it was discovered that the mice have multiple inserts of the transgene and were heterozygous at all loci, resulting in non-transgenic pups upon inbreeding in a stochastic manner. To ensure homogeneity of cultures and reproducibility of results, the mice were bred to stable homozygosity as confirmed by quantitative PCR and outbreeding. The genotype of all animals used for culture was confirmed by quantitative PCR. We cultured primary hippocampal neurons from the G2019S LRRK2 (G2019S) or C57BL/6 J (NTG) control animals. G2019S neurons express ~ 25-fold elevated LRRK2, resulting in ~ 50-fold increase in phosphorylated LRRK2 at residue Ser935 (pS935), a readout for LRRK2 activity [6, 7, 26] (Fig. 1a, b). Despite dramatic elevation in LRRK2 expression and activity, soluble α-synuclein levels were unchanged (Fig. 1a, b). We induced α-synuclein pathology in these cultures as described previously [12] by adding 2.5 μg/mL recombinant mouse α-synuclein pre-formed fibrils (PFFs) to the cultures at 7 days in vitro (DIV) and allowing the neurons to develop pathology for a further 14 days post-transduction (DPT). The protein from neurons was then sequentially extracted in 1% TX-100 followed by 2% SDS, allowing the separation of pathological, insoluble α-synuclein from soluble α-synuclein. Both NTG and G2019S neurons accumulated insoluble α-synuclein phosphorylated at residue Ser129 (pS129) to a similar extent (Fig. 1a, c). Additionally, the autophagy receptor p62, which decorates pathological inclusions, including Lewy bodies in PD, accumulates to a similar extent in both genotypes (Fig. 1a, c). Thus, a dramatic elevation in LRRK2 activity does not alter pathological α-synuclein accumulation at 14 DPT.

G2019S LRRK2 hippocampal neurons show mild, reversible elevation in α-synuclein pathology at 21 DPT

However, it has recently been demonstrated that G2019S neurons may show time-dependent changes in α-synuclein pathology that don't become apparent until 18 DPT [32]. Therefore, we cultured NTG and G2019S neurons, treated at 7 DIV with 1 μg/mL α-synuclein PFFs, and allowed the neurons to develop pathology for 21 DPT. In addition, we treated the neurons 2 days prior to transduction with two validated LRRK2 inhibitors, PF-06447475 (PF-475) and PF-06685360 (PF-360) at 5, 30, and 120 nM. At 21 DPT, the neurons were fixed and stained for pS129 α-synuclein, MAP2 (a somatodendritic marker), and NeuN (a marker of neuronal nuclei). Both NTG and G2019S neurons develop robust neuritic and cell body pathology in comparison to neurons treated with PBS as a vehicle control which never develop pS129 α-synuclein inclusions (Fig. 2a, b). We were able to detect a mild elevation of α-synuclein pathology in the G2019S neurons, which was reversible with 30 and 120 nM PF-360 (Fig. 2a, b, c). In every other respect measured, NTG and G2019S neurons responded similarly to α-synuclein PFF treatment. The area covered by MAP2 and the number of neurons were not different between the two genotypes (Fig. 2d, e), and the mild elevation in pathology did not induce further toxicity. In addition, at no concentration did the LRRK2 inhibitors affect α-synuclein pathology, MAP2 area or neuron

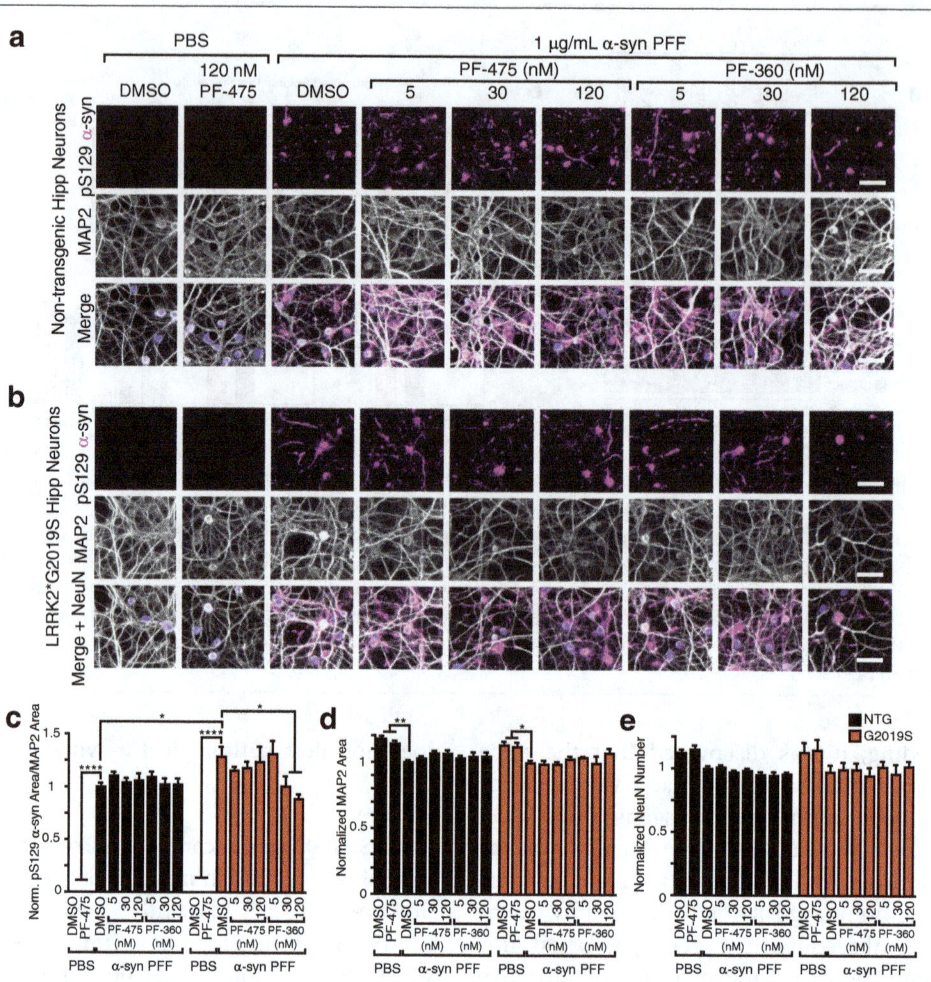

Fig. 2 G2019S LRRK2 hippocampal neurons show mild, reversible elevation in induced α-synuclein pathology 21 days post-transduction. Primary hippocampal neurons from NTG (**a**) or G2019S (**b**) pups were transduced with α-synuclein PFFs and allowed to age a further 21 days prior to fixation and staining for pS129 α-synuclein (magenta), MAP2 (gray) and NeuN (blue). The neurons were additionally treated with LRRK2 inhibitors PF-475 and PF-360 2 days prior to transduction and fed with media containing inhibitors each week thereafter. No large differences can be observed in the type or abundance of α-synuclein pathology. **c** Quantification of α-synuclein pathology reveals a mild elevation in G2019S neurons, which is reversible with 30 or 120 nM PF-360. *$P < 0.05$ by Dunnett's multiple comparison test between NTG and G2019S neurons or Sidak's multiple comparisons test between G2019S neurons treated with LRRK2 inhibitors. **d** MAP2 area is reduced with 21 days α-synuclein PFF treatment in both NTG and G2019S neurons, and is not significantly affected by LRRK2 inhibitor treatment. *$P < 0.05$ by 2-way ANOVA with Dunnett's multiple comparison test for comparison within genotype. **e** The number of neurons, as quantified by NeuN number, is reduced with 21 days α-synuclein PFF treatment in both NTG and G2019S neurons, although not significantly by 2-way ANOVA followed by Dunnett's multiple comparison test and is not significantly affected by LRRK2 inhibitor treatment. ($N = 12$ biological replicates). Means + s.e.m.; all values are normalized to NTG neurons treated with α-synuclein PFFs and DMSO. Scale bars = 50 μm

number in the NTG neurons indicating that there is no apparent relationship between LRRK2 activity in NTG neurons and α-synuclein pathology. We conclude that, while interesting, the observed elevation in α-synuclein pathology in the G2019S neurons is too mild to make this a valuable screening tool for LRRK2-dependent phenotypes.

LRRK2 inhibitors do not alter α-synuclein pathology in wildtype neurons

The lack of an effect of LRRK2 inhibitors on α-synuclein pathology in NTG neurons was surprising given previous publications showing a reduction of α-synuclein pathology in response to both LRRK2 inhibition [32] and knockdown with anti-sense oligonucleotides [38]. While LRRK2 inhibitors are initially being tested in patients with LRRK2 mutations, there is speculation that if LRRK2 is a fundamental protein in PD pathogenesis, LRRK2 inhibitors may provide clinical benefit for those without LRRK2 mutations. Therefore, we sought to investigate LRRK2 in wildtype neurons from a second, distinct strain of mice (CD1). We first sought to validate the effect of LRRK2 inhibitors on LRRK2 activity in these neurons and further test these

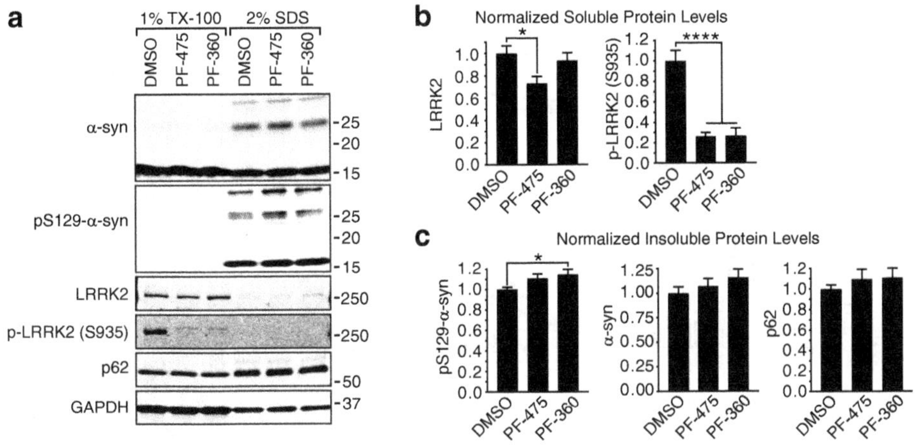

Fig. 3 LRRK2 inhibition does not reduce insoluble α-synuclein in wildtype hippocampal neurons. **a** Primary hippocampal neurons from CD1 pups were treated with 30 nM LRRK2 inhibitors PF-475, PF-360 or DMSO as a vehicle control, then transduced with 2.5 μg/mL α-synuclein PFFs and allowed to age a further 14 days prior to sequential detergent fractionation. TX-100-insoluble α-synuclein and p62 are similar in both LRRK2 inhibitor treated and untreated neurons. **b** Quantification of soluble proteins show some reduction of LRRK2 protein levels PF-475 treatment and ~ 75% inhibition of LRRK2 activity (as assayed by pS935 LRRK2) by both PF-475 and PF-360. **c** Insoluble pS129 α-synuclein was slightly, but significantly elevated by PF-360 treatment, while α-synuclein and p62 were unchanged by one-way ANOVA. ($N = 5$ biological replicates for each protein). Means + s.e.m.; *$P < 0.05$, ****$p < 0.0001$ by one-way ANOVA with Dunnett's multiple comparison test. All values are normalized first to GAPDH, as a loading control, then to DMSO-treated neurons

inhibitors on insoluble, pathological α-synuclein accumulation. CD1 hippocampal neurons were treated with LRRK2 inhibitors at 5 DIV and transduced with 2.5 μg/mL α-synuclein PFFs at 7 DIV. Neurons were harvested by sequential detergent fractionation at 14 DPT. We were able to confirm a robust ~ 75% inhibition of LRRK2 S935 phosphorylation with 30 nM PF-475 or PF-360 (Fig. 3a, b). PF-475 also modestly reduced total LRRK2 levels (Fig. 3a, b). However, inhibition of LRRK2 resulted in no reduction in insoluble α-synuclein, pS129 α-synuclein, or p62 (Fig. 3a, c). Instead, pS129 α-synuclein was slightly, but significantly elevated by LRRK2 inhibitor treatment (Fig. 3a, c).

We sought to further validate this finding with a larger family of LRRK2 inhibitors at increased concentrations that would leave no residual LRRK2 activity. We chose an additional, validated LRRK2 inhibitor (MLi-2) for further investigation and added these inhibitors at concentrations ranging from 30 to 300 nM to CD1 neurons. Use of these inhibitors resulted in near complete depletion of pS935 LRRK2 (Fig. 4a, b). The neurons were then transduced with α-synuclein PFFs and fixed at 14 DPT. No LRRK2 inhibitor, at any concentration, altered α-synuclein pathology (Fig. 4c, d), MAP2 area (Fig. 4c, e) or neuron number (Fig. 4c, f).

We then tested whether inhibition of LRRK2 activity can alter α-synuclein pathology induced by a means other than PFFs. We have recently demonstrated the ability of LB α-synuclein purified from human brain to induce pS129 α-synuclein pathology in WT neurons [24]. Cortical gray matter from brains with high LB burden were sequentially extracted with high salt, Triton X-100, sucrose, and sarkosyl buffers, yielding a final pellet enriched in LB α-synuclein. This pellet was then suspended in phosphate-buffered saline by sonication, yielding a final concentration of α-synuclein from 7.5–22.4 μg/mL, Fig. 5a, Table 1). As before, primary hippocampal neurons were treated with LRRK2 inhibitors at 5 DIV followed by treatment with 40 ng/mL LB α-synuclein two days later. This is the maximum concentration that neurons can be treated with due to the relatively low concentration of α-synuclein in these preps. Neurons were fixed and stained 14 days after the addition of LB α-synuclein. The induced pathology is sparser than that induced by PFFs due to the lower concentration of α-synuclein (Fig. 5b). The pathology induced by LB α-synuclein and neuron health were not meaningfully altered by LRRK2 inhibition (Fig. 5b, c, d, e), consistent with PFF treatment.

Dopaminergic neurons show no change in α-synuclein pathology in response to G2019S LRRK2 overexpression or LRRK2 inhibition

All the experiments to this point were performed in primary hippocampal neuron cultures. These cultures develop robust α-synuclein pathology and can be obtained in an abundance suitable for both immunocytochemistry and biochemistry. However, they are not the neurons most affected in PD patients. In order to address whether we were missing a phenotype that is dependent on expression of mutant LRRK2 in dopaminergic neurons, we developed ventral midbrain and striatum primary neuron co-cultures. When treated

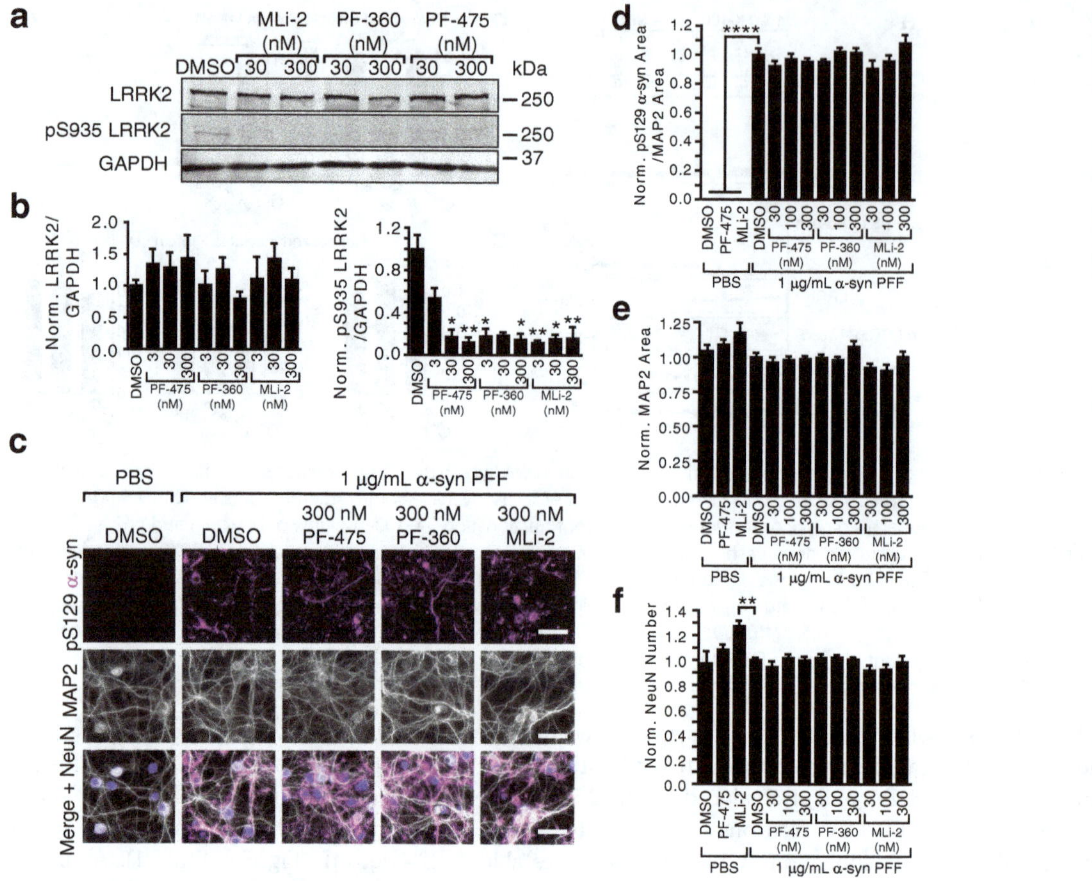

Fig. 4 LRRK2 inhibition does not reduce pathological α-synuclein in wildtype hippocampal neurons. **a** Primary cortical neurons were treated with LRRK2 inhibitors PF-475, PF-360, or MLi-2, at 5 DIV and fed with media containing inhibitors each week for 16 days. Cell lysate was run by Western blot to detect LRRK2 and pS935 LRRK2, which is indicative of LRRK2 activity. Images shown are representative of $n = 4–12$ biological replicates. **b** Quantification of Western blot of LRRK2 and pS935 LRRK2. LRRK2 levels were not significantly altered by one-way ANOVA, but pS935 levels were reduced to near undetectable levels (*$p < 0.05$, **$p < 0.01$, Kruskal-Wallis test with Dunn's multiple comparison test). **c** Primary hippocampal neurons from CD1 pups were transduced with α-synuclein PFFs and allowed to age a further 14 days prior to fixation and staining for pS129 α-synuclein (magenta), MAP2 (gray) and NeuN (blue). The neurons were additionally treated with LRRK2 inhibitors PF-475, PF-360, or MLi-2, 2 days prior to transduction and fed with media containing inhibitors each week thereafter. No large differences can be observed in the type or abundance of α-synuclein pathology. **d** Quantification of α-synuclein pathology reveals no change in response to LRRK2 inhibition, while PBS-treated neurons have no pathology (****$p < 0.0001$ by Dunnett's multiple comparison test). MAP2 area (**e**) and neuron number (**f**) are also not altered in response to LRRK2 inhibition. No significant response was seen when compared with vehicle-treated neurons by one-way ANOVA with Dunnett's multiple comparison test (**d**) or by Kruskal-Wallis test followed by Dunn's multiple comparison test (**e**) and (**f**). ($N = 9$ biological replicates). Means + s.e.m.; all values are normalized to neurons treated with α-synuclein PFFs and DMSO. Scale bars = 50 μm

with α-synuclein PFFs at 7 DIV and allowed to age 14 DPT, dopaminergic neurons positive for TH develop cell body and neuritic pS129 α-synuclein pathology (Fig. 6a). We treated midbrain/striatum co-cultures from NTG and G2019S pups with 30 nM LRRK2 inhibitors or vehicle control at 5 DIV. The neurons were then treated with α-synuclein PFFs at 7 DIV and fixed 14 DPT and stained for pS129 α-synuclein and TH. Both cultures develop a similar amount of α-synuclein pathology in TH+ neurons, and none of the LRRK2 inhibitors changed the level of pathology in either NTG or G2019S neurons (Fig. 6a, b). Further, α-synuclein PFFs were not more toxic to G2019S dopaminergic neurons, and LRRK2 inhibitors did not significantly improve survival of TH+ neurons (Fig. 6c).

Discussion

In this study, we utilized primary neuron cultures to assess the status of α-synuclein pathology in relation to LRRK2 activity. We performed biochemical and immunocytochemical analysis of primary hippocampal and midbrain neurons cultured from two strains of wildtype mice and a mouse expressing LRRK2 with the familial G2019S mutation. To further manipulate LRRK2 activity, we used three validated LRRK2 inhibitors.

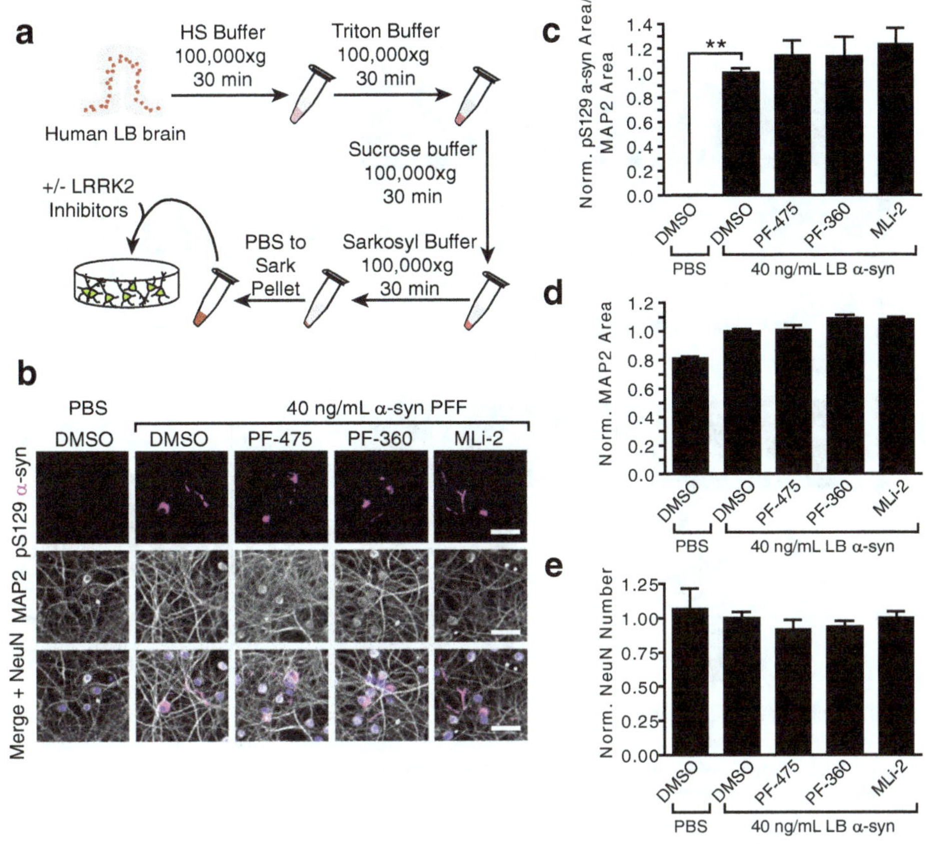

Fig. 5 LRRK2 inhibition does not alter pathology induced by human Lewy body α-synuclein. **a** A schematic representation of pathological α-synuclein purification from human cortical tissue. **b** Primary hippocampal neurons from CD1 pups were treated with 100 nM LRRK2 inhibitors or a vehicle control. Two days later, neurons were treated with 40 ng/mL human LB α-synuclein and allowed to age a further 14 days prior to fixation and staining for pS129 α-synuclein (magenta), MAP2 (gray) and NeuN (blue). No large differences can be observed in the type or abundance of α-synuclein pathology. **c** Quantification of α-synuclein pathology reveals an increase in neurons treated with LB α-synuclein compared to those treated with PBS (**$p < 0.01$), but no change in response to LRRK2 inhibition. MAP2 area (**d**) and neuron number (**e**) are also not altered meaningfully in response to LRRK2 inhibition. ($N = 11–12$ biological replicates treated with LB α-synuclein from 4 separate cases (2 AD, 1 PDD, 1 DLB). Means + s.e.m.; all values are normalized to neurons treated with LB α-synuclein and DMSO. Scale bars = 50 μm

In none of these assays did we observe more than a mild LRRK2-dependent alteration in α-synuclein pathology.

The LRRK2*G019S neurons we describe have ~ 25-fold elevated LRRK2 levels and ~ 50-fold elevated kinase activity (Fig. 1a, b). Despite this dramatic overexpression of LRRK2, there is no apparent effect on the neuron health or viability (Figs. 2, 4, 5, and 6). This is in contrast with early research using viral overexpression of LRRK2 [8, 18], but in keeping with the many transgenic models of LRRK2 that have since been generated [3, 19, 20, 37]. While there is strong support that overexpression of LRRK2 does not dramatically alter cell health, the effect of LRRK2 on α-synuclein has been unclear.

We induced pathological α-synuclein inclusion formation in NTG and G2019S neurons through addition of recombinant α-synuclein PFFs or human brain-derived

Table 1 Clinical Information of the cases used for the Extraction of Pathological alpha-synuclein

Case No.	Clinical Diagnosis	Pathological Diagnosis	Race	Sex	Age of Disease onset	Age at Death	PMI (h)	Brain Region Used	α-Synuclein (μg/ml)
1	AD Probable	AD/DLB	White	Female	52	62	11	Middle Frontal Gyrus	20.86
2	CBS	AD/DLB	White	Female	45	55	15	Middle Frontal Gyrus	22.43
3	DLB	DLB	White	Male	76	83	6	Cingulate Gyrus	7.55
4	PDD	PDD	White	Male	60	72	19	Cingulate Gyrus	8.28

PMI postmortem interval

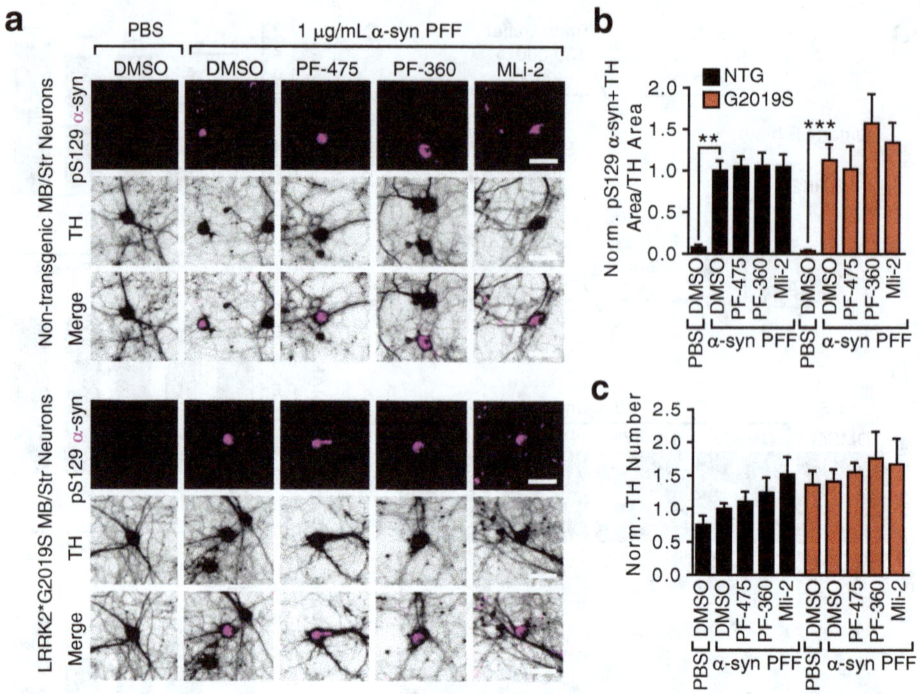

Fig. 6 Neither G2019S LRRK2 expression nor LRRK2 inhibition alters α-synuclein pathology in midbrain neurons. **a** Primary midbrain/striatum cultures from NTG or G2019S pups were transduced with α-synuclein PFFs and allowed to age a further 14 days prior to fixation and staining for pS129 α-synuclein (magenta) and TH (gray). The neurons were additionally treated with 30 nM LRRK2 inhibitors PF-475, PF-360, or MLi-2 2 days prior to transduction and fed with media containing inhibitors each week thereafter. **b** Quantification of α-synuclein pathology in TH+ neurons shows no effect of G2019S LRRK2 expression or LRRK2 inhibitor treatments by 2-way ANOVA (**$p < 0.01$, ***$p < 0.001$ for PBS- compared to PFF-treated neurons by Dunnett's multiple comparison test). **c** The number of TH+ neurons showed no significant response to treatment by Kruskal-Wallis test followed by Dunn's multiple comparison test. ($N = 6$–9 biological replicates). Means + s.e.m.; all values are normalized to NTG neurons treated with α-synuclein LB material and DMSO. Scale bars = 50 μm

LB α-synuclein. We designed our initial experiments to test the relationship between LRRK activity and α-synuclein at 14 DPT, before the onset of neurodegeneration. We found that there was no alteration of α-synuclein pathology in G2019S neurons. A recent publication using a similar model showed a mild elevation in α-synuclein in G2019S hippocampal neurons at 18 DPT, while detecting no difference at 7 DPT [32]. We found that at 21 DPT, we did observe a mild enhancement of α-synuclein pathology in G2019S neurons that was responsive to LRRK2 inhibition (Fig. 2). At this timepoint, neurons have begun degenerating, and while we see no LRRK2-dependent difference in degeneration, it is unclear if it is the neurodegenerative process that results in a mild elevation of α-synuclein pathology in G2019S neurons.

To further explore the role of endogenous LRRK2 in α-synuclein pathogenesis, we cultured wildtype hippocampal and midbrain neurons, and showed using biochemistry and immunocytochemistry that LRRK2 kinase inhibition is unable to alter induced α-synuclein pathology (Figs. 3, 4, 5, and 6). These findings are in sharp contrast to recent reports that LRRK2 inhibitors [32] or LRRK2 protein reduction by anti-sense oligonucleotides [38] are able to ameliorate α-synuclein pathology in wildtype neurons. To ensure the validity of our results, we used both biochemical extraction of pathological α-synuclein as well as immunocytochemistry. Pathology induced by both recombinant α-synuclein PFFs and human LB α-synuclein were resistant to alteration by LRRK2 inhibition. We also used three validated LRRK2 inhibitors, representing different classes of compounds. All immunocytochemical quantification of α-synuclein was normalized to MAP2 to ensure no effect of cell density. Our results in wildtype hippocampal neurons generated from two strains of mice in addition to dopaminergic midbrain neurons give us increased confidence that the lack of LRRK2-dependent phenotypes we see are valid.

LRRK2 is the most common cause of inherited PD. Even so, only around 30% of those with G2019S mutation in LRRK2 will go on to develop PD [22]. It is therefore probable that LRRK2 mutations exacerbate an extant predisposition to PD. Another hypothesized determinant of susceptibility to PD is the misfolding of α-synuclein within aging brains. It is logical to assume that challenging neurons with both misfolded α-synuclein and mutated LRRK2 would be sufficient to drive an enhanced pathogenic process. While there is compelling evidence that this may be true in mouse models [3, 5, 32], we are unable to generate a robust model of LRRK2-dependent α-synuclein pathogenesis in primary neuron cultures. There are several possible reasons that in vivo models cannot be recapitulated in cell culture. Neuron cultures are inherently closed systems. Therefore, if LRRK2 activity can affect the spread of α-synuclein pathology through the brain, this effect would not be captured in a dish. Primary neuron cultures also lack all the cell types and complex synaptic organization present in vivo. Indeed, LRRK2 is highly expressed in astrocytes [13] and neuroinflammation has been implicated in LRRK2-dependent phenotypes [3]. It is also possible that LRRK2 is not critical in the early stages of pathology formation, and only during later stages of disease progression does LRRK2 activity become important. This is supported by our finding that α-synuclein pathology is only elevated in G2019S neurons 21 days after transduction, after the onset of neurodegeneration. In addition, patients with LRRK2 mutations do not have an earlier onset of disease than patients with sporadic onset [11], suggesting that LRRK2 does not speed the disease process, as triplication of α-synuclein does [27]. While α-synuclein inclusions are common in PD patients with LRRK2 mutations, not all LRRK2 patients have α-synuclein pathology and a substantial portion of LRRK2 patients also have tau inclusions [25]. Future studies of the pathological spread of α-synuclein and tau in vivo are warranted to better understand the underlying etiology of LRRK2 mutations in PD.

Conclusions

There is substantial genetic and pathological data indicating that mutations in LRRK2 lead to an increased susceptibility to PD, and LRRK2 inhibitors are currently in clinical trials for the treatment of PD. Yet, how mutations in LRRK2 predispose patients to PD is still unclear. In this study, we show that in primary neurons, only after the onset of neurodegeneration does G2019S LRRK2 elevate α-synuclein pathology. Further, while LRRK2 inhibitors can rescue this elevated pathology, they show no benefit to wildtype neurons. Future studies of the link between LRRK2 mutations and the pathophysiology of PD will be critical to inform clinical studies of LRRK2 inhibitors.

Acknowledgements

We would like to thank our patients and their families who made this study possible and members of our laboratories for critical discussions related to this paper. We would like to thank the University of Pennsylvania Neuron Culture Service Center for their assistance procuring CD1 hippocampal neuron cultures.

Funding

This study was supported by the Michael J. Fox Foundation and National Institute of Health grants: T32-AG000255, P30-AG10124, P50-NS053488.

Authors' contributions

Conception and design: MXH, CP, JQT, VMYL; Acquisition and analysis of data: MXH and CP; Drafting of the article: MXH, VMYL. All authors read and approved the final manuscript.

Competing interests

The authors declare that they have no competing interests.

References

1. Baba M, Nakajo S, Tu PH, Tomita T, Nakaya K, Lee VM, Trojanowski JQ, Iwatsubo T (1998) Aggregation of alpha-synuclein in Lewy bodies of sporadic Parkinson's disease and dementia with Lewy bodies. Am J Pathol 152:879–884
2. Covell DJ, Robinson JL, Akhtar RS, Grossman M, Weintraub D, Bucklin HM, Pitkin RM, Riddle D, Yousef A, Trojanowski JQ, Lee VM (2017) Novel conformation-selective alpha-synuclein antibodies raised against different in vitro fibril forms show distinct patterns of Lewy pathology in Parkinson's disease. Neuropathol Appl Neurobiol 43:604–620. https://doi.org/10.1111/nan.12402
3. Daher JP, Abdelmotilib HA, Hu X, Volpicelli-Daley LA, Moehle MS, Fraser KB, Needle E, Chen Y, Steyn SJ, Galatsis P, Hirst WD, West AB (2015) Leucine-rich repeat kinase 2 (LRRK2) pharmacological inhibition abates alpha-Synuclein gene-induced neurodegeneration. J Biol Chem 290:19433–19444. https://doi.org/10.1074/jbc.M115.660001
4. Daher JP, Pletnikova O, Biskup S, Musso A, Gellhaar S, Galter D, Troncoso JC, Lee MK, Dawson TM, Dawson VL, Moore DJ (2012) Neurodegenerative phenotypes in an A53T alpha-synuclein transgenic mouse model are independent of LRRK2. Hum Mol Genet 21:2420–2431. https://doi.org/10.1093/hmg/dds057
5. Daher JP, Volpicelli-Daley LA, Blackburn JP, Moehle MS, West AB (2014) Abrogation of alpha-synuclein-mediated dopaminergic neurodegeneration in LRRK2-deficient rats. Proc Natl Acad Sci U S A 111:9289–9294. https://doi.org/10.1073/pnas.1403215111
6. Dzamko N, Deak M, Hentati F, Reith AD, Prescott AR, Alessi DR, Nichols RJ (2010) Inhibition of LRRK2 kinase activity leads to dephosphorylation of Ser(910)/Ser(935), disruption of 14-3-3 binding and altered cytoplasmic localization. Biochem J 430:405–413. https://doi.org/10.1042/BJ20100784
7. Fell MJ, Mirescu C, Basu K, Cheewatrakoolpong B, DeMong DE, Ellis JM, Hyde LA, Lin Y, Markgraf CG, Mei H, Miller M, Poulet FM, Scott JD, Smith MD, Yin Z, Zhou X, Parker EM, Kennedy ME, Morrow JA (2015) MLi-2, a potent, selective, and centrally active compound for exploring the therapeutic potential and safety of LRRK2 kinase inhibition. J Pharmacol Exp Ther 355:397–409. https://doi.org/10.1124/jpet.115.227587
8. Greggio E, Jain S, Kingsbury A, Bandopadhyay R, Lewis P, Kaganovich A, van der Brug MP, Beilina A, Blackinton J, Thomas KJ, Ahmad R, Miller DW, Kesavapany S, Singleton A, Lees A, Harvey RJ, Harvey K, Cookson MR (2006) Kinase activity is required for the toxic effects of mutant LRRK2/dardarin. Neurobiol Dis 23:329–341. https://doi.org/10.1016/j.nbd.2006.04.001
9. Guerreiro PS, Huang Y, Gysbers A, Cheng D, Gai WP, Outeiro TF, Halliday GM (2013) LRRK2 interactions with alpha-synuclein in Parkinson's disease brains and in cell models. J Mol Med (Berl) 91:513–522. https://doi.org/10.1007/s00109-012-0984-y
10. Guo JL, Covell DJ, Daniels JP, Iba M, Stieber A, Zhang B, Riddle DM, Kwong LK, Xu Y, Trojanowski JQ, Lee VM (2013) Distinct alpha-synuclein strains differentially promote tau inclusions in neurons. Cell 154:103–117. https://doi.org/10.1016/j.cell.2013.05.057
11. Healy DG, Falchi M, O'Sullivan SS, Bonifati V, Durr A, Bressman S, Brice A, Aasly J, Zabetian CP, Goldwurm S, Ferreira JJ, Tolosa E, Kay DM, Klein C, Williams DR, Marras C, Lang AE, Wszolek ZK, Berciano J, Schapira AH, Lynch T, Bhatia KP, Gasser T, Lees AJ, Wood NW (2008) Phenotype, genotype, and

worldwide genetic penetrance of LRRK2-associated Parkinson's disease: a case-control study. The Lancet Neurology 7:583–590. https://doi.org/10.1016/S1474-4422(08)70117-0
12. Henderson MX, Chung CH, Riddle DM, Zhang B, Gathagan RJ, Seeholzer SH, Trojanowski JQ, Lee VMY (2017) Unbiased proteomics of early Lewy body formation model implicates active microtubule affinity-regulating kinases (MARKs) in synucleinopathies. J Neurosci 37:5870–5884. https://doi.org/10.1523/JNEUROSCI.2705-16.2017
13. Henry AG, Aghamohammadzadeh S, Samaroo H, Chen Y, Mou K, Needle E, Hirst WD (2015) Pathogenic LRRK2 mutations, through increased kinase activity, produce enlarged lysosomes with reduced degradative capacity and increase ATP13A2 expression. Hum Mol Genet 24:6013–6028. https://doi.org/10.1093/hmg/ddv314
14. Herzig MC, Bidinosti M, Schweizer T, Hafner T, Stemmelen C, Weiss A, Danner S, Vidotto N, Stauffer D, Barske C, Mayer F, Schmid P, Rovelli G, van der Putten PH, Shimshek DR (2012) High LRRK2 levels fail to induce or exacerbate neuronal alpha-synucleinopathy in mouse brain. PLoS One 7:e36581. https://doi.org/10.1371/journal.pone.0036581
15. Irwin DJ, Lee VM, Trojanowski JQ (2013) Parkinson's disease dementia: convergence of alpha-synuclein, tau and amyloid-beta pathologies. Nat Rev Neurosci 14:626–636. https://doi.org/10.1038/nrn3549
16. Irwin DJ, White MT, Toledo JB, Xie SX, Robinson JL, Van Deerlin V, Lee VM, Leverenz JB, Montine TJ, Duda JE, Hurtig HI, Trojanowski JQ (2012) Neuropathologic substrates of Parkinson disease dementia. Ann Neurol 72:587–598. https://doi.org/10.1002/ana.23659
17. Kang UB, Marto JA (2017) Leucine-rich repeat kinase 2 and Parkinson's disease. Proteomics 17. https://doi.org/10.1002/pmic.201600092
18. Lee BD, Shin JH, VanKampen J, Petrucelli L, West AB, Ko HS, Lee YI, Maguire-Zeiss KA, Bowers WJ, Federoff HJ, Dawson VL, Dawson TM (2010) Inhibitors of leucine-rich repeat kinase-2 protect against models of Parkinson's disease. Nat Med 16:998–1000. https://doi.org/10.1038/nm.2199
19. Li X, Patel JC, Wang J, Avshalumov MV, Nicholson C, Buxbaum JD, Elder GA, Rice ME, Yue Z (2010) Enhanced striatal dopamine transmission and motor performance with LRRK2 overexpression in mice is eliminated by familial Parkinson's disease mutation G2019S. J Neurosci 30:1788–1797. https://doi.org/10.1523/JNEUROSCI.5604-09.2010
20. Lin X, Parisiadou L, Gu XL, Wang L, Shim H, Sun L, Xie C, Long CX, Yang WJ, Ding J, Chen ZZ, Gallant PE, Tao-Cheng JH, Rudow G, Troncoso JC, Liu Z, Li Z, Cai H (2009) Leucine-rich repeat kinase 2 regulates the progression of neuropathology induced by Parkinson's-disease-related mutant alpha-synuclein. Neuron 64:807–827. https://doi.org/10.1016/j.neuron.2009.11.006
21. Luk KC, Song C, O'Brien P, Stieber A, Branch JR, Brunden KR, Trojanowski JQ, Lee VM (2009) Exogenous alpha-synuclein fibrils seed the formation of Lewy body-like intracellular inclusions in cultured cells. Proc Natl Acad Sci U S A 106:20051–20056. https://doi.org/10.1073/pnas.0908005106
22. Monfrini E, Di Fonzo A (2017) Leucine-rich repeat kinase (LRRK2) genetics and Parkinson's disease. Advances in neurobiology 14:3–30. https://doi.org/10.1007/978-3-319-49969-7_1
23. Orenstein SJ, Kuo SH, Tasset I, Arias E, Koga H, Fernandez-Carasa I, Cortes E, Honig LS, Dauer W, Consiglio A, Raya A, Sulzer D, Cuervo AM (2013) Interplay of LRRK2 with chaperone-mediated autophagy. Nat Neurosci 16:394–406. https://doi.org/10.1038/nn.3350
24. Peng C, Gathagan RJ, Covell DJ, Medellin C, Stieber A, Robinson JL, Zhang B, Pitkin RM, Olufemi MF, Luk KC, Trojanowski JQ, Lee VM (2018) Cellular milieu imparts distinct pathological alpha-synuclein strains in alpha-synucleinopathies. Nature. https://doi.org/10.1038/s41586-018-0104-4
25. Poulopoulos M, Levy OA, Alcalay RN (2012) The neuropathology of genetic Parkinson's disease. Movement disorders : official journal of the Movement Disorder Society 27:831–842. https://doi.org/10.1002/mds.24962
26. Sheng Z, Zhang S, Bustos D, Kleinheinz T, Le Pichon CE, Dominguez SL, Solanoy HO, Drummond J, Zhang X, Ding X, Cai F, Song Q, Li X, Yue Z, van der Brug MP, Burdick DJ, Gunzner-Toste J, Chen H, Liu X, Estrada AA, Sweeney ZK, Scearce-Levie K, Moffat JG, Kirkpatrick DS, Zhu H (2012) Ser1292 autophosphorylation is an indicator of LRRK2 kinase activity and contributes to the cellular effects of PD mutations. Sci Transl Med 4:164ra161. https://doi.org/10.1126/scitranslmed.3004485
27. Singleton AB, Farrer M, Johnson J, Singleton A, Hague S, Kachergus J, Hulihan M, Peuralinna T, Dutra A, Nussbaum R, Lincoln S, Crawley A, Hanson M, Maraganore D, Adler C, Cookson MR, Muenter M, Baptista M, Miller D, Blancato J, Hardy J, Gwinn-Hardy K (2003) Alpha-Synuclein locus triplication causes Parkinson's disease. Science 302:841. https://doi.org/10.1126/science.1090278
28. Skibinski G, Nakamura K, Cookson MR, Finkbeiner S (2014) Mutant LRRK2 toxicity in neurons depends on LRRK2 levels and synuclein but not kinase activity or inclusion bodies. J Neurosci 34:418–433. https://doi.org/10.1523/JNEUROSCI.2712-13.2014
29. Spillantini MG, Crowther RA, Jakes R, Hasegawa M, Goedert M (1998) Alpha-Synuclein in filamentous inclusions of Lewy bodies from Parkinson's disease and dementia with lewy bodies. Proc Natl Acad Sci U S A 95:6469–6473
30. Spillantini MG, Schmidt ML, Lee VM, Trojanowski JQ, Jakes R, Goedert M (1997) Alpha-synuclein in Lewy bodies. Nature 388:839–840. https://doi.org/10.1038/42166
31. Steger M, Tonelli F, Ito G, Davies P, Trost M, Vetter M, Wachter S, Lorentzen E, Duddy G, Wilson S, Baptista MA, Fiske BK, Fell MJ, Morrow JA, Reith AD, Alessi DR, Mann M (2016) Phosphoproteomics reveals that Parkinson's disease kinase LRRK2 regulates a subset of Rab GTPases. eLife 5. https://doi.org/10.7554/eLife.12813
32. Volpicelli-Daley LA, Abdelmotilib H, Liu Z, Stoyka L, Daher JP, Milnerwood AJ, Unni VK, Hirst WD, Yue Z, Zhao HT, Fraser K, Kennedy RE, West AB (2016) G2019S-LRRK2 expression augments alpha-Synuclein sequestration into inclusions in neurons. J Neurosci 36:7415–7427. https://doi.org/10.1523/JNEUROSCI.3642-15.2016
33. Volpicelli-Daley LA, Luk KC, Lee VM (2014) Addition of exogenous alpha-synuclein preformed fibrils to primary neuronal cultures to seed recruitment of endogenous alpha-synuclein to Lewy body and Lewy neurite-like aggregates. Nat Protoc 9:2135–2146. https://doi.org/10.1038/nprot.2014.143
34. Volpicelli-Daley LA, Luk KC, Patel TP, Tanik SA, Riddle DM, Stieber A, Meaney DF, Trojanowski JQ, Lee VM (2011) Exogenous alpha-synuclein fibrils induce Lewy body pathology leading to synaptic dysfunction and neuron death. Neuron 72:57–71. https://doi.org/10.1016/j.neuron.2011.08.033
35. West AB, Cowell RM, Daher JP, Moehle MS, Hinkle KM, Melrose HL, Standaert DG, Volpicelli-Daley LA (2014) Differential LRRK2 expression in the cortex, striatum, and substantia nigra in transgenic and nontransgenic rodents. J Comp Neurol 522:2465–2480. https://doi.org/10.1002/cne.23583
36. West AB, Moore DJ, Biskup S, Bugayenko A, Smith WW, Ross CA, Dawson VL, Dawson TM (2005) Parkinson's disease-associated mutations in leucine-rich repeat kinase 2 augment kinase activity. Proc Natl Acad Sci U S A 102:16842–16847. https://doi.org/10.1073/pnas.0507360102
37. Yue M, Hinkle KM, Davies P, Trushina E, Fiesel FC, Christenson TA, Schroeder AS, Zhang L, Bowles E, Behrouz B, Lincoln SJ, Beevers JE, Milnerwood AJ, Kurti A, McLean PJ, Fryer JD, Springer W, Dickson DW, Farrer MJ, Melrose HL (2015) Progressive dopaminergic alterations and mitochondrial abnormalities in LRRK2 G2019S knock-in mice. Neurobiol Dis 78:172–195. https://doi.org/10.1016/j.nbd.2015.02.031
38. Zhao HT, John N, Delic V, Ikeda-Lee K, Kim A, Weihofen A, Swayze EE, Kordasiewicz HB, West AB, Volpicelli-Daley LA (2017) LRRK2 antisense oligonucleotides ameliorate alpha-Synuclein inclusion formation in a Parkinson's disease mouse model. Molecular therapy Nucleic acids 8:508–519. https://doi.org/10.1016/j.omtn.2017.08.002

8

Neuroimaging-pathological correlations of $[^{18}F]$THK5351 PET in progressive supranuclear palsy

Aiko Ishiki[1], Ryuichi Harada[1,2,9*], Hideaki Kai[3], Naomi Sato[4], Tomoko Totsune[5], Naoki Tomita[1], Shoichi Watanuki[6], Kotaro Hiraoka[6], Yoichi Ishikawa[6], Yoshihito Funaki[6], Ren Iwata[6], Shozo Furumoto[6], Manabu Tashiro[6], Hironobu Sasano[4], Tetsuyuki Kitamoto[3], Yukitsuka Kudo[1], Kazuhiko Yanai[2,6], Katsutoshi Furukawa[7], Nobuyuki Okamura[2,6,8] and Hiroyuki Arai[1]

Abstract

Recent positron emission tomography (PET) studies have demonstrated the accumulation of tau PET tracer in the affected region of progressive supranuclear palsy (PSP) cases. To confirm the binding target of radiotracer in PSP, we performed an imaging-pathology correlation study in two autopsy-confirmed PSP patients who underwent $[^{18}F]$THK5351 PET before death. One patient with PSP Richardson syndrome showed elevated tracer retention in the globus pallidus and midbrain. In a patient with PSP-progressive nonfluent aphasia, $[^{18}F]$THK5351 retention also was observed in the cortical areas, particularly the temporal cortex. Neuropathological examination confirmed PSP in both patients. Regional $[^{18}F]$THK5351 standardized uptake value ratio (SUVR) in antemortem PET was significantly correlated with monoamine oxidase-B (MAO-B) level, reactive astrocytes density, and tau pathology at postmortem examination. In in vitro autoradiography, specific THK5351 binding was detected in the area of antemortem $[^{18}F]$THK5351 retention, and binding was blocked completely by a reversible selective MAO-B inhibitor, lazabemide, in brain samples from these patients. In conclusion, $[^{18}F]$THK5351 PET signals reflect MAO-B expressing reactive astrocytes, which may be associated with tau accumulation in PSP.

Keywords: PSP, Monoamine oxidase, Reactive astrocyte, Tau, PET, $[^{18}F]$THK5351

Introduction

Tau positron emission tomography (PET), which provides the topographic distribution of tau aggregates in the brain, would be useful for the diagnosis of Alzheimer's disease (AD) and for the assessment of tau burden in the clinical trials of antidementia drugs. Most studies on a tau PET radiopharmaceutical ($[^{18}F]$AV1451) showed a robust difference between the control subjects and the patients with AD [16]. Regional distribution of $[^{18}F]$AV1451 was correlated with tau neuropathology in *MAPT* R406W mutation carriers [37]. Tau PET also has been considered potentially useful for antemortem assessment of non-AD tauopathies, such as progressive supranuclear palsy (PSP), corticobasal degeneration (CBD), and some variants of frontotemporal lobar degeneration (FTLD) [44]. $[^{18}F]$AV1451 PET studies have shown elevated tracer retention where tau pathology was observed frequently in patients with PSP and CBD. However, several reports have highlighted the discrepancies between antemortem PET and postmortem in vitro binding studies, particularly in non-AD tauopathies. In vitro autoradiography validation studies demonstrated that $[^{18}F]$AV1451 failed to bind to 4-repeat tau lesions in PSP and CBD [18, 24, 38]. Recent progress in the development of second-generation tau tracers successfully reduced the off-target binding in the basal ganglia and brainstem. However, to our knowledge, no tau PET radiopharmaceutical has been fully validated against neuropathology to date [23, 43]. $[^{18}F]$THK5351 was one

* Correspondence: ryuichi.harada.c8@tohoku.ac.jp
[1]Department of Geriatrics and Gerontology, Division of Brain Science, Institute of Development, Aging and Cancer, Tohoku University, 4-1 Seiryo-machi, Aoba-ku, Sendai, Miyagi, Japan
[2]Department of Pharmacology, Tohoku University School of Medicine, 2-1 Seiryo-machi, Aoba-ku, Sendai, Miyagi, Japan
Full list of author information is available at the end of the article

of the first-generation tau PET radiotracers that was designed originally to detect tau aggregates in the form of PHF-tau in AD [11]. Clinical PET studies in PSP and CBS patients have demonstrated prominent [^{18}F]THK5351 retention [2, 14, 19] in the midbrain and basal ganglia where tau pathology was observed frequently at autopsy [20, 45]. [^{18}F]THK5351 binding in these areas is associated closely with disease progression because the amount of tracer retention was correlated positively with clinical severity of PSP [2]. However, recent studies have suggested the existence of off-target binding to monoamine oxidase-B (MAO-B). A single oral dose of selegiline, a selective irreversible MAO-B inhibitor, substantially reduced [^{18}F]THK5351 binding in the brain of patients with PSP as well as AD [29]. In an autopsy case of AD, regional [^{18}F]THK5351 binding was correlated significantly with MAO-B density as well as tau level. Therefore, [^{18}F]THK5351 PET signal reflects the combination of tau pathology and reactive astrocytes in the AD brain [10]. However, what an [^{18}F]THK5351 PET signal reflects in the PSP brain remains unclear.

We examined imaging-pathology correlation in two autopsy-confirmed PSP patients who showed prominent tracer retention on an antemortem [^{18}F]THK5351 PET scan.

Materials and methods

The ethics committee of the Tohoku University Graduate School of Medicine approved this study, and informed consent for neuroimaging and autopsy was obtained for each subject.

PET and MRI scans and image analyses

PET images were acquired using an Eminence STARGATE PET scanner (Shimadzu, Kyoto, Japan). After intravenous injection of [^{18}F]THK5351 (185 MBq) or [^{11}C]PiB (296 MBq), dynamic PET images were obtained for 60 ([^{18}F]THK5351) or 70 ([^{11}C]PiB) minutes. T1-weighted magnetic resonance images (MRI) were obtained using a SIGNA 1.5-Tesla machine (General Electric, Milwaukee, WI, USA) according to a previously described method [14]. Standardized uptake value (SUV) images of [^{18}F]THK5351 (40–60 min after injection) and [^{11}C]PiB (50–70 min after injection) were obtained by normalizing tissue radioactivity concentration by injected dose and body weight. The regional SUV-to-cerebellar cortex SUV ratio (SUVR) was used as an index of tracer retention. SPM12 software (SPM12; Wellcome Department of Imaging Neuroscience, UCL, London, UK) was used to coregister the PET images on the MRI image. PMOD Ver. 3.7 software (PMOD Technologies GmbH, Zurich, Switzerland) was used to draw regions of interest (ROIs) on the coregistered MRI image.

Brain tissue samples

The left hemisphere was immersed in 10% formalin for histology. The brain portions were frozen on powdered dry ice for biochemical analyses and unfixed tissue-based assays. Tissue sections of paraffin-embedded blocks were stained with Luixol fast blue and hematoxylin-eosin. Selected sections were stained with anti-tau AT8 (1:20; Innogenetics, Ghent, Belgium), anti-β-amyloid 4G8 (1:10,000; BioLegend [Signet], San Diego, CA USA), anti-α-synuclein P-syn/81A (1:100, BioLegend [Covance]), anti-TDP43 pS409/410–1 (1:5000; Cosmo Bio, Tokyo, Japan), and anti-GFAP 6F2 (1:100; Agilent [Dako], Santa Clara, CA, USA) antibodies. Brain slices 12 μm thick were generated with a cryostat (Microm HM560; Thermo Scientific, Waltham, MA, USA) using − 20 °C chamber and − 15 °C object temperatures. The sections were transferred to Matsunami Adhesive Slide (MAS)–coated glass slides (Matsunami Glass Ind., Ltd., Osaka, Japan). After drying, the sections were stored at − 80 °C. In subject 1, brain homogenates (0.1 mg/mL) additionally were prepared in phosphate-buffered saline (PBS) and stored at − 80°C until experimental use.

Quantification of tau and glial fibrillary acidic protein (GFAP) immunoreactivity

Microscopic images from each section of paraffin-embedded blocks were captured and a threshold of optical density was obtained by Image J software (National Institutes of Health [NIH], Bethesda, MD, USA). Tau and GFAP immunoreactivity was defined as total percentage of area covered by tau and GFAP immunostaining in each ROI.

In vitro autoradiography of [^{18}F]THK5351

The brain sections were dried and were dipped in PBS for a total of 25 min and, then, preincubated in PBS containing 1% bovine serum albumin (BSA). Then, the brain sections were incubated for 30 min at room temperature with [^{18}F]THK5351 (370 kBq/mL). After incubation, the sections were washed sequentially with PBS containing 1% BSA for 5 min, followed by PBS for 5 min twice. The dried sections were exposed to an imaging plate (BAS IP MS 2025 E; GE Healthcare, Little Chalfont, UK) overnight. Autoradiographic images were obtained from Typhoon FLA-9500 (GE Healthcare). To account for the binding to MAO-B in brain tissues, the reaction was incubated in the presence of MAO-B inhibitor, Lazabemide (1 μM). After post-fixation in 4% paraformaldehyde for 30 min, adjacent frozen sections were immunostained with anti-tau AT8, anti-MAO-B (1:400, Sigma-Aldrich Corp., St. Louis, MO, USA), and anti-GFAP 6F2 antibodies.

In vitro binding assay of [^{3}H]THK5351

The reaction mixture contained [^{3}H]THK5351 (1 nM; specific activity, 2.96 TBq/mmol; radiochemical purity, 98.9%; Sekisui Medical, Inc., Tokyo, Japan) and brain homogenates (0.5 μg), in a final volume 200 μL. Nonspecific binding was defined in the presence of 2 μM unlabeled THK5351. The mixture was incubated at room temperature for 2 h, and separation of bound from free radioactivity was achieved by filtration under reduced pressure (Multiscreen HTS Vaccum Manifold, Multiscreen HTS 96-well 0.65 μm filtration plate; Millipore, Billerica, MA, USA), followed by three washes with PBS containing 0.1% BSA. The filters were incubated in 2 mL scintillation fluid (Emulsifier-Safe; Perkin Elmer, Boston, MA, USA), and a β counter (LS6500 liquid scintillation counter; Beckman Coulter, Brea, CA, USA) was used to count the radioactivity.

Semiquantification of PHF-tau by immunoblotting

Immunoblotting for PHF-tau was performed according to a previously reported protocol [39]. After centrifugation (20,000 *g*, 15 min, 4 °C) of brain homogenates, the resulting pellet was dissolved in extraction buffer containing 10 mM Tris-HCl (pH 7.5), 0.8 M NaCl, 10% sucrose, 1 mM ethylene glycol-bis β-aminoethyl ether (EGTA), 2% sarkosyl, and then incubated for 30 min at 37 °C. The supernatants were collected after centrifugation at 20,000 *g* for 10 min at 25 °C. After ultracentrifugation (100,000 *g*, 20 min, 25 °C), the pellets were washed with 0.5 mL sterile saline and solubilized in sodium dodecyl sulfate (SDS)–sample buffer and, then, run on a 5–20% gradient polyacrylamide gel (SuperSep™ Ace; Wako, Osaka, Japan). Proteins were transferred to polyvinylidine fluoride (PVDF) membrane, blocked by incubation with 3% gelatin (Wako) for 10 min at 37 °C, followed by overnight incubation at room temperature with the anti-tau monoclonal antibody T46 (1:2000, Thermo Fisher Scientific), biotinylated anti-mouse secondary antibody, ABC complex (Vector Laboratories, Burlingame, CA, USA) and developed with diaminobenzidine and nickel chloride. For semiquantification of sarkosyl-insoluble tau, the three dominant bands (68, 64, and 60 kDa) were quantified by ImageJ software (Additional file 1: Figure S1). Sarkosyl-insoluble tau (PHF-tau) was expressed as ratio using cerebellum as reference.

Quantification of MAO-B and GFAP by enzyme-linked immunosorbent assay (ELISA)

Brain MAO-B levels were quantified using a human MAO-B ELISA kit (Ab157393, Abcam, Cambridge, UK) with MAO-B standard (M7441, Sigma-Aldrich Corp.). Extraction of MAO-B was performed according to the manufacturer's instructions. For the quantification of GFAP, brain homogenates were extracted with Tris-HCl buffer containing 0.1% Triton-X as described previously [13]. A human GFAP ELISA kit (BioVendor, Asheville, NC, USA) was used to quantify the GFAP levels.

Statistical analysis

Spearman rank correlation coefficients were calculated to examine the association between radiotracer binding, histopathology, and biochemical data. Statistical significance was defined at $P < 0.05$. GraphPad Prism software (GraphPad, San Diego, CA, USA) was used to perform this analysis.

Results

Case reports

Subject 1

An 84-year-old right-handed male presented with memory disturbance and disorientation. One year later, standing and gait became unstable with progression of extrapyramidal signs and PSP was diagnosed clinically. PET scans were performed 2 years after the diagnosis of PSP. At the time of the PET scan, he was bedridden and the Mini-Mental State Examination (MMSE) score was 1 of 30. Neurologic examinations revealed limited vertical eye movement. The PSP rating scale score was 82. A brain MRI showed significant midbrain atrophy. A typical "hummingbird sign" was observed in the sagittal section. He died of aspiration pneumonia 295 days after the PET scan. Detailed clinical information has been described previously [14].

Subject 2

A 73-year-old right-handed male presented with memory disturbance. Mild cognitive impairment was diagnosed clinically 3 years after the first symptoms appeared. He gradually presented with speech impairment, stereotypical behavior, and change of food preference, and progressive nonfluent aphasia (PNFA) was diagnosed. We did not perform DNA sequencing to confirm a mutation in the *MAPT* gene. One year later, he presented with unstable gait and was prone to falls. At the PET scan, he was bedridden and the MMSE score was 1 of 30. An MRI showed diffuse brain atrophy prominent in the right anterior temporal, hippocampus, amygdala, and caudate nuclei. He died of aspiration pneumonia 79 days after PET scan.

[^{18}F]THK5351 and [^{11}C]PiB PET scans

Figure 1 shows the [^{18}F]THK5351 PET images from the two subjects. Images from a cognitively normal individual are shown for comparison at the bottom (Fig. 1). Subject 1 showed significant [^{18}F]THK5351 retention in the globus pallidus and midbrain. Mild tracer retention was observed also in the other cortices, including

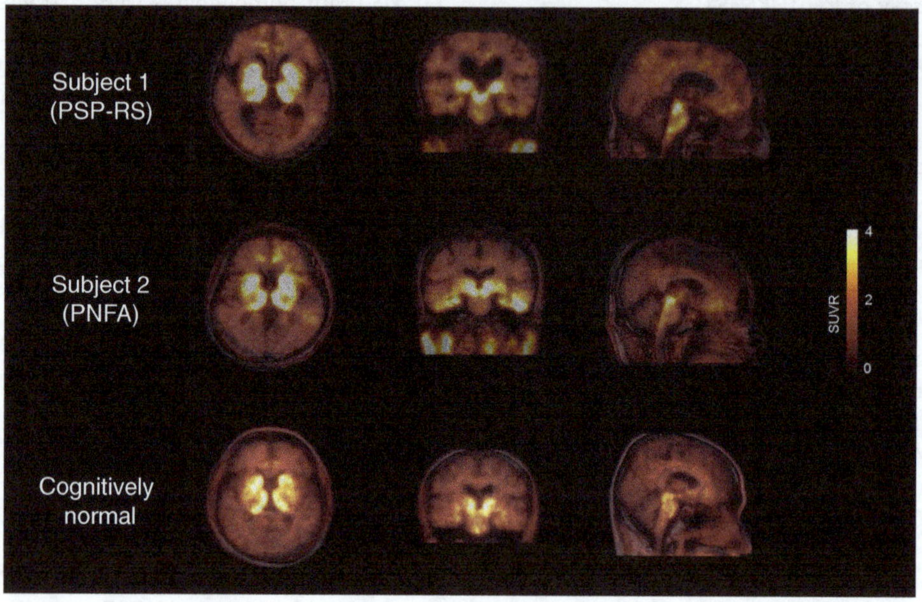

Fig. 1 [18F]THK5351 PET images from two study subjects and a cognitively normal subject. The scale indicates SUVR range from 0 to 4

parahippocampal and inferior temporal gyri. Subject 2 showed prominent [^{18}F]THK5351 retention in the parahippocampal and inferior temporal gyri, as well as the globus pallidus and midbrain. No remarkable retention of [^{11}C]PiB was observed in the neocortex in both of the subjects (data not shown).

Neuropathological examination

Brain weight in subject 1 was 1580 g. Autopsy revealed severe atrophy in the midbrain tegmetum and pons, and subthalamic nucleus, and relatively mild atrophy in the frontal cortex, but not in the basal ganglia. Neuropathological examination revealed tau pathology in neuronal and glial cells consistent with PSP. Globose tangles were observed in the midbrain, pons, medulla, subthalamic nucleus, and nucleus basalis of Meynert. Moderate numbers of tufted astrocytes were observed also in the amygdala, motor cortex, and superior frontal gyrus. Neurofibrillary tangles were observed in the entorhinal cortex and subiculum, which corresponded to age-related Braak stage II [1]. The tau immunoreactivity density appeared greatest in the medial temporal regions, followed by the basal ganglia and frontal cortex. Small cerebral infarctions were observed in the putamen and the cerebellum. Gliosis and neuronal loss were observed also in the substantia nigra. However, amyloid-β, α-synuclein, and TDP-43 pathology were absent in this case. These characteristics were consistent with the diagnosis of definite PSP.

Brain weight in subject 2 was 920 g. Autopsy revealed severe atrophy in bilateral temporal lobes, including the hippocampus and amygdala. Brain atrophy was obviously observed in the tegmentum of the midbrain and pons. There was neuronal loss in the pigmented neurons of the substantia nigra and locus coeruleus. Brain atrophy was observed also in the globus pallidus, hypothalamic nucleus, and cerebellar dentate nucleus. AT8 immunostaining revealed abundant tau burden, including neurofibrillary tangles, globose tangles, tufted astrocytes, coiled bodies, and neuropil threads in the temporal, cingulate, frontal, striatum, globus pallidus, and subthalamic nucleus. In addition, thorn-shaped astrocytes, typical in aging-related tau astrogliopathy, were observed in the temporal lobe gray and white matter [21]. Sparse amyloid plaques were observed in the cerebral cortex (Thal phase for Aβ plaques: 2, CERAD: Sparse). Both α-synuclein and TDP-43 pathology were absent in this case. Gliosis was severe in the bilateral hippocampus and amygdala. Astrocytosis with neuronal loss was prominent in the temporal cortex, followed by the frontal and cingulate cortices. Three- and four-repeat tau-immunohistochemistry studies, respectively, revealed that these tau lesions were composed of four-repeat tau. The distribution, isoform, and morphology of tau immunoreactive lesions were consistent with atypical PSP [17], which was diagnosed as PSP-FTD.

In vivo–in vitro correlation analyses

Biochemical analysis revealed the presence of sarkosyl-insoluble tau (68 and 64 kDa), corresponding to 4-repeat tau protein in both cases (Additional file 1: Figure S1). In subject 1, sarkosyl-insoluble tau was high in the parahippocampal gyrus and hippocampus, moderate in the globus pallidus and putamen, and low in other areas (Fig. 2a). The parahippocampal gyrus contained 3- (60 kDa band) and 4-repeat tau, suggesting that they are age-related tau. AT8 immunohistochemistry was positive in the brain sections from the same tissue (data not shown). In subject 1, in vivo [^{18}F]THK5351 binding was correlated significantly with sarkosyl-insoluble tau levels determined by Western blot analysis ($r = 0.67$, $P = 0.039$; Fig. 2b). In addition, we found a strong correlation between in vivo [^{18}F]THK5351 binding and MAO-B levels ($r = 0.78$, $P = 0.0096$; Fig. 2c). A significant positive correlation was observed also between in vivo [^{18}F]THK5351 binding and GFAP level ($r = 0.67$, $P = 0.039$; Fig. 2d). In vitro [^{3}H]THK5351 binding assay using brain homogenates also demonstrated a strong correlation between in vivo [^{18}F]THK5351 retention and in vitro tracer binding in subject 1 ($r = 0.92$, $P = 0.005$; Fig. 2e). Tau and GFAP immunoreactivities in the brain sections were measured quantitatively for correlation analysis between in vivo tracer retention and histopathology (Fig. 3). We observed positive correlation trends between in vivo [^{18}F]THK5351 retention and tau loads ($r = 0.48$, $P = 0.06$), and between in vivo [^{18}F]THK5351 retention and GFAP immunoreactivity ($r = 0.49$, $P = 0.05$).

In subject 2, in vivo [^{18}F]THK5351 binding was correlated significantly with tau-immunohistochemistry using AT8 antibody ($r = 0.48$, $P = 0.037$; Fig. 4b). Furthermore, in vivo [^{18}F]THK5351 retention was correlated positively with the density of GFAP immunoreactive astrocytes ($r = 0.64$, $P = 0.0033$).

In vitro autoradiography

In vitro autoradiography of [^{18}F]THK5351 in frozen sections demonstrated high tracer binding in the globus pallidus as well as putamen in subject 1 and in the frontal cortex in subject 2 (Fig. 5), which was consistent with in vivo PET results (Fig. 1). These bindings were displaced completely after treatment with MAO-B inhibitor, Lazabemide [10]. The spatial pattern of [^{18}F]THK5351 binding was similar to that of MAO-B immunostaining, suggesting that the target of [^{18}F]THK5351 binding was MAO-B–positive astrogliosis rather than the tau aggregates in the PSP brain.

Discussion

Tremendous efforts have been made to develop tau-selective PET radiopharmaceuticals. The first-generation tau PET tracers, such as [^{11}C]PBB3, [^{18}F]AV1451, and [^{18}F]THK5351, have shown accumulation in the predilection site for tau deposition. Tau PET imaging recapitulated topographical regional distribution patterns similar to those reported by Braak staging of tau pathology at autopsy [44]. However, they showed nonnegligible off-target

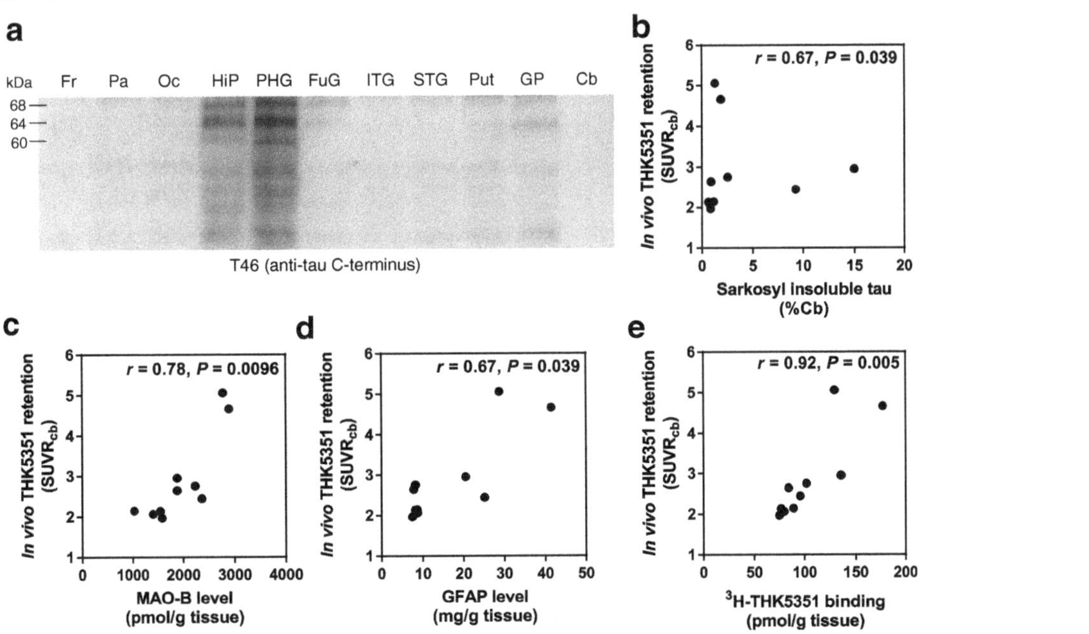

Fig. 2 Neuroimaging, biochemical, in vitro binding correlations in subject 1 (PSP-RS). **a** Immunoblot analysis of sarkosyl-insoluble tau; 11 regions (Fr, frontal cortex; Pa, parietal cortex; Oc, occipital cortex; HiP, hippocampus; PHG, parahippocampal gyrus; FuG, fusiform gyrus; ITG, inferior temporal gyrus; STG, superior temporal gyrus; Put, putamen; GP, globus pallidus; Cb, Cerebellum) detected by T46 (anti-tau C-terminus). **b** [^{18}F]THK5351 SUVR plotted against sarkosyl-insoluble tau level (%cerebellum). **c** [^{18}F]THK5351 SUVR plotted against MAO-B level. **d** [^{18}F]THK5351 SUVR plotted against GFAP level. **e** [^{18}F]THK5351 SUVR plotted against in vitro [^{3}H]THK5351 binding

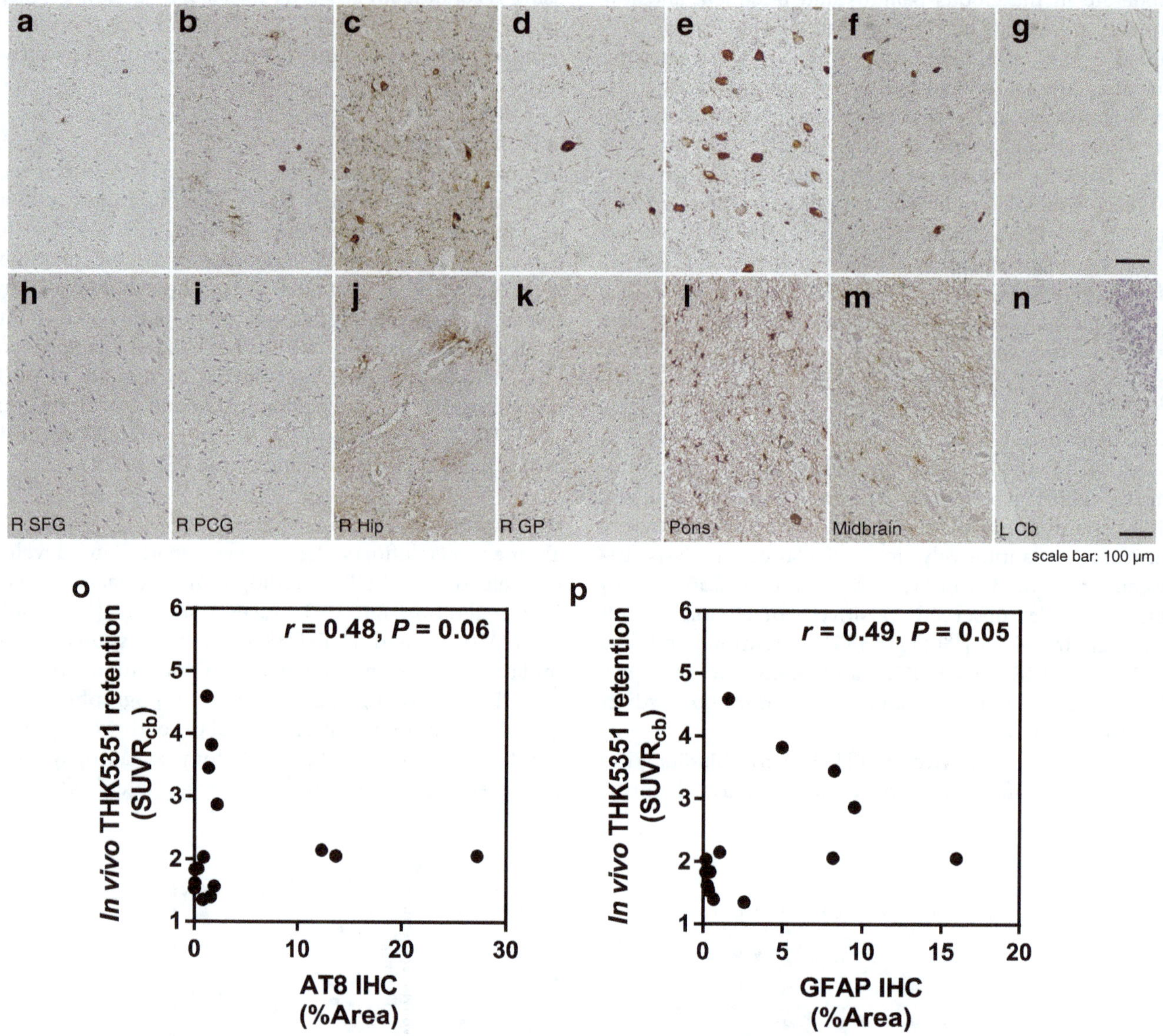

Fig. 3 Neuroimaging-histopathologic correlations in subject 1 (PSP-RS). **a–n** Microscopic examination of tau pathology (**a–g**) and astrogliosis (**h–n**). R SFG, right superior frontal gyrus (**a, n**); R PCG, right posterior cingulate gyrus (**b, i**); R HiP, right hippocampus (**c, j**); R GP, right globus pallidus (**d, k**); Pons (**e, l**); Midbrain (**f, m**); and L Cb, left cerebellar cortex (**g, n**). [^{18}F]THK5351 SUVR plotted against AT8 tau–positive areas (**o**) and GFAP-positive areas (**p**)

binding [4, 11, 27]. A recent human blocking study using selegiline demonstrated binding of [^{18}F]THK5351 to MAO-B [29]. Furthermore, the regional [^{18}F]THK5351 binding was correlated significantly with density of MAO-B in our autopsy case of AD [10]. In this study, we expanded the imaging-pathology correlation analysis to autopsy-confirmed PSP cases showing two different clinical phenotypes, Richardson syndrome (PSP-RS) and PNFA.

A patient with PSP-RS showed remarkable [^{18}F]THK5351 retention in the globus pallidus and midbrain [2, 14]. The spatial distribution of [^{18}F]THK5351 retention in this patient was similar to the topographical distribution of tau pathology in cases of classic PSP-RS [45]. Postmortem examination of this patient confirmed the existence of 4-repeat tau aggregates in these regions. However, imaging-pathology correlation analysis indicated a significant correlation between in vivo [^{18}F]THK5351 retention and MAO-B level. Furthermore, in vitro autoradiography demonstrated that [^{18}F]THK5351 binding in the globus pallidus was displaced by the MAO-B inhibitor, suggesting that [^{18}F]THK5351 mainly binds to the MAO-B rather than the 4-repeat tau aggregates. In our previous study using paraffin-embedded fixed brain sections, we observed specific binding of [^{18}F]THK5351 to tufted astrocytes

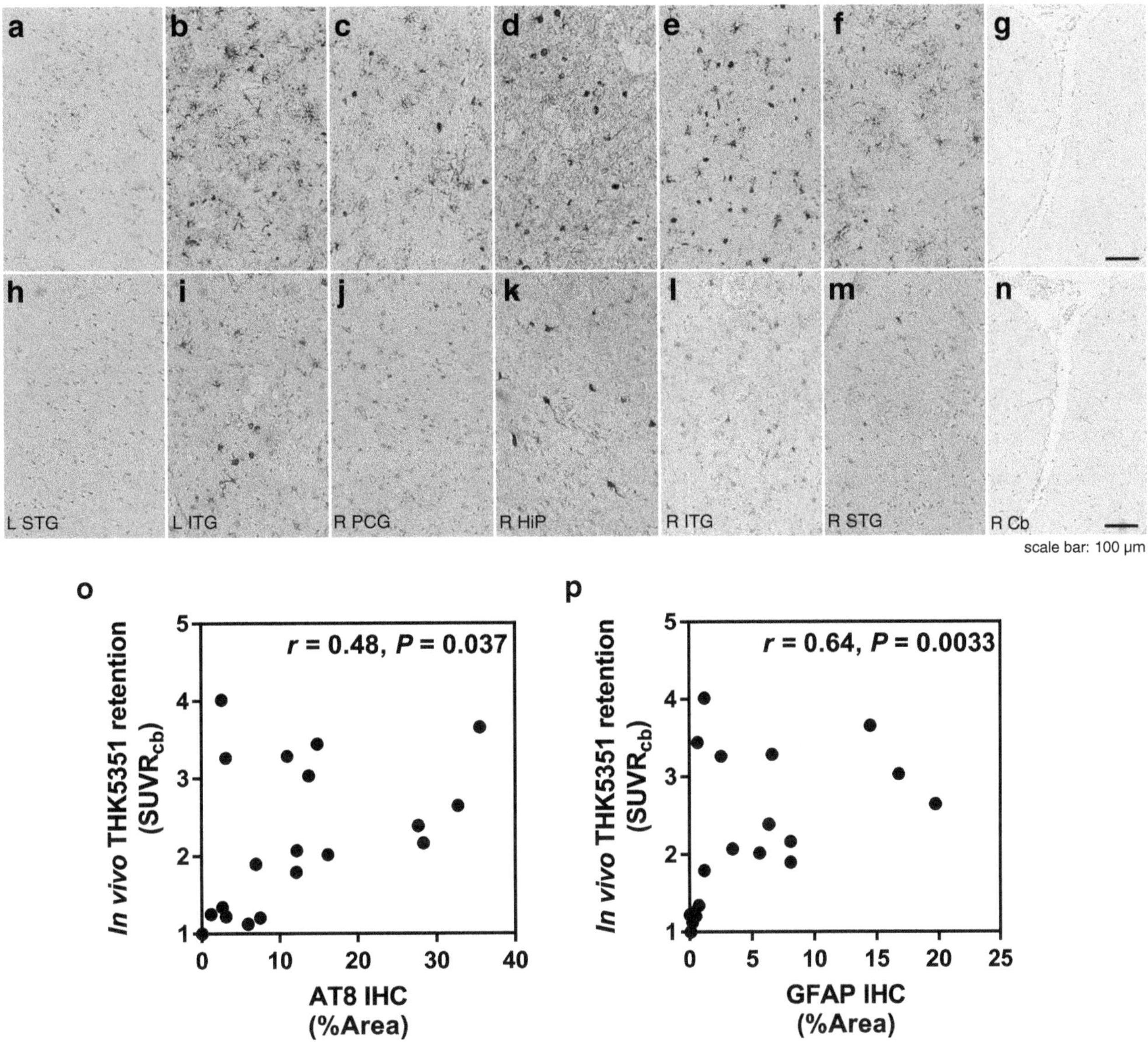

Fig. 4 Neuroimaging-histopathologic correlations in subject 2 (PNFA). **a–n** Microscopic examination of tau pathology (**a–g**) and astrogliosis (**h–n**). L STG, left superior temporal gyrus (**a, n**); L ITG, left inferior temporal gyrus (**b, i**); R PCG, right posterior cingulate gyrus (**c, j**); R HiP, right hippocampus (**d, k**); R ITG, right inferior temporal gyrus (**e, l**); R STG, right superior temporal gyrus (**f, m**); and L Cb, left cerebellar cortex (**g, n**). [^{18}F]THK5351 SUVR plotted against AT8 tau-positive areas (**o**) and GFAP-positive areas (**p**)

and neurofibrillary tangles in the PSP brain [14]. However, the fixation of tissues and use of alcohol in the differentiation process may affect the tracer binding (i.e.,., diminishing the natural binding sites and/or yielding artificial binding sites) in in vitro autoradiography experiments. In this study, we performed in vitro autoradiographs of fresh-frozen sections without using alcohol and found a substantial amount of tracer binding to MAO-B. Fresh-frozen section results showed good agreement with antemortem [^{18}F]THK5351 PET analysis. These results highlighted the importance of appropriate experimental procedures in the validation of PET radiopharmaceuticals.

[^{18}F]AV1451 PET studies in PSP cases have shown high tracer retention in the globus pallidus and midbrain, as observed in [^{18}F]THK5351 PET. However, the postmortem in vitro autoradiography did not show any significant binding of [^{18}F]AV1451 in these brain regions [18, 24, 38]. The discrepancy between in vitro and in vivo PET results may be explained also by the same technical problems as those observed in THK5351. Most of these studies used high concentrations of ethanol in the differentiation process of autoradiography [5, 25, 33, 46]. High binding affinity of [^{18}F]AV1451 to monoamine oxidases (MAO-A and MAO-B for $K_d = 1.6$ nM and 21 nM, respectively) was observed in in vitro binding

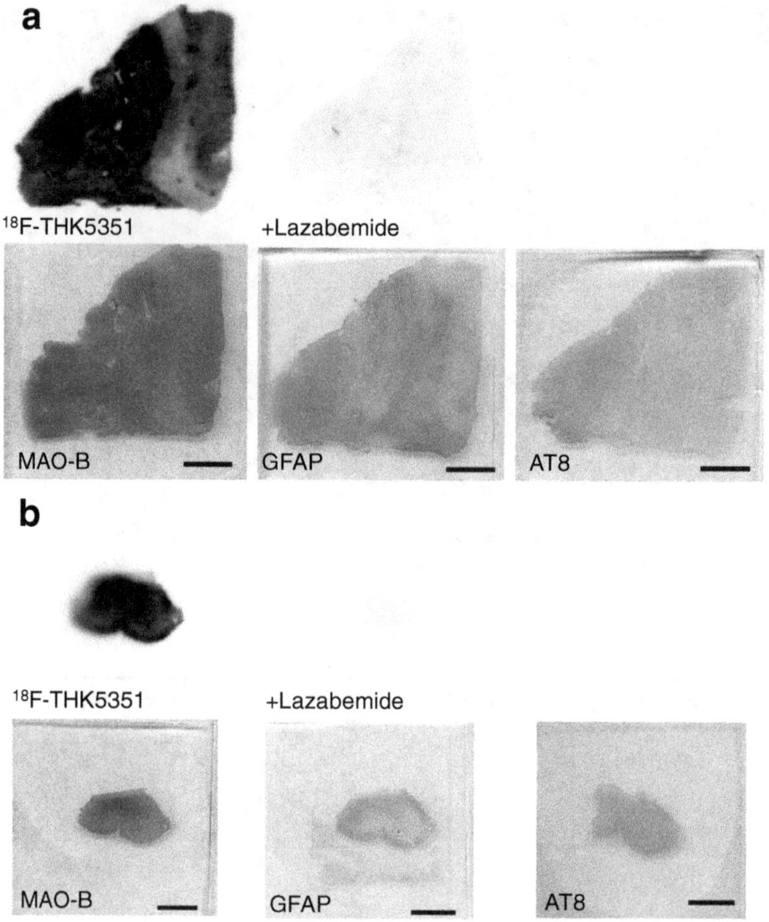

Fig. 5 In vitro autoradiography of [^{18}F]THK5351 and immunohistochemistry (MAO-B, GFAP, AT8-tau) in frozen sections from subjects. **a** Basal ganglia from subject 1 and **b** frontal cortex from subject 2. The specific binding to MAO-B was confirmed by a reversible MAO-B inhibitor, Lazabemide. *Scale bars*: 5 mm

assay [42]. [^{18}F]AV1451 binding to MAO may be overlooked by the use of ethanol. Retrospective investigation of [^{18}F]AV1451 PET in patients with Parkinson's disease showed no significant difference between conditions before and after treatment with irreversible MAO-B inhibitors (selegiline and rasagiline) [9]. Therefore, the dominant off-target binding substrates of [^{18}F]AV1451 would be MAO-A or other unknown molecules.

We observed a significant correlation between tau pathology and GFAP in both of our subjects. Tau pathology in PSP includes neurofibrillary tangles, tufted astrocytes, coiled bodies, and threads pathology [45]. A postmortem study reported that the density of GFAP correlated with that of neurofibrillary tangles, but not with tufted astrocytes in PSP, suggesting the greater contribution of neurofibrillary tangles to astrogliosis in PSP [40]. MAO-B is expressed dominantly in the mitochondrial outer membrane of astrocytes. Since elevation of MAO-B levels in the brain has been implicated in several neurodegenerative diseases, MAO-B is an attractive target as a molecular imaging marker of astrogliosis [7]. Recently, a postmortem study in parkinsonian conditions, including PSP, demonstrated that MAO-B levels elevated remarkably in the midbrain of PSP and positively correlated with astroglial markers, such as GFAP, vimentin, and Hsp27 [41], which was consistent with our observation. MAO-B PET imaging using [^{11}C]L-deprenyl-D2 showed elevated tracer retention in the brain of several neurodegenerative diseases including AD [6, 15, 34]. Other investigators have reported the elevation of tracer binding in prodromal AD, but not in symptomatic AD [3, 30, 36]. However, many postmortem studies have shown the elevation of MAO-B levels in the postmortem brains of AD [8, 26, 35]. As discussed previously [41], this discrepancy might be explained by the low sensitivity of [^{11}C]L-deprenyl-D2 PET. Recently, second-generation MAO-B PET tracers, such as [^{11}C]SL25.1188, have been developed and showed reversible binding to MAO-B [31, 32]. Furthermore, the development of [^{18}F]labeled PET tracers is ongoing [12, 28].

Our study strongly supported that [^{18}F]THK5351 PET dominantly reflected the binding to MAO-B in patients with PSP. Therefore, [^{18}F]THK5351 PET would be useful for in vivo assessment of astrogliosis in PSP. Future research should proceed with development of PET tracers for selective detection of astrogliosis and sensitive detection of 4-repeat tau in the human brain. -

In PSP-RS cases, ischemic changes observed in the putamen might induce reactive astrocytes. Recently, reactive astrocytes have been categorized into two different types depending on the gene expression: A1 astrocytes highly upregulated many classical complement cascades and are toxic as observed in neuroinflammation; A2 astrocytes upregulated many neurotrophic factors and are protective as observed in ischemia [22]. The GFAP showed elevated expression in both reactive astrocytes. [^{18}F]THK5351 PET signal in the putamen of PSP-RS cases may reflect elevation of MAO-B levels induced by ischemia. Further studies are required to clarify MAO-B expression profiles in reactive astrocytes subtypes.

Conclusions

Our imaging-pathology validation study demonstrated the binding of [^{18}F]THK5351 to MAO-B–positive astrogliosis in the PSP brain. Therefore, [^{18}F]THK5351 PET may be useful to assess astrocytosis in non-AD tauopathies.

Abbreviations

3R: 3 repeat; 4R: 4 repeat; AD: Alzheimer's disease; BSA: Bovine serum albumin; Cb: Cerebellum; CBD: Corticobasal degeneration; CBS: Corticobasal syndrome; ELISA: Enzyme-linked immunosorbent assay; Fr: Frontal cortex; FTLD: Frontemporal lobar degeneration; FuG: Fusiform gyrus; GFAP: Glial fibrillar acid protein; GP: Globus pallidus; HiP: Hippocampus; ITG: Inferior temporal gyrus; L Cb: Left cerebellar cortex; MAO-B: Monoamine oxidase-B; MRI: Magnetic resonance imaging; Oc: Occipital cortex; Pa: Parietal cortex; PBS: Phosphate-buffered saline; PET: Positron emission tomography; PHF: Paired helical filament; PHG: Parahippocampal gyrus; PNFA: Progressive nonfluent aphasia; PSP: Progressive supranuclear palsy; PSP-RS: Progressive supranuclear palsy Richardson syndrome; Put: Putamen; R GP: Right globus pallidus; R PCG: Right posterior cingulate gyrus; R SFG: Right superior frontal gyrus; STG: Superior temporal gyrus; SUV: Standardized uptake value; SUVR: Standardized uptake value ratio

Acknowledgements

We are grateful to the study subjects and the staffs for Cyclotron and Radioisotope Center, Tohoku University.

Funding

This study was supported by research funds from GE Healthcare, the SEI (Sumitomo Electric Industries, Ltd.) Group CSR Foundation, Grant-in-Aid for Research Activity Start-up (16H06621), Grant-in-Aid for Young Scientists (B) (15 K19767), Grant-in-Aid for Scientific Research (B) (15H04900), Grant-in-Aid for Scientific Research on Innovative Areas (Brain Protein Aging and Dementia Control) (26117003) from MEXT and Shimazu Science Foundation. This work is partially supported by the Initiative for Realizing Diversity in the Research Environment (Tohoku University Morinomiyako Project for Empowering Women in Research) from Japan Science and Technology Agency, JST.

Authors' contributions

AI, RH, KF, and NO conceived the study and participated in its design and coordination. AI, SW, KH, MT, and NO acquired PET images. AI, TT, NT, KF, and AH performed clinical examination. AI and NO carried out PET image analysis. RH carried out biochemical analysis, immunostaining, and autoradiography. AI, RH, and NO carried out neuroimaging-pathological correlations and performed statistical analysis and drafted the manuscript. YI, YF, SF, and RI carried out radiosynthesis. HK, NS, HS, and TK carried out autopsy, preparing tissues, immunostaining, and neuropathologic examination. YK, KY, KF, and HA supervised the study. All the authors read and approved the final manuscript.

Competing interests

NO, SF, and YK received the research funding from GE Healthcare. NO and YK own stock of CLINO Ltd.

Author details

[1]Department of Geriatrics and Gerontology, Division of Brain Science, Institute of Development, Aging and Cancer, Tohoku University, 4-1 Seiryo-machi, Aoba-ku, Sendai, Miyagi, Japan. [2]Department of Pharmacology, Tohoku University School of Medicine, 2-1 Seiryo-machi, Aoba-ku, Sendai, Miyagi, Japan. [3]Department of Neurological Science, Tohoku University School of Medicine, 2-1 Seiryo-machi, Aoba-ku, Sendai, Miyagi, Japan. [4]Department of Pathology, Tohoku University School of Medicine, 4-1 Seiryo-machi, Aoba-ku, Sendai, Miyagi, Japan. [5]Department of Nuclear Medicine and Radiology, Institute of Development, Aging and Cancer, Tohoku University, 4-1 Seiryo-machi, Aoba-ku, Sendai, Miyagi, Japan. [6]Cyclotron and Radioisotope Center, Tohoku University, 6-3 Aoba, Aramaki, Aoba-ku, Sendai, Miyagi, Japan. [7]Division of Community Medicine, Faculty of Medicine, Tohoku Medical and Pharmaceutical University, 1-15-1 Fukumuro, Miyagino-ku, Sendai, Miyagi, Japan. [8]Division of Pharmacology, Faculty of Medicine, Tohoku Medical and Pharmaceutical University, 1-15-1 Fukumuro, Miyagino-ku, Sendai, Miyagi, Japan. [9]Department of Pharmacology, Tohoku University School of Medicine 2-1, Seiryo-machi, Aoba-ku, Sendai 9808575, Japan.

References

1. Braak H, Alafuzoff I, Arzberger T, Kretzschmar H, Del Tredici K (2006) Staging of Alzheimer disease-associated neurofibrillary pathology using paraffin sections and immunocytochemistry. Acta Neuropathol 112:389–404
2. Brendel M, Schonecker S, Hoglinger G, Lindner S, Havla J, Blautzik J et al (2017) [^{18}F]-THK5351 PET correlates with topology and symptom severity in progressive supranuclear palsy. Front Aging Neurosci 9:440
3. Carter SF, Scholl M, Almkvist O, Wall A, Engler H, Langstrom B et al (2012) Evidence for astrocytosis in prodromal Alzheimer disease provided by ^{11}C-deuterium-L-deprenyl: a multitracer PET paradigm combining ^{11}C-Pittsburgh compound B and ^{18}F-FDG. J Nucl Med 53:37–46
4. Chien DT, Bahri S, Szardenings AK, Walsh JC, Mu F, Su MY et al (2013) Early clinical PET imaging results with the novel PHF-tau radioligand [F-18]-T807. J Alzheimers Dis 34:457–468
5. Declercq L, Celen S, Lecina J, Ahamed M, Tousseyn T, Moechars D et al (2016) Comparison of new tau PET-tracer candidates with [^{18}F]T808 and [^{18}F]T807. Mol Imaging 15:1-15.
6. Engler H, Nennesmo I, Kumlien E, Gambini JP, Lundberg P, Savitcheva I et al (2012) Imaging astrocytosis with PET in Creutzfeldt-Jakob disease: case report with histopathological findings. Int J Clin Exp Med 5:201–207
7. Fowler JS, Logan J, Shumay E, Alia-Klein N, Wang GJ, Volkow ND (2015) Monoamine oxidase: radiotracer chemistry and human studies. J Labelled Comp Radiopharm 58:51–64
8. Gulyas B, Pavlova E, Kasa P, Gulya K, Bakota L, Varszegi S et al (2011) Activated MAO-B in the brain of Alzheimer patients, demonstrated by [^{11}C]-L-deprenyl using whole hemisphere autoradiography. Neurochem Int 58:60–68
9. Hansen AK, Brooks DJ, Borghammer P (2018) MAO-B inhibitors do not block in vivo flortaucipir([^{18}F]-AV-1451) binding. Mol Imaging Biol 20:356–360
10. Harada R, Ishiki A, Kai H, Sato N, Furukawa K, Furumoto S et al (2017) Correlations of ^{18}F-THK5351 PET with post-mortem burden of tau and astrogliosis in Alzheimer's disease. J Nucl Med 59:671–674

11. Harada R, Okamura N, Furumoto S, Furukawa K, Ishiki A, Tomita N et al (2016) ^{18}F-THK5351: a novel PET radiotracer for imaging neurofibrillary pathology in Alzheimer disease. J Nucl Med 57:208–214
12. Hicks JW, Sadovski O, Parkes J, Houle S, Hay BA, Carter RL et al (2015) Radiosynthesis and ex vivo evaluation of [^{18}F]-(S)-3-(6-(3-fluoropropoxy)benzo[d]isoxazol-3-yl)-5-(methoxymethyl)oxazoli din-2-one for imaging MAO-B with PET. Bioorg Med Chem Lett 25:288–291
13. Ingelsson M, Fukumoto H, Newell KL, Growdon JH, Hedley-Whyte ET, Frosch MP (2004) Early Abeta accumulation and progressive synaptic loss, gliosis, and tangle formation in AD brain. Neurology 62:925–931
14. Ishiki A, Harada R, Okamura N, Tomita N, Rowe CC, Villemagne VL et al (2017) Tau imaging with [^{18}F]THK-5351 in progressive supranuclear palsy. Eur J Neurol 24:130–136
15. Johansson A, Engler H, Blomquist G, Scott B, Wall A, Aquilonius SM et al (2007) Evidence for astrocytosis in ALS demonstrated by [^{11}C](L)-deprenyl-D2 PET. J Neurol Sci 255:17–22
16. Johnson KA, Schultz A, Betensky RA, Becker JA, Sepulcre J, Rentz D et al (2016) Tau positron emission tomographic imaging in aging and early Alzheimer disease. Ann Neurol 79:110–119
17. Josephs KA, Boeve BF, Duffy JR, Smith GE, Knopman DS, Parisi JE et al (2005) Atypical progressive supranuclear palsy underlying progressive apraxia of speech and nonfluent aphasia. Neurocase 11:283–296
18. Josephs KA, Whitwell JL, Tacik P, Duffy JR, Senjem ML, Tosakulwong N et al (2017) [^{18}F]AV-1451 tau-PET uptake does correlate with quantitatively measured 4R-tau burden in autopsy-confirmed corticobasal degeneration. Acta Neuropathol 132:931–933
19. Kikuchi A, Okamura N, Hasegawa T, Harada R, Watanuki S, Funaki Y et al (2016) In vivo visualization of tau deposits in corticobasal syndrome by ^{18}F-THK5351 PET. Neurology 87:2309–2316
20. Kouri N, Murray ME, Hassan A, Rademakers R, Uitti RJ, Boeve BF et al (2017) Neuropathological features of corticobasal degeneration presenting as corticobasal syndrome or Richardson syndrome. Brain 134:3264–3275
21. Kovacs GG, Ferrer I, Grinberg LT, Alafuzoff I, Attems J, Budka H et al (2016) Aging-related tau astrogliopathy (ARTAG): harmonized evaluation strategy. Acta Neuropathol 131:87–102
22. Liddelow SA, Guttenplan KA, Clarke LE, Bennett FC, Bohlen CJ, Schirmer L et al (2017) Neurotoxic reactive astrocytes are induced by activated microglia. Nature 541:481–487
23. Lois C, Gonzalez I, Johnson KA, Price JC (2018) PET imaging of tau protein targets: a methodology perspective. Brain Imaging Behav 1:1–2
24. Marquie M, Normandin MD, Meltzer AC, Siao Tick Chong M, Andrea NV, Anton-Fernandez A et al (2017) Pathological correlations of [F-18]-AV-1451 imaging in non-alzheimer tauopathies. Ann Neurol 81:117–128
25. Marquie M, Normandin MD, Vanderburg CR, Costantino IM, Bien EA, Rycyna LG et al (2015) Validating novel tau positron emission tomography tracer [F-18]-AV-1451 (T807) on postmortem brain tissue. Ann Neurol 78:787–800
26. Marutle A, Gillberg PG, Bergfors A, Yu W, Ni R, Nennesmo I et al (2013) ^{3}H-deprenyl and ^{3}H-PIB autoradiography show different laminar distributions of astroglia and fibrillar beta-amyloid in Alzheimer brain. J Neuroinflammation 10:90
27. Maruyama M, Shimada H, Suhara T, Shinotoh H, Ji B, Maeda J et al (2013) Imaging of tau pathology in a tauopathy mouse model and in Alzheimer patients compared to normal controls. Neuron 79:1094–1108
28. Nag S, Fazio P, Lehmann L, Kettschau G, Heinrich T, Thiele A et al (2016) In vivo and in vitro characterization of a novel MAO-B inhibitor Radioligand, ^{18}F-labeled deuterated Fluorodeprenyl. J Nucl Med 57:315–320
29. Ng KP, Pascoal TA, Mathotaarachchi S, Therriault J, Kang MS, Shin M et al (2017) Monoamine oxidase B inhibitor, selegiline, reduces ^{18}F-THK5351 uptake in the human brain. Alzheimers Res Ther 9:25
30. Rodriguez-Vieitez E, Saint-Aubert L, Carter SF, Almkvist O, Farid K, Scholl M et al (2016) Diverging longitudinal changes in astrocytosis and amyloid PET in autosomal dominant Alzheimer's disease. Brain 139:922–936
31. Rusjan PM, Wilson AA, Miler L, Fan I, Mizrahi R, Houle S et al (2014) Kinetic modeling of the monoamine oxidase B radioligand [^{11}C]SL25.1188 in human brain with high-resolution positron emission tomography. J Cereb Blood Flow Metab 34:883–889
32. Saba W, Valette H, Peyronneau MA, Bramoulle Y, Coulon C, Curet O et al (2010) [^{11}C]SL25.1188, a new reversible radioligand to study the monoamine oxidase type B with PET: preclinical characterisation in nonhuman primate. Synapse 64:61–69
33. Sander K, Lashley T, Gami P, Gendron T, Lythgoe MF, Rohrer JD et al (2016) Characterization of tau positron emission tomography tracer [^{18}F]AV-1451 binding to postmortem tissue in Alzheimer's disease, primary tauopathies, and other dementias. Alzheimers Dement 12:1116–1124
34. Santillo AF, Gambini JP, Lannfelt L, Langstrom B, Ulla-Marja L, Kilander L et al (2011) In vivo imaging of astrocytosis in Alzheimer's disease: an ^{11}C-L-deuteriodeprenyl and PIB PET study. Eur J Nucl Med Mol Imaging 38: 2202–2208
35. Saura J, Luque JM, Cesura AM, Da Prada M, Chan-Palay V, Huber G et al (1994) Increased monoamine oxidase B activity in plaque-associated astrocytes of Alzheimer brains revealed by quantitative enzyme radioautography. Neuroscience 62:15–30
36. Scholl M, Carter SF, Westman E, Rodriguez-Vieitez E, Almkvist O, Thordardottir S (2015) Early astrocytosis in autosomal dominant Alzheimer's disease measured in vivo by multi-tracer positron emission tomography. Sci Rep 5:16404
37. Smith R, Puschmann A, Scholl M, Ohlsson T, van Swieten J, Honer M et al (2016) [^{18}F]AV-1451 tau PET imaging correlates strongly with tau neuropathology in MAPT mutation carriers. Brain 139:2372–2379
38. Smith R, Scholl M, Honer M, Nilsson CF, Englund E, Hansson O (2017) Tau neuropathology correlates with FDG-PET, but not AV-1451-PET, in progressive supranuclear palsy. Acta Neuropathol 133:149–151
39. Taniguchi-Watanabe S, Arai T, Kametani F, Nonaka T, Masuda-Suzukake M, Tarutani A et al (2016) Biochemical classification of tauopathies by immunoblot, protein sequence and mass spectrometric analyses of sarkosyl-insoluble and trypsin-resistant tau. Acta Neuropathol 131:267–280
40. Togo T, Dickson DW (2012) Tau accumulation in astrocytes in progressive supranuclear palsy is a degenerative rather than a reactive process. Acta Neuropathol 104:398–402
41. Tong J, Rathitharan G, Meyer JH, Furukawa Y, Ang LC, Boileau I et al (2017) Brain monoamine oxidase B and a in human parkinsonian dopamine deficiency disorders. Brain 140:2460–2474
42. Vermeiren C, Motte P, Viot D, Mairet-Coello G, Courade JP, Citron M et al (2018) The tau positron-emission tomography tracer AV-1451 binds with similar affinities to tau fibrils and monoamine oxidases. Mov Disord 33: 273–281
43. Villemagne VL (2018) Selective tau imaging: der stand der dinge. J Nucl Med 59:175–176
44. Villemagne VL, Dore V, Burnham SC, Masters CL, Rowe CC (2018) Imaging tau and amyloid-beta proteinopathies in Alzheimer disease and other conditions. Nat Rev Neurol 14:225
45. Williams DR, Holton JL, Strand C, Pittman A, de Silva R, Lees AJ et al (2007) Pathological tau burden and distribution distinguishes progressive supranuclear palsy-parkinsonism from Richardson's syndrome. Brain 130: 1566–1576
46. Xia CF, Arteaga J, Chen G, Gangadharmath U, Gomez LF, Kasi D et al (2013) [^{18}F]T807, a novel tau positron emission tomography imaging agent for Alzheimer's disease. Alzheimers Dement 9:666–676

9

Neuropathology and cognitive performance in self-reported cognitively healthy centenarians

Andrea B. Ganz[1,2,3], Nina Beker[3], Marc Hulsman[4], Sietske Sikkes[3], Netherlands Brain Bank[5], Philip Scheltens[3], August B. Smit[1], Annemieke J. M. Rozemuller[2], Jeroen J. M. Hoozemans[2†] and Henne Holstege[3,4*†]

Abstract

With aging, the incidence of neuropathological hallmarks of neurodegenerative diseases increases in the brains of cognitively healthy individuals. It is currently unclear to what extent these hallmarks associate with symptoms of disease at extreme ages. Forty centenarians from the 100-plus Study cohort donated their brain. Centenarians self-reported to be cognitively healthy at baseline, which was confirmed by a proxy. Objective ante-mortem measurements of cognitive performance were associated with the prevalence, distribution and quantity of age- and AD-related neuropathological hallmarks. Despite self-reported cognitive health, objective neuropsychological testing suggested varying levels of ante-mortem cognitive functioning. Post-mortem, we found that neuropathological hallmarks related to age and neurodegenerative diseases, such as Aβ and Tau pathology, as well as atherosclerosis, were abundantly present in most or all centenarians, whereas Lewy body and pTDP-43 pathology were scarce. We observed that increased pathology loads correlated across pathology subtypes, and an overall trend of higher pathology loads to associate with a lower cognitive test performance. This trend was carried especially by the presence of neurofibrillary tangles (NFTs) and granulovacuolar degeneration (GVD) and to a lesser extent by Aβ-associated pathologies. Cerebral Amyloid Angiopathy (CAA) specifically associated with lower executive functioning in the centenarians. In conclusion, we find that while the centenarians in this cohort escaped or delayed cognitive impairment until extreme ages, their brains reveal varying levels of disease-associated neuropathological hallmarks, some of which associate with cognitive performance.

Keywords: Healthy aging, Cognitively healthy centenarians, 100-plus Study, Neuropathology, Alzheimer's disease, Clinicopathological correlation

Introduction

The increase in average life expectancy warrants insight into healthy aging. In particular, the study of centenarians might reveal new leads towards healthy aging and potential clues to overcome age-related diseases. Alzheimer's disease (AD) is the most common age-related neurodegenerative disease for which increasing age is the most important risk factor. The prevalence of AD is estimated to double every 5 years after the age of 65, resulting in a population prevalence of roughly 40% for western Europeans aged 90 years and older [11, 31, 35]. The two most prominent neuropathological hallmarks of AD are (1) the intracellular accumulation of hyperphosphorylated Tau protein (pTau) in Neurofibrillary tangles (NFTs) and (2) the accumulation of extracellular Amyloid-β (Aβ) fibrils into senile plaques [27, 33]. Additional AD-associated neuropathological changes are: neuritic plaques (NPs), where Aβ plaques and dystrophic neurites occur in the same structures, cerebral amyloid angiopathy (CAA), characterized by the deposition of Aβ in the endothelial cells of blood vessels, and granulovacuolar degeneration (GVD), which is characterized by the accumulation of stress proteins in

* Correspondence: h.holstege@vumc.nl
†Jeroen J. M. Hoozemans and Henne Holstege contributed equally to this work.
[3]Alzheimer Centre, Department of Neurology, Amsterdam Neuroscience, VU University Medical Center, Postbus 7057, 1007 MB Amsterdam, The Netherlands
[4]Department of Clinical Genetics, Amsterdam Neuroscience, VU University Medical Center, de Boelelaan, 1118 1081 HV Amsterdam, The Netherlands
Full list of author information is available at the end of the article

intracellular granules. Whereas Lewy body and phosphorylated TAR DNA-binding protein 43 (pTDP-43) proteinopathies are usually associated with other neurodegenerative diseases, they often are also observed in late-onset AD cases [42].

Clinicopathologic correlation studies revealed that the severity of cognitive impairment in AD correlates best with the burden of neocortical NFTs [31]. The presence of Aβ is a prerequisite for AD and may catalyze the pathological process that ultimately leads to clinical dementia [42]. However, the concurrent accumulation of individual pathologies, like CAA, GVD, LB, and pTDP-43, may have an additive effect on the rate of cognitive decline, and contribute to the apparent decrease of the association between NFTs, Aβ and dementia symptoms in older ages [42]. Brains of older dementia patients commonly show less NFT and Aβ pathology compared to younger AD patients [9, 17, 18, 38]. This suggests that, while disease-associated proteinopathies distinguish well between brains from young AD cases and age-matched non-demented controls, this appears more complicated for brains from older individuals. So far, post-mortem brain assessments of cognitively healthy individuals who reached > 110 years revealed various results: some cognitively healthy centenarians did not accumulate significant pathology, while others appeared to have relatively high levels of pathology [13, 32, 43].

Strengths and weaknesses, and the unique aspects of the 100-plus Study

Ideally, to assess the unique aspects of maintained cognitive health during extreme longevity, one would like to assess brain tissues of cognitively healthy centenarians from individuals who were recruited at much younger ages and followed up until death, i.e. in the context of a longitudinal population study. However, this is complicated as only a small subset of individuals reaches ages older than 100 and of these, only a small subset remains cognitively healthy. To overcome this problem, most studies collected tissues retrospectively, and often, no extensive and consistent set of neuropsychological measurements before death is available [6, 12–14, 16, 20]. Furthermore, we found that most studies dichotomize the disease label (case or control) based on post-mortem findings or on neuropsychological assessments and/or clinical diagnosis of dementia (e.g. CDR scale), that were collected relatively long prior to death [2, 4, 6, 10, 13, 16, 17, 19, 21, 25]. Some studies provide only (semi-)quantitative scores of selected hallmarks in selected brain regions [8, 9, 15]. Together, this complicates the neuropathological assessment of resilience against cognitive decline despite extreme longevity [6, 12–14, 16, 20].

In the 100-plus Study, we focus specifically on this aspect by including only cognitively healthy centenarians in our cohort [19]. The longitudinal set-up of our study allows us to focus specifically on the neuropsychological changes prior to death and the levels and distribution of neuropathology throughout the brain. For this, a unique aspect of the 100-plus Study is the longitudinal administering of a comprehensive set of neuropsychological tests between 100 years and death. After death, we invest in a complete characterization of brain tissues, using an elaborate set of neuropathological hallmarks across several brain areas. The 100-plus Study is relatively young, and while 91 centenarians have agreed to post-mortem brain donation, we can now present the initial data of the first 40 brains.

The aim of this study is to investigate how neuropathological changes relate with performance on neuropsychological tests in centenarians. Prospective neuropsychological testing of these individuals allowed us to correlate ante-mortem cognitive functioning of selected tests with the occurrence of pathological hallmarks of neurodegenerative diseases in the post-mortem brain. For this, we focused on inclusions of pTau as NFTs [4] and aging-related tau astrogliopathy (ARTAG) [24]; the distribution of Aβ protein as diffuse [46], classical or NPs [26], and CAA [45]; the distribution of casein kinase 1 delta (CK1δ) as a marker of GVD [44]; and the distribution Lewy bodies [7] and pTDP-43 accumulations [28]. Furthermore, for an individual case, we report on the in-vivo assessment of pathology using an MRI and amyloid PET scan, and the occurrence of post-mortem neuropathological changes.

Material and methods

100-plus Study cohort

The 100-plus Study is a prospective centenarian cohort study. Inclusion criteria for the study are, next to being able to provide proof of being 100 years or older, that centenarians "self-report to be cognitively healthy, which is confirmed by a proxy" [19]. Although it is not a requirement for study participation, almost 30% of all participants agree to post-mortem brain donation. Here we compare the ante- and post-mortem status of the first 40 participants of the 100-plus Study that came to autopsy.

The 100-Plus Study was approved by the Medical Ethical Committee of the VU University Medical Center. Informed consent was obtained from all study participants. The detailed study protocol is described elsewhere [19].

Post-mortem brain autopsy procedures

Autopsies were performed in collaboration with the Netherlands Brain Bank (NBB, Amsterdam, The Netherlands). Brain weight was recorded, and we macroscopically determined levels of atrophy and atherosclerosis of the intracranial vessels. Atrophy was subjectively staged by an experienced neuropathologist according to severity (none (0), mild (1), moderate (2) or strong (3)). Atherosclerosis was scored as mild (1), if only some parts of the circle of Willis and the basal arteries were affected; moderate (2), if the circle of Willis and the basal arteries were severely affected and the arteria cerebri media was not affected beyond the first cm; and severe (3), if also the deeper part of the arteria cerebri media was affected. The right hemisphere of the brain was formalin fixed, and the left hemisphere was dissected and the pieces were snap frozen in liquid nitrogen.

Neuropathology: Immunohistochemistry

Neuropathological characterization of centenarian brains was performed by Haematoxylin and Eosin (H&E) stain, Gallyas silver stain [34, 48] and immunohistochemistry (IHC). For IHC, brain tissues were formalin fixed and paraffin embedded (FFPE), then sectioned into 6 μm slices and mounted on microscope slides (Leica Xtra adhesive slides, Leica Microsystems, Rijswijk, The Netherlands). After deparaffinization and rehydration, endogenous peroxidase activity was blocked in 0.3% H_2O_2 in phosphate buffered saline, pH 7.0 (PBS) for 30 min. Antigen retrieval was performed with heated sodium-citrate buffer (10 mM/L, pH 6.0). For the staining of α-synuclein, pretreatment included only heated sodium citrate without endogenous peroxidase blocking. All primary antibodies were diluted in normal antibody diluent (Immunologic, VWR company, Duiven, The Netherlands) (Table 1). Primary antibody incubation was performed overnight at 4 ° C. Subsequently, sections were incubated with the EnVision detection system (goat anti-mouse/rabbit horseradish peroxidase (HRP), DAKO, Heverlee, Belgium) for 40 min at room temperature. Between incubation steps, sections were rinsed with PBS. Sections were incubated for 5 min with the chromogen 3,3′-diaminobenzidine (DAB, EnVision Detection system/HRP, DAKO, Heverlee, Belgium) to visualize immunoreactivity. Nuclei were counterstained with haematoxylin. Hereafter, slides were dehydrated and mounted using the non-aqueous mounting medium Quick-D (Klinipath, Duiven, The Netherlands). Negative controls were obtained by performing the same procedures while omitting the primary antibody.

Neuropathological evaluation

Distribution of Aβ and pTau in NFTs and NPs was determined by immunohistochemical staining (IHC) with respectively IC-16 and AT-8 antibodies on the frontal cortex (F2), temporal pole cortex, parietal cortex (superior and inferior lobule), occipital pole cortex and the hippocampus (CA1 and entorhinal area of the parahippocampal gyrus). NFTs and NPs were identified using a combination of Gallyas silver staining and IHC for AT-8. Aβ distribution was evaluated according to the Thal staging ranging from 0 to 5 [47]. The temporal-spatial distribution of NFTs was evaluated according to the Braak stages ranging from 0 to VI [3–5]. NPs were evaluated according to CERAD scores ranging from 0 to 3 [26].

The presence of ARTAG was assessed using IHC for pTau in the frontal cortex (F2), temporal pole cortex, parietal cortex (superior and inferior lobule), occipital pole cortex and the hippocampus (CA1 and entorhinal area of the parahippocampal gyrus).

GVD was assessed by IHC using CK1δ as a marker, and scored based on the staging system from Thal et al., 2011 (Thal stage GVD*) [44], ranging from 0 to 5. The presence of CK1δ positive accumulations was assessed in the hippocampal areas CA1/Subiculum and CA4, entorhinal cortex, temporal pole cortex, amygdala, cingulate gyrus, frontal (F2) and parietal lobe. GVD stage was classified as 1, if only the subiculum and CA1 region of the hippocampal formation were affected. In stage 2, the CA4 and/or entorhinal cortex were additionally affected. Additional CK1δ granules in the temporal pole cortex were classified as stage 3. Cases were scored as stage 4 if the amygdala was affected, but neither the cingulate gyrus or the frontal or parietal cortex were affected. If either cingulate gyrus, frontal cortex or parietal cortex showed additional depositions of CK1δ, cases were classified as stage 5.

pTDP-43 pathology was assessed by IHC and stages ranged from 0 to 3 according to Nag et al., 2015 [28]. Immunohistochemistry with the pTDP-43 antibody was performed on slices of the amygdala (stage 1), hippocampal areas CA1/Subiculum and dentate gyrus, entorhinal cortex (stage 2), frontal and temporal pole cortex

Table 1 Overview of primary antibodies

Antibody	Antigen	Species	Dilution (FFPE material)	Manufacturer
IC-16	N-terminal amino acids 1–6 of the Aβ peptide	mouse	1:800	Kind gift of Prof. Dr. Korth, Heinrich Heine University, Düsseldorf, Germany [50]
AT-8	Tau phosphorylated at Ser202 and Thr205	mouse	1:800	Pierce Biotechnology, Rockford, IL, USA
CK1δ	casein kinase 1 delta	mouse	1:100	Santa Cruz Biotechnology, Heidelberg, Germany
pTDP-43	Transactive response DNA binding protein 43	mouse	1:8000	Cosmo Bio, Tokyo, Japan
LB509	alpha-synuclein	mouse	1:200	Zymed, Thermo Fisher Scientific, Bleiswijk, The Netherlands

(stage 3), in which the presence of cytoplasmic inclusions was assessed.

Lewy body pathology was assessed according to Braak [2, 7] by IHC for α-synuclein in the hippocampus, amygdala, medulla oblongata, substantia nigra and locus coeruleus. For a case with high amounts of α-synuclein inclusions, the frontal and precentral gyrus were additionally assessed.

Neuropsychological tests and educational attainment

All study participants were visited at home by a trained researcher at baseline inclusion, and when available and willing, at yearly follow-up visits. During these visits, we objectively assessed cognitive functioning using an elaborate test battery described elsewhere [19]. Here we report the performance on the Mini-Mental State Examination (MMSE), Visual Association Test (VAT) and the Clock Drawing Test (CDT), as they are well known and often used for dementia screening. The MMSE is an 11-item test evaluating overall cognitive functioning with a scoring range of 0–30 (bad-good) [16]; missing items were imputed as described before [19], provided no more than 6 items were missing. The VAT is a test for episodic memory with a 0–12 (trial 1 + 2) range (bad-good) [25], and the CDT is a test for visuospatial and executive functioning, with a 0–5 range (bad-good) [39, 40]. When sensory impairments, fatigue, or lack of motivation impeded test administration, no score was reported (N/A). We report test scores at baseline and at last visit before death. For cases with only one visit, baseline- and last visit are the same. Number of visits and time between last visit and death per case is listed in Additional file 1: Table S1. Educational attainment was assessed by self-report and categorized according to the International Standard Classification of Education 1997 (ISCED) [49], as well as years of education.

Correlation of cognitive performance with post-mortem brain pathology

To determine whether performance on cognitive tests of centenarians correlated with post-mortem brain pathologies, we correlated pre-mortem neuropsychological test scores and demographic descriptives with levels of post-mortem neuropathological hallmarks of aging and disease. For this, we used MMSE, VAT and CDT test scores, both at baseline and last visit. A secondary measure of cognitive performance was "the ability to complete testing" as a proxy of fatigue or non-willingness; scores were 2 (all tests completed, or tests not applied due to sensory problems), 1 (MMSE completed, which was administered first, but not VAT and/or CDT), and 0 (no tests completed). After each study visit, the impression of cognitive health of the participant was subjectively estimated by a trained researcher as 0 (symptoms of impairment), 1 (possible symptoms of impairment), or 2 (no symptoms of impairment) (see [19] for protocol). The scored impression of cognitive health closest to death was used for analysis. ApoE genotypes were ranked according to their association with increased AD-risk (odds ratios) as reported previously [8]: E2/2 (OR 0.24); E2/3 (OR 0.5); E3/3 (OR 1.0); E2/4 (OR 3.2); E3/4 (OR 5.5), E4/4 (OR 20.6). Education was categorized by years of formal education. Sex: female, 0; male, 1. As post-mortem characteristics of all 40 brains, we used brain weights, corrected for sex by linear regression and the levels of atrophy and atherosclerosis, scored as described above. For a subset of 35 brains, Thal stage GVD* and pTDP-43 staging was available, and for 26 brains Braak stage for Lewy bodies, Thal stage for CAA, Thal stage for Aβ, CERAD score for NPs, Braak stage for NFT distribution, infarct occurrence and hippocampal sclerosis presence was available. Overview of all variables is provided in Additional file 2: Tables S2 and Additional file 1: Table S1.

Statistical analyses

Correlations between neuropsychological test performance and neuropathology were determined using Pearson correlation. We calculated *p*-values and false discovery rates (fdr) for all correlations (Additional file 3: Tables S3b and S3c). In Fig. 3, strength of the Pearson correlation coefficient is indicated by the size and color of each dot (Additional file 3: Table S3a), the fdr is indicated as asterisks (* < 20%, ** < 10%, *** < 5%). All calculations were performed in R (version 3.3) [36].

PET/MRI scan in case report

Scanning was performed 1 month after study inclusion for case 100069. The participant was injected with 383 MBq 11C-PIB. Sixty minutes after injection, dynamic images of the brain were captured on the Philips TF PET-MRI scanner in 6 frames of 5 min duration. Due to extensive movement, only the activity in the first frame could be used. The PET scan was visually assessed by an experienced nuclear medicine physician.

Results

We analyzed brain tissue from 40 centenarians, (72.5% female), aged between 100 and 111 years (Additional file 1: Table S1).

Neuropathological characteristics in centenarian brains

The mean post-mortem interval for all 40 donated brains was 6h44min (range: 3.5–12 h). At autopsy the median brain weight was 1195 g (IQR 1060 g–1355 g) in males and 1115 g (IQR 965 g–1320 g) in females. ApoE genotypes were: E2/3 (15.8%), E3/3 (73.7%), E2/4 (5.3%), and E3/4 (7.9%). Full neuropathological characterization was present for 26 brains, partial characterization with staging for pTDP-43 stage and Thal stage GVD* was present for 35 cases. We observed varying levels of atherosclerosis in all 40 brains. Mild or moderate atrophy was present in 50% of all cases, while severe atrophy was not observed in any of the 40 brains. All 26 centenarian-brains with full neuropathological assessment revealed known age-related pathologies such as ARTAG [24] (Fig. 1c and Additional file 1: Table S1), and were scored with high stages of GVD: only GVD stages between 3 and 5 were observed (Fig. 1i). According to the NIA-AA guidelines, 8% of the centenarians had no AD-associated neuropathological changes, 42% had low neuropathological changes, 50% had intermediate changes, and none had high level of changes (Fig. 1g). Levels of Aβ deposits cover all possible Thal stages (mean Thal stage for Aβ: 2.6). The NFT distribution ranged from Braak stage I to IV, (mean Braak stage: III). None of the centenarians had Braak stage 0, or Braak stage V or VI. The level of NPs ranged from CERAD scores 0 to 2, CERAD score 3 was not observed (mean CERAD score: 0.8). In 20 of the 26 centenarians we observed CAA pathology (77%, mean Thal stage for CAA: 1), always in combination with Aβ plaques. We observed pTDP-43 pathology in 13 of 35 centenarians (37%, mean pTDP-43 stage: 0.9), and 5 cases showed additional hippocampal sclerosis (19.2%). Hippocampal sclerosis was exclusively observed in combination with pTDP-43 pathology (Additional file 1: Table S1). Lewy body pathology was observed in 4 of 26 cases (15.4%, mean Braak stage for Lewy bodies: 0.4), 3 of which co-occurred with pTDP-43 pathology. Despite high cognitive test performance (baseline score on the MMSE: 27), one case was clinically diagnosed with Parkinson's disease years before entering the study. The brain included many Lewy bodies at post-mortem neuropathological evaluation (Braak stage for Lewy bodies VI). Additionally, we detected infarcts in 14 (54%) of the 26 centenarians.

Overall, the centenarians in our cohort showed moderate levels of AD related pathology. Centenarians rarely showed the highest score for any of the AD associated

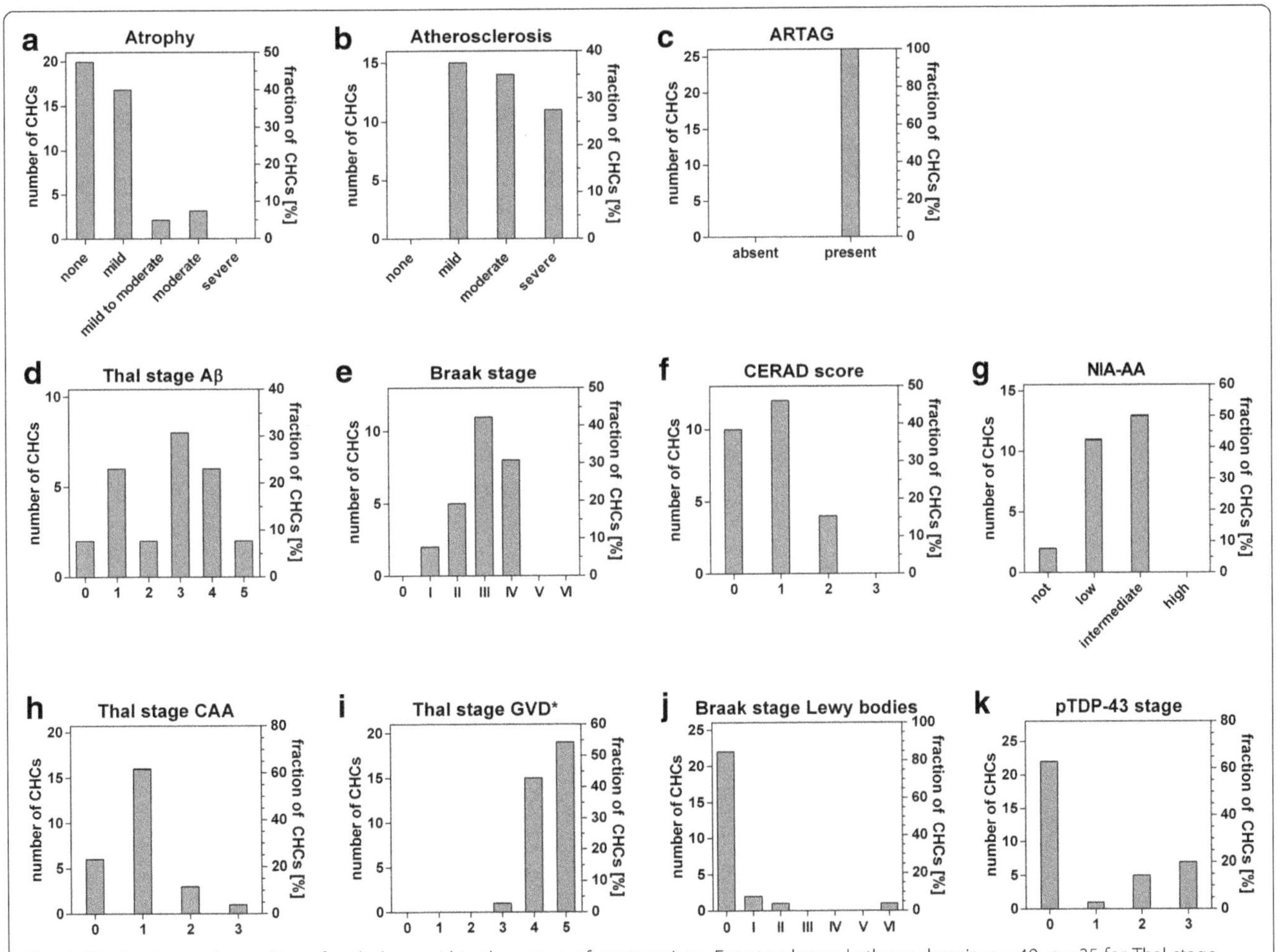

Fig. 1 Distribution and severities of pathology within the group of centenarians. For atrophy and atherosclerosis, $n = 40$. $n = 35$ for Thal stage GVD* and pTDP-43 stage, for all other pathologies, $n = 26$. Thal stage GVD* indicates a staging system adapted from Thal et al., 2011 [44]

pathologies, with the exception of GVD. Overall scores for Lewy bodies and pTDP-43 appeared relatively low in centenarians.

Performance on neuropsychological tests of 40 centenarian brain donors

The aim of this study is to investigate how neuropathological changes are associated with performance on neuropsychological tests in centenarians. The last visit occurred on average 10 ± 7 months prior to brain donation. 18 centenarians were available for at least one follow-up visit; follow-up for two additional centenarians was performed by questionnaire. Centenarians had a variable educational attainment (median years of education: 8, range 6 - 20y). MMSE, VAT and CDT scores were available for respectively 95, 67.5 and 65% of centenarians at baseline (Fig. 2a). At last visit, MMSE, VAT and CDT scores were available for respectively 87.5, 57.5 and 52.5% of centenarians. The mean (±SD) score on the MMSE was 24 ± 4.5 at baseline and 23.7 ± 4.6 at last visit. Mean scores for the VAT were 7.7 ± 3.2 at baseline and 6.9 ± 3.6 at last visit respectively (Fig. 2b), while CDT scores were on average 2.9 ± 1.3 at baseline and 3.3 ± 1.5 at last visit (Fig. 2c). Detailed demographics, neuropsychological and neuropathological measurements at the individual level are listed in Additional file 1: Table S1.

Correlations between different neuropathological hallmarks

The levels of neuropathological hallmarks of AD are inter-correlated (Fig. 3 and Additional file 3: Table S3). Particularly, Braak stage for NFTs correlated significantly with GVD levels (false discovery rate (fdr = 0.002), and to a lesser extent with CERAD scores (fdr = 0.196). Thal stage for Aβ correlated significantly with levels of CAA and Braak stages (fdr = 0.8; and fdr = 0.16 respectively), and as expected with CERAD scores (fdr = 4.46E-16). pTDP-43 stage is strongly correlated with hippocampal sclerosis (fdr = 0.044). In contrast, the levels of alpha-synuclein were not associated with the levels of any other assessed neuropathology.

Correlations between test performance, demographic characteristics and pathology

We observed an overall trend that performance correlates among cognitive tests. For the centenarians who completed cognitive tests at baseline and at last visit, we find a strong correlation between performances (Fig. 3). The ability to complete testing was associated with lower ages at death, researcher impression of cognitive health and higher baseline MMSE scores. Likewise, we observed that pathology loads correlate among some pathology subtypes. We also observe an overall trend that lower pathology loads correlate with better performance on tests (Fig. 3). This trend is mainly carried by the association of Braak stages for NFTs and higher GVD stages with lower cognitive performance across all tests. Higher Thal stages for Aβ pathology and higher CERAD scores also show this trend with lower test performance, but to a much lesser extent. Two specific associations stand out: First, increased loads of CAA correlated significantly with a low CDT performance at baseline (fdr = 0.156) and, despite a smaller group-size, this association was intensified for CDT performance at last visit (fdr = 0.02). Second, the presence and severity of hippocampal sclerosis correlated with a decreased ability to complete testing at follow up visits (fdr = 0.03) and non-significantly with a lower performance on the MMSE, both at baseline (fdr = 0.46), and last visit (fdr = 0.24). GVD stage only correlated with a low MMSE performance at baseline (fdr = 0.16). This correlation was lost at last visit (fdr = 0.25).

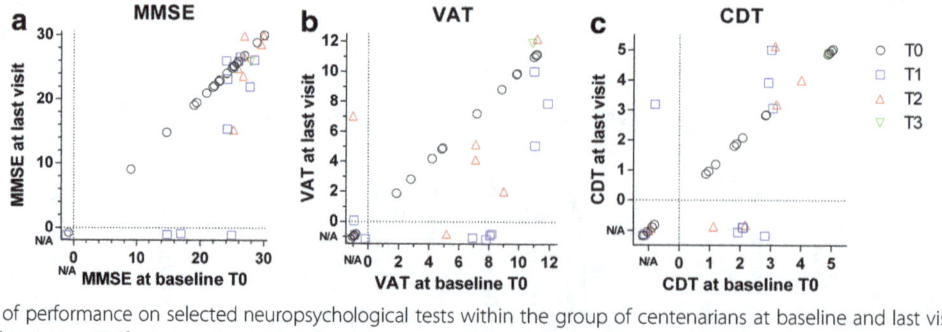

Fig. 2 Distribution of performance on selected neuropsychological tests within the group of centenarians at baseline and last visit. For all neuropsychological tests, $n = 40$. If a test was not administered or not completed, the score was indicated as not available (N/A), set apart from the scores by a dashed line. Dots are scattered to ensure visibility of all points. Cases for which only baseline data is available (T0) are shown as black circles, cases with one (T1), two (T2) or three (T3) follow-up visit are shown as blue squares and red or green triangles respectively

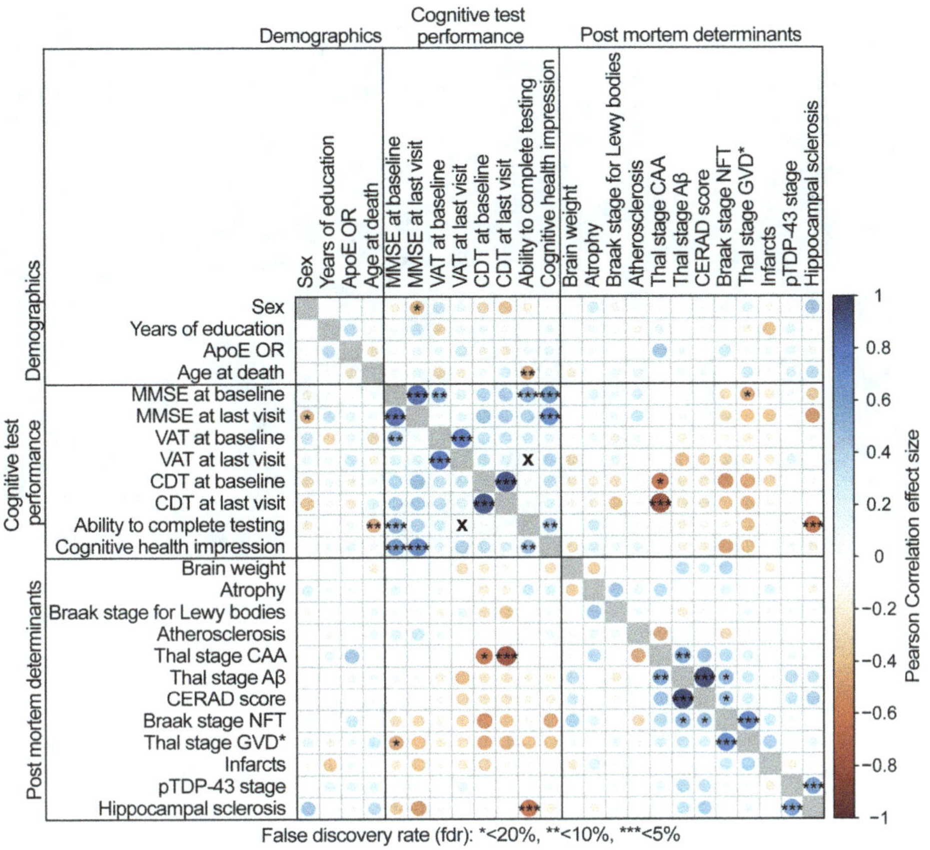

Fig. 3 Pearson correlation plot with false discovery rate (fdr). Color and size of the circles indicate the strength of the Pearson correlation coefficient (for Pearson correlation coefficient, *p*-value and numerical fdr see Additional file 3: Table S3a-c), asterisks indicate the false discovery rate (* < 20%, ** < 10%, *** < 5%), X indicates no correlation. Correlations between the same test at baseline and last visit were performed for 20 cases with at least one follow up visit. Thal stage GVD* indicates that we utilized a staging system for GVD adapted from Thal et al., 2011 [44]

Case report of 103 year old female

Case 100069 was a female centenarian with a fit physique included in the 100-plus Study at the age of 102. She finished the first stage of tertiary education, and had enjoyed a total of 18 years of education (ISCED level 5). At baseline she scored 27 points on the MMSE and 3/5 points on the CDT. She volunteered to undergo an MRI and PIB-PET scan 1 month after inclusion into the study. The MRI scan revealed moderate hippocampal atrophy (MTA score 2), white matter abnormalities (Fazekas score II), and few microbleeds. The PET scan using [^{11}C]PiB as an amyloid tracer was positive throughout the brain, with the highest signal in the frontal area (Fig. 4). The centenarian died 10 months after inclusion of cachexia. Proxies reported maintained cognitive health until the terminal phase. Brain autopsy was performed with a post mortem delay of 8.5 h. Overall, no major abnormalities were observed at the macroscopic level. Mild atrophy of the temporal lobe was observed and arteries were mildly atherosclerotic. Two small meningeomas were observed in the left part of the scull, as well as a small (0.6 cm) old cortical infarct in the medial frontal gyrus. The substantia nigra appeared relatively pale. Neuropathological evaluation revealed intermediate AD neuropathologic changes (A3B2C1). Consistent with the positive amyloid PET scan in vivo, we observed Aβ pathology in the form of classical and diffuse plaques (Thal stage Aβ 4), as well as capillary CAA-type 1 (capCAA) (Thal stage CAA 2) (Fig. 5 panel d-f) during the post-mortem neuropathological analysis. Diffuse Aβ deposits were detected in the frontal, frontobasal, occipital, temporal and parietal cortex, the molecular layer, CA1 and subiculum of the hippocampus, as well as the caudate nucleus, putamen and nucleus accumbens. A relatively low number of classic senile plaques with a dense core was observed throughout the neocortex. Prominent presence of CAA was observed in the parietal cortex and the leptomeninges. Capillary CAA (type 1) was observed in moderate levels in the frontal cortex (Fig. 5, panel f), the cerebellum, sporadically in the occipital cortex, and was absent in the temporal cortex. Together, the relatively high levels of

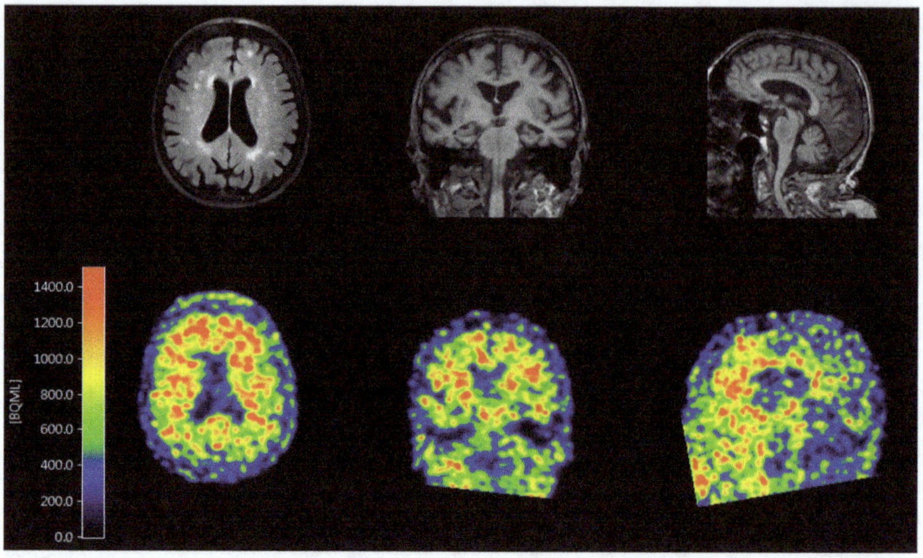

Fig. 4 Dynamic [^{11}C]PiB-PET and MRI scan of case 100069. The scan was performed by the ECAT EXACT HR1 scanner (Siemens/CTI) 1 month after study inclusion. PET scan for amyloid is positive in the frontal area, MRI shows moderate hippocampal atrophy (MTA score 2) as well as vascular lesions in the white matter (Fazekas score II), suggesting amyloid angiopathy

CAA might explain the high signal of the [^{11}C]PiB-PET, as CAA is also known to be detected by this tracer (Farid et al., 2017 [15]), as well as the abnormalities observed on the MRI.

Immunostaining for pTau showed prominent occurrence of dystrophic neurites, neurofibrillary tangles and pretangles in the hippocampal areas CA1, subiculum and transentorhinal cortex. Moderate numbers of pretangles and threads were observed in the frontal cortex and occipital cortex. Severe presence of pTau immunoreactive neuropil threads and (pre)tangles was observed in the temporal cortex. Additionally, we observed pTau positive glial cells in the temporal cortex and subcortical white matter. In the anterior part of the hippocampus, pTau positive glial cells were observed associated with blood vessels, also indicative of ARTAG [24]. pTau positive neurons and glial cells were also observed in the amygdala and insula. In summary, immuno-positive pTau was observed as NFTs (Braak stage IV) and NP like structures (CERAD score 1), as well as in the form of ARTAG (Fig. 5, panel g-i). GVD (CK1δ positive granules) was present in high numbers in the hippocampal subfields CA1 and subiculum, CA4, entorhinal cortex, temporal cortex, amygdala and gyrus cinguli (Thal stage GVD* 5) (Fig. 5, panel j-k). Accumulations of pTDP-43 pathology were widespread, including the amygdala, hippocampus and temporal pole cortex (pTDP-43 stage 3) (Fig. 5, panel a-c). No α-synuclein inclusions were observed in hippocampus, substantia nigra, amygdala, locus coeruleus, and in the nuclei of the medulla oblongata. A relatively moderate decrease of Purkinje cells was observed in the cerebellum.

Discussion

In a unique cohort of 40 centenarians, in which individual cognitive functioning was assessed shortly before death, we investigated the post-mortem brain for disease- and aging-associated neuropathological changes. At baseline, cognitive performance varied: neuropsychological test performance suggested that some centenarians had no symptoms of cognitive impairment, while others showed considerable impairment in several cognitive domains. Furthermore, a small subset of centenarians with multiple follow-up visits showed some decline after study inclusion, while others remained cognitively stable until death. We also observed an overall trend that higher pathology loads associate amongst each other, but also with a lower performance on cognitive tests: this trend is carried especially by the NFT and GVD loads and to a lesser extent by Aβ-associated pathologies. Whereas previous findings indicated that many elderly individuals with CAA remain asymptomatic [15], our results suggested that the severity of amyloid accumulation in the vessel walls (CAA), but not Aβ accumulation in the form of plaques, significantly associated with lower executive functioning, as measured by the Clock Drawing Test (CDT).

To indicate the uniqueness of each centenarian and the importance of studying clinicopathological correlations in this special group we present a selected centenarian who appeared lively and healthy upon visiting our hospital with no signs of cognitive impairment, judged independently by a trained researcher and a neurologist. Both her hearing and visual abilities were good. While she scored 27 points on the MMSE, which is well above the age-groups

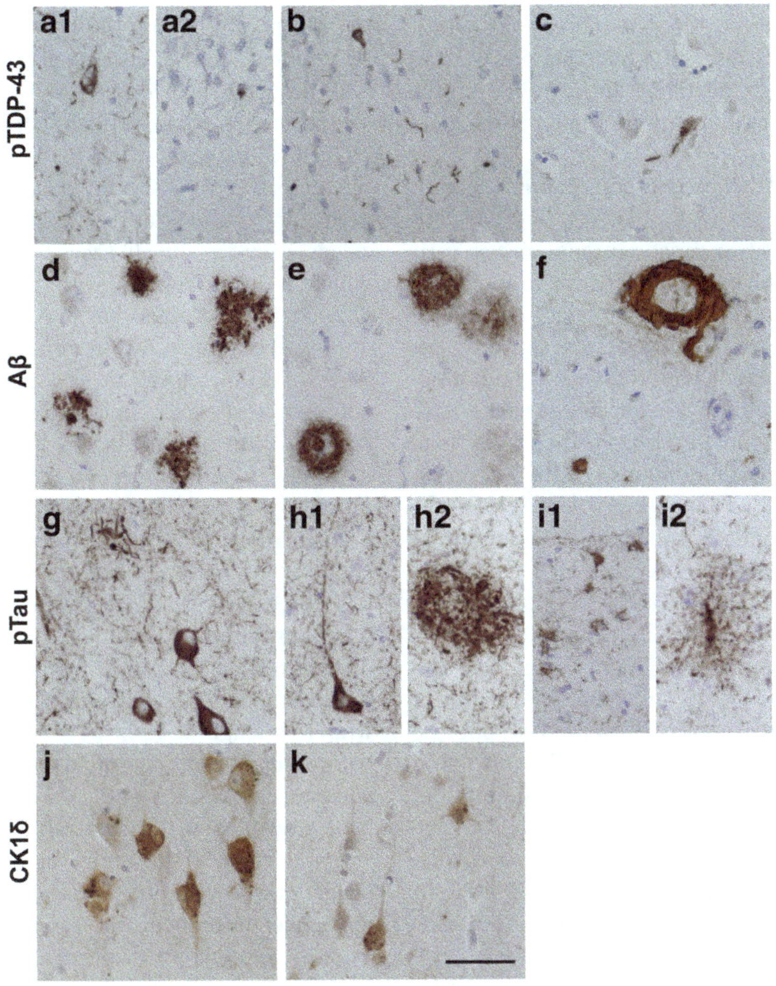

Fig. 5 Representative neuropathological lesions found in the hippocampus (**a**, **d**, **g**, **j**), middle temporal lobe cortex (**b**, **e**, **h**, **i**, **k**), amygdala (**c**) and frontal lobe cortex (**f**) of case 100069. Shown are exemplary pTDP-43 accumulations (**a-c**) in the hippocampal subregion CA1 (**a1**) and dentate gyrus (DG) (**a2**), temporal pole cortex (T) (**b**) and Amygdala (Amy) (**c**), Aβ positivity (**d-f**) in the form of diffuse and classical plaques in the hippocampal CA1 region (**d**) and temporal pole cortex (**e**), as well as CAA of large vessels and capillaries in the frontal lobe (F2) (**f**). pTau immuno-staining (**g-i**) is shown as (pre)tangles and neuritic plaque like structures in the hippocampal CA1 region (**g**) and temporal pole cortex (**h1** and **h2**), as well as astroglial pTau in ARTAG in the temporal pole cortex (**i1** and **i2**). GVD (CK1δ granules) (**j-k**) is shown in the hippocampus (**j**) and temporal pole cortex (**k**). Scale bar 25 μm

cut-off score to indicate dementia [21], she did not attain maximum scores on the VAT (9/12) and the CDT (3/5). Scoring 3 points on the CDT indicates that while the visuospatial organization of the clock was correct, the centenarian had difficulties to place the hands of the clock correctly to 10 past 11. This might suggest some difficulties with visuo-spatial and/or executive functioning. She died 9 months later of cachexia. Despite her overall and cognitive well-being, a PiB-PET scan performed in the same week as the neuropsychological assessment was positive for amyloid Aβ, and we observed abnormalities in the MRI scan. During post-mortem neuropathological characterization, we found a prominent presence of diffuse Aβ deposits, relatively few classical and neuritic plaques, and a moderate level of CAA type 1, especially in the frontal lobe. Together, the relatively few diffuse Aβ deposits but relatively high levels of CAA might explain the high signal of the PiB-PET, as CAA is also known to be detected by this tracer [15]. The presented case was carrier of the ApoE2/4 genotype, which has been associated with a higher chance of developing AD relative to ApoE3/3 carriers [8], and possibly with an increased occurrence of CAA [32]. Pre-mortem imaging is at present not able to replace thorough post-mortem characterization of pathology. The combination of both techniques and cognitive testing in the present case allows us to confirm pre-mortem scan observations post-mortem and to rule out that a considerable amount of the post-mortem observed pathology built up after the cognitive testing and brain scans. Together, our findings suggest that cognitive performance of self-reported cognitively healthy centenarians is, at least in part, sensitive to the increase of neuropathological hallmarks of disease, while individual cases manage to maintain high cognitive functioning in the presence of considerable amounts of multiple pathologies.

Accumulation of neuropathologies is common in centenarians

Aβ pathology was present in most centenarians at variable levels, and Braak stages for NFT were found in all centenarians. Distribution occurred up to stage IV, and we did not observe Braak stages 0, V or VI. Similarly, we detected significant accumulations of NPs, which did not exceed CERAD score 2. In fact, several centenarians have exceptionally good brain function with a high NFT load (Braak stage IV) and NP accumulations (CERAD scores 1 or 2), as well as high Aβ load (Thal stages 3–5). This is intriguing, since most younger individuals with similar amounts of pathology, namely Braak stage NFT III and IV, have at least some symptoms of AD [6, 31, 42]. An apparent dissociation of the association between Braak stage NFT and cognitive status at higher ages has also been reported previously [9, 31]. Overall, the cognitive function of these centenarians was conserved despite the presence of neuropathological hallmarks. We also find that several centenarians have no or only low amounts of Aβ pathology and intermediate levels of NFT loads, corresponding with the neuropathological description of primary age-related tauopathy (PART) [12]. The relation between PART and the occurrence of dementia is still elusive and its implications for cognition are still debated [14, 20]. The centenarians with PART in this cohort show variable performance on neuropsychological tests.

Thus far, many neuropathological changes such as ARTAG, atherosclerosis, hippocampal sclerosis, pTDP-43, GVD and Lewy bodies, are reported to accumulate with age independently of cognitive decline [1, 23, 24, 30, 42], while the simultaneous occurrence of multiple pathologies in elderly cases has previously been associated with increased dementia risk [22]. All centenarians presented high stages of GVD pathology, as well as atherosclerosis and ARTAG. GVD is known to accompany Tau pathology [34] and its occurrence and distribution throughout the brain in AD has been first described in 2011[61]. To our knowledge, there are no reports regarding GVD levels at extreme ages. Hunter and colleagues have described GVD in the hippocampal tissue of a cohort with the mean age of 90 and found associations of severe GVD with dementia status similar to that of severe NFTs [28]. In line with the findings by Hunter and colleagues, our findings illustrate that GVD is universal in extremely aged individuals and that in non-demented elderly, the associations of GVD with cognitive test performance is of similar strength as that observed with Braak stages [28]. In contrast, the accumulation of pTDP-43 is usually observed in cases with FTD or ALS, but has also been described to occur in AD patients and non-demented elderly [28, 29, 42, 51]. The occurrence in centenarians was limited and we observed no association with cognitive test performance. pTDP-43 aggregation has been suggested to be facilitated by Aβ pathology [42], for which we find only weak evidence in centenarians. We find that higher pTDP-43 stages occurred in all cases with hippocampal sclerosis, which is in agreement with previous observations [28]. Hippocampal sclerosis has previously been associated with lower performance on neuropsychological tests [30], and here we find a significant association with the inability to complete tests, a possible proxy for fatigue. Likewise, the accumulation of α-synuclein (Lewy bodies) was also limited in centenarians, despite the reported increased occurrence of this pathology with age [42]. We did not observe a correlation between the presence of Lewy bodies and cognitive function. The overall low occurrence of pTDP-43 and Lewy body pathologies in this group of centenarians implies that these pathologies are more likely disease-related and not aging-related. In addition, we found one odd case with a Braak stage 6 for Lewy bodies, who was diagnosed with Parkinson's disease many years before death, but performed well on the MMSE. The occurrence of strokes and other vascular pathologies has been shown to be a major risk factor of dementia in individuals over 85 [10]. However, brain infarcts of any size have not shown good correlation to cognitive test performance in the current sample. We found very weak negative association of occurrence of infarcts with lower MMSE scores at last visit and CDT at baseline.

In our cohort of centenarians, increased levels of pathology in general correlate with lower cognitive performance. Apart from the strong association of CAA severity with performance on the CDT, Thal stage GVD* specifically associates with lower performance on the MMSE, and hippocampal sclerosis is associated with the ability to complete testing. The two pathological hallmarks that associate with most cognitive measures are Thal stage GVD* and the Braak stage NFT, although most associations are weak, suggesting that the presence of one or two neuropathological hallmarks is not sufficient to evoke cognitive symptoms. This observation is in agreement with the idea that the simultaneous accumulation of different neuropathological hallmarks of AD could collectively account for the cognitive decline that is associated with aging [20–22, 31, 42]. It should however be kept in mind that the present study does not include any cases with clinically overt dementia and that the reported associations between pathological hallmarks and cognitive test performance describe very subtle changes in cognition. It remains elusive whether these centenarians retained their cognitive health to extreme ages because they delayed the accumulation of pathologies to much later ages, or because build-up of pathology was slower. Additionally, cognitively healthy centenarians might possess compensatory mechanisms, e.g. to maintain synapse numbers and health, as synaptic loss has previously been implicated as the main driver of cognitive impairment [37]. More in-depth molecular analysis, such as quantitative immunohistochemical analysis and proteomic characterization, will be necessary to gain new insights into the molecular changes and possible compensatory mechanisms underlying cognitive decline or maintained cognitive health at old age.

Thus far, we present the findings in a sample of 40 centenarians. With the continuation of this prospective study, we will be able to validate these findings in a larger sample in due time. Also, as of yet we did not observe a cognitively healthy centenarian who was free of atherosclerosis or AD-associated pathologies, as reported previously for a 115 year old woman [13]. In line with reports that cognitive performance is highly correlated with survival in the oldest old [41], we find that the centenarians who score highest on cognitive tests in the ongoing prospective study are underrepresented among the first centenarians in the 100-plus Study who came to autopsy (data not shown). We therefore speculate, that individuals with a low burden of pathology might survive until extreme ages, and will come to autopsy at a later time after inclusion.

Conclusions

In conclusion, we find that AD associated neuropathology is common in centenarians, albeit within limits for specific neuropathological hallmarks. Furthermore, we find that although the centenarians in this cohort escaped or delayed cognitive impairment until extreme ages, the accumulation of overall pathologies relate with lower cognitive performance. It remains unclear whether pathology accumulation was slower compared to others, or whether accumulation started later. Overall, the registration of ante-mortem cognitive performance combined with thorough post-mortem brain analysis provides a unique window of opportunity for the association of cognitive function with the occurrence of neuropathological changes in centenarians.

Acknowledgements
We thank and acknowledge all participating centenarians and their family members and the persons who contributed to this work as part of their bachelors' and masters' thesis: Neline van Woerden, Elleke Tissink, Melissa de Reus, Rianne Koeling, Ramon Bettings and Julia Letschert.

Funding
This work was funded by Stichting Alzheimer Nederland (WE09.2014–03), Stichting Diorapthe (VSM 14 04 14 02) and Stichting VUmc Fonds.

Authors' contributions
ABG performed the experiments. NB and SS have performed and interpreted the neuropsychological tests. NBB collected and performed part of the neuropathological characterization of the brain tissues donated to the 100-plus Study. ABG and MH have performed the data analysis. ABG, JJMH and HH have written the manuscript. ABS, AJMR, JJMH and HH supervised the research. PS, JJMH and HH were involved in designing the study. All authors read and approved the final manuscript.

Competing interests
The authors declare that they have no competing interest.

Author details
[1]Department of Molecular and Cellular Neuroscience, Center for Neurogenomics and Cognitive Research, Amsterdam Neuroscience, Vrije Universiteit Amsterdam, De Boelelaan 1085, 1081 HV Amsterdam, The Netherlands. [2]Department of Pathology, Amsterdam Neuroscience, VU University Medical Center, PO Box 7057, 1007 MB Amsterdam, The Netherlands. [3]Alzheimer Centre, Department of Neurology, Amsterdam Neuroscience, VU University Medical Center, Postbus 7057, 1007 MB Amsterdam, The Netherlands. [4]Department of Clinical Genetics, Amsterdam Neuroscience, VU University Medical Center, de Boelelaan, 1118 1081 HV Amsterdam, The Netherlands. [5]Netherlands Institute for Neuroscience, Meibergdreef 47, 1105 BA Amsterdam, The Netherlands.

References

1. Alafuzoff I, Gelpi E, Al-Sarraj S, Arzberger T, Attems J, Bodi I, Bogdanovic N, Budka H, Bugiani O, Englund E, Ferrer I, Gentleman S, Giaccone G, Graeber MB, Hortobagyi T, Höftberger R, Ironside JW, Jellinger K, Kavantzas N, King A, Korkolopoulou P, Kovács GG, Meyronet D, Monoranu C, Parchi P, Patsouris E, Roggendorf W, Rozemuller A, Seilhean D, Streichenberger N, Thal DR, Wharton SB, Kretzschmar H (2012) The need to unify neuropathological assessments of vascular alterations in the ageing brain. Multicentre survey by the BrainNet Europe consortium. Exp Gerontol 47: 825–833. https://doi.org/10.1016/j.exger.2012.06.001
2. Alafuzoff I, Ince PG, Arzberger T, Al-Sarraj S, Bell J, Bodi I, Bogdanovic N, Bugiani O, Ferrer I, Gelpi E, Gentleman S, Giaccone G, Ironside JW, Kavantzas N, King A, Korkolopoulou P, Kovács GG, Meyronet D, Monoranu C, Parchi P, Parkkinen L, Patsouris E, Roggendorf W, Rozemuller A, Stadelmann-Nessler C, Streichenberger N, Thal DR, Kretzschmar H (2009) Staging/typing of Lewy body related α-synuclein pathology: a study of the BrainNet Europe consortium. Acta Neuropathol 117:635–652. https://doi.org/10.1007/s00401-009-0523-2
3. Braak H, Alafuzoff I, Arzberger T, Kretzschmar H, Tredici K (2006) Staging of Alzheimer disease-associated neurofibrillary pathology using paraffin sections and immunocytochemistry. Acta Neuropathol 112:389–404. https://doi.org/10.1007/s00401-006-0127-z
4. Braak H, Braak E (1991) Neuropathological stageing of Alzheimer-related changes. Acta Neuropathol 82:239–259. https://doi.org/10.1007/BF00308809
5. Braak H, Braak E (1995) Staging of Alzheimer's disease-related neurofibrillary changes. Neurobiol Aging 16:271–278. https://doi.org/10.1016/0197-4580(95)00021-6
6. Braak H, Braak E (1997) Frequency of stages of Alzheimer-related lesions in different age categories. Neurobiol Aging 18:351–357. https://doi.org/10.1016/S0197-4580(97)00056-0
7. Braak H, Del Tredici K, Rüb U, Vos RAI De, Jansen Steur ENH, Braak E (2003) Staging of brain pathology related to sporadic Parkinson ' s disease 24:197–211
8. Corneveaux JJ, Myers AJ, Allen AN, Pruzin JJ, Ramirez M, Engel A, Nalls MA, Chen K, Lee W, Chewning K, Villa SE, Meechoovet HB, Gerber JD, Frost D, Benson HL, O'Reilly S, Chibnik LB, Shulman JM, Singleton AB, Craig DW, Van Keuren-Jensen KR, Dunckley T, Bennett DA, de Jager PL, Heward C, Hardy J, Reiman EM, Huentelman MJ (2010) Association of CR1, CLU and PICALM with Alzheimer's disease in a cohort of clinically characterized and neuropathologically verified individuals. Hum Mol Genet 19:3295–3301. https://doi.org/10.1093/hmg/ddq221
9. Corrada MM, Berlau DJ, Kawas CH (2012) A population-based clinicopathological study in the oldest-old: the 90+ study. Curr Alzheimer

Res 9:709–717 doi: CAR-EPUB-20120402-004

10. Corrada MM, Mozaffar F, Evans MA, Bullain SS, Brookmeyer R, Kawas CH (2016) History of vascular disease and risk of dementia in the oldest-old: the 90+ study. Alzheimers Dement 12:P249–P250. https://doi.org/10.1016/j.jalz.2016.06.447
11. Corrada MM, Brookmeyer R, Paganini-Hill A, Berlau D, Kawas CH (2010) Dementia Incidence Continues to Increase with Age in the Oldest Old The 90+ Study. 67:114–121. https://doi.org/10.1002/ana.21915.Dementia
12. Crary JF, Trojanowski JQ, Schneider JA, Abisambra JF, Abner EL, Alafuzoff I, Arnold SE, Attems J, Beach TG, Bigio EH, Cairns NJ, Dickson DW, Gearing M, Grinberg LT, Hof PR, Hyman BT, Jellinger K, Jicha GA, Kovacs GG, Knopman DS, Kofler J, Kukull WA, Mackenzie IR, Masliah E, McKee A, Montine TJ, Murray ME, Neltner JH, Santa-Maria I, Seeley WW, Serrano-Pozo A, Shelanski ML, Stein T, Takao M, Thal DR, Toledo JB, Troncoso JC, Vonsattel JP, White CL, Wisniewski T, Woltjer RL, Yamada M, Nelson PT (2014) Primary age-related tauopathy (PART): a common pathology associated with human aging. Acta Neuropathol 128:755–766. https://doi.org/10.1007/s00401-014-1349-0
13. den Dunnen WFA, Brouwer WH, Bijlard E, Kamphuis J, van Linschoten K, Eggens-Meijer E, Holstege G (2008) No disease in the brain of a 115-year-old woman. Neurobiol Aging 29:1127–1132. https://doi.org/10.1016/j.neurobiolaging.2008.04.010
14. Duyckaerts C, Braak H, Brion J, Buée L, Del Tredici K, Goedert M, Halliday G, Neumann M, Spillantini MG, Tolnay M, Uchihara T (2015) PART is part of Alzheimer disease. Acta Neuropathol 129:749–756. https://doi.org/10.1007/s00401-015-1390-7
15. Farid K, Charidimou A, Baron JC (2017) Amyloid positron emission tomography in sporadic cerebral amyloid angiopathy: a systematic critical update. NeuroImage Clin 15:247–263. https://doi.org/10.1016/j.nicl.2017.05.002
16. Folstein MF, Folstein SE, McHugh PR (1975) "Mini-mental state". A practical method for grading the cognitive state of patients for the clinician. J Psychiatr Res 12:189–198. https://doi.org/10.1016/0022-3956(75)90026-6
17. Gardner RC, Valcour V, Yaffe K (2013) Dementia in the oldest old: a multi-factorial and growing public health issue. Alzheimers Res Ther 5:27. https://doi.org/10.1186/alzrt181
18. Haroutunian V, Schnaider-Beeri M, Schmeidler J, Wysocki M, Purohit DP, Perl DP, Libow LS, Lesser GT, Maroukian M, Grossman HT (2008) Role of the neuropathology of Alzheimer disease in dementia in the oldest-old. Arch Neurol 65:1211–1217. https://doi.org/10.1001/archneur.65.9.1211
19. Holstege H, Beker N, Dijkstra T, Pieterse K, Wemmenhove E, Schouten K, van Poppel FWA, Meijers-Heijboer H, Hulsman M, Scheltens P (2018) The 100-plus study of Dutch cognitively healthy centenarians: rationale, design and cohort description. BioRxiv doi: https://doi.org/10.1101/295287
20. Jellinger KA, Attems J (2015) Challenges of multimorbidity of the aging brain : a critical update. J Neural Transm:505–521. https://doi.org/10.1007/s00702-014-1288-x
21. Kapasi A, DeCarli C, Schneider JA (2017) Impact of multiple pathologies on the threshold for clinically overt dementia. Acta Neuropathol 134:1–16. https://doi.org/10.1007/s00401-017-1717-7
22. Kawas CH, Kim RC, Sonnen JA, Bullain SS, Trieu T, Corrada MM (2015) Multiple pathologies are common and related to dementia in the oldest-old: the 90+ study. Neurology 85:535–542. https://doi.org/10.1212/wnl.0000000000001831
23. Köhler C (2016) Granulovacuolar degeneration: a neurodegenerative change that accompanies tau pathology. Acta Neuropathol 132:339–359. https://doi.org/10.1007/s00401-016-1562-0
24. Kovacs GG, Ferrer I, Grinberg LT, Alafuzoff I, Attems J, Budka H, Cairns NJ, Crary JF, Duyckaerts C, Ghetti B, Halliday GM, Ironside JW, Love S, Mackenzie IR, Munoz DG, Murray ME, Nelson PT, Takahashi H, Trojanowski JQ, Ansorge O, Arzberger T, Baborie A, Beach TG, Bieniek KF, Bigio EH, Bodi I, Dugger BN, Feany M, Gelpi E, Gentleman SM, Giaccone G, Hatanpaa KJ, Heale R, Hof PR, Hofer M, Hortobágyi T, Jellinger K, Jicha GA, Ince P, Kofler J, Kövari E, Kril JJ, Mann DM, Matej R, McKee AC, McLean C, Milenkovic I, Montine TJ, Murayama S, Lee EB, Rahimi J, Rodriguez RD, Rozemüller A, Schneider JA, Schultz C, Seeley W, Seilhean D, Smith C, Tagliavini F, Takao M, Thal DR, Toledo JB, Tolnay M, Troncoso JC, Vinters HV, Weis S, Wharton SB, White CL, Wisniewski T, Woulfe JM, Yamada M, Dickson DW (2016) Aging-related tau astrogliopathy (ARTAG): harmonized evaluation strategy. Acta Neuropathol 131:87–102. https://doi.org/10.1007/s00401-015-1509-x
25. Lindeboom J, Schmand B, Tulner L, Walstra G (2002) Visual association test to detect early dementia of the Alzheimer type. J Neurol Neurosurg Psychiatry 73:126–133. https://doi.org/10.1136/jnnp.73.2.126
26. Mirra S, Heyman A, McKeel D, Sumi S, Crain B, Brownlee L, Vogel F, Hughes J, van Belle G, Berg L (1991) The consortium to establish a registry for Alzheimer's disease (CERAD). Part II Stand Neuropathologic Assessment Alzheimer's Dis 41:479–486
27. Montine TJ, Phelps CH, Beach TG, Bigio EH, Cairns NJ, Dickson DW, Duyckaerts C, Frosch MP, Masliah E, Mirra SS, Nelson PT, Schneider JA, Thal DR, Trojanowski JQ, Vinters HV, Hyman BT (2012) National institute on aging-Alzheimer's association guidelines for the neuropathologic assessment of Alzheimer's disease: a practical approach. Acta Neuropathol 123:1–11. https://doi.org/10.1007/s00401-011-0910-3
28. Nag S, Yu L, Capuano AW, Wilson RS, Leurgans SE, Bennett DA, Schneider JA (2015) Hippocampal sclerosis and TDP-43 pathology in aging and Alzheimer disease. Ann Neurol 77:942–952. https://doi.org/10.1002/ana.24388
29. Nag S, Yu L, Wilson RS, Chen EY, Bennett DA, Schneider JA (2017) TDP-43 pathology and memory impairment in elders without pathologic diagnoses of AD or FTLD. Neurology 88:653–660. https://doi.org/10.1212/WNL.0000000000003610
30. Nelson PT, Schmitt FA, Lin Y, Abner EL, Jicha GA, Patel E, Thomason PC, Neltner JH, Smith CD, Santacruz KS, Sonnen JA, Poon LW, Gearing M, Green RC, Woodard JL, Van Eldik LJ, Kryscio RJ (2011) Hippocampal sclerosis in advanced age: clinical and pathological features. Brain 134:1506–1518. https://doi.org/10.1093/brain/awr053
31. Nelson P. T. et al (2012) Correlation of alzheimer disease neuropathologic changes with cognitive status: a review of the literature. J Neuropathol Exp Neurol 2012 May; 71(5) 362–381 https://doi.org/10.1097/NEN.0b013e31825018f7.Correlation
32. Neltner JH, Abner EL, Jicha GA, Schmitt FA, Patel E, Poon LW, Marla G, Green RC, Davey A, Johnson MA, Jazwinski SM, Kim S, Davis D, Woodard JL, Kryscio RJ, Van Eldik LJ, Nelson PT (2015) Brain pathologies in extreme old age. Neurobiol Aging. https://doi.org/10.1016/j.neurobiolaging.2015.10.009
33. NIA (1997) Consensus recommendations for the postmortem diagnosis of Alzheimer's disease. The National Institute on Aging, and Reagan institute working group on diagnostic criteria for the Neuropathological assessment of Alzheimer's disease. Neurobiol Aging 18:S1–S2. https://doi.org/10.1016/S0197-4580(97)00057-2
34. Pascual G, Wadia JS, Zhu X, Keogh E, Kükrer B, van Ameijde J, Inganäs H, Siregar B, Perdok G, Diefenbach O, Nahar T, Sprengers I, Koldijk MH, van d LECB, Peferoen LA, Zhang H, Yu W, Li X, Wagner M, Moreno V, Kim J, Costa M, West K, Fulton Z, Chammas L, Luckashenak N, Fletcher L, Holland T, Arnold C, Anthony Williamson R, Hoozemans JJ, Apetri A, Bard F, Wilson IA, Koudstaal W, Goudsmit J (2017) Immunological memory to hyperphosphorylated tau in asymptomatic individuals. Acta Neuropathol 133:767–783. https://doi.org/10.1007/s00401-017-1705-y
35. Prince M, Wimo A, Guerchet M, Gemma-Claire A, Wu Y-T, Prina M (2015) World Alzheimer report 2015: the global impact of dementia - an analysis of prevalence, incidence, cost and trends. Alzheimer's Dis Int 84. https://doi.org/10.1111/j.0963-7214.2004.00293.x
36. R Core Team, R Foundation for Statistical Computing, Vienna A (2016) R: A Language and Environment for Statistical Computing
37. Robinson JL, Molina-Porcel L, Corrada MM, Raible K, Lee EB, Lee VMY, Kawas CH, Trojanowski JQ (2014) Perforant path synaptic loss correlates with cognitive impairment and Alzheimer's disease in the oldest-old. Brain 137:2578–2587. https://doi.org/10.1093/brain/awu190
38. Savva GM, Wharton SB, Ince PG (2009) Age, neuropathology, and dementia — NEJM. N Engl J Med 361:1118. https://doi.org/10.1056/NEJMoa0806142
39. Shulman KI (2000) Clock drawing: is it the ideal cognitive screening test? Int J Geriatr Psychiatry 15:548–561. https://doi.org/10.1002/1099-1166(200006)15:6<548::AID-GPS242>3.0.CO;2-U
40. Shulman KI, Pushkar Gold D, Cohen CA, Zucchero CA (1993) Clock-drawing and dementia in the community: a longitudinal study. Int J Geriatr Psychiatry 8:487–496. https://doi.org/10.1002/gps.930080606
41. Skoog J, Backman K, Ribbe M, Falk H, Gudmundsson P, Thorvaldsson V, Borjesson-Hanson A, Ostling S, Johansson B, Skoog I (2017) A longitudinal study of the mini-mental state examination in late nonagenarians and its relationship with dementia, mortality, and education. J Am Geriatr Soc 65:

1296–1300. https://doi.org/10.1111/jgs.14871

42. Spires-Jones TL, Attems J, Thal DR (2017) Interactions of pathological proteins in neurodegenerative diseases. Acta Neuropathol 134:1–19. https://doi.org/10.1007/s00401-017-1709-7
43. Takao M, Hirose N, Arai Y, Mihara B, Mimura M (2016) Neuropathology of supercentenarians - four autopsy case studies. Acta Neuropathol Commun 4:97. https://doi.org/10.1186/s40478-016-0368-6
44. Thal DR, Del Tredici K, Ludolph AC, Hoozemans JJM, Rozemuller AJ, Braak H, Knippschild U (2011) Stages of granulovacuolar degeneration: their relation to Alzheimer's disease and chronic stress response. Acta Neuropathol 122: 577–589. https://doi.org/10.1007/s00401-011-0871-6
45. Thal DR, Ghebremedhin E, Rüb U, Yamaguchi H, Del Tredici K, Braak H (2002) Two types of sporadic cerebral amyloid angiopathy. J Neuropathol Exp Neurol 61:282–293. https://doi.org/10.1093/jnen/61.3.282
46. Thal DR, Rüb U, Orantes M, Braak H (2002) Phases of a beta-deposition in the human brain and its relevance for the development of AD. Neurology 58:1791–1800. https://doi.org/10.1212/WNL.58.12.1791
47. Thal DR, Rüb U, Schultz C, Sassin I, Ghebremedhin E, Del Tredici K, Braak E, Braak H (2000) Sequence of Abeta -protein deposition in the human medial temporal lobe. J Neuropathol Exp Neurol 59:733–748
48. Uchihara T (2007) Silver diagnosis in neuropathology: principles, practice and revised interpretation. Acta Neuropathol 113:483–499. https://doi.org/10.1007/s00401-007-0200-2
49. UNESCO. International Standard Classification of Education ISCED 1997 http://www.unesco.org/education/information/nfsunesco/doc/isced_1997.htm
50. Verwey NA, Hoozemans JJM, Korth C, van Royen MR, Prikulis I, Wouters D, Twaalfhoven HAM, van Haastert ES, Schenk D, Scheltens P, AJM R, Blankenstein MA, Veerhuis R (2013) Immunohistochemical characterization of novel monoclonal antibodies against the N-terminus of amyloid β-peptide. Amyloid 20:179–187. https://doi.org/10.3109/13506129.2013.797389
51. Wilson RS, Yu L, Trojanowski JQ, Chen E-Y, Boyle PA, Bennett DA, Schneider JA (2013) TDP-43 pathology, cognitive decline, and dementia in old age. JAMA Neurol 70:1418. https://doi.org/10.1001/jamaneurol.2013.3961

10

The age of onset and evolution of Braak tangle stage and Thal amyloid pathology of Alzheimer's disease in individuals with Down syndrome

Yvonne S. Davidson[1], Andrew Robinson[1], Vee P. Prasher[2,3] and David M. A. Mann[1*]

Abstract

While post mortem studies have identified the major cell types and functional systems affected in Alzheimer's disease (AD) the initial sites and molecular characteristics of pathology are still unclear. Because individuals with Down syndrome (DS) (trisomy 21) develop the full pathological changes of AD in a predictable way by the time they reach middle to late age, a study of the brains of such persons at different ages makes an ideal 'model system' in which the sites of earliest onset of pathology can be detected and the subsequent progression of changes be monitored. In the present study we have examined the brains of 56 individuals with DS ranging from new-born to 76 years for the presence of amyloid and tau pathology in key cortical and subcortical regions. Amyloid pathology was found to commence in the late teens to twenties as a deposition of diffuse plaques initially within the temporal neocortex, quickly involving other neocortical regions but only reaching subcortical regions and cerebellum by the late forties. Cerebral amyloid angiopathy did not regularly commence until after 45–50 years of age. Tau pathology usually commenced after 35 years of age, initially involving not only entorhinal areas and hippocampus but also subcortical regions such as locus caeruleus (LC) and dorsal raphe nucleus (DRN). Later, tau pathology spread throughout the neocortex reaching occipital lobes in most instances by mid-50 years of age. Such a pattern of spread is consistent with that seen in typical AD. We found no evidence that tau pathology might commence within the brain in DS before amyloid deposition had occurred, but there was limited data that suggests tau pathology in LC or DRN might predate that in entorhinal areas and hippocampus or at least be coincident.

Keywords: Alzheimer's disease, Down syndrome, Amyloid, Tau

Introduction

Alzheimer's disease (AD) is characterised pathologically by the abundant presence of deposits of amyloid β protein (Aβ) in the brain parenchyma in the form of amyloid plaques, and in blood vessel walls as cerebral amyloid angiopathy (CAA), and neurofibrillary tangles (NFT) composed of hyperphosphorylated tau proteins [19, 35]. While post mortem studies based on established cases of AD have identified the major cell types and functional systems affected by the disorder, the initial sites of pathology are still unclear. According to the original and modified Braak stageing protocols [4, 7], the earliest sites of tau pathology lie within the entorhinal and transentorhinal cortex (stage I), spreading to hippocampus (stage II), temporal cortex (stage III) and eventually to other regions of cerebral cortex (stage IV), finally reaching visual association cortex (stage V) and primary visual cortex (stage VI). Conversely, the order of amyloid plaque deposition [46] commences within neocortical regions, particularly within the temporal lobe (phase 1), and spreads to involve allocortical regions such as the hippocampus and amygdala (phase 2), then into subcortical regions (phase 3), brain stem (phase 4) and finally cerebellum (phase 5).

However, this concept of the primacy and spread of tau pathology in AD has recently been questioned. From

* Correspondence: david.mann@manchester.ac.uk
[1]Institute of Brain, Behaviour and Mental Health, Faculty of Medical and Human Sciences University of Manchester, Salford Royal Hospital, Stott Lane, Salford M6 8HD, England
Full list of author information is available at the end of the article

a study of 42 cognitively normal individuals under 30 years of age, Braak and Del Tredici suggested that the earliest site of tau pathology in AD might actually occur within certain subcortical nuclei, notably the locus caeruleus (LC), predating that within the entorhinal area [6]. Of these 42 individuals, deposits of Aβ were present in only 1 person, a 17-year old with Down Syndrome (DS), simultaneously challenging the concept of the amyloid cascade hypothesis of AD [14]. Another study by this same research group of 2332 unselected post mortems ranging from 1 to 100 years of age [8] found tau pathology in 58 cases, in the absence of Aβ deposition in all but one instance (again the same case of DS as included in [6]). Tau pathology was essentially restricted to those individuals aged 30 years or less, and occurred in LC and certain other non-cortical nuclei such as the upper raphe in the brainstem and the nucleus basalis of Meynert in the basal forebrain, without there being any entorhinal/cortical involvement. These data were interpreted as providing evidence for there being stages in the pathological process of AD that predate those affecting entorhinal/transentorhinal areas, and that changes in these subcortical nuclei may represent the very earliest sites of damage to the brain in AD. Nevertheless, from these kinds of observational studies it is not possible to predict whether any of the affected individuals would have gone on to develop AD had they survived longer. Moreover, the lack of an (inducible) animal model that fully recapitulates the pathological process of AD precludes experimental studies of the time course of the development of AD pathology.

On the other hand, it has long been known that individuals with Down syndrome (DS) associated with an additional copy of chromosome 21 (trisomy 21) develop the full pathological changes of AD by the time they reach middle age, and sometimes as young as 40 years [9, 13, 16, 18, 28–30, 38, 42, 50]. Hence, a study of the brains of such persons at different ages makes an ideal 'model system' in which the earliest sites of Alzheimer-type pathology can be observed and the subsequent progression of such changes be monitored. As with individuals with duplications in *APP*, DS is associated with an overexpression of APP protein, and therefore it might be argued that DS represents a model of Aβ hyperproduction rather than AD per se. Nonetheless, it still remains closer in pathological terms to AD than any other human condition or experimental paradigm. In the present study we have examined the brains of 56 individuals with DS ranging from new-born to 76 years for the presence of amyloid and tau pathology in certain cortical and subcortical regions and have charted the onset and progression of these, and other, pathologies in each brain region with age, and in relationship to each other.

Material and methods

Serial wax sections were cut at 6 μm thickness from formalin fixed tissue blocks from the brains of 56 individuals with DS (34 males, 22 females) ranging from new-born to 76 years (mean 48.0 ± 20.2 years). There was no significant difference in mean age between males and females (males, 48.3 ± 20.7 years; females, 47.4 ± 19.8 years). Thirteen of the 56 cases were drawn from the Manchester Brain Bank (MBB), 7 were obtained from Institute of Psychiatry (IOP) Brain Bank, London, 22 from the Thomas Willis Brain Bank (TWBB), Oxford, with the remaining 14 being obtained through Professor V P Prasher at University of Birmingham. All brains had been obtained at autopsy through appropriate consenting procedures with Local Ethical Committee approval. Selected case details are provided in Table 1. Details concerning karyotyping were only available for 13 individuals, but all 13 were a full trisomy 21 (Table 1).

Brain regions investigated were frontal cortex (BA8/9), temporal cortex (BA 21/22) to include the entorhinal cortex and hippocampus (at the level of the geniculate bodies), occipital cortex (BA17/18), cerebellar cortex, and brainstem to include substantia nigra (SN), LC and DRN (where available) and corpus striatum (CS) (caudate nucleus and putamen). Adjacent sections were routinely stained by haematoxylin and eosin, and immunostained for tau (using mouse monoclonal antibody, AT8 (Innogenetics, Antwerp, Belgium, 1:750)) and Aβ (using mouse monoclonal antibody, 4G8 (Covance Research Products Inc., Dedham MA, USA, 1:3000). Following 4G8 and AT8 immunostaining, all cases were staged as to Thal phase of Aβ deposition [46] and Braak stage of neurofibrillary degeneration using the revised Braak criteria for AT8 immunostained paraffin sections [7]. Further sets of sections of brainstem (substantia nigra ($n = 27$) and/or locus caeruleu ($n = 56$)) and temporal lobe with entorhinal cortex and hippocampus were immunostained for phosphorylated α-synuclein using a polyclonal anti-psyn1175 antibody [36] at 1:1000 dilution (kind gift of Dr. Masato Hasegawa at Tokyo Metropolitan Institute of Medical Science, Japan), and an additional set of sections of temporal cortex with hippocampus was immunostained for phosphorylated and non-phosphorylated TDP-43 using a polyclonal antibody (10782–2-AP Proteintech, Manchester, 1:1000). Those sections immunostained for tau, α-synuclein and TDP-43 underwent antigen retrieval by pressure cooking in citrate buffer for 30 min, reaching 120 degrees Celsius and > 15 kPa pressure whereas sections immunostained for Aβ were subject to incubation in 90% formic acid for 5 min as pretreatment.

Sections were also examined microscopically for the appearance, severity and topographical distribution of immunostaining of Aβ within brain parenchyma (as amyloid plaques) and cerebral vessels (as CAA). A five-point

Table 1 Selected demographic, genetic and neuropathological details for 56 individuals with Down syndrome

Case ID#	UKBBN ID#	gender	age	karyotype	*APOE*	Thal	Braak	Allen CAA	Thal CAA
1	na	M	0.01	na	na	0	0	0	0
2	na	F	0.1	na	na	0	0	0	0
3	na	M	1.6	na	na	0	0	0	0
4	na	M	1.6	na	na	0	0	0	0
5	na	F	3	na	na	0	0	0	0
6	na	M	11	na	na	0	0	0	0
7	na	F	13	na	na	0	0	0	0
8	BBN_2966	M	13	47XY21	3,3	1	0	0	0
9	na	M	23	na	na	0	0	0	0
10	na	F	27	na	na	1	0	0	0
11	na	M	35	na	na	2	0	0	0
12	na	M	36	na	na	5	II	0	0
13	BBN_2963	F	37	47XX21	3,4	5	I	0	0
14	na	F	39	na	na	2	b*	0	0
15	na	M	42	na	na	5	V	1	1
16	BBN_17186	F	47	na	na	5	VI	3	2
17	BBN_17189	M	47	na	na	5	III	1	1
18	BBN_17178	F	49	na	3,4	4	III	1	1
19	BBN_2981	M	50	47XY21	3,4	3	II	1	1
20	na	F	50	na	na	0	b*	0	0
21	na	M	51	na	na	5	VI	1	1
22	BBN_2968	M	53	47XY21	3,3	5	III	1	1
23	BBN_3356	F	53	na	3,4	5	VI	2	1
24	BBN_16954	M	54	na	2,4	5	VI	3	2
25	BBN_3365	M	55	na	3,4	5	VI	2	1
26	na	M	55	na	na	5	V	1	1
27	BBN_3438	F	56	na	3,3	5	VI	1	1
28	BBN_16273	F	56	na	3,4	5	VI	1	1
29	BBN_2978	M	57	47XY21	3,3	5	V	3	2
30	na	M	57	na	na	5	VI	1	1
31	BBN_3020	F	58	47XX21	3,3	5	V	1	1
32	BBN_3355	M	58	na	3,4	5	VI	3	2
33	BBN_3358	F	58	na	3,3	5	VI	2	1
34	BBN_3437	F	58	na	2,3	5	V	1	1
35	BBN_3353	M	59	na	2,3	5	VI	3	2
36	BBN_3363	M	59	na	3,3	5	VI	2	1
37	BBN_2990	M	60	47XY21	3,3	5	VI	2	1
38	BBN_3364	M	60	na	3,3	5	VI	2	1
39	na	F	60	na	na	5	0	0	0
40	na	M	60	na	na	5	VI	2	1
41	BBN_16835	M	60	na	3,3	5	III	2	1
42	BBN_3352	F	61	na	2,3	5	VI	3	2
43	BBN_3439	F	61	na	3,4	5	VI	2	1
44	BBN_2964	F	62	47XX21	3,3	5	V	3	2

Table 1 Selected demographic, genetic and neuropathological details for 56 individuals with Down syndrome *(Continued)*

Case ID#	UKBBN ID#	gender	age	karyotype	*APOE*	Thal	Braak	Allen CAA	Thal CAA
45	BBN_2965	M	62	47XY21	3,3	5	V	1	1
46	BBN_2967	F	62	47XX21	3,3	5	IV	3	2
47	BBN_3354	M	62	na	3,3	5	VI	3	2
48	BBN_3441	M	62	na	2,3	5	VI	3	2
49	na	M	63	na	na	5	VI	1	1
50	BBN_2969	M	64	47XY21	3,3	5	IV	1	1
51	BBN_3440	F	64	na	3,3	5	VI	2	1
52	BBN_2975	M	65	47XY21	3,3	5	V	1	1
53	BBN_17004	M	65	na	3,3	5	V	1	1
54	na	M	66	na	na	5	V	1	1
55	na	F	69	na	na	5	VI	1	1
56	BBN_2985	M	76	47XY21	2,3	5	III	3	2

Thal = Thal phase of amyloid deposition and Braak = Braak tau stage. CAA phenotype was assessed in accordance with Allen et al. (2014) and Thal et al. (2010). UKBBN = UK Brain Bank Network ID number, na = not available/applicable

scoring system [31, 37] was employed to separately grade the severity of plaques and CAA.

Plaques

Grade 0 - no amyloid plaques in present.
Grade 1 - A few amyloid plaques in each low power (× 10 microscope objective) field.
Grade 2 - A moderate number of amyloid plaques in each low power field.
Grade 3 - Many dispersed amyloid plaques in each low power field.
Grade 4 - Very many, densely packed amyloid plaques in each low power field.

CAA

Grade 0 - No CAA in blood vessel walls in leptomeninges or brain parenchyma.
Grade 1 - Occasional blood vessels with CAA in leptomeninges and/or brain parenchyma, usually not occupying the full thickness of the wall.
Grade 2 - A moderate number of blood vessels with CAA in leptomeninges and/or brain parenchyma, some occupying the full thickness of the wall.
Grade 3 - Many blood vessels with CAA in leptomeninges and/or brain parenchyma, some occupying the full thickness of the wall.
Grade 4 - Most or all blood vessels with severe CAA in leptomeninges and/or brain parenchyma, occupying the full thickness of the wall.

CAA subtype, based on examination of frontal, temporal and occipital cortex in sections immunostained for Aβ, was assigned to all cases. Two classification systems were employed, as previously described [2, 47]. According to Allen et al. [2], Type 1 describes cases predominantly with many diffuse and cored Aβ plaques, throughout the cerebral cortex, in which CAA is confined within leptomeningeal vessels. Type 2 describes cases where, along with many diffuse and cored Aβ plaques, CAA is present in both leptomeningeal and deeper penetrating arteries, especially within occipital cortex. Type 3 describes cases where capillary CAA is present along with arterial CAA, especially within primary visual cortex, but with relatively few Aβ plaques. Type 4 describes a predominantly vascular phenotype, where Aβ deposition is much more prevalent in and around blood vessels throughout the brain and Aβ plaques are scarce or absent. According to Thal et al. [47] type 1 CAA includes both leptomeningeal and parenchymal vascular involvement and type 2 additionally involves capillaries.

The severity of overall tau (AT8) pathology (which included neurofibrillary tangles, neuritic plaques and neuropil threads) was assessed as:

Grade 0 - no tau pathology present.
Grade 1 - few, widely scattered neurofibrillary tangles and/or neuropil threads in each low power (× 10 microscope objective) field.
Grade 2 - a moderate number of clustered neurofibrillary tangles and/or neuropil threads in each low power field.
Grade 3 - many clustered neurofibrillary tangles and/or neuropil threads in each low power field.
Grade 4 - many densely packed neurofibrillary tangles and/or neuropil threads in each low power field.

A similar system was employed to score α-synuclein immunostained Lewy body and Lewy neurite pathology in SN and LC, entorhinal and temporal cortex, and for TDP-43 immunopositive neuronal cytoplasmic inclusions in the dentate gyrus of the hippocampus and fusiform gyrus of the temporal lobe.

APOE genotyping

DNA was extracted from frozen cerebellum (or frontal cortex when cerebellum was not available) by routine methods; frozen tissues were not available for genotyping in 24 cases (Table 1). *APOE* genotyping was performed on all samples using method of Wenham et al. [49].

Statistical analysis

All data analysis was performed using SPSS v 21.0. Levels of significance were two-tailed and set at $p < 0.05$.

Results

Histological changes

Amyloid pathology

Of the 56 individuals, 8 (cases #1–7 and 9) showed no amyloid plaques whatsoever in any brain region examined. Five of these (cases #1–5) were aged 3 years or under, two (cases #6 and 7) were aged 11 and 13 years, and one (case #9) was 23 years of age. Of the remaining 48 individuals, three, aged 13, 27, and 50 years (cases #8, 10 and 20, respectively), showed only rare to moderate numbers of diffuse amyloid plaques (Fig. 1a). In the 27 and 50-year olds these occurred within the temporal cortex alone, but were also present in frontal and occipital cortex in the 13-year old. None were present in the hippocampus, corpus striatum, cerebellum or brainstem of any of these 3 individuals. The other 45 individuals all showed either a moderate number of, or many, amyloid plaques (Fig. 2). However, in 5 of these (cases #11–14 and 19, aged 35, 36, 37, 39 and 50 years, respectively) plaques were mostly diffuse with only few cored, neuritic amyloid plaques being seen within the temporal neocortex and hippocampus, whereas in all other individuals over 50 years of age plaque density and morphology was similar to that typically seen in AD. Hence, cases #1–7 and #9 (where no amyloid plaques were present) corresponded to Thal phase 0, cases #8, 10 and 20 to Thal phase 1, cases #11 and 14 to Thal phase 2, case #19 to Thal phase 3, case #18 to Thal phase 4 with all other cases corresponding to Thal phase 5 (Fig. 2).

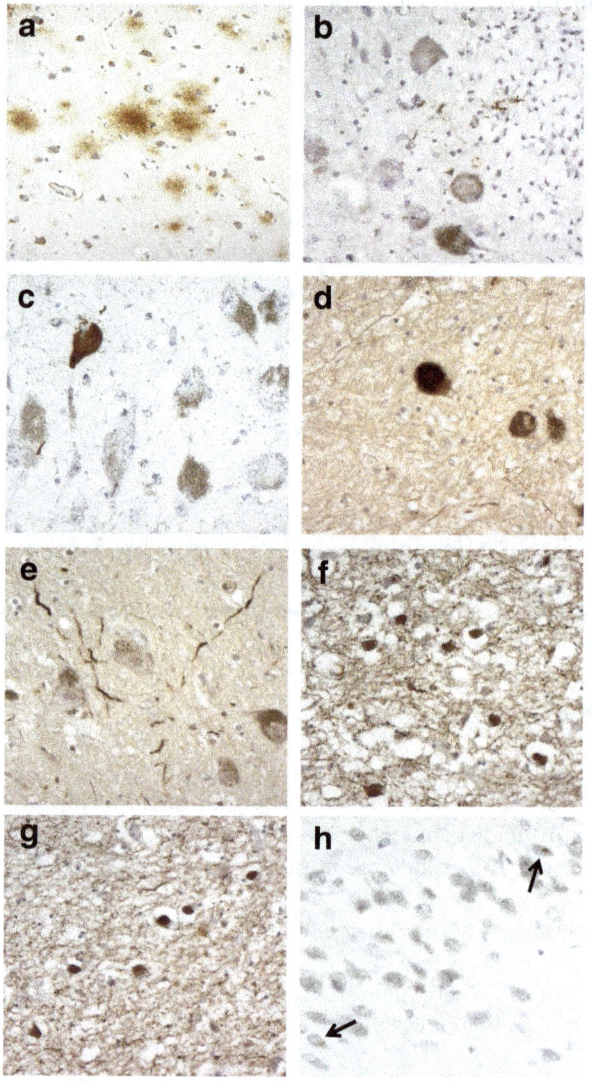

Fig. 1 Pathological changes in Down syndrome. In case #8, aged 13 years, amyloid deposits are present in the temporal cortex as diffuse plaques in the absence of any tau pathology (**a**). A few tau positive neurites are present in locus caeruleus in case #14 (**b**) and a single tau positive neurofibrillary tangle is seen, again in locus caeruleus, in case #20 (**c**), in the absence of any tau pathology elsewhere in the brain. A few α-synuclein positive Lewy bodies (**d**) and Lewy neurites (**e**) are present in the substantia nigra in case #45, aged 62 years, but these are more densely present in entorhinal cortex (**f**) and temporal neocortex (**g**) of the same case. Sparse TDP-43 neuronal cytoplasmic inclusions (arrowed) are seen in dentate gyrus granule cells in case #43, aged 61 years (**h**). Immunoperoxidase-haematoxylin; × 250 microscope magnification (**a**) × 400 microscope magnification (**b**–**h**)

Cerebral amyloid angiopathy

Fifteen (of twenty) individuals aged 50 years or below showed no CAA at all. CAA was seen only in 5 individuals (cases #15–19) (Fig. 2). In case #15 (aged 42 years) CAA sparsely affected leptomeningeal arteries in the temporal and occipital cortex, but CAA was also present in a few leptomeningeal arteries of the frontal, temporal and occipital cortex and cerebellum in case #19. In the other 3 individuals (cases #16–18, aged 47, 47 and 49 years) CAA was moderate to severe and was present in leptomeningeal arteries in the frontal (except case #16), temporal and occipital cortex and cerebellum (all 3 cases). Cases #15, 18 and 19 therefore displayed type 1 CAA [2]. In case #17 (aged 47 years) CAA also involved parenchymal arteries

Case ID#	1 to 7	8	9	10	11	12	13	14	15	16	17	18	19	20	21	22	23	24	25	26	27	28	29
Age	0-13	13	23	27	35	36	37	39	42	47	47	49	50	50	51	53	53	54	55	55	56	56	57
Ab (Tcx)	0	1	0	2	3	3	4	2	4	3	4	3	3	1	4	4	4	4	3	4	3	3	3
Ab (Fcx)	0	1	0	1	3	0	0	2	4	0	3	3	2	0	4	4	3	4	3	4	3	3	3
Ab (Ocx)	0	1	0	1	3	3	4	1	3	3	3	3	3	0	4	2	4	3	4	4	3	3	3
Ab (mol layer)	0	0	0	0	2	3	3	1	3	2	3	3	2	0	3	3	3	3	3	3	3	3	2
Ab ECX	0	0	0	0	2	3	3	2	3	3	4	2	2	0	3	3	3	3	3	3	3	3	2
Ab CA1	0	0	0	0	2	3	3	1	3	2	4	2	2	0	3	3	3	3	3	3	3	3	2
Ab DG	0	0	0	0	2	3	3	1	3	2	3	2	2	0	3	3	3	3	2	3	3	3	2
Ab (CS)	0	0	0	0	0	0	1	0	0	2	1	3	1	0	3	3	3	3	2	3	4	2	3
Ab (LC/DRN)	0	0	0	0	0	1	1	0	0	1	3	1	1	0	3	1	1	2	2	1	2	1	1
Ab (CBM)	0	0	0	0	0	0	3	0	0	4	4	1	0	0	0	2	3	3	2	1	2	4	4
Thal phase	0	1	0	1	2	5	5	2	5	5	5	4	3	1	5	5	5	5	5	5	5	5	5
CAA (Tcx)	0	0	0	0	0	0	0	0	2	1	3	3	1	0	3	1	2	4	2	2	1	3	1
CAA (Fcx)	0	0	0	0	0	0	0	0	0	0	3	3	1	0	3	0	4	3	3	2	1	3	4
CAA (Ocx)	0	0	0	0	0	0	0	0	2	2	3	2	1	0	3	1	4	4	3	3	2	1	4
CAA (CS)	0	0	0	0	0	0	0	0	0	0	0	0	0	0	0	1	2	0	1	0	0	0	0
CAA (CBM)	0	0	0	0	0	0	0	0	0	4	4	1	1	0	0	0	1	4	3	3	1	2	4
CAA subtype	0	0	0	0	0	0	0	0	1	3	2	1	1	0	1	1	2	3	2	1	1	1	3
tau (Ecx)	0	0	0	0	0	3	2	0	3	4	3	3	3	0	4	2	4	4	3	4	4	4	3
tau (CA1)	0	0	0	0	0	2	1	0	3	4	3	3	2	0	4	2	4	4	3	4	4	4	3
tau (Tcx)	0	0	0	0	0	0	0	0	1	4	3	3	1	0	4	2	4	3	3	4	4	3	3
tau (Fcx)	0	0	0	0	0	0	0	0	1	4	1	0	0	0	4	2	4	4	4	4	4	4	2
tau (Ocx)	0	0	0	0	0	0	0	0	1	4	1	0	0	0	4	2	4	3	3	4	4	4	2
tau (LC)	0	0	0	0	0	1	1	1	2	3	1	1	1	1	3	1	3	2	3	2	3	1	1
tau (DRN)	0	0	0	0	0	1	1	1	2	3	1	1	1	1	3	1	3	2	2	3	2	1	1
tau (SN)	na	0	na	na	na	na	0	na	na	na	na	na	0	na	na	2	2	na	1	na	2	na	2
tau (CS)	0	0	0	0	0	0	0	0	0	1	0	0	0	0	1	0	1	0	0	1	1	1	0
tau (CBM)	0	0	0	0	0	0	0	0	0	0	0	0	0	0	0	0	0	0	0	0	0	0	0
Braak stage	0	0	0	0	0	II	I	a	V	VI	III	III	II	b	VI	IV	VI	VI	VI	V	VI	VI	V
Lewy bodies	0	0	0	0	0	0	0	0	0	0	0	0	0	0	3	0	0	0	0	0	0	0	0
TDP-43	0	0	0	0	0	0	0	0	0	0	0	0	0	0	0	0	0	1	0	0	0	0	0

Case ID#	30	31	32	33	34	35	36	37	38	39	40	41	42	43	44	45	46	47	48	49	50	51	52	53	54	55	56
Age	57	58	58	58	58	59	59	60	60	60	60	60	61	61	62	62	62	62	62	63	64	64	65	65	66	69	76
Ab (Tcx)	3	4	4	4	3	3	3	4	3	4	3	4	4	3	3	3	3	3	4	4	3	3	3	3	3	4	3
Ab (Fcx)	3	3	3	3	3	3	3	3	3	3	3	3	3	3	4	3	3	3	3	3	3	3	2	3	3	3	3
Ab (Ocx)	3	3	3	3	3	3	3	3	3	3	3	3	3	2	3	3	3	4	3	3	3	3	3	3	3	3	3
Ab (mol layer)	3	3	3	3	3	3	3	3	3	3	3	3	4	2	2	3	2	3	3	3	2	3	2	3	3	3	3
Ab ECX	3	3	3	3	2	3	3	3	3	3	3	3	3	2	3	3	3	3	3	4	3	3	2	3	3	3	3
Ab CA1	3	3	3	3	2	2	2	3	3	3	2	3	4	2	3	3	3	4	3	3	3	4	3	3	3	3	3
Ab DG	3	3	3	3	2	3	2	3	3	3	3	3	4	2	2	3	3	3	4	3	3	3	3	3	3	3	3
Ab (CS)	3	3	4	4	3	3	4	2	3	3	3	3	3	2	4	3	2	2	4	4	3	2	3	3	3	3	4
Ab (LC/DRN)	2	2	2	1	2	1	1	1	1	1	1	2	1	1	2	1	1	1	2	1	1	1	1	1	1	1	2
Ab (CBM)	3	3	4	4	2	3	2	2	3	3	3	3	3	2	4	3	3	2	4	3	2	2	2	2	3	3	4
Thal phase	5	5	5	5	5	5	5	5	5	5	5	5	5	5	5	5	5	5	5	5	5	5	5	5	5	5	5
CAA (Tcx)	0	2	3	3	0	3	1	3	2	0	4	3	3	1	2	0	2	0	3	1	1	0	1	1	1	1	0
CAA (Fcx)	0	1	3	3	1	3	3	3	3	0	3	3	3	3	4	3	3	3	4	1	1	1	3	4	1	1	3
CAA (Ocx)	0	1	3	4	1	2	4	2	4	0	4	3	4	2	4	3	2	3	4	2	1	1	2	2	2	3	4
CAA (CS)	0	0	0	1	0	1	0	0	1	0	0	0	3	0	0	0	2	0	0	0	0	0	0	0	0	0	1
CAA (CBM)	0	1	4	4	1	1	4	2	3	0	4	2	3	2	4	4	3	3	4	2	1	0	3	3	2	2	4
CAA subtype	0	1	3	2	1	3	2	2	2	0	2	2	3	2	3	1	3	3	3	1	1	2	1	1	1	1	3
tau (Ecx)	4	3	4	4	4	4	3	3	4	0	4	4	3	3	3	3	3	3	4	3	3	4	3	4	4	4	3
tau (CA1)	4	3	4	4	4	4	3	3	4	0	4	3	4	3	3	3	3	4	4	3	3	4	3	4	4	4	3
tau (Tcx)	4	3	4	4	3	4	3	3	4	0	4	3	4	3	3	3	3	4	4	3	3	3	3	4	4	4	3
tau (Fcx)	4	3	4	4	4	4	3	4	4	0	4	1	4	4	3	3	2	4	4	3	2	4	3	4	4	4	2
tau (Ocx)	4	2	3	4	3	3	3	3	4	0	4	1	4	4	2	3	1	4	4	3	1	3	3	4	4	4	1
tau (LC)	3	2	2	2	3	3	3	3	3	0	3	3	3	2	2	3	3	3	3	3	3	3	3	3	2	2	3
tau (DRN)	3	2	3	2	3	3	1	3	3	0	3	3	3	2	2	3	3	1	1	3	1	3	3	3	2	3	3
tau (SN)	na	1	3	3	2	1	3	3	1	na	na	na	3	1	3	3	2	2	2	na	3	2	3	na	na	na	1
tau (CS)	0	0	0	1	1	0	1	0	1	0	0	0	1	1	0	0	1	1	1	0	0	1	0	1	1	1	0
tau (CBM)	0	0	0	0	0	0	0	0	0	0	0	0	0	0	0	0	0	0	0	0	0	0	0	0	0	0	0
Braak stage	VI	V	VI	VI	V	VI	VI	VI	VI	0	VI	IV	VI	VI	V	V	IV	VI	VI	VI	IV	VI	V	VI	V	VI	IV
Lewy bodies	0	0	0	0	0	0	0	0	0	0	0	0	0	3	0	2	0	0	3	3	0	2	0	0	0	0	0
TDP-43	0	0	0	0	0	0	1	0	0	0	0	0	1	1	0	0	0	0	1	0	0	0	0	0	0	0	0

Fig. 2 'Heat map' illustrating the onset and progression of amyloid plaque, CAA and tau pathology across the different brain regions for the 56 cases of Down syndrome. Box colours indicate increasing severity of pathological change from blue through to red. Numbers in boxes are derived from scoring systems described in the text. Tcx = temporal cortex, Fcx = frontal cortex, Ocx = occipital cortex, Ecx = entorhinal cortex, h = molecular layer of hippocampus, CA1 = CA1 region of hippocampus, DG = dentate gyrus of hippocampus, CS = corpus striatum, LC = locus coeruleus, DRN = dorsal raphe nucleus, SN = substantia nigra, CBM = cerebellum, Ab = amyloid deposits (plaques), CAA = cerebral amyloid angiopathy, tau = tau tangles

(type 2) and parenchymal arteries and capillaries (type 3 CAA) in case #16.

All 36 individuals over 50 years of age (except cases #30 and 39, aged 57 and 60 years) showed some degree of CAA (Fig. 2). In 14 individuals this was confined to leptomeningeal arteries (CAA type 1), being only mild to moderate in 10 of these, but severe or very severe in the other 6. In 10 individuals, CAA involved intraparenchymal arteries as well as leptomeningeal arteries (CAA type 2), at least in occipital cortex, often also in frontal and/or temporal cortex, but not in cerebellum. In the remaining 10 individuals there was capillary involvement as well as leptomeningeal and parenchymal artery involvement, again always in the occipital cortex, but occasionally also in the frontal cortex.

Overall, therefore, CAA was present in 39 individuals. According to Allen et a criterial [2] this was present as type 1 CAA in 17 of these (44%), type 2 in 11 individuals (28%) and type 3 in 11 individuals (28%) (Table 1, Fig. 2). According to Thal et al. criteria [47], CAA was present as type 1 in 72% individuals and type 2 in 28% individuals (Table 1).

Mild CAA was seen in small arteries in CS in only 9 individuals (Fig. 2).

Tau pathology

Of the 56 individuals, 14 showed no tau tangles or neuropil threads whatsoever in entorhinal cortex, hippocampus or neocortex. Eleven of these (cases #1–11) were aged 35 years or under, one (case #14) was aged 39 years, one (case #20) was 50 years of age and one (case #39 was 60 years of age. Interestingly, in cases #14 and #20, there was scant tau neuritic (Fig. 1b) or neurofibrillary (Fig. 1c) pathology in LC, but without any involvement of cortical or other subcortical structures. Such cases might be classed as pretangle/prodromal stage 'a' or 'b', respectively (see [6, 8] – a stage recently postulated to predate Stage I in earlier stageing systems [4, 7]. In case #39 no tau pathology at all was seen in any brain region.

Of the other 42 individuals, 10 (cases # 12, 13, 17–19, 22, 41, 46, 50 and 56 aged 36, 37, 47, 47, 50, 53, 60, 62, 64 and 76 years, respectively) showed only a moderate number of, or many tangles within the hippocampus (and entorhinal cortex), with only rare, or a moderate number of, tangles in the temporal, frontal or occipital cortex. These were considered to be at Braak stages II-IV. The remaining 32 individuals (30 of whom were over 50 years of age) showed a moderate number of, many, or very many, tangles in all neocortical regions and hippocampus, similar in appearance, distribution and degree to that typically seen in AD, and were assessed as being at Braak stages V or VI (Fig. 2).

Tau pathology was also investigated in SN in 27 cases where this region was available. No tau pathology was present in any case under 50 years of age, but rapidly developed thereafter such that this was present as neurofibrillary tangles and neuropil threads in all cases examined who were older than 50 years of age, ranging from moderate numbers of both through to there being very many present (Fig. 2).

No tau pathologies consistent with Ageing Related Tau Astrogliopathy (ARTAG) [22] or Argyrophilic Grain Disease [5] were seen in any of the studied cases.

α-Synuclein pathology

a few to a moderate number of α-synuclein immunopositive Lewy bodies (Fig. 1d) and Lewy neurites (Fig. 1e) were present in SN and/or LC in 5 cases (#21, 43, 45, 48 and 49), all over 50 years of age, but both pathologies were numerous in the entorhinal cortex (Fig. 1f) and moderately present in the temporal cortex (Fig. 1g), in the same 5 cases and also in case #51 where none were present in the SN or LC. Loss of neurones from SN was generally absent or sparse, even in those cases where Lewy body pathology was present.

TDP-43 pathology

TDP-43 pathology was absent from hippocampus and fusiform gyrus/temporal cortex in all but 5 cases (cases #24, 36, 42, 43 and 48, aged 54, 59, 61, 61 and 62 years, respectively). In these latter 5 cases sparse granular neuronal cytoplasmic inclusions were present in cells of the dentate gyrus of the hippocampus (Fig. 1h), but none were seen in fusiform gyrus or temporal cortex. In 3 cases (cases #42, 43 and 47) hippocampal sclerosis of CA1 was also present.

Other pathologies

We carefully examined routine haematoxylin eosin stained sections for evidence of small vessel disease, microinfarctions, overt microbleeds or intracerebral haemorrhage but found none to be consistently present in any patient or CAA subtype.

Early sites of pathological changes

Figure 2 shows a 'heat map' illustrating the earliest sites, and progression, of amyloid plaque, CAA and tau pathology across the different brain regions for the 56 cases.

Amyloid pathology commences in late teens to late twenties as a deposition of diffuse plaques initially within temporal lobe (Thal phase 1), quickly involving other neocortical regions and hippocampus (Thal phase 2), but only reaching subcortical regions (Thal phases 3 and 4) and cerebellum (Thal phase 5) by the late forties. After 50 years of age, every region of the brain, including cerebellum and corpus striatum, is moderately or heavily invested with amyloid plaques (Thal phase 5). Interestingly, CAA does not regularly commence until after 45–50 years of age. In terms of tau pathology and Braak stageing, there is a progressive 'spread' of neurofibrillary pathology throughout the brain, usually commencing after the age of 35 years. This initially involves not only entorhinal areas and hippocampus but also subcortical regions such as LC and DRN, sometimes in the absence of entorhinal involvement. Later, tau pathology spreads throughout the neocortex reaching occipital lobes (Braak stages V or VI) in most instances by mid-50 years of age. Lewy body pathology and TDP-43 pathological changes were infrequently present and generally only seen in individuals over 50–60 years of age.

APOE genotyping

APOE genotypes are given in Table 1. There were 5 individuals bearing ε2ε3 genotype, 18 bearing ε3ε3 genotype, 8 bearing ε3ε4 genotype and 1 bearing ε2ε4 genotype. There were no ε2 or ε4 homozygotes. These genotypes provided *APOE* ε2 and ε4 allele frequencies of 7.8 and 14.0%, respectively. However, age at death was earlier in those individuals bearing one *APOE* ε4 allele (52.6 ± 6.9 years) compared to those bearing only *APOE* ε3 alleles (57.8 ± 11.6 years, $p = 0.158$) and those with *APOE* ε2 alleles (63.2 ± 7.3 years, $p = 0.019$), the latter, in turn, being later than in those individuals bearing only *APOE* ε3 alleles ($p = 0.232$). There were no associations between *APOE* ε2 or ε4 alleles and the severity of Aβ plaque deposition (Thal phase), CAA subtype or severity of tau pathology (Braak stage).

Discussion

Although post mortem studies of established cases of AD have identified the major cell types and functional systems affected by the disorder, the initial sites of pathology are still unclear. According to the 2006 Braak stageing protocol [7], the earliest sites of tau pathology lie within the entorhinal and transentorhinal cortex (stage I), spreading to hippocampus (stage II), temporal cortex (stage III) and eventually to other regions of cerebral cortex (stage IV), finally reaching visual association cortex (stage V) and primary visual cortex (stage VI). However, this classification has recently been modified and stages prior to the entorhinal involvement affecting subcortical nuclei such as LC and DRN (pre-tangle/prodromalstages a-c) in isolation from any cortical involvement have been proposed [6, 8]. Conversely, the order of amyloid plaque deposition [46] commences within neocortical regions, particularly within the temporal lobe (phase 1), and spreads to involve allocortical regions such as the hippocampus and amygdala (phase 2), then into subcortical regions (phase 3), brain stem (phase 4) and finally cerebellum (phase 5). However, even though both of these protocols were based on a reasonably large number of demented and non-demented individuals (83 individuals were included in the original Braak tau stageing in 1991, and again in 2006 in the modified criteria, with 47 being employed for Thal phase protocols) the data generated still represents an assimilation of single time point, cross sectional observations into a continuum of change. The stageing protocols are therefore based on the presumption that 'normal' cases with limited, and presumed early, non-clinical pathological changes would have progressed into ones with dementia and fully developed pathology had they lived longer, and conversely those with full blown AD pathology would have flowed through the same, more limited, stages earlier in the development of disease. While this is a reasonable presumption, it still remains as such given the fact that the data are generated from a heterogeneous collection of heathy and demented individuals where the same risk factors for disease onset and progression may not necessarily apply. The advantage of studying individuals with DS lies mainly in the fact that they are a more homogenous study group who largely share the same genetic (and to some extent environmental) risk of disease, and are therefore a more predictable 'model' of disease onset and progression than are (selected) members of the general population.

Consequently, when comparing the origin and spread of tau and amyloid pathology (see Fig. 2) in this series of individuals with DS, it is clear that amyloid pathology occurred in the absence of tau pathology in 3 of 4 individuals aged between 13 and 35 years; neither were present in one 23-year old. Initially, this was present broadly to a similar extent in all regions of cerebral cortex, progressing with time into hippocampus, striatum and cerebellum. A pattern typical of AD [46] was reached by 50–55 years of age. These findings bear out our previous studies on more limited numbers of cases [28, 29] and are consistent with those of other workers where cases showing amyloid deposits in the absence of tau can be seen in individuals as young as 8 years of age [23, 24]. Early deposits of amyloid (Aβ) are seen as diffuse plaques and to be composed of the longer form $A\beta_{42(3)}$, with the shorter form, $A\beta_{40}$, only appearing later in (more advanced) cored plaques [20]. It has been suggested that deposition of amyloid in very young individuals with DS may have occurred in relationship to an institutionalized residential background [23]. In these present study, a mix of institutionalised and community based individuals were studied though no clear difference in pattern of amyloid deposition was seen between such individuals where this information was definitely available.

Interestingly, in the present study, amyloid deposition in blood vessel walls (CAA) did not commence before 42 years of age, some 30 years after initial deposition of Aβ as plaques. Similar findings have recently been reported by Head et al. [15]. It has been postulated that the strong association between age, CAA and AD pathology in the general population is driven, at least partially, by an impaired efficiency of cerebral vessels in later life in expelling extracellular fluid containing soluble forms of Aβ as a consequence of atherosclerosis/arteriosclerosis within such vessels [48]. However, individuals with DS appear to be protected against hypertension [1] and show less cerebrovascular pathology typically associated with cardiovascular risk factors, including atherosclerotic lesions and arteriolosclerosis [15, 27]. Paradoxically, this ought to result in a better preservation of perivascular drainage channels in DS, and consequently less severe CAA compared to aged persons in the general population with AD. Potential inefficiencies in perivascular drainage might only appertain to those few very elderly individuals with DS who might survive to an age bordering on those in the general population. However, Aβ can also be cleared from the brain through several other routes, involving endocytosis by microglia and astrocytes, or enzymatic degradation. It is therefore possible that failures in these latter pathways in younger persons with DS might foster an inability to expel Aβ and result in CAA.

As previously reported [18, 43, 44], *APOE* alleles and genotypes were similar to those in the general population, and in contrast to AD, there was no elevation of *APOE* ε4 allele (or reduction in ε2 allele) frequency. Nonetheless, again as reported previously [18, 41, 43, 51], age at death was earlier in ε4 allele bearers than in those without ε4 allele and was later in ε2 allele bearers than in those without ε2 allele suggesting that possession of *APOE* ε4 allele may hasten the onset of dementia and mortality by promoting an earlier formation, or a more rapid accumulation, of plaques and tangles. Although possession of *APOE* ε4 allele, and particularly homozygosity for this, has been reported to favour CAA at capillary level in persons with AD [37, 45, 47] we found no association in DS between *APOE* ε4 allele and type 3 CAA [2] (or type 2 CAA as in [47]).

On the other hand, tau pathology did not commence anywhere in the brain until after 35 years of age, though its onset in most cases appeared synchronous within both entorhinal/transentorhinal areas and subcortical nuclei (LC and DRN), with hippocampus and neocortical regions only becoming involved after 45–50 years of age. However, in two instances (cases #14 and 20) there was scant neuritic/neurofibrillary pathology in LC without any involvement of other cortical or subcortical structures. Such cases might be classed as 'prodromal stages 'a' or 'b' [6, 8]. Nonetheless, thereafter pattern of spread of tau pathology in DS is similar to that seen in typical AD [4, 7]. Hence, observations in DS strongly validate present staging protocols for tau and amyloid pathology, and provide the clearest 'model' yet for investigation the origins and progress of pathological changes typical of AD.

While most cases studied fitted in well with this age-increase pattern of spread of amyloid and tau pathology, though there were 2 notable exceptions, cases #20 and #39, which did not conform to pathological expectations given their chronological age. In case #20, aged 50 years, virtually no amyloid, and no tau pathology, was present, while in case #39 there was abundant amyloid pathology, though tau pathology was absent. It is possible that these individuals bore a karyotype other than full trisomy 21 since it is known that cases bearing only partial trisomy excluding the *APP* locus, but covering the obligate DS region, show little or no Alzheimer type pathology, even at advanced age [12, 40]. Unfortunately, a karyotype was not available for these 2 cases.

The low prevalence (9% cases) of TDP-43 pathological changes in hippocampus and fusiform gyrus is consistent with previous studies and parallels that seen in cases of sporadic and inherited early onset AD [11, 26]. This type of TDP-43 proteinopathy is much more common in late onset cases of AD [11, 34] at a time beyond the lifespan of people with DS. The higher prevalence of TDP-43 pathology in late onset AD compared to early onset AD and DS may be triggered as part of an age-associated process operating in conjunction with AD at a later time of life. Nonetheless, it is also possible that the presence of AD pathology per se initiates and promotes TDP-43 pathology. However, if this were so then a higher prevalence of TDP-43 pathology might be expected in DS than that which is seen given the severity of AD pathology occurring in older persons with DS.

A previous study has reported that α-synuclein immunopositive Lewy bodies and Lewy neurites are common in older individuals with DS, especially within the amygdaloid nucleus where as many as half of cases can show such changes [25]. In the present report, Lewy bodies and Lewy neurites were present in SN or LC or both in only 5 cases (9%) and were generally few or moderate in number. In these cases, no clear loss of nigral neurones had occurred. On the other hand, Lewy bodies and Lewy neurites were much more common in the entorhinal cortex and, to a lesser extent, temporal cortex, but again occurred only in 6 (11%) cases (which included the 5 cases where SN or LC was affected). Unfortunately, the amygdaloid nucleus was not available for investigation in the present study, though given the absence of Lewy body pathology in entorhinal cortex in most cases it is unlikely that these negative cases would have shown (at least florid) changes in the amygdala. The reason for the apparent lower frequency of Lewy body pathology in the present series of cases compared to that reported by Lippa and colleagues [25] is not clear given that both series examined individuals of a similar age range and employed α-synuclein immunostaining, albeit with different antibodies, though may be explained by the lack of investigation of the amygdala in our own study.

We did obtain some evidence (from cases #14 and 20) supporting the view [6, 11] that tau pathology in subcortical nuclei might predate that within entorhinal/transentorhinal areas, and that there might be stages in the tau pathological process before these latter cerebral cortical regions become affected. On the other hand, we observed that in 3 of the youngest individuals amyloid pathology preceded that of tau, and conversely that tau pathology was never seen in the absence of Aβ deposition – findings again consistent with the amyloid cascade hypothesis of AD [14]. Such findings accord with the view that pathological changes in tau might in some way be induced by damage to nerve terminals at the sites of amyloid plaque formation, with retrograde responses in the perikaryon leading to NFT formation. In the case of LC and DRN neurons this would occur at plaque sites within the cerebral cortex (and particularly the temporal cortex), since it is known that these nerve cell types project diffusely, but topographically, all cortical regions. Indeed, in DS and AD nerve cells of LC which project to cortical regions rich in plaques are lost whereas those projecting to relatively plaque free regions such as cerebellum, and plaque free spinal cord, are preserved [32, 33]. In entorhinal/transentorhinal areas induction of damage would take place at plaque sites within the molecular layer of the hippocampus where such neurons project via the perforant pathway [17]. The observations that tau pathology only became prevalent in SN after the age of 50 years – some 10–15 years after LC and DRN – would accord with the later deposition (relative to the cerebral cortex) of Aβ within the caudate nucleus and putamen, regions where these neurons make their principal connections.

On the other hand, it is possible that tau aggregation precedes and induces amyloid deposition in some way. Indeed, previous work based on cognitively normal young individuals suggests that areas such as LC might be the initial site of tau pathology in AD [6, 8]. However, the absence of amyloid deposits in the brains of such normal individuals implies a pathological process at work other than one that leads to AD, unless it is accepted that tau pathology in some way induces amyloid pathology at a later stage in persons other than those with DS. It is also possible that the tau pathology seen in these very young individuals is indicative of primary age related tauopathy (PART), where tau pathology occurs, especially in entorhinal/transentorhinal regions, in the relative or complete absence of amyloid deposition [10]. However, PART is generally associated with aged individuals, and an onset of this tau pathology in youth with maintenance through into old age seems unlikely. Tau pathological changes in LC and entorhinal cortex, in the absence of significant amyloid deposits, can also be seen in many patients with other neurodegenerative disorders such as Amyotrophic Lateral Sclerosis [3] or Huntington's disease [21]. Furthermore, it is known that a reversible PHF-like pattern of tau pathology can be induced under certain physiological conditions such as hypothermia and anaesthesia [39]. Therefore, it remains possible that neurons of LC (as well as others such as those in DRN and nucleus of Meynert) are exquisitely vulnerable to a range of physiological or neurotoxic changes that induce tau pathology, and that these putative early changes in tau in LC in healthy young people in the absence of amyloid deposits [6, 8] might simply be serendipitous or even transient, never progressing into a pathological process culminating in AD.

Finally, it is possible that the initiation of tau and amyloid pathologies occur independently but once started each process might act synergistically to promote the progression of the other. It might even be the case that onset of tau pathology in persons with DS represents early onset of aging processes since it is well known that such individuals display other aspects of 'precocious aging' involving skin, hair or cardiac changes at an earlier time of life compared to people within the general population.

Conclusion

In conclusion, a study of the brains of individuals with DS at different ages reinforces the concepts underlying the amyloid cascade hypothesis of AD and supports present stageing protocols for the onset and spread of both amyloid and tau pathology.

Acknowledgements

We acknowledge the support of the Manchester Brain Bank by Alzheimer's Research UK and Alzheimer's Society through their funding of the Brains for Dementia Research (BDR) Programme. Manchester Brain Bank also receives Service Support costs from Medical Research Council.

Funding

Manchester Brain Bank receives funding from Alzheimer's Research UK and Alzheimer's Society, through the Brains for Dementia Research (BDR) Programme, and also receives Service Support Costs from Medical Research Council of UK.

Authors' contributions

Study concept, design and manuscript preparation (DM, VP), microscopic assessments (DM), technical support and data analysis (AR, YD).

Competing interests

The authors declare that they have no competing interests.

Author details

[1]Institute of Brain, Behaviour and Mental Health, Faculty of Medical and Human Sciences University of Manchester, Salford Royal Hospital, Stott Lane, Salford M6 8HD, England. [2]South Birmingham Community NHS Trust, Birmingham, UK. [3]Liverpool John Moores University, Liverpool, UK.

References

1. Alexander M, Petri H, Ding Y, Wandel C, Khwaja O, Foskett N (2016) Morbidity and medication in a large population of individuals with Down syndrome compared to the general population. Dev Med Child Neurol 58:246–254
2. Allen N, Robinson AC, Snowden S, Davidson YS, Mann DMA (2014) Patterns of cerebral amyloid angiopathy define histopathological phenotypes in Alzheimer's disease. Neuropathol Appl Neurobiol 40:136–148
3. Behrouzi R, Liu X, Wu D, Robinson AC, Tanaguchi-Watanabe S, Rollinson S et al (2016) Pathological tau deposition in motor Neurone disease and frontotemporal lobar degeneration associated with TDP-43 proteinopathy. Acta Neuropathol Commun 4:33
4. Braak H, Braak E (1991) Neuropathological stageing of Alzheimer-related changes. Acta Neuropathol 82:239–259
5. Braak H, Braak E (1998) Argyrophilic grain disease: frequency of occurrence in different age categories and neuropathological diagnostic criteria. J Neural Transm 105:801–819
6. Braak H, Del Tredici K (2011) The pathological process underlying Alzheimer's disease in individuals under thirty. Acta Neuropathol 12:171–181
7. Braak H, Alafuzoff I, Arzberger T, Kretzschmar H, Del Tredici K (2006) Staging of Alzheimer disease-associated neurofibrillary pathology using paraffin sections and immunocytochemistry. Acta Neuropathol 112:389–404
8. Braak H, Thal DR, Ghebremedhin E, Del Tredici K (2011) Stages of the pathologic process in Alzheimer disease: age categories from 1 to 100 years. J Neuropathol Exp Neurol 70:960–969
9. Burger PC, Vogel FS (1973) The development of the pathological changes of Alzheimer's disease and senile dementia in patients with Down's syndrome. Am J Pathol 73:457–476
10. Crary JF, Trojanowski JQ, Schneider JA, Abisambra JF, Abner EL, Alafuzoff I et al (2014) Primary age-related tauopathy (PART): a common pathology associated with human aging. Acta Neuropathol 128:755–766
11. Davidson YS, Raby S, Foulds PG, Robinson A, Thompson JC, Sikkink S et al (2011) TDP-43 pathological changes in early onset familial and sporadic Alzheimer's disease, late onset Alzheimer's disease and Down's syndrome: association with age, hippocampal sclerosis and clinical phenotype. Acta Neuropathol 122:703–713
12. Doran E, Keator D, Head E, Phelan MJ, Kim R, Totoiu M et al (2017) Down syndrome, partial trisomy 21, and absence of Alzheimer's disease: the role of APP. J Alzheimers Dis 56:459–470
13. Ellis WG, McCulloch JR, Corley CL (1974) Presenile dementia in Down's syndrome. Ultrastructural identity with Alzheimer's disease. Neurology 24:101–106
14. Hardy J, Allsop D (1991) Amyloid deposition as the central event in the aetiology of Alzheimer's disease. Trends Pharmacol Sci 12:383–388
15. Head E, Phelan MJ, Doran E, Kim RC, Poon WW, Schmidt FA et al (2017) Cerebrovascular pathology in Down syndrome and Alzheimer disease. Acta Neuropathol Comm 5:93
16. Hof PR, Bouras C, Perl DP, Sparks DL, Mehta N, Morrison JH (1995) Age-related distribution of neuropathologic changes in the cerebral cortex of patients with Down's syndrome. Quantitative regional analysis and comparison with Alzheimer's disease. Arch Neurol 52:379–391
17. Hyman BT, Van Hoesen GW, Damasio AR, Barnes CL (1984) Alzheimer's disease: cell-specific pathology isolates the hippocampal formation. Science 225:1168–1170
18. Hyman BT, West HL, Rebeck GW, Lai F, Mann DM (1995) Neuropathological changes in Down's syndrome hippocampal formation. Effect of age and apolipoprotein E genotype. Arch Neurol 52:373–378
19. Hyman BT, Phelps CH, Beach TG, Bigio EH, Cairns NJ, Carrillo MC et al (2012) National Institute on Aging–Alzheimer's association guidelines for the neuropathologic assessment of Alzheimer's disease. Alzheimers Dement 8:1–13
20. Iwatsubo T, Mann DMA, Odaka A, Suzuki N, Ihara Y (1995) Amyloid ß-protein (Aß) deposition: $Aß_{42(43)}$ precedes $Aß_{(40)}$ in Down's syndrome. Ann Neurol 37:294–299
21. Jellinger KA (1998) Alzheimer-type lesions in Huntington's disease. J Neural Transm 105:787–799
22. Kovacs GG, Ferrer I, Grinberg LT, Alafuzoff I, Attems J, Budka H et al (2016) Aging-related tau astrogliopathy (ARTAG): harmonized evaluation strategy. Acta Neuropathol 131:87–102
23. Lemere CA, Blusztajn JK, Yamaguchi H, Wisniewski T, Saido TC, Selkoe DJ (1996) Sequence of deposition of heterogeneous amyloid beta-peptides and APOE in Down syndrome: implications for initial events in amyloid plaque formation. Neurobiol Dis 3:16–32

24. Leverenz JB, Raskind MA (1998) Early amyloid deposition in the medial temporal lobe of young Down syndrome patients: a regional quantitative analysis. Exp Neurol 150:296–304
25. Lippa CF, Schmidt ML, Lee VM, Trojanowski JQ (1999) Antibodies to alpha-synuclein detect Lewy bodies in many Down's syndrome brains with Alzheimer's disease. Ann Neurol 45:353–357
26. Lippa CF, Rosso AL, Stutzbach LD, Neumann M, Lee VM, Trojanowski JQ (2009) Transactive response DNA-binding protein 43 burden in familial Alzheimer disease and Down syndrome. Arch Neurol 66:1483–1488
27. Lott IT, Head E (2005) Alzheimer disease and Down syndrome: factors in pathogenesis. Neurobiol Aging 26:383–389
28. Mann DMA (1988) The pathological association between Down syndrome and Alzheimer disease. Mech Ageing Dev 43:99–136
29. Mann DMA, Esiri MM (1988) The site of the earliest lesions of Alzheimer's disease. New Eng J Med 318:789–790
30. Mann DMA, Younis N, Jones D, Stoddart RW (1992) The time course of pathological events concerned with plaque formation in Down's syndrome with particular reference to the involvement of microglial cells. Neurodegeneration 1:201–215
31. Mann DMA, Davidson YS, Robinson AC, Allen N, Hashimoto T, Richardson A et al (2018) Patterns and severity of vascular amyloid in Alzheimer's disease associated with duplications and missense mutations in APP gene, Down syndrome and sporadic Alzheimer's disease. Acta Neuropathol. https://doi.org/10.1007/s00401-018-1866-3
32. Marcyniuk B, Mann DM, Yates PO (1986) The topography of cell loss from locus caeruleus in Alzheimer's disease. J Neurol Sci 76:335–345
33. Marcyniuk B, Mann DM, Yates PO, Ravindra CR (1988) Topography of nerve cell loss from the locus caeruleus in middle aged persons with Down's syndrome. J Neurol Sci 83:15–24
34. McAleese KE, Walker L, Erskine D, Thomas AJ, McKeith IG, Attems J (2017) TDP-43 pathology in Alzheimer's disease, dementia with Lewy bodies and ageing. Brain Pathol 20:472–479
35. Montine TJ, Phelps CH, Beach TG, Bigio EH, Cairns NJ, Dickson DW et al (2012) National Institute on Aging-Alzheimer's association guidelines for the neuropathologic assessment of Alzheimer's disease: a practical approach. Acta Neuropathol 123:1–11
36. Obi K, Akiyama H, Kondo H, Shimomura Y, Hasegawa M, Iwatsubo T (2008) Relationship of phosphorylated α-synuclein and tau accumulation to Aβ deposition in the cerebral cortex of dementia with Lewy bodies. Expl Neurol 210:409–420
37. Olichney JM, Hansen LA, Galasko D, Saitoh T, Hofstetter CR, Katzman R et al (1996) The apolipoprotein E epsilon 4 allele is associated with increased neuritic plaques and cerebral amyloid angiopathy in Alzheimer's disease and Lewy body variant. Neurology 47:190–196
38. Olson MI, Shaw CM (1969) Presenile dementia and Alzheimer's disease in mongolism. Brain 92:147–156
39. Planel E, Richter KE, Nolan CE, Finley JE, Liu L, Wen Y et al (2007) Anaesthesia leads to tau hyperphosphorylation through inhibition of phosphatase activity by hypothermia. J Neurosci 27:3090–3097
40. Prasher VP, Farrer MJ, Kessling AM, Fisher EM, West RJ, Barber PC et al (1998) Molecular mapping of Alzheimer-type dementia in Down's syndrome. Ann Neurol 43:380–383
41. Prasher VP, Schupf N, Sajith SG, Zigman WB, Rees S, Patel A et al (2008) Significant effect of APOE epsilon 4 genotype on the risk of Alzheimer's disease and mortality in persons with Down syndrome. Int J Geriatr Psychiatry 23:1134–1140
42. Ropper AH, Williams RS (1980) Relationship between plaques and tangles and dementia in Down's syndrome. Neurology 30:639–644
43. Royston MC, Mann D, Pickering-Brown S, Owen F, Perry R, Raghavan R et al (1994) Apolipoprotein E epsilon 2 allele promotes longevity and protects patients with Down's syndrome from dementia. Neuroreport 5:2583–2585
44. Saunders AM, Schmader K, Breitner JC, Benson MD, Brown WT, Goldfarb L et al (1993) Apolipoprotein E epsilon 4 allele distributions in late-onset Alzheimer's disease and in other amyloid-forming diseases. Lancet 342:710–711
45. Shinohara M, Murray ME, Frank RD, Shinohara M, DeTure M, Yamazaki Y et al (2016) Impact of sex and APOE4 on cerebral amyloid angiopathy in Alzheimer's disease. Acta Neuropathol 132:225–234
46. Thal DR, Rüb U, Orantes M, Braak H (2002) Phases of a beta-deposition in the human brain and its relevance for the development of AD. Neurology 58:1791–1800
47. Thal DR, Papassotiropoulos A, Saido TC, Griffin WS, Mrak RE, Kölsch H et al (2010) Capillary cerebral amyloid angiopathy identifies a distinct APOE epsilon4-associated subtype of sporadic Alzheimer's disease. Acta Neuropathol 120:169–183
48. Weller RO, Boche D, Nicoll JA (2009) Microvasculature changes and cerebral amyloid angiopathy in Alzheimer's disease and their potential impact on therapy. Acta Neuropathol 118:87–102
49. Wenham PR, Price WH, Blandell G (1991) Apolipoprotein E genotyping by one-stage PCR. Lancet 337:1158–1159
50. Wisniewski KE, Wisniewski HM, Wen GY (1985) Occurrence of neuropathological changes and dementia of Alzheimer's disease in Down's syndrome. Ann Neurol 17:278–282
51. Zigman WB, Jenkins EC, Tycko B, Schupf N, Silverman W (2005) Mortality is associated with apolipoprotein E ε4 in non-demented adults with Down syndrome. Neurosci Lett 390:93–97

11

A53T-α-synuclein overexpression in murine locus coeruleus induces Parkinson's disease-like pathology in neurons and glia

Martin Timo Henrich[1], Fanni Fruzsina Geibl[1], Bolam Lee[1], Wei-Hua Chiu[1], James Benjamin Koprich[2], Jonathan Michael Brotchie[2], Lars Timmermann[1], Niels Decher[3], Lina Anita Matschke[1,3] and Wolfgang Hermann Oertel[1*]

Abstract

Degeneration of noradrenergic locus coeruleus neurons occurs during the prodromal phase of Parkinson's disease and contributes to a variety of non-motor symptoms, e.g. depression, anxiety and REM sleep behavior disorder. This study was designed to establish the first locus coeruleus α-synucleinopathy mouse model, which should provide sufficient information about the time-course of noradrenergic neurodegeneration, replicate cardinal histopathological features of the human Parkinson's disease neuropathology and finally lead to robust histological markers, which are sufficient to assess the pathological changes in a quantitative and qualitative way. We show that targeted viral vector-mediated overexpression of human mutant A53T-α-synuclein in vivo in locus coeruleus neurons of wild-type mice resulted in progressive noradrenergic neurodegeneration over a time frame of 9 weeks. Observed neuronal cell loss was accompanied by progressive α-synuclein phosphorylation, formation of proteinase K-resistant α-synuclein-aggregates, accumulation of Ubi-1- and p62-positive inclusions in microglia and induction of progressive micro- and astrogliosis. Apart from this local pathology, abundant α-synuclein-positive axons were found in locus coeruleus output regions, indicating rapid anterograde axonal transport of A53T-α-synuclein. Taken together, we present the first model of α-synucleinopathy in the murine locus coeruleus, replicating essential morphological features of human Parkinson's disease pathology. This new model may contribute to the research on prodromal Parkinson's disease, in respect to pathophysiology and the development of disease-modifying therapy.

Keywords: Parkinson's disease, Locus coeruleus, Alpha-synuclein, Adeno-associated viral vectors, Prodromal mouse model, Microglia, noradrenergic neurons

Introduction

Parkinson's disease (PD) is the second most common neurodegenerative disorder [2] characterized by progressive degeneration of dopaminergic (DA) substantia nigra (SN) neurons and their striatal axon terminals [40, 68]. One characteristic neuropathological hallmark of PD are intracytoplasmic eosinophilic inclusions, the so-called Lewy bodies, which develop in specific brain regions in a spatio-temporal pattern and consist predominantly of misfolded α-synuclein (aSYN) [11, 83]. The finding that duplications, triplications or missense mutations (e.g. A53T, A30P or G46 L) of the aSYN gene (SNCA) cause familial forms of PD [46, 67] has justified the assumption that aSYN plays a crucial role in the pathogenesis of PD.

Only within the last 20 years it is accepted that PD cannot solely be understood as a disease associated with the degeneration of DA SN neurons, as the PD pathology involves the central, peripheral, autonomic and enteric nervous system [11, 12, 16, 79, 95]. The degeneration of DA SN neurons and the onset of motor dysfunction are preceded by a latency of several years, if not decades, in which the PD pathology develops in brain regions outside the DA SN. This phase, termed prodromal PD, is clinically characterized by the occurrence

* Correspondence: oertelw@med.uni-marburg.de
Lina Anita Matschke and Wolfgang Hermann Oertel are shared senior authors.
Martin Timo Henrich and Fanni Fruzsina Geibl contributed equally to this work.
[1]Department of Neurology, Philipps University Marburg, Baldingerstraße 1, 35043 Marburg, Germany
Full list of author information is available at the end of the article

of certain non-motor symptoms, e.g. hyposmia, constipation, depression and idiopathic REM sleep behavior disorder [31, 53, 84]. Since the prodromal phase is seen as the ideal time window for applying disease-modifying therapy [60, 92], it is of high importance to establish animal models, which allow testing of new and future therapeutic approaches on brain structures that are affected during prodromal PD. The noradrenergic locus coeruleus (LC), a monoaminergic nucleus located in the pontine brainstem [3, 8], plays a crucial role during the prodromal phase of PD and represents therefore an ideal brain structure for such in-depth characterization in an experimental animal model [97]. Dysfunction and degeneration of neurons in the LC region are associated with several of the above listed non-motor symptoms, including depression, signs of reduced arousal, anxiety and REM sleep behavior disorder (RBD) [17, 27, 93]. Neuropathological analysis of human PD brain samples revealed up to 80% LC neuronal cell loss in PD patients, thereby exceeding the degree of SN neurodegeneration in the same individuals [58, 99]. Moreover, experimental evidence indicates that toxin-induced LC cell loss sensitized DA SN neurons for neurodegeneration [9, 22], whereas noradrenergic hyperinnervation resulted in neuroprotective effects [41]. This data implies that LC neurodegeneration itself plays a double role by firstly being responsible for several non-motor symptoms and secondly for accelerating the progression of PD at the nigral level [27]. LC cells exhibit a common at-risk phenotype compared to other neuronal populations such as the DA nigral neurons and the cholinergic neurons of the dorsal motor nucleus of the vagal nerve which undergo neurodegeneration in PD [6, 78]. LC neurons integrate information from a broad range of different brain regions and broadcast information with extensively branched and thinly myelinated axons throughout the complete neuroaxis [8, 75]. Furthermore, they exhibit an intrinsic pacemaking activity, generating action potentials continuously [55] thereby raising their basal metabolic stress level [78].

In this study, we have characterized the first model of α-synucleinopathy in the murine LC. We show that targeted viral vector-mediated overexpression of human mutant A53T-aSYN in vivo in LC neurons of wild-type mice resulted in progressive LC neurodegeneration over a time frame of 9 weeks. Observed LC cell loss was accompanied by prominent and over time increasing micro- and astrogliosis. In addition, our data revealed accumulation of phosphorylated aSYN, progressive aggregation of aSYN as demonstrated by proteinase K-resistant aSYN aggregates and Ubi-1- and p62-positive inclusions comparable with findings from human PD samples. Co-staining with different cellular markers revealed that the p62- and Ubi-1-positive aggregates were found exclusively in microglial cells, while being absent in neurons, astrocytes and oligodendrocytes. Beside this local LC pathology, we observed abundant aSYN-positive axons in a high number of LC output regions, indicating rapid anterograde axonal transport of the human aSYN. In conclusion, our new murine LC model replicated cardinal morphological features of human PD pathology.

Materials and methods

Animals

A total of 70 wild-type male C57BL/6 N mice (Charles River, Sulzfeld, Germany), 8 weeks old at the beginning of the experiment, were used. Mice were housed in individually ventilated cages with ad libitum access to food and water under a 12 h/12 h light-dark cycle. All procedures performed in studies involving animals were in accordance with the ethical standards of the institution at which the studies were conducted (Regierungspräsidium Giessen, Germany V54–19 c 20 15 h 01 MR 20/15 Nr. 66/2015).

Recombinant adeno-associated viral (rAAV) vectors and stereotactic injection

Two different recombinant adeno-associated viral (rAAV) vectors of a mixed 1/2 serotype were used to overexpress human mutant-A53T-aSYN (rAAV1/2-CMV/CBA-human-A53T-aSYN-WPRE-BGH-pA (rAAV1/2-A53T-aSYN); viral titer 5.1×10^{12} gp/ml, purchased from GeneDetect) or luciferase (rAAV1/2-CMV/CBA-luciferase-WPRE-BGH-pA (rAAV1/2-Luc), viral titer 5.0×10^{12} gp/ml, purchased from GeneDetect). Each of the two vectors was driven by a chicken beta actin (CBA) promoter combined with a cytomegalovirus (CMV) immediate early enhancer sequence and a woodchuck post-transcriptional regulatory element (WPRE) to assess a high transcription rate [38, 44]. For stereotactic delivery of the rAAV vectors, mice were anesthetized with 100 mg/kg ketamine and 5 mg/kg xylazine via intraperitoneal injection. A volume of 1.25 µl of rAAV1/2-A53T-aSYN or rAAV1/2-Luc was stereotactically injected in the right LC region using a microinjector (UltraMicro Pump UMP3, World Precision Instruments) with a velocity of 125 nl/min based on the following coordinates: ML – 0.9 mm, AP -5.4 mm and DV -3.65 mm relative to Bregma [66].

Tissue preparation

Mice were sacrificed through transcardial perfusion with 0.1 M phosphate-buffered saline (PBS) for 5 min followed by 4% ice-cold paraformaldehyde (PFA) in 0.1 M phosphate buffer (PB) (pH 7.4) for 5 min using a supply pump at a rate of 10 ml/min. Brains were carefully removed and post-fixed in 4% PFA for 3 days and then transferred to 30% sucrose solution for 3 days for cryoprotection. Brains were cut into 20 µm thick coronal sections using a cryostat microtome (Leica CM3050 S, Nussloch, Germany). Sections were then stored at 4 °C in cryoprotect-solution (1:1:3 volume ratio of ethylenglycol, glycerol and 0.1 M PB) until further processing.

Immunohistochemistry with 3,3-diaminobenzidine (DAB)

Free-floating sections containing the LC/SN region were washed in 0.1 M PB and quenched with 3% H_2O_2 and 10% methanol for 15 min. After a second wash, sections were blocked in 5% normal donkey serum with 0.3% Triton X-100 in 0.1 M PB for 1 h before incubating them overnight with primary antibodies against TH, p-aSYN, Ubi-1 or p62 (Table 1) at 4 °C in the same blocking solution. On the second day, sections were washed in 0.1 M PB for 20 min and then incubated with the appropriate biotinylated secondary antibody (Table 1) for 1 h, followed by incubation in avidin-biotin-peroxidase solution (ABC Elite, Vector Laboratories) for 1 h before initiating the color reaction with 5% DAB (Serva), diluted in 0.1 M PB with 0.02% H_2O_2. All DAB-stained sections were mounted, dried, counterstained with cresyl-violet and coverslipped with mounting gel (Corbit-Balsam, Eukitt). Brightfield images were acquired using an AxioImager M2 microscope (Zeiss) equipped with an Axiocam 506 color camera (Zeiss).

Immunofluorescence staining

Sections were washed in 0.1 M PB, then blocked in 10% normal donkey serum with 0.3% Triton X-100 in 0.1 M PB for 1 h before incubating them with primary antibodies (Table 1) at 4 °C in the same blocking solution overnight. On the second day, sections were washed in 0.1 M PB containing 0.3% Triton X-100 and then incubated with fluorophore-conjugated, species-specific secondary antibodies (Table 1) for 2 h at room temperature in 0.1 M PB containing 0.3% Triton X-100 and 10% normal donkey serum. Before mounting sections were washed for 25 min in 0.1 M PB containing 0.3% Triton X-100. Exceptions from this general protocol were made for staining luciferase, p-aSYN, IbA1 and Olig2, where after primary antibody incubation a biotinylated species-specific secondary antibody was used to further improve signal to noise by conjugation with streptavidin. Images were acquired using an AxioImager M2 microscope (Zeiss) equipped with an ORCA-Flash4.0 LT CMOS camera (Hamamatsu C11440-42 U). For confocal images, a TCS SP8 microscope (Leica) was used. Images were processed with FIJI image software [81] to enhance signal-to-noise. Image data for 3D reconstructions were obtained with a Zeiss Spinning Disc Microscope (Axio Observer Z1)

Table 1 Characteristics of the primary and secondary antibodies

Antigen	Host	Cat. No.	Manufacturer	Dilution
Tyrosine Hydroxylase	Rabbit	AB152	Merck Millipore	1:1000
Tyrosine Hydroxylase	Sheep	AB1542	Merck Millipore	1:1000
AAV VP1/VP2/VP3	Rabbit	61,084	Progen	1:250
Alpha-synuclein (p-S129)	Rabbit	ab51253	Abcam	1:2000
Alpha-synuclein (syn211)	Mouse	AHB0261	ThermoFisher	1:1000
Luciferase	Goat	NB100–1677	Novus Biologicals	1:250
GFAP	Chicken	ab4674	Abcam	1:2000
IbA1	Rabbit	019–19,741	Wako	1:500
Ubiquitin (Ubi-1)	Mouse	ab7254	Abcam	1:2000
SQSTM1/p62	Mouse	ab56416	Abcam	1:2000
Olig2	Rabbit	ab109186	Abcam	1:500
MAP2	Chicken	ab5392	Abcam	1:2000
Anti-rabbit AlexaFluor488	Donkey	A-21206	Invitrogen	1:1000
Anti-goat AlexaFluor488	Donkey	A-11055	Invitrogen	1:1000
Anti-mouse AlexaFluor488	Donkey	A-2102	Invitrogen	1:1000
Anti-chicken Cy3	Donkey	703–165-155	Jackson ImmunoResearch	1:1000
Anti-mouse Cy3	Donkey	715–165-150	Jackson ImmunoResearch	1:1000
Anti-goat Cy3	Donkey	705–165-147	Jackson ImmunoResearch	1:1000
Biotinylated anti-rabbit	Donkey	711–065-152	Jackson ImmunoResearch	1:1000
Biotinylated anti-mouse	Donkey	715–065-151	Jackson ImmunoResearch	1:1000
Biotinylated anti-goat	Donkey	705–065-147	Jackson ImmunoResearch	1:1000
Streptavidin AlexaFluor647	Donkey	016–600-084	Jackson ImmunoResearch	1:1000

equipped with an Axiocam MRm (Zeiss) and an Evolve 512 EMCCD Camera (Photometrics) and post-processed with ZEN 2012 software (Zeiss).

Proteinase K treatment

To analyze the formation of insoluble aggregates, sections were digested with Proteinase K (PK) using a modified protocol described elsewhere [21, 86]. 20 µm thick sections with 120 µm interslice distance containing the complete LC region were washed in 0.1 M PB and subsequently digested in 0.1 M PB containing 0.3% Triton X-100 and 12 µg/ml PK (Cat. No. 4333793, Invitrogen) at 65 °C for 10 min. To visualize insoluble aggregates, digested sections were double stained against human aSYN, p62, Ubi-1 or luciferase in combination with TH (Table 1), following the fluorescence staining protocol described above. Complete absence of TH immunoreactivity served as an indicator for successful PK digestion, thus sections in which TH immunoreactivity was still visible were excluded from analysis implicating an incomplete protein digestion. Images were acquired using an AxioImager M2 microscope (Zeiss) equipped with an ORCA-Flash4.0 LT CMOS camera (Hamamatsu C11440-42 U).

Stereology

To quantify TH-positive LC and SN neurons, the optical fractionator workflow (StereoInvestigator version 9, MicroBrightField Biosciences) was used. Therefore, tissue sections were stained against TH with DAB and counterstained with cresyl-violet as described above. To quantify LC cell numbers, five sections per animal containing the complete rostro-caudal extent of the LC region, separated by 120 µm, were selected. Contours including all TH-positive neurons of the LC were drawn, excluding neurons of the SubLC region. For quantification of TH-positive SN neurons, seven sections separated by 240 µm covering the complete caudo-rostral extent of the SN were used. Contours were drawn based on the cytoarchitectonic distribution of SN neurons [24] including SN pars compacta but excluding SN pars reticulata or ventral tegmental area neurons. Parameters used for counting were: grid size 100 × 100 µm, counting frame 85 × 85 µm, and 2 µm guard zones.

Quantification of reactive micro- and astrogliosis

Triple immunofluorescence stainings were performed to visualize astro- and microgliosis using antibodies directed against GFAP for astroglia, IbA1 for microglia and TH to label LC neurons (Table 1). To quantify signs of reactive gliosis, we evaluated 5 LC sections of 6 animals per time point by measuring the optical density (OD) of the injected versus the non-injected side using FIJI. First, greyscale images were converted to 8 bit and the LC region was outlined with a rectangular contour (1200px x 800px). Then, OD was measured and lastly a background correction was performed by subtracting the mean background signal for every section. The background corrected OD values of all 5 sections of the injected side were summed and compared to the summed value of the non-injected side.

Quantification of S129-phosphorylated aSYN

To analyze the degree of p-aSYN, a triple immunofluorescence staining against p-aSYN, human aSYN and TH was performed (Table 1). Five sections of 4 animals per time point, containing the complete rostro-caudal extent of the LC region, were selected for analysis. First, images were converted to 8 bit before making them binary. By using a preset intensity threshold, pixels were given either an intensity value of 255 (when positive for p-aSYN) or 0 (when negative for p-aSYN). The resulting p-aSYN signal intensity value was then divided by the area positive for non-phosphorylated aSYN. This ratio was calculated for all five sections and averaged per animal.

Quantification of aSYN transport

Seven coronal sections (Bregma: + 4.28, + 2.86, + 1.18, + 0.38, − 0.58, − 3.16 and − 7.56) covering the complete mouse brain were stained against human aSYN (Syn 211) or Luc (Table 1) and the degree of aSYN accumulation was assessed by scoring human aSYN positive axons/cell bodies as follows: – no positive axons; + sparse (few positive axons); ++ mild (more positive axons); +++ moderate (many positive axons, covering almost the complete brain region) and ++++ severe pathology (large number of positive axons densely covering the complete brain region). (+) describes an intermediate state. Six animals per time point were analyzed and the scores for each brain region were averaged.

Statistical analyses

In general, all data values are expressed as mean ± SEM or mean ± min/max. Differences were considered significant at $p < 0.05$. Multiple comparisons were made by one-way or two-way ANOVA analysis followed by Tukey's or Sidak's multiple comparisons test. To calculate correlations, Pearson's correlation coefficient with 95% confidence interval was used. All statistical analyses were performed using GraphPad Prism version 7.00 (GraphPad Software, La Jolla California USA). Figures were created with Adobe Illustrator version 21.1 (Adobe Systems).

Results

rAAV vector-mediated overexpression of human A53T-aSYN in LC neurons

To determine whether and in which time frame aSYN overexpression induces PD-like pathology in LC neurons we chose to overexpress human mutant A53T-aSYN by injecting rAAV1/2-A53T-aSYN [38, 44] unilaterally in the right LC region of wild-type mice (Fig. 1a, b). To verify that the resulting cellular effects were attributable to the aSYN protein itself, luciferase (Luc) was used as a control protein. To investigate time-dependent effects, animals were consecutively sacrificed after 3 days, 1, 3, 6 and 9 weeks (Fig. 1b).

By analyzing the first set of animals 3 days after viral injection, we confirmed that both vectors entered LC neurons equally (Fig. 1c, d), resulting in infection rates of 85.17 ± 2.53% for A53T-aSYN and 83.87 ± 3.31% for Luc (unpaired t-test, $p = 0.77$) (Fig. 1d). Double immunofluorescence stainings against TH and human aSYN or TH and Luc (Fig. 1e, f) revealed that both vectors induced protein expression already at this early time point with similar strength (A53T-aSYN 59.89 ± 2.95% and Luc 54.39 ± 3.57%, unpaired t-test, $p = 0.30$). Protein expression was mainly restricted to the LC covering the whole nucleus (Fig. 1g, h). In addition, a variable number of immuno-reactive cells were observed in the adjacent regions (ncl. Parabrachialis, Barrington's nucleus, mesencephalic trigeminal nucleus and vestibular nuclei) (Fig. 1g). In LC neurons, cell bodies, as well as axons and dendrites were robustly labeled, indicating strong protein expression. Similar findings were observed for rAAV1/2-Luc injected animals. Notably, there was no aSYN or Luc signal in LC cells on the non-injected side at any time point (Fig. 1g). This allowed us to use the non-injected (left) side as an internal control.

A53T-aSYN overexpression causes LC neurodegeneration

In the first set of experiments, the extent of aSYN induced LC cell loss was assessed with unbiased stereological quantification of TH-positive LC cells 1, 3, 6 and 9 weeks after viral vector delivery. In the A53T-aSYN group, significant degeneration of TH-positive LC cells was measured already 3 weeks post-injection, with 15.86 ± 2.09% cell loss compared to control side. Neurodegeneration increased progressively reaching 34.84 ± 3.39% after 6 weeks and 56.25 ± 5.19% after 9 weeks (Fig. 2a, b). Cell loss was homogenously distributed over the complete rostro-caudal extent of the LC. No cellular pathology was observed in the Luc control group at any investigated time point, confirming that neither the viral vector nor overexpression of a cytoplasmic protein was able to induce neurodegeneration in our model (Fig. 2a, b).

Moreover, immunofluorescent TH-stainings and subsequent confocal imaging revealed that A53T-aSYN, but not Luc overexpression was accompanied by qualitative changes of neuronal morphology, including dystrophic axons and pyknotic perikarya (Fig. 2c).

Accumulation of phosphorylated-aSYN in the LC region

Phosphorylation of aSYN at amino acid serine 129 (p-aSYN) is a commonly observed phenomenon in human PD brain tissue and in animal models artificially overexpressing aSYN [1, 25, 52, 72, 98]. In these models, the S129 phosphorylation is frequently used as an indicator for aSYN aggregation. In our current study, we measured the signal intensity of p-aSYN systematically via double immunofluorescence stainings for TH and p-aSYN. Our data revealed that A53T-aSYN overexpression led to strong and progressive phosphorylation of aSYN in LC neurons (Fig. 3a, b). Accumulation of p-aSYN started early with positive cells being observable already 1 week post-injection, reaching highest levels at the latest time point. Generally, the p-aSYN signal was homogenously distributed in the cytoplasm of TH-positive LC cells. In addition, robust labeling of the nucleus was observed (Fig. 3d, e). To exclude the possibility of non-specific antibody labeling we analyzed rAAV-Luc injected animals, which showed no signal for p-aSYN at any time point (Fig. 3d, e). Next, we wanted to quantify if the degree of phosphorylation correlated with the degree of noradrenergic cell loss. Therefore, the p-aSYN signal intensity values were plotted and correlated with the percentage of LC cell loss (Fig. 3c). The strong correlation ($r = 0.67$, $p < 0.05$) indicates that the degree of aSYN phosphorylation can be used as a predictor of aSYN toxicity in our model.

Formation of proteinase K (PK)-resistant, p62-, Ubi-1- and aSYN-positive aggregates

Lewy bodies in human PD brain tissue are characterized by immunoreactivity for insoluble (PK-resistant) aSYN, but also for a variety of other proteins, such as ubiquitin-1 (Ubi-1) and p62/SQSTM1/sequestosome-1 (p62) [33, 47]. Both of the latter proteins are implicated in the cellular clearance of aSYN. Occurrence of PK-resistant Ubi-1-positive aggregates indicates an overburdened proteasomal clearing system, while dysfunction of the lysosomal system can result in accumulation of p62-positive aggregates [73]. To test whether proteasomal and/or lysosomal clearance might be impaired in our model, we systematically screened A53T-aSYN and Luc overexpressing animals for p62- and Ubi-1-immunoreactivity. A53T-aSYN, but not Luc injected mice showed abundant p62- and Ubi-1-positive aggregates starting 3 weeks after viral vector delivery reaching highest numbers at the latest time point (Fig. 4a, b). Ubi-1-, as well as p62-positive inclusions appeared as small circular objects surrounding the nuclei of the cells (Fig. 4b) and were restricted to the ipsilateral side of injection. As in the previous experiments most of the p-aSYN signal was seen in TH-positive neurons

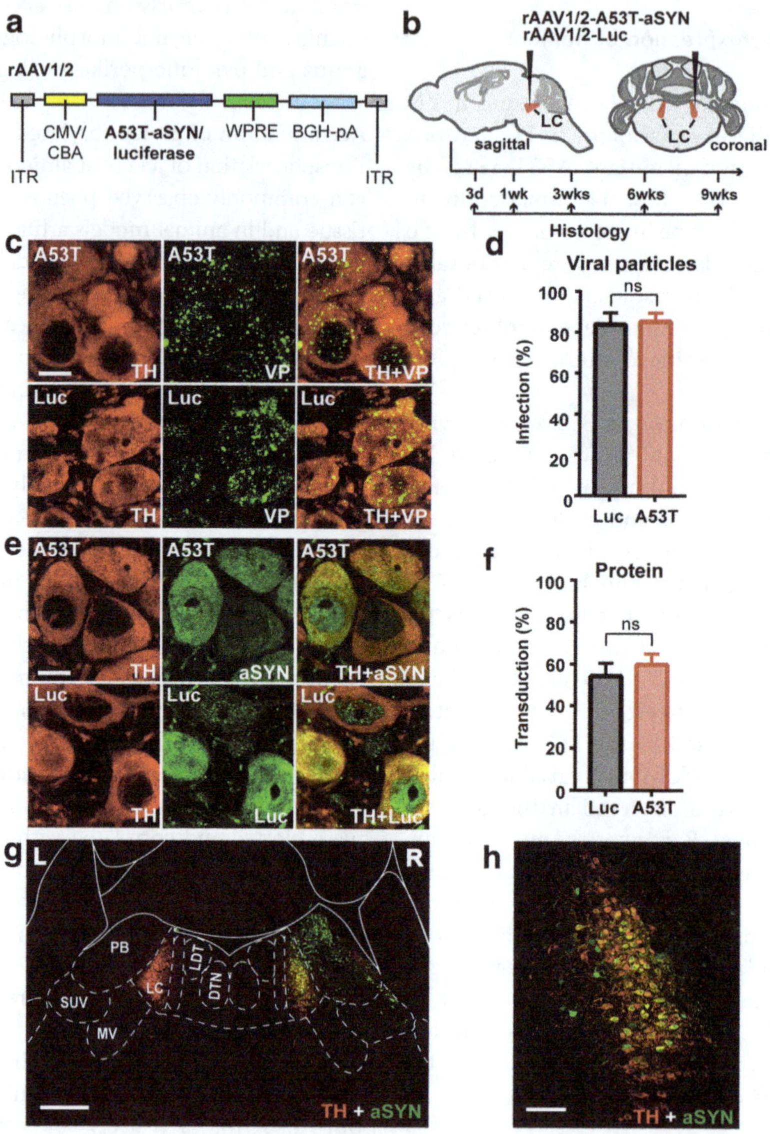

Fig. 1 Locally induced protein overexpression via injection of rAAV vectors in the LC region. **a** rAAV1/2 vectors contain a chicken β-actin promoter hybridized with a CMV immediate early enhancer sequence (CMV/CBA) to drive expression of either A53T-aSYN or luciferase (control). ITR, inverted terminal repeat; WPRE, woodchuck hepatitis virus posttranscriptional regulatory element; BGH-pA, bovine growth hormone polyadenylation sequence. **b** Experimental design and schematic illustration of the injection site. Animals were consecutively sacrificed after 3 days, 1, 3, 6 and 9 weeks for immunohistochemical evaluation. **c-f** Analysis of the infection or transduction rates via double immunofluorescence staining for TH (red) and viral coating proteins (VP, green) (**c**, **d**) or TH (red) and human A53T-aSYN (green) or luciferase (green) (**e**, **f**), respectively. Co-localization of TH and VP indicates successful entry of viral particles, whereas co-localization of TH and A53T-aSYN/luciferase indicates successful protein expression. Student's t-test revealed no significant difference between the transduction rates of the two vectors ($p > 0.05$, $n = 3$ animals per protein) (**d**, **f**). Values (mean ± SEM) represent the percentage (%) of TH-positive neurons that were also positive for VP, aSYN or Luc. **g** Overview of the pontine brainstem (Bregma: – 5.30 mm) stained against TH (red) and human aSYN (green) depicting the transduced area 3 days post-injection. Abbreviations: L, left; R, right; PB, parabrachial nucl.; SUV, superior vestibular nucl.; MV, medial vestibular nucl.; DTN, dorsal tegmental nucl.; LDT, laterodorsal tegmental nucl. **h** Higher magnification overview image of the TH-positive LC region (red) transduced with human A53T-aSYN (green). Scale bars 25 μm in **c**, **e**; 500 μm in **g** and 100 μm in **h**

(Fig. 3a, d), we expected a high rate of co-localization for p62 and Ubi-1 with the LC marker TH. However, the majority of p62 and Ubi-1 immunoreactivity was located next to TH-positive LC cells, suggesting that other cells are involved in this process (Fig. 4a). To elucidate in which cell type the p62-positive aggregates were located, double immunofluorescence stainings for p62 with MAP2 (neuronal marker), Olig2 (oligodendroglial marker), GFAP (astrocytic marker) or IbA1 (microglial marker) were performed. While p62 did not co-localize with MAP2 (Fig. 5a), Olig2 (Fig. 5b) or GFAP (Fig. 5c), we observed clear co-localization with IbA1 (Fig. 5d), indicating that

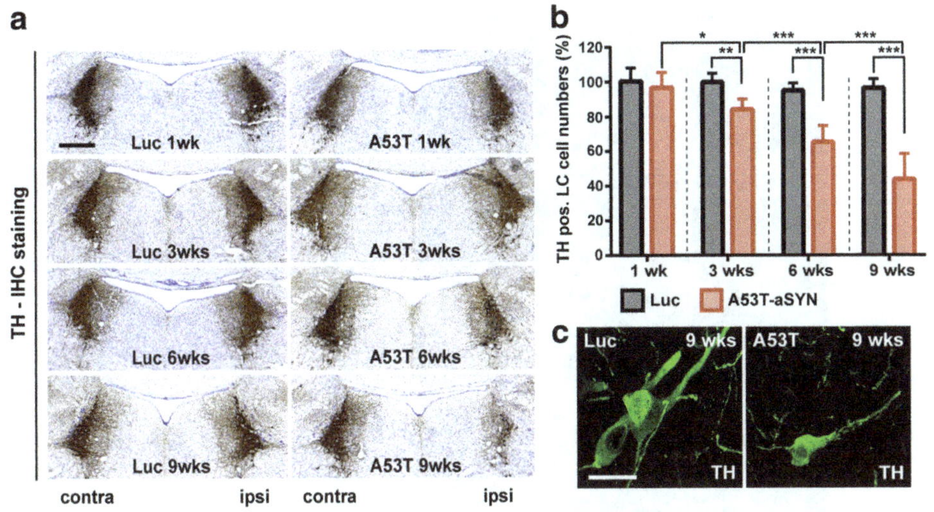

Fig. 2 Progressive loss of TH-immunoreactive LC cells after rAAV1/2-A53T-aSYN injection. **a**, **b** Representative images (Bregma – 5.40 mm) and unbiased stereology of TH-positive LC-neurons in A53T-aSYN (*red bars, right column*) or Luc (*black bars, left column*) overexpressing animals. Values (mean ± SEM) are expressed as cell numbers on the injected side compared to non-injected side (%). $n = 8$ per time point and group, two-way ANOVA analysis followed by Tukey's post-hoc test, $^{*}p < 0.05$, $^{**}p < 0.01$, $^{***}p < 0.001$. **c** Representative confocal images of neuronal morphology after 9 weeks of protein overexpression. Pyknotic cell bodies and dystrophic axons were observed in A53T-aSYN, but not in Luc overexpressing animals. Scale bars 250 μm in **a**, 50 μm in **c**

the p62-positive inclusions were located in microglial cells. Moreover, we further confirmed that Ubi-1-positive aggregates were also located in microglia (Fig. 5e). Double immunofluorescence stainings for IbA1 and aSYN (Syn211) (Fig. 5f, arrow) and GFAP and aSYN (Syn211) (Fig. 5g, arrow) revealed that microglia, as well as astroglia exhibited human aSYN after 3 weeks of aSYN overexpression.

Next, we aimed to investigate if the observed p62- and Ubi-1-positive inclusions indeed consisted of insoluble aggregated proteins. Since PK resistance is accepted as a valid marker for the formation of insoluble aggregates in human PD samples and animal models [5, 38, 86], we digested tissue samples of A53T-aSYN and Luc injected mice of all time points with PK. As a result, numerous PK-resistant insoluble aggregates positive for p62, Ubi-1 and aSYN were found in A53T-aSYN injected mice (Fig. 4c). Notably, PK-resistant aSYN aggregates had the same shape and size as Ubi-1- and p62-inclusions. Further, all three kinds of aggregates started to appear 3 weeks after initiation of A53T-aSYN overexpression and were restricted to the site of viral injection. PK digestion and subsequent analysis of rAAV-Luc injected animals revealed no signal for aSYN, p62, Ubi-1 or Luc in any analyzed section.

Targeted α-synucleinopathy induces reactive micro- and astrogliosis in the LC region

Microglia activation and reactive astrocytes have been observed by respective PET imaging in human prodromal and manifest PD patients [26, 63], post-mortem PD brain samples [56, 62] and aSYN animal models [4, 87, 88]. Most of the studies using animal models focused on the impact of microglia activation following nigrostriatal degeneration. In the current study, we aimed to investigate whether a focally induced α-synucleinopathy in the LC region would lead to reactive micro- and astrogliosis. Therefore, a triple immunofluorescence staining for IbA1 (microglial marker), GFAP (astroglial marker) and TH was carried out and the intensity of fluorescence signal was quantified (Fig. 6a-c). Already 3 weeks of A53T-aSYN overexpression were sufficient to induce a 3.5-fold increase of astroglial signal intensity in the injected LC region compared to Luc control. The astrogliosis further progressed up to a 6-fold increase after 9 weeks (Fig. 6b). Simultaneously, a 3-fold signal increase for microglia was measured after 3 weeks of A53T-aSYN overexpression and a 5-fold increase after 9 weeks, compared to Luc (Fig. 6c). 3D reconstructed high magnification confocal images revealed a dense glial network in A53T-aSYN overexpressing animals, in which the remaining TH-positive LC neurons were embedded already 3 weeks after viral vector delivery (Fig. 6d). Abundant direct physical contacts between TH-positive LC neurons and astro- and microglia could be resolved. In addition, numerous LC cells appeared to be nearly completely engulfed by microglial processes (Fig. 6d, arrows). In contrast, overexpression of Luc did not lead to any significant increase of astro- or microglia intensity values (Fig. 6a-d). Besides the interaction of astro- and microglia with LC neurons, we also observed direct physical contacts between astrocytes and microglial cells (Fig. 6e, arrow).

To underline our hypothesis that the degree of aSYN-induced pathology is closely associated with the degree

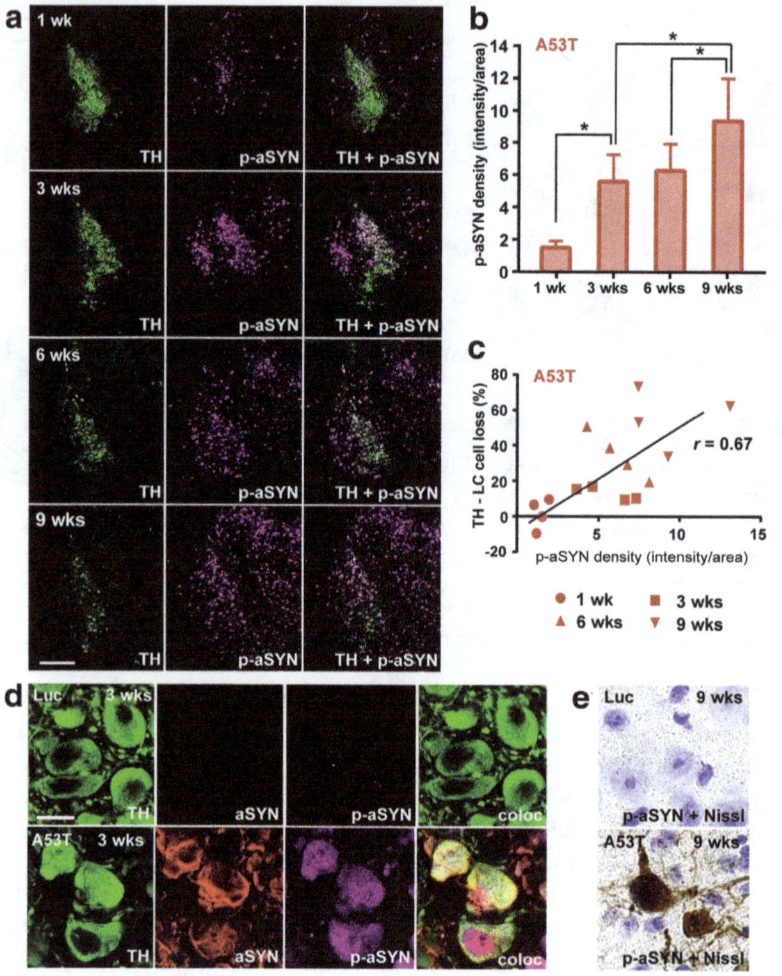

Fig. 3 Progressive accumulation of phosphorylated aSYN (p-aSYN) in the LC region. **a**, **b** Representative images (Bregma – 5.40 mm) and quantification of p-aSYN in the LC region via double immunofluorescence staining for TH (green) and p-aSYN (magenta). Values are presented as mean ± SEM, $n = 4$ per time point and group, one-way ANOVA analysis followed by Tukey's post-hoc test, $*p < 0.05$. **c** Robust correlation was observed between loss of TH-positive LC cells and accumulation of p-aSYN ($r = 0.67$, $p < 0.05$). **d** Confocal microscopy confirmed accumulation of p-aSYN (magenta) in TH-positive LC cells (green) 3 weeks post injection in A53T-aSYN (red) overexpressing animals (*lower row*). **e** p-aSYN immunoreactivity in the LC-region of A53T-aSYN overexpressing animals (*lower row*) 9 weeks post injection. No A53T-aSYN or p-aSYN immunoreactivity was observed in Luc overexpressing animals (*upper row*) at any time point. Scale bars 250 μm in **a**, 25 μm in **d-e**

of microgliosis, we correlated the microglial intensity values with the percentage of LC neurodegeneration (Fig. 6f, g). This revealed a correlation coefficient of $r = 0.80$ ($p < 0.05$) for A53T-aSYN, whereas for the Luc overexpressing animals no significant correlation was found ($r = 0.09$, $p > 0.05$).

Extensive transport of human A53T-aSYN to efferent brain regions

After investigating the local effects of A53T-aSYN overexpression, we addressed the question whether the aSYN pathology can propagate to anatomically connected brain regions. A variety of studies using overexpression of rAAV-aSYN or injection of preformed aSYN fibrils (PFF's) have described transport or spread of aSYN to anatomically connected brain regions [35, 52, 54, 70, 77, 91]. To investigate the propagation of human A53T-aSYN after inducing the α-synucleinopathy in LC neuronal somata, we stained predetermined brain sections against human aSYN (Syn211) or Luc and rated the occurrence of aSYN- or Luc-positive axons or cell bodies (Table 2). While overexpression of Luc resulted in a staining pattern, which was limited to the injection site and absent in distant brain regions, we observed aSYN signal in a high number of brain regions in A53T-aSYN injected mice (Fig. 7). One week after injection of rAAV-A53T-aSYN in the right LC region, abundant aSYN-positive axons were observed in various brain regions which are known output regions of LC neurons [85]. The human aSYN signal was solely axonal and no aSYN-positive cell bodies were

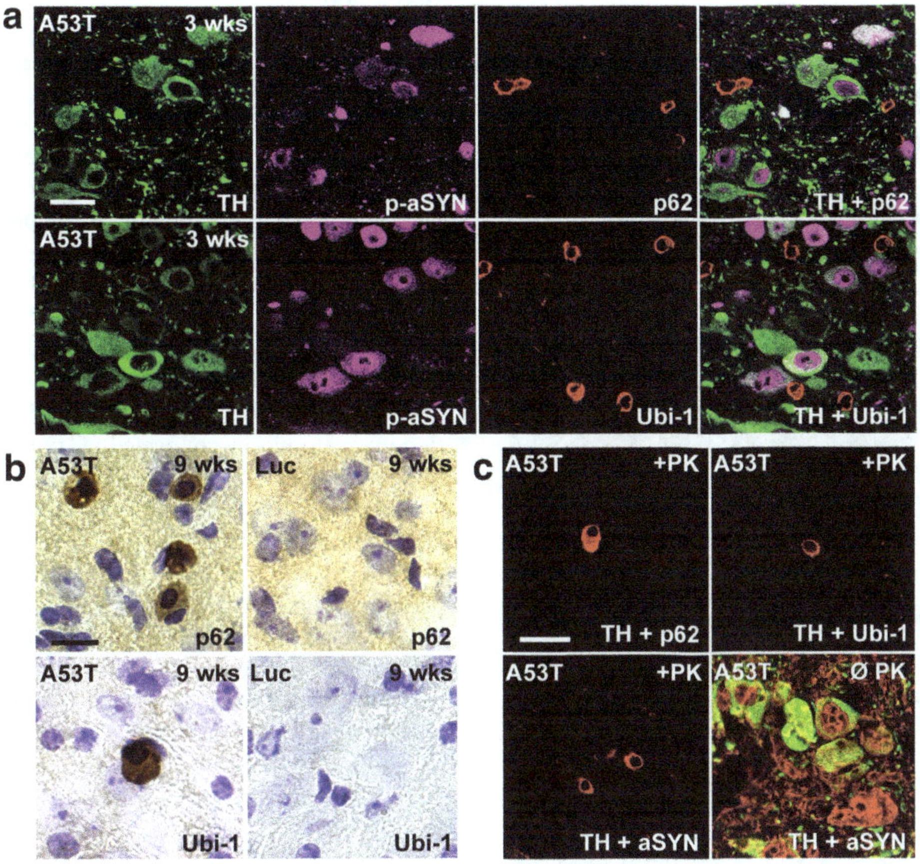

Fig. 4 Formation of insoluble protein aggregates in A53T-aSYN overexpressing animals. **a** Staining for p62 (red, *upper row*) and Ubi-1 (red, *lower row*) revealed abundant p62- and Ubi-1-positive aggregates in the LC-region. These aggregates were found in close proximity to, but did not co-localize with TH-positive (green) LC cells, which were positive for p-aSYN (magenta). **b** Representative images of p62- (*upper left*) and Ubi-1 (*lower left*) positive aggregates in A53T-aSYN animals. No aggregates were observed in Luc overexpressing animals at any time point (*right column*). **c** p62-, Ubi-1 and aSYN stainings after proteinase K (PK) digestion or without digestion (Ø PK, *lower right*) confirmed that p62- (*upper left*), Ubi-1- (*upper right*) and human aSYN-positive (*lower left*) aggregates were insoluble. Scale bars 50 μm in **a** and **c**, 25 μm in **b**

detected. Regions showing the strongest aSYN signal included the main olfactory bulb, lateral septal nucleus, diagonal band nucleus, bed nuclei of the stria terminalis, central amygdalar nucleus, periaqueductal gray, midbrain reticular nucleus, substantia nigra (SN) pars compacta and the ventral tegmental area (Table 2). We counted 36 brain regions, which contained human aSYN-positive axons after one week, indicating that human A53T-aSYN was transported rapidly along the axons towards the synaptic terminals in an anterograde direction. Despite the increase of axonal aSYN signal, no aSYN-positive cell bodies were detected outside of the LC region at any investigated time point, arguing against the hypothesis that human A53T-aSYN is released in LC output regions and taken up by synaptically connected cells in the short time frame of 9 weeks. This is highlighted by the finding that staining against p-aSYN revealed no signs of phosphorylation or aggregation of endogenous aSYN in distant brain regions after 9 weeks whereas the axons containing human (non-phosphorylated) A53T-aSYN stained positive for TH (Fig. 8c).

No substantia nigra (SN) cell loss after 9 weeks of human A53T-aSYN overexpression in LC neurons

Already after 1 week of A53T-aSYN overexpression in LC neurons, human aSYN positive axons passing by DA SN neurons could be detected. After 9 weeks, SN neurons were densely surrounded by aSYN containing axons (Fig. 8a) but no human aSYN signal was observed in the somata of SN cells. Stereological quantification of TH-positive SN neurons (Fig. 8b) revealed no significant difference of TH-immunoreactive neurons between A53T-aSYN compared to Luc overexpressing mice neither for the left nor for the right SN (One-way ANOVA; $p > 0.05$). This result points out that LC degeneration, in combination with profound local axonal aSYN accumulation was not sufficient to induce degeneration of DA SN neurons within the relatively short period of 9 weeks.

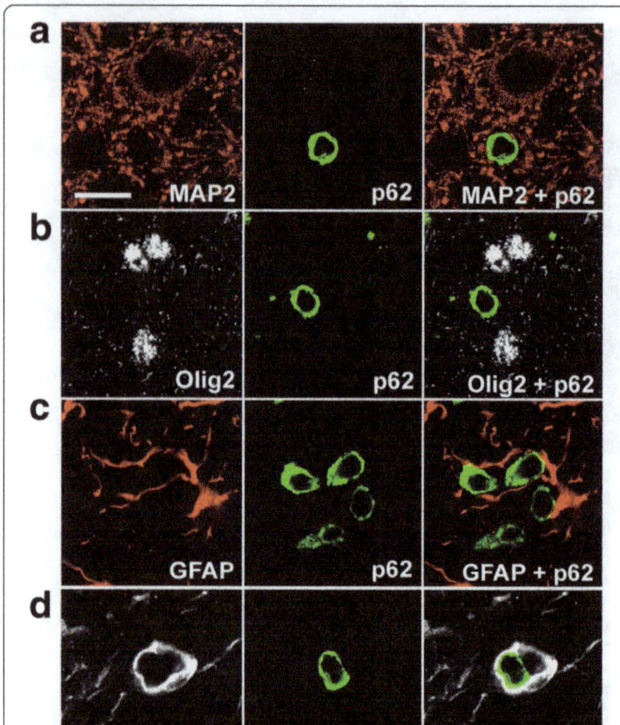

Fig. 5 p62- and Ubi-1 positive aggregates co-localize with IbA1-positive microglia. **a-c** Representative confocal microscopy images of p62 (green, *second column*) and MAP2 (**a**, red, *first row*), Olig2 (**b**, gray, *second row*), or GFAP (**c**, red, *third row*) show no co-localization of p62 and the different cellular markers. In contrast, co-staining p62 (green) and IbA1 (**d**, gray, *fourth row*) or Ubi-1 (green) and IbA1 (**e**, gray, *fifth row*) revealed clear co-localization. IbA1 positive microglial cells (**f**, gray, *sixth row*) and GFAP-positive astroglia (**g**, red, *seventh row*) also co-stained for aSYN (*arrows* in **f**, **g**). Scale bar for **a-g** 25 μm

Discussion

Degeneration of the LC noradrenergic system is a key event during PD pathogenesis in the prodromal phase of the disease. In this study, we present the first targeted LC α-synucleinopathy mouse model, which replicated cardinal features of human PD pathology. We have designed our rAAV vector-based overexpression model to generate robust and rapid induction of aSYN pathology, including phosphorylation and aggregation of aSYN, noradrenergic neurodegeneration, development of dystrophic axon morphology, signs of proteasomal and lysosomal dysfunction and prominent neuron-glial interactions. Furthermore, the herein characterized aSYN transport pattern allows investigating the effects of aSYN-induced LC neurodegeneration on anatomically connected LC output structures.

Progressive S129 phosphorylation and formation of PK-resistant aSYN-positive aggregates

Phosphorylation of aSYN at amino acid S129 is a dominant pathological modification of aSYN [1] since approximately 90% of aSYN in human Lewy bodies is phosphorylated at this position, whereas only 4% of soluble aSYN exhibits this posttranslational modification [25]. In PD animal models, phosphorylation at S129 is used as a key marker to investigate an induced α-synucleinopathy and its occurrence has often been interpreted as formation of aSYN aggregates [10, 52, 65, 72, 87]. In our current study, we show abundant and over time increasing S129-phosphorylation of aSYN in the cytoplasm and nucleus of LC cells (Fig. 3a, d). Previous studies have pointed out that aSYN has different cellular localizations. Beside the presynaptic and cytoplasmic localization, a nuclear occurrence of aSYN is known [80]. Nuclear p-aSYN has been observed in previous studies where aSYN was overexpressed [30, 96] and it could be shown that nuclear aSYN interacts with histone molecules. It was even suggested that the S129-phosphorylation may play an important role for the nuclear translocation of aSYN [64]. To confirm that phosphorylation of aSYN was accompanied by formation of high molecular weight aSYN aggregates we performed PK digestion experiments that revealed small circular aSYN positive inclusion bodies restricted to the injection site (Fig. 4c). Our model thereby reproduces a key feature of the LC pathology observed in human PD patients. Importantly, since PK digestion led to the destruction of all soluble proteins it did not allow us to investigate if the developing aSYN-positive inclusions are located in neurons or glial cells. The observed discrepancy between a high amount of p-aSYN-positive cells and a relatively limited number of aSYN-positive PK-resistant inclusions raises the question whether aSYN S129-phosphorylation can solely be used as a sufficient marker for aSYN aggregation. Our data indicate that S129-phosphorylation is an important indicator for aSYN pathology, but immunohistochemistry for other aggregation

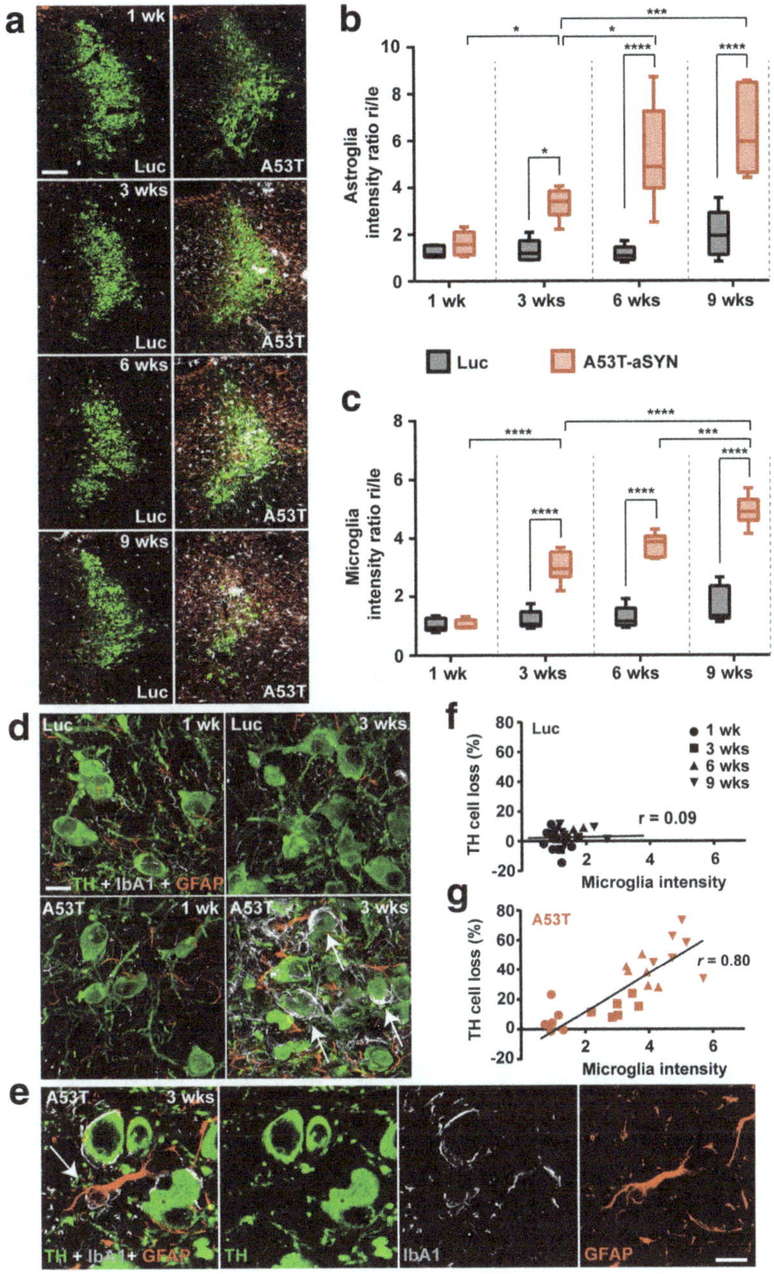

Fig. 6 A53T-aSYN overexpression leads to a pronounced reactive micro- and astrogliosis in the LC-region. **a** Representative images of the LC region of Luc (*left column*) or A53T-aSYN (*right column*) injected animals stained for TH (green), IbA1 (gray) and GFAP (red) display a marked increase of micro- and astroglia over time in A53T-aSYN overexpressing mice. Quantification of GFAP (**b**) and IbA1 (**c**) signal intensity revealed a progressive increase of astro- and microglia signal in A53T-aSYN injected animals (*red boxes*) compared to Luc control (*black boxes*). Values (mean ± min/max) are expressed as the signal intensity ratio of the injected side compared to the non-injected side. $n = 6$ animals per time point and group. Two-way ANOVA analysis followed by Tukey's post-hoc test, *$p < 0.05$, **$p < 0.01$, ***$p < 0.001$, ****$p < 0.0001$. **d** Reconstructed high magnification confocal images of the LC region showing physical contacts between TH-positive (green) LC cells and IbA1-positive micro- (gray) and GFAP-positive astroglia (red) after 3 weeks of A53T-aSYN overexpression (*lower right*). Engulfment (arrow) of TH-positive neurons by glial cells was only observed in A53T-aSYN expressing animals and not in Luc control mice (*upper row*). **e** Direct physical contacts were also observed between micro- and astroglia (arrow). **f**, **g** Correlating TH cell loss with the microglia intensity values indicates a strong association between increase of microglia and severity of TH cell loss in A53T-aSYN overexpressing animals ($r = 0.80$, $p < 0.05$), whereas there was no correlation in Luc expressing animals ($r = 0.09$, $p > 0.05$). Pearson's correlation coefficient with 95% confidence interval. Scale bars 100 μm in **a**, 25 μm in **d** and **e**

Table 2 Semiquantitative analysis of human aSYN-pathology in distant brain regions

		Injected (right) hemisphere Time of A53T-aSYN overexpression				Non-injected (left) hemisphere Time of A53T-aSYN overexpression			
		1 wk	3 wks	6 wks	9 wks	1 wk	3 wks	6 wks	9 wks
Bregma	Main olf. Bulb, gr. layer	+	++	++(+)	++	(+)	+	+	(+)
+4.28 mm	Inner plexiform layer	–	+(+)	+(+)	+	–	(+)	(+)	(+)
	Outer plexiform layer	(+)	+	+	+	–	(+)	(+)	(+)
Bregma	Cortex	+	++	++(+)	++	(+)	+	+	(+)
+ 2.96 mm	Main olf. Bulb	+	++	++(+)	++	(+)	(+)	+	(+)
	Ant. olf. Nucleus	+	+(+)	+(+)	+	–	(+)	(+)	(+)
	Lateral olf. Tract	(+)	+(+)	+	+	–	–	–	–
Bregma	Cortex	+	++(+)	++(+)	++(+)	–	+	+	+
+ 1.18 mm	Taenia tecta, dors. Part	+	++	++	+(+)	–	+	+	(+)
	Corpus callosum	(+)	+(+)	+	+	–	(+)	(+)	(+)
	Lateral septal nucleus	+(+)	++(+)	+++	++(+)	(+)	+	+(+)	+(+)
	Diagonal band nucleus	+(+)	++(+)	+++	++(+)	(+)	+	+(+)	+(+)
	Nucleus accumbens	+	+	+	+	–	(+)	(+)	(+)
	Caudoputamen	(+)	+	+	(+)	–	(+)	(+)	(+)
Bregma	Medial septal nucleus	+	+(+)	++	+(+)	(+)	+	+(+)	+
+ 0.38 mm	Cortex	(+)	++(+)	++(+)	++	–	+	+	+
	Bed ncl. of stria term.	++	+++	+++(+)	+++	(+)	+	++	++
	Magnocellular ncl.	(+)	+	++	++	–	(+)	+	+
	Hypothalamus	+	++(+)	++(+)	+++	–	+(+)	+(+)	++
	Lateral septal nucleus	(+)	++	++(+)	++(+)	–	+	+(+)	+(+)
	Caudoputamen	(+)	+	+	(+)	–	(+)	(+)	(+)
	Subst. innominata	+	+	+(+)	+(+)	(+)	(+)	+	+
Bregma	Central amygdalar ncl.	+	++	+++	+++(+)	(+)	+(+)	++	++
−0.58 mm	Subst. innominata	+(+)	++	++(+)	+++	+	+(+)	++	++
	Globus pallidus	(+)	+	+	+	–	(+)	(+)	(+)
	Hypothalamus	+	++	++(+)	++	(+)	+	+(+)	+(+)
	Lat. hypothalamic area	+(+)	++	+++	++(+)	(+)	+	++	++
	Fimbria	(+)	+	(+)	(+)	(+)	+	(+)	(+)
	Stria terminalis	+	+(+)	+(+)	+(+)	–	(+)	+	+
	Corpus callosum	–	+	+	+	–	–	(+)	(+)
	Cortex	(+)	++(+)	++(+)	++	–	+	+	+
Bregma	Cortex	–	+(+)	+(+)	+	–	(+)	(+)	(+)
−3.16 mm	Sup. colliculus, sens.	–	+(+)	+(+)	+	–	+	+	+
	Sup. colliculus, motor	(+)	+(+)	++	++	(+)	+(+)	++	++
	Periaqueductal gray	+(+)	++	++(+)	++(+)	(+)	+(+)	++	++
	Midbrain reticular ncl.	+(+)	++	++	++(+)	+	+(+)	++	++
	Red nucleus	(+)	+	+(+)	+	+	++	++(+)	++
	Ventral tegmental area	+	+(+)	++	++(+)	+(+)	++	++(+)	++(+)
	Subst. nigra, pars compacta	+(+)	+(+)	++	++	(+)	+	+(+)	+(+)
	Subst. nigra, pars reticulata	(+)	+	+	(+)	(+)	(+)	(+)	(+)
	Hippocampus	–	+	+(+)	+	–	(+)	+	+
	Interpeduncular ncl.	(+)	+(+)	++	++(+)	(+)	+(+)	++(+)	++(+)
	Thalamus	(+)	+(+)	++	++	(+)	+	+(+)	+(+)

Table 2 Semiquantitative analysis of human aSYN-pathology in distant brain regions *(Continued)*

		Injected (right) hemisphere Time of A53T-aSYN overexpression				Non-injected (left) hemisphere Time of A53T-aSYN overexpression			
		1 wk	3 wks	6 wks	9 wks	1 wk	3 wks	6 wks	9 wks
Bregma	Dorsal motor ncl. of n. X	–	+	+(+)	+(+)	–	(+)	+	+
–7.56 mm	Hypoglossal ncl.	–	+	+	+	(+)	(+)	+	(+)
	Parvicell. reticular ncl.	+(+)	+(+)	+(+)	+(+)	(+)	(+)	+	+
	Intermediate ret. ncl.	+	+	++	+(+)	–	(+)	+	+
	Medullary reticular ncl.	+	+(+)	+(+)	+(+)	–	+	+	+
	Lateral ret. ncl.	–	(+)	+	(+)	–	(+)	(+)	(+)
	Ncl. of the solitary tract	–	(+)	+	+(+)	–	(+)	+	+
	Spinal ncl. of the n. V	–	(+)	(+)	(+)	–	–	(+)	(+)
	Area postrema	(+)	(+)	+	+	(+)	(+)	+	+
	Arbor vitae	–	+	+	+	–	+	+	+
	Gr. layer (cerebellum)	+	+(+)	+(+)	+(+)	(+)	+	+	+
	Mol. layer (cerebellum)	–	+	+	+	–	+	+	+

Occurrence of human aSYN-positive axons was graded out of seven coronal brain sections as follows: – no positive axons; + sparse (few positive axons); ++ mild (more positive axons); +++ moderate (many positive axons, covering almost the complete brain region) and ++++ severe pathology (large number of positive axons densely covering the complete brain region); (+) describes an intermediate state between two categories to allow a more accurate description. $n = 6$ per time point. Abundance of aSYN-positive axons increased over time and was more prominent in the injected (right) hemisphere. The signal for human aSYN was solely axonal and no aSYN-positive cell bodies were detected

markers should be added to confirm the occurrence of aSYN aggregates [69, 90].

Formation of p62- and Ubi-1-positive proteinaceous inclusions in microglia

Additional markers, which are also commonly accepted to investigate protein aggregation and simultaneously serve as indicators for dysfunction of the proteasomal or lysosomal protein degradation system include Ubi-1 and p62 [33, 47]. Based on previous reports, which showed close co-localization of p-aSYN and Ubi-1 or p62 [54, 74], we expected to find overlap of these markers in our model. But notably, all p62 and Ubi-1 aggregates were located next to p-aSYN positive LC cells (Fig. 4a). Co-staining p62 and Ubi-1 with different glial and neuronal markers revealed that the p62 and Ubi-1 inclusions were located in IbA1-positive microglial cells (Fig. 5d, e). Further, we also show that microglia exhibited human aSYN, probably as a result of local aSYN uptake or phagocytosis of aSYN containing cellular debris. (Fig. 5f). The possibility that the microglial cells were transduced by rAAV1/2-A53T seems to be unlikely, since the used rAAV1/2 vector possesses a high neuronal tropism [44] and triple stainings for IbA1 (microglia), GFAP (astroglia) and aSYN revealed no aSYN-immunoreactivity 3 days after viral vector delivery within micro- or astroglial cells. Despite this, we cannot completely exclude the possibility of microglia transduction by the initial injection of rAAV1/2-A53T. Deposition of internalized aSYN aggregates in microglia has already been observed in vitro [49], but our study represents (to our knowledge) the first in vivo evidence of inclusion formation in microglial cells. We hypothesize that these p62- und Ubi-1-positive aggregates develop de novo in microglial cells possibly because of massive human aSYN uptake, which exceeds the lysosomal degradation capacities and leads to protein aggregation.

Currently we can only speculate why p62 and Ubi-1 reactivity was observed in microglia but absent in LC neurons. Previous studies have shown that p62-positive inclusions co-localize with Ubi-1 not only in neuronal but also in glial cells in neurodegenerative diseases including Alzheimer's disease, dementia with Lewy bodies and PD [47]. Furthermore, it has been shown that microglia rapidly internalize aSYN thereby representing the most efficient scavengers of neuronal released aSYN [48, 71]. By clearing aSYN, microglia might actively delay accumulation of aSYN and maturation of aSYN aggregates in LC neurons. One could hypothesize that in our model aSYN is rapidly released from LC neurons and taken up by microglia, which in turn leads to microglial but not neuronal accumulation of p62 und Ubi-1 aggregates. A longer duration of the experiment may clarify the question, whether Ubi-1- and p62-positive inclusions might also develop in LC neurons.

Reactive astro- and microglia and their implication in aSYN-induced LC pathology

Another key aspect in several animal models in which aSYN was injected or overexpressed [87, 88, 100] is the profound involvement of reactive astro- and microgliosis during the development of the aSYN pathology. It has been shown that activated microglial cells, besides their implication in clearing aSYN, are able to trigger the

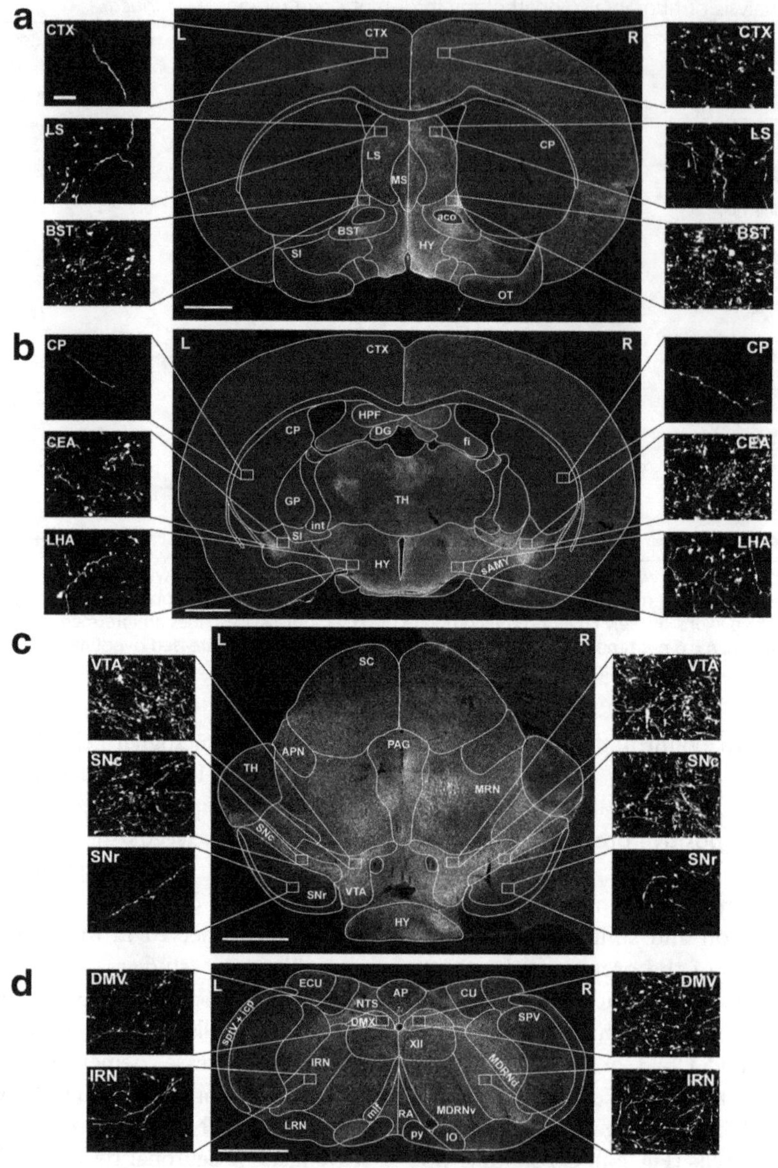

Fig. 7 Widespread transport of human A53T-aSYN to interconnected brain regions. **a-d** Representative images of analyzed brain sections stained against human aSYN (Syn211) (Bregma + 0.50 mm **a**, Bregma − 0.94 mm **b**, Bregma − 3.16 mm **c**, Bregma − 7.56 mm **d**). *Scale bars* 1 mm in **a-d**, 25 μm in all high magnification images. Abbreviations: CTX, cortex; CP, caudoputamen; LS, lateral septal nucleus; MS, medial septal nucleus; aco, anterior commissure; BST, bed nuclei of stria terminalis; HY, hypothalamus; SI, substantia innominata; OT, olfactory tubercle; HPF, hippocampal formation; DG, dentate gyrus; fi, fimbria hippocampi; int, internal capsule; TH, thalamus; GP, globus pallidus; sAMY, striatum-like amygdalar nuclei; LHA, lateral hypothalamic area; CEA, central amygdalar nucleus; SC, superior colliculus; APN, anterior pretectal nucleus; PAG, periaqueductal gray; MRN, midbrain reticular nucleus; VTA, ventral tegmental area; SNc, substantia nigra pars compacta; SNr, substantia nigra pars reticulata; AP, area postrema; NTS, nucleus of the solitary tract; CU, cuneate nucleus; ECU, external cuneate nucleus; DMX, dorsal motor nucleus of the vagus nerve; XII, hypoglossal nucleus; SPV, spinal nucleus of the trigeminal; MDRNd, medullary reticular nucleus, dorsal part; MDRNv, medullary reticular nucleus, ventral part; IRN, intermediate reticular nucleus; IO, inferior olivary complex; py, pyramid; RA, raphe nuclei; mlf, medial longitudinal fascicle; LRN, lateral reticular nucleus; sptV, spinal tract of the trigeminal nerve; icp, inferior cerebellar peduncle; L, left (contralateral); R, right (ipsilateral)

release of inflammatory cytokines and accelerate the production of reactive oxygen species, thereby likely contributing to the process of neurodegeneration [32, 42, 100]. In our model, LC cells were surrounded by a massive network of astro- and microglia already after 3 weeks of aSYN overexpression, with many microglial cells almost completely engulfing the surviving LC neurons (Fig. 6d, arrows). This early induction of microgliosis (Fig. 6c) is in line with previous findings where microgliosis even preceded the onset of neurodegeneration [4, 13]. Furthermore, we observed a strong correlation between the increase of microglial signal and LC cell loss (Fig. 6g),

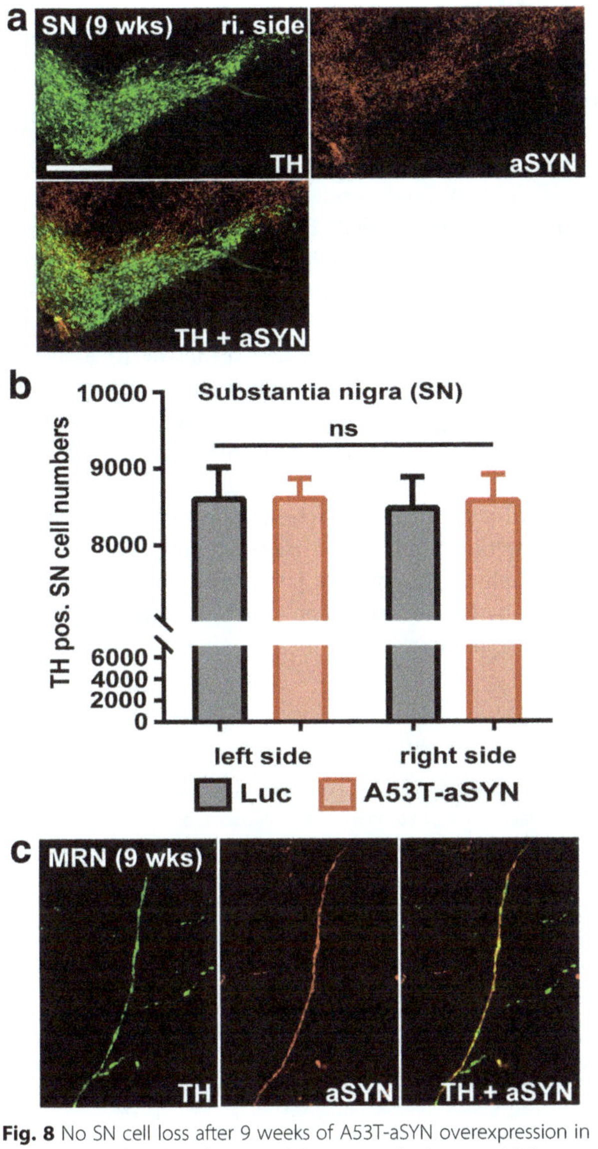

Fig. 8 No SN cell loss after 9 weeks of A53T-aSYN overexpression in LC region. **a** Abundant human aSYN-positive (red, *upper right*) axons were observed in the TH-positive SN region (green, *upper left*) after 9 weeks of A53T-aSYN overexpression in the LC. In contrast, no aSYN-positive cell bodies could be detected. **b** Quantification of TH-positive SN neurons 9 weeks post injection revealed no significant difference between A53T-aSYN group (*red bars*) and Luc control group (*black bars*) for either side. Values are presented as mean ± SEM, $n = 8$ per group and side. One-way ANOVA analysis ($p > 0.05$). **c** Representative image of TH and human aSYN axonal co-localization in distant brain regions, exemplified for midbrain reticular nucleus (MRN). The majority of aSYN positive axons co-stained for TH indicating that they origin from the LC. Scale bars 250 μm in **a**, 25 μm in **c**

implying the conclusion that reactive microglial cells are important modulators of aSYN-induced toxicity not only in the dopaminergic SN but also in the noradrenergic LC. Microgliosis was accompanied by severe and progressively increasing astrogliosis. Reactive astrocytes surrounded and partially engulfed LC neurons. Furthermore, they formed direct physical contacts with reactive microglia (Fig. 6e, arrow) and exhibited clear signal for human aSYN (Fig. 5g). Importantly, reactive astrocytes can also take part in clearing aSYN by endocytosis and degradation in their lysosomal system [50, 76]. Furthermore, they interact closely with microglia and release pro- and anti-inflammatory molecules [18, 57]. Our LC model exemplifies this close interdependency between neurons, micro- and astroglia. We show that glial cells are highly involved in the process of aSYN degradation and that glial dysfunction or failure could be a factor of PD progression. However, it should also be considered that the LC itself plays a central role in decreasing neuroinflammation [20]. Noradrenaline is able to suppress the expression of pro-inflammatory cytokines in glial cells while simultaneously elevating the expression of anti-inflammatory markers [19, 59]. Hence, it is reasonable to assume that loss of LC neurons additionally increases the neuroinflammatory response and contributes to the progressive increase of micro- and astroglial activity seen in our model.

Anterograde axonal transport of aSYN to LC output regions

To slow or prevent the progression of PD, it is essential to investigate if and how the α-synucleinopathy propagates within the brain. Recent evidence [36, 45, 52, 54, 70] suggests that toxic aSYN species formed in a small number of cells can spread trans-synaptically to distant but anatomically connected brain regions where they act as seeds to trigger the formation of insoluble aSYN aggregates [29, 54]. Furthermore, cell culture experiments have demonstrated that aSYN can be taken up by cells and transported in both the retrograde and anterograde direction [15, 23, 94]. The noradrenergic LC has a broad input-output connectome [82, 85] making this brain region suitable to investigate trans-neuronal spread. Moreover, Iba and colleagues [37] have demonstrated in a tauopathy model that injections of synthetic tau fibrils were able to induce tau pathology in LC neurons which then propagated to LC afferents and efferents. To investigate if this also translates into our LC aSYN overexpression model we systematically analyzed and scored the aSYN pathology after 1, 3, 6 and 9 weeks (Fig. 7, Table 2). Our results indicate that the overexpressed human A53T-aSYN, once produced in the cytoplasm of LC neurons, is only transported in the anterograde direction towards the synaptic terminals, as abundant aSYN-positive axons and terminals in efferent LC regions co-stained for TH (Fig. 7, Fig. 8c, Table 2). The broad LC output connectome [85] likely explains this high amount of aSYN-positive axons in distant brain regions of the ipsilateral but also contralateral hemisphere. The mild aSYN pathology of the contralateral (non-injected) side can be explained by LC projections crossing the midline and innervating brain structures of the contralateral hemisphere [39]. In contrast to the profound axonal aSYN immunoreactivity, we found no aSYN-positive cell bodies outside of the LC region, arguing against trans-neuronal spread of aSYN in the relatively short time frame of 9 weeks. The absence of Luc-positive axons in LC output regions might be explained on one hand by protein size (Luc 62 kDa vs. aSYN 15 kDa) and on the other hand by the naturally presynaptic localization of aSYN [7, 89]. We therefore conclude that the aggregation prone aSYN species created by overexpression of human A53T-aSYN in the LC region are not transferred to other neuronal populations within the investigated 9 weeks. A longer time period and subsequently higher aSYN burden in the LC system may be necessary to enable such a transfer at later time points. This is in line with the finding that despite the severe degree of axonal aSYN accumulation in the SN region after 9 weeks of A53T-aSYN overexpression in the LC region, no statistically significant SN neurodegeneration was observed (Fig. 8).

Open questions and limitations

In this study, we have decided to overexpress human mutant A53T-aSYN by injection of a previously well-established rAAV vector. The vector used in this study has proven effective in inducing progressive neurodegeneration of SN neurons by several groups in several PD animal models [28, 34, 38, 43, 44]. In this context, it would be of relevance to investigate whether overexpression of wild-type aSYN in the LC would have led to a different histopathological phenotype. Considering the lower rate of β-sheet and fibril formation of wild-type aSYN compared to the A53T-aSYN variant [14, 51], one could hypothesize that overexpression of wild-type aSYN might lead to milder histopathological alterations. However, this has to be demonstrated in the LC model in a further study. For this initial study we have focused on a relatively short time frame of up to 9 weeks which allowed us to characterize the initial, local and time-dependent histopathological alterations of LC neurons caused by A53T-aSYN. Since 9 weeks is likely too short to observe the full neuropathology, a future study containing longer observation times of up to 52 weeks or even longer would be suggested. This would allow to further investigate whether trans-synaptic spread of aSYN and subsequent degeneration of dopaminergic SN neurons occur at a later time-point. As our study primarily aims to address the histopathological consequences of A53T-aSYN overexpression in LC neurons, we have not carried out a behavioral assessment. Nevertheless, the model would benefit from a thoroughly carried out behavioral characterization, including sleep recordings covering the possible occurrence of any non-motor or subtle motor symptoms.

Conclusions

In a time, in which on one hand the clinical research focus shifts away from the neurodegeneration of the dopaminergic nigrostriatal pathway towards the prodromal stages of PD and on the other hand the first potentially disease modifying therapies enter clinical testing [61], animal models mimicking the prodromal phase of PD are needed. In this study, we have reproduced cardinal histopathological features of the human LC PD-pathology, delineated the time-course of noradrenergic neurodegeneration and characterized robust histological markers, which are sufficient to assess the pathological changes in a quantitative and qualitative way. Taken together, this animal model may contribute to the research on the pathophysiology of the prodromal stage of PD. Further studies with longer observation times and additional characterization (e.g. behavioral assessment, biochemical analyses) are required to determine whether the herein presented model will prove helpful in the development and testing of disease-modifying therapy.

Abbreviations

aSYN: α-synuclein; DA: Dopaminergic; LC: Locus coeruleus; Luc: Luciferase; p-aSYN: Phosphorylated α-synuclein; PB: Phosphate buffer; PBS: Phosphate buffered saline; PD: Parkinson's disease; PFA: Paraformaldehyde; PK: Proteinase K; rAAV: Recombinant adeno-associated viral; RBD: REM sleep behavior disorder; SN: Substantia nigra; TH: Tyrosine hydroxylase

Acknowledgements

We thank Sabine Anfimov and Christine Höft for technical assistance regarding the experiments. We also gratefully acknowledge the Core Facility Cellular Imaging of Philipps University-Marburg for the use of the Leica TCS SP8 confocal microscope and Zeiss Axio Observer Z1 spinning disc microscope. We thank Katrin Roth for the assistance with microscopy. WHO is a Hertie-Senior-Research Professor supported by the Charitable Hertie Foundation, Frankfurt/Main, Germany. LAM and WHC have received a grant from the intramural research fund of the Rhön-Klinikum Aktiengesellschaft. BL is a fellow of Deutscher Akademischer Austauschdienst.

Funding

WHO is supported by the Charitable Hertie Foundation, Frankfurt/Main, Germany. LAM and WHC have received a grant from the Rhön-Klinikum Aktiengesellschaft. BL is a fellow of DAAD.

Authors' contributions

WHO, LAM and WHC designed the study. MTH, FFG and BL performed experiments, conducted immunohistochemical analysis and analyzed data. WHO, LAM and ND supervised the project. MTH, FFG, LAM and WHO wrote the manuscript. ND, LT, JBK and JMB critically revised the manuscript. All authors read and approved the final manuscript.

Competing interests

The authors declare no competing financial interests. JBK and JMB have equity stakes in, and have received consultancy fees from, Atuka Inc., outside of the submitted work. WHO received personal fees for educational talks and/or consultancy, outside of the submitted work, from Abbvie, Adamas, Bristol-Myer-Squibb, Desitin, Mundipharma, Neuropore, Novartis, Roche and UCB Pharma and grants from the Deutsche Forschungsgemeinschaft, the International Parkinson-Fonds The Netherlands, the Michael J. Fox

Foundation, USA, the National Research Fond Luxembourg and from Novartis Pharma, Germany.

Author details
[1]Department of Neurology, Philipps University Marburg, Baldingerstraße 1, 35043 Marburg, Germany. [2]Krembil Research Institute, Toronto Western Hospital, University Health Network, Toronto, ON, Canada. [3]Department of Physiology and Pathophysiology, Philipps University Marburg, 35043 Marburg, Germany.

References

1. Anderson JP, Walker DE, Goldstein JM, de Laat R, Banducci K, Caccavello RJ et al (2006) Phosphorylation of Ser-129 is the dominant pathological modification of alpha-synuclein in familial and sporadic Lewy body disease. J Biol Chem 281(40):29739–29752. https://doi.org/10.1074/jbc.M600933200
2. Ascherio A, Schwarzschild MA (2016) The epidemiology of Parkinson's disease: risk factors and prevention. Lancet Neurol 15(12):1257–1272. https://doi.org/10.1016/S1474-4422(16)30230-7
3. Aston-Jones G, Cohen JD (2005) An integrative theory of locus coeruleus-norepinephrine function: adaptive gain and optimal performance. Annu Rev Neurosci 28:403–450. https://doi.org/10.1146/annurev.neuro.28.061604.135709
4. Barkholt P, Sanchez-Guajardo V, Kirik D, Romero-Ramos M (2012) Long-term polarization of microglia upon alpha-synuclein overexpression in nonhuman primates. Neuroscience 208:85–96. https://doi.org/10.1016/j.neuroscience.2012.02.004
5. Beach TG, Adler CH, Sue LI, Vedders L, Lue L, White Iii CL et al (2010) Multi-organ distribution of phosphorylated alpha-synuclein histopathology in subjects with Lewy body disorders. Acta Neuropathol 119(6):689–702. https://doi.org/10.1007/s00401-010-0664-3
6. Benarroch EE (2017) Locus coeruleus. Cell Tissue Res. https://doi.org/10.1007/s00441-017-2649-1
7. Bendor JT, Logan TP, Edwards RH (2013) The function of alpha-synuclein. Neuron 79(6):1044–1066. https://doi.org/10.1016/j.neuron.2013.09.004
8. Berridge CW, Waterhouse BD (2003) The locus coeruleus–noradrenergic system: modulation of behavioral state and state-dependent cognitive processes. Brain Res Rev 42(1):33–84. https://doi.org/10.1016/S0165-0173(03)00143-7
9. Bing G, Zhang Y, Watanabe Y, McEwen BS, Stone EA (1994) Locus coeruleus lesions potentiate neurotoxic effects of MPTP in dopaminergic neurons of the substantia nigra. Brain Res 668(1–2):261–265. https://doi.org/10.1016/0006-8993(94)90534-7
10. Bourdenx M, Dovero S, Engeln M, Bido S, Bastide MF, Dutheil N et al (2015) Lack of additive role of ageing in nigrostriatal neurodegeneration triggered by alpha-synuclein overexpression. Acta Neuropathol Commun 3:46. https://doi.org/10.1186/s40478-015-0222-2
11. Braak H, Del Tredici K, Rüb U, Vos D, Rob AI, Steur J, Ernst NH, Braak E (2003) Staging of brain pathology related to sporadic Parkinson's disease. Neurobiol Aging 24(2):197–211
12. Cersosimo MG, Benarroch EE (2012) Pathological correlates of gastrointestinal dysfunction in Parkinson's disease. Neurobiol Dis 46(3):559–564. https://doi.org/10.1016/j.nbd.2011.10.014
13. Chung CY, Koprich JB, Siddiqi H, Isacson O (2009) Dynamic changes in presynaptic and axonal transport proteins combined with striatal neuroinflammation precede dopaminergic neuronal loss in a rat model of AAV alpha-synucleinopathy. J Neurosci 29(11):3365–3373. https://doi.org/10.1523/JNEUROSCI.5427-08.2009
14. Coskuner O, Wise-Scira O (2013) Structures and free energy landscapes of the A53T mutant-type alpha-synuclein protein and impact of A53T mutation on the structures of the wild-type alpha-synuclein protein with dynamics. ACS Chem Neurosci 4(7):1101–1113. https://doi.org/10.1021/cn400041j
15. Desplats P, Lee H-J, Bae E-J, Patrick C, Rockenstein E, Crews L et al (2009) Inclusion formation and neuronal cell death through neuron-to-neuron transmission of alpha-synuclein. Proc Natl Acad Sci U S A 106(31):13010–13015. https://doi.org/10.1073/pnas.0903691106
16. Doppler K, Jentschke H-M, Schulmeyer L, Vadasz D, Janzen A, Luster M et al (2017) Dermal phospho-alpha-synuclein deposits confirm REM sleep behaviour disorder as prodromal Parkinson's disease. Acta Neuropathol 133(4):535–545. https://doi.org/10.1007/s00401-017-1684-z
17. Espay AJ, LeWitt PA, Kaufmann H (2014) Norepinephrine deficiency in Parkinson's disease: the case for noradrenergic enhancement. Mov Disord 29(14):1710–1719. https://doi.org/10.1002/mds.26048
18. Farina C, Aloisi F, Meinl E (2007) Astrocytes are active players in cerebral innate immunity. Trends Immunol 28(3):138–145. https://doi.org/10.1016/j.it.2007.01.005
19. Feinstein DL, Heneka MT, Gavrilyuk V, Dello Russo C, Weinberg G, Galea E (2002) Noradrenergic regulation of inflammatory gene expression in brain. Neurochem Int 41(5):357–365
20. Feinstein DL, Kalinin S, Braun D (2016) Causes, consequences, and cures for neuroinflammation mediated via the locus coeruleus: noradrenergic signaling system. J Neurochem 139(Suppl 2):154–178. https://doi.org/10.1111/jnc.13447
21. Fernagut PO, Hutson CB, Fleming SM, Tetreaut NA, Salcedo J, Masliah E et al (2007) Behavioral and histopathological consequences of paraquat intoxication in mice: effects of alpha-synuclein over-expression. Synapse 61(12):991–1001. https://doi.org/10.1002/syn.20456
22. Fornai F, Torracca MT, Bassi L, D'Errigo DA, Scalori V, Corsini GU (1996) Norepinephrine loss selectively enhances chronic nigrostriatal dopamine depletion in mice and rats. Brain Res 735(2):349–353
23. Freundt EC, Maynard N, Clancy EK, Roy S, Bousset L, Sourigues Y et al (2012) Neuron-to-neuron transmission of alpha-synuclein fibrils through axonal transport. Ann Neurol 72(4):517–524. https://doi.org/10.1002/ana.23747
24. Fu Y, Yuan Y, Halliday G, Rusznak Z, Watson C, Paxinos G (2012) A cytoarchitectonic and chemoarchitectonic analysis of the dopamine cell groups in the substantia nigra, ventral tegmental area, and retrorubral field in the mouse. Brain Struct Funct 217(2):591–612. https://doi.org/10.1007/s00429-011-0349-2
25. Fujiwara H, Hasegawa M, Dohmae N, Kawashima A, Masliah E, Goldberg MS et al (2002) Alpha-Synuclein is phosphorylated in synucleinopathy lesions. Nat Cell Biol 4(2):160–164. https://doi.org/10.1038/ncb748
26. Gerhard A, Pavese N, Hotton G, Turkheimer F, Es M, Hammers A et al (2006) In vivo imaging of microglial activation with 11C(R)-PK11195 PET in idiopathic Parkinson's disease. Neurobiol Dis 21(2):404–412. https://doi.org/10.1016/j.nbd.2005.08.002
27. Gesi M, Soldani P, Giorgi FS, Santinami A, Bonaccorsi I, Fornai F (2000) The role of the locus coeruleus in the development of Parkinson's disease. Neurosci Biobehav Rev 24(6):655–668. https://doi.org/10.1016/S0149-7634(00)00028-2
28. Gleave JA, Arathoon LR, Trinh D, Lizal KE, Giguere N, Barber JHM et al (2017) Sirtuin 3 rescues neurons through the stabilisation of mitochondrial biogenetics in the virally-expressing mutant alpha-synuclein rat model of parkinsonism. Neurobiol Dis 106:133–146. https://doi.org/10.1016/j.nbd.2017.06.009
29. Goedert M (2015) NEURODEGENERATION. Alzheimer's and Parkinson's diseases: the prion concept in relation to assembled Aβ, tau, and α-synuclein. Science 349(6248): 1255555. https://doi.org/10.1126/science.1255555
30. Goers J, Manning-Bog AB, McCormack AL, Millett IS, Doniach S, Di Monte DA et al (2003) Nuclear localization of alpha-synuclein and its interaction with histones. Biochemistry 42(28):8465–8471. https://doi.org/10.1021/bi0341152
31. Goldman JG, Postuma R (2014) Premotor and nonmotor features of Parkinson's disease. Curr Opin Neurol 27(4):434–441. https://doi.org/10.1097/WCO.0000000000000112
32. Harms AS, Cao S, Rowse AL, Thome AD, Li X, Mangieri LR et al (2013) MHCII is required for alpha-synuclein-induced activation of microglia, CD4 T cell proliferation, and dopaminergic neurodegeneration. J Neurosci 33(23):9592–9600. https://doi.org/10.1523/JNEUROSCI.5610-12.2013
33. Hasegawa M, Fujiwara H, Nonaka T, Wakabayashi K, Takahashi H, Lee VM-Y et al (2002) Phosphorylated alpha-synuclein is ubiquitinated in alpha-synucleinopathy lesions. J Biol Chem 277(50):49071–49076. https://doi.org/10.1074/jbc.M208046200
34. He Q, Koprich JB, Wang Y, Yu W-B, Xiao B-G, Brotchie JM et al (2015) Treatment with Trehalose prevents behavioral and neurochemical deficits produced in an AAV α-Synuclein rat model of Parkinson's disease. Mol Neurobiol. https://doi.org/10.1007/s12035-015-9173-7
35. Helwig M, Klinkenberg M, Rusconi R, Musgrove RE, Majbour NK, El-Agnaf OMA

et al (2016) Brain propagation of transduced α-synuclein involves non-fibrillar protein species and is enhanced in α-synuclein null mice. Brain 139(3):856–870. https://doi.org/10.1093/brain/awv376

36. Holmqvist S, Chutna O, Bousset L, Aldrin-Kirk P, Li W, Björklund T et al (2014) Direct evidence of Parkinson pathology spread from the gastrointestinal tract to the brain in rats. Acta Neuropathol 128(6):805–820. https://doi.org/10.1007/s00401-014-1343-6
37. Iba M, McBride JD, Guo JL, Zhang B, Trojanowski JQ, Lee VM-Y (2015) Tau pathology spread in PS19 tau transgenic mice following locus coeruleus (LC) injections of synthetic tau fibrils is determined by the LC's afferent and efferent connections. Acta Neuropathol 130(3):349–362. https://doi.org/10.1007/s00401-015-1458-4
38. Ip CW, Klaus L-C, Karikari AA, Visanji NP, Brotchie JM, Lang AE et al (2017) AAV1/2-induced overexpression of A53T-alpha-synuclein in the substantia nigra results in degeneration of the nigrostriatal system with Lewy-like pathology and motor impairment: a new mouse model for Parkinson's disease. Acta Neuropathol Commun 5(1):11. https://doi.org/10.1186/s40478-017-0416-x
39. Jones BE, Moore RY (1977) Ascending projections of the locus coeruleus in the rat. II. Autoradiographic study. Brain Res 127(1):25–53
40. Kalia LV, Lang AE (2015) Parkinson's disease. Lancet 386(9996):896–912. https://doi.org/10.1016/S0140-6736(14)61393-3
41. Kilbourn MR, Sherman P, Abbott LC (1998) Reduced MPTP neurotoxicity in striatum of the mutant mouse tottering. Synapse 30(2):205–210. https://doi.org/10.1002/(SICI)1098-2396(199810)30:2<205:AID-SYN10>3.0.CO;2-0
42. Kim C, Ho D-H, Suk J-E, You S, Michael S, Kang J et al (2013) Neuron-released oligomeric alpha-synuclein is an endogenous agonist of TLR2 for paracrine activation of microglia. Nat Commun 4:1562. https://doi.org/10.1038/ncomms2534
43. Koprich JB, Johnston TH, Huot P, Reyes MG, Espinosa M, Brotchie JM (2011) Progressive neurodegeneration or endogenous compensation in an animal model of Parkinson's disease produced by decreasing doses of alpha-synuclein. PLoS One 6(3):e17698. https://doi.org/10.1371/journal.pone.0017698
44. Koprich JB, Johnston TH, Reyes MG, Sun X, Brotchie JM (2010) Expression of human A53T alpha-synuclein in the rat substantia nigra using a novel AAV1/2 vector produces a rapidly evolving pathology with protein aggregation, dystrophic neurite architecture and nigrostriatal degeneration with potential to model the pathology of Parkinson's disease. Mol Neurodegener 5:43. https://doi.org/10.1186/1750-1326-5-43
45. Kordower JH, Chu Y, Hauser RA, Olanow CW, Freeman TB (2008) Transplanted dopaminergic neurons develop PD pathologic changes: a second case report. Mov Disord 23(16):2303–2306. https://doi.org/10.1002/mds.22369
46. Kruger R, Kuhn W, Leenders KL, Sprengelmeyer R, Muller T, Woitalla D et al (2001) Familial parkinsonism with synuclein pathology: clinical and PET studies of A30P mutation carriers. Neurology 56(10):1355–1362
47. Kuusisto E, Salminen A, Alafuzoff I (2001) Ubiquitin-binding protein p62 is present in neuronal and glial inclusions in human tauopathies and synucleinopathies. Neuroreport 12(10):2085–2090
48. Lee H-J, Suk J-E, Bae E-J, Lee J-H, Paik SR, Lee S-J (2008) Assembly-dependent endocytosis and clearance of extracellular alpha-synuclein. Int J Biochem Cell Biol 40(9):1835–1849. https://doi.org/10.1016/j.biocel.2008.01.017
49. Lee H-J, Suk J-E, Bae E-J, Lee S-J (2008) Clearance and deposition of extracellular alpha-synuclein aggregates in microglia. Biochem Biophys Res Commun 372(3):423–428. https://doi.org/10.1016/j.bbrc.2008.05.045
50. Lee H-J, Suk J-E, Patrick C, Bae E-J, Cho J-H, Rho S et al (2010) Direct transfer of alpha-synuclein from neuron to astroglia causes inflammatory responses in synucleinopathies. J Biol Chem 285(12):9262–9272. https://doi.org/10.1074/jbc.M109.081125
51. Li J, Uversky VN, Fink AL (2001) Effect of familial Parkinson's disease point mutations A30P and A53T on the structural properties, aggregation, and fibrillation of human alpha-synuclein. Biochemistry 40(38):11604–11613
52. Luk KC, Kehm V, Carroll J, Zhang B, O'Brien P, Trojanowski JQ et al (2012) Pathological α-synuclein transmission initiates Parkinson-like neurodegeneration in nontransgenic mice. Science 338(6109):949–953. https://doi.org/10.1126/science.1227157
53. Mahlknecht P, Seppi K, Poewe W (2015) The concept of prodromal Parkinson's disease. J Parkinsons Dis 5(4):681–697. https://doi.org/10.3233/JPD-150685
54. Masuda-Suzukake M, Nonaka T, Hosokawa M, Oikawa T, Arai T, Akiyama H et al (2013) Prion-like spreading of pathological alpha-synuclein in brain. Brain 136(Pt 4):1128–1138. https://doi.org/10.1093/brain/awt037
55. Matschke LA, Bertoune M, Roeper J, Snutch TP, Oertel WH, Rinné S et al (2015) A concerted action of L- and T-type ca(2+) channels regulates locus coeruleus pacemaking. Mol Cell Neurosci 68:293–302. https://doi.org/10.1016/j.mcn.2015.08.012
56. McGeer PL, Itagaki S, Boyes BE, McGeer EG (1988) Reactive microglia are positive for HLA-DR in the substantia nigra of Parkinson's and Alzheimer's disease brains. Neurology 38(8):1285–1291
57. McGeer PL, McGeer EG (2008) Glial reactions in Parkinson's disease. Mov Disord 23(4):474–483. https://doi.org/10.1002/mds.21751
58. McMillan PJ, White SS, Franklin A, Greenup JL, Leverenz JB, Raskind MA et al (2011) Differential response of the central noradrenergic nervous system to the loss of locus coeruleus neurons in Parkinson's disease and Alzheimer's disease. Brain Res 1373:240–252. https://doi.org/10.1016/j.brainres.2010.12.015
59. Mori K, Ozaki E, Zhang B, Yang L, Yokoyama A, Takeda I et al (2002) Effects of norepinephrine on rat cultured microglial cells that express alpha1, alpha2, beta1 and beta2 adrenergic receptors. Neuropharmacology 43(6):1026–1034
60. Oertel W, Schulz JB (2016) Current and experimental treatments of Parkinson disease: a guide for neuroscientists. J Neurochem 139(Suppl 1):325–337. https://doi.org/10.1111/jnc.13750
61. Oertel WH (2017) Recent advances in treating Parkinson's disease. F1000Res 6: 260. Doi: https://doi.org/10.12688/f1000research.10100.1
62. Orr CF, Rowe DB, Mizuno Y, Mori H, Halliday GM (2005) A possible role for humoral immunity in the pathogenesis of Parkinson's disease. Brain 128(Pt 11):2665–2674. https://doi.org/10.1093/brain/awh625
63. Ouchi Y, Yoshikawa E, Sekine Y, Futatsubashi M, Kanno T, Ogusu T et al (2005) Microglial activation and dopamine terminal loss in early Parkinson's disease. Ann Neurol 57(2):168–175. https://doi.org/10.1002/ana.20338
64. Oueslati A (2016) Implication of alpha-Synuclein phosphorylation at S129 in Synucleinopathies: what have we learned in the last decade? J Parkinsons Dis 6(1):39–51. https://doi.org/10.3233/JPD-160779
65. Paumier KL, Luk KC, Manfredsson FP, Kanaan NM, Lipton JW, Collier TJ et al (2015) Intrastriatal injection of pre-formed mouse alpha-synuclein fibrils into rats triggers alpha-synuclein pathology and bilateral nigrostriatal degeneration. Neurobiol Dis 82:185–199. https://doi.org/10.1016/j.nbd.2015.06.003
66. Paxinos G, Franklin KBJ (2013) Paxinos and Franklin's the mouse brain in stereotaxic coordinates, 4th edn. Elsevier Acad. Press, Amsterdam
67. Polymeropoulos MH, Lavedan C, Leroy E, Ide SE, Dehejia A, Dutra A et al (1997) Mutation in the alpha-synuclein gene identified in families with Parkinson's disease. Science 276(5321):2045–2047
68. Postuma RB, Berg D, Stern M, Poewe W, Olanow CW, Oertel W et al (2015) MDS clinical diagnostic criteria for Parkinson's disease. Mov Disord 30(12):1591–1601. https://doi.org/10.1002/mds.26424
69. Recasens A, Ulusoy A, Kahle PJ, Di Monte DA, Dehay B (2017) In vivo models of alpha-synuclein transmission and propagation. Cell Tissue Res. https://doi.org/10.1007/s00441-017-2730-9
70. Rey NL, George S, Steiner JA, Madaj Z, Luk KC, Trojanowski JQ et al (2018) Spread of aggregates after olfactory bulb injection of alpha-synuclein fibrils is associated with early neuronal loss and is reduced long term. Acta Neuropathol 135(1):65–83. https://doi.org/10.1007/s00401-017-1792-9
71. Rey NL, Petit GH, Bousset L, Melki R, Brundin P (2013) Transfer of human alpha-synuclein from the olfactory bulb to interconnected brain regions in mice. Acta Neuropathol 126(4):555–573. https://doi.org/10.1007/s00401-013-1160-3
72. Rey NL, Steiner JA, Maroof N, Luk KC, Madaj Z, Trojanowski JQ et al (2016) Widespread transneuronal propagation of alpha-synucleinopathy triggered in olfactory bulb mimics prodromal Parkinson's disease. J Exp Med 213(9):1759–1778. https://doi.org/10.1084/jem.20160368
73. Richter-Landsberg C, Leyk J (2013) Inclusion body formation, macroautophagy, and the role of HDAC6 in neurodegeneration. Acta Neuropathol 126(6):793–807. https://doi.org/10.1007/s00401-013-1158-x
74. Rieker C, Dev KK, Lehnhoff K, Barbieri S, Ksiazek I, Kauffmann S et al (2011) Neuropathology in mice expressing mouse alpha-synuclein. PLoS One 6(9):e24834. https://doi.org/10.1371/journal.pone.0024834
75. Robertson SD, Plummer NW, de Marchena J, Jensen P (2013) Developmental origins of central norepinephrine neuron diversity. Nat Neurosci 16(8):1016–1023. https://doi.org/10.1038/nn.3458

76. Rostami J, Holmqvist S, Lindstrom V, Sigvardson J, Westermark GT, Ingelsson M et al (2017) Human astrocytes transfer aggregated alpha-Synuclein via tunneling nanotubes. J Neurosci 37(49):11835–11853. https://doi.org/10.1523/JNEUROSCI.0983-17.2017
77. Rusconi R, Ulusoy A, Aboutalebi H, Di Monte DA (2018) Long-lasting pathological consequences of overexpression-induced alpha-synuclein spreading in the rat brain. Aging Cell. https://doi.org/10.1111/acel.12727
78. Sanchez-Padilla J, Guzman JN, Ilijic E, Kondapalli J, Galtieri DJ, Yang B et al (2014) Mitochondrial oxidant stress in locus coeruleus is regulated by activity and nitric oxide synthase. Nat Neurosci 17(6):832–840. https://doi.org/10.1038/nn.3717
79. Schapira AHV, Chaudhuri KR, Jenner P (2017) Non-motor features of Parkinson disease. Nat Rev Neurosci 18(8):509. https://doi.org/10.1038/nrn.2017.91
80. Schell H, Hasegawa T, Neumann M, Kahle PJ (2009) Nuclear and neuritic distribution of serine-129 phosphorylated alpha-synuclein in transgenic mice. Neuroscience 160(4):796–804. https://doi.org/10.1016/j.neuroscience.2009.03.002
81. Schindelin J, Arganda-Carreras I, Frise E, Kaynig V, Longair M, Pietzsch T et al (2012) Fiji: an open-source platform for biological-image analysis. Nat Methods 9(7):676–682. https://doi.org/10.1038/nmeth.2019
82. Schwarz LA, Miyamichi K, Gao XJ, Beier KT, Weissbourd B, DeLoach KE et al (2015) Viral-genetic tracing of the input–output organization of a central noradrenaline circuit. Nature 524(7563):88–92. https://doi.org/10.1038/nature14600
83. Spillantini MG, Schmidt ML, Lee VM, Trojanowski JQ, Jakes R, Goedert M (1997) Alpha-synuclein in Lewy bodies. Nature 388(6645):839–840. https://doi.org/10.1038/42166
84. Stiasny-Kolster K, Doerr Y, Moller JC, Hoffken H, Behr TM, Oertel WH et al (2005) Combination of 'idiopathic' REM sleep behaviour disorder and olfactory dysfunction as possible indicator for alpha-synucleinopathy demonstrated by dopamine transporter FP-CIT-SPECT. Brain 128(Pt 1):126–137. https://doi.org/10.1093/brain/awh322
85. Szabadi E (2013) Functional neuroanatomy of the central noradrenergic system. J Psychopharmacol (Oxford) 27(8):659–693. https://doi.org/10.1177/0269881113490326
86. Taschenberger G, Garrido M, Tereshchenko Y, Bahr M, Zweckstetter M, Kugler S (2012) Aggregation of alphaSynuclein promotes progressive in vivo neurotoxicity in adult rat dopaminergic neurons. Acta Neuropathol 123(5):671–683. https://doi.org/10.1007/s00401-011-0926-8
87. Thakur P, Breger LS, Lundblad M, Wan OW, Mattsson B, Luk KC et al (2017) Modeling Parkinson's disease pathology by combination of fibril seeds and alpha-synuclein overexpression in the rat brain. Proc Natl Acad Sci U S A 114(39):E8284–E8293. https://doi.org/10.1073/pnas.1710442114
88. Theodore S, Cao S, McLean PJ, Standaert DG (2008) Targeted overexpression of human alpha-synuclein triggers microglial activation and an adaptive immune response in a mouse model of Parkinson disease. J Neuropathol Exp Neurol 67(12):1149–1158. https://doi.org/10.1097/NEN.0b013e31818e5e99
89. Thorne N, Inglese J, Auld DS (2010) Illuminating insights into firefly luciferase and other bioluminescent reporters used in chemical biology. Chem Biol 17(6):646–657. https://doi.org/10.1016/j.chembiol.2010.05.012
90. Uchihara T, Giasson BI (2016) Propagation of alpha-synuclein pathology: hypotheses, discoveries, and yet unresolved questions from experimental and human brain studies. Acta Neuropathol 131(1):49–73. https://doi.org/10.1007/s00401-015-1485-1
91. Ulusoy A, Phillips RJ, Helwig M, Klinkenberg M, Powley TL, Di Monte DA (2017) Brain-to-stomach transfer of alpha-synuclein via vagal preganglionic projections. Acta Neuropathol 133(3):381–393. https://doi.org/10.1007/s00401-016-1661-y
92. Vekrellis K, Xilouri M, Emmanouilidou E, Rideout HJ, Stefanis L (2011) Pathological roles of α-synuclein in neurological disorders. Lancet Neurol 10(11):1015–1025. https://doi.org/10.1016/S1474-4422(11)70213-7
93. Vermeiren Y, de Deyn PP (2017) Targeting the norepinephrinergic system in Parkinson's disease and related disorders: the locus coeruleus story. Neurochem Int 102:22–32. https://doi.org/10.1016/j.neuint.2016.11.009
94. Volpicelli-Daley LA, Luk KC, Patel TP, Tanik SA, Riddle DM, Stieber A et al (2011) Exogenous alpha-synuclein fibrils induce Lewy body pathology leading to synaptic dysfunction and neuron death. Neuron 72(1):57–71. https://doi.org/10.1016/j.neuron.2011.08.033
95. Wakabayashi K, Takahashi H (1997) Neuropathology of autonomic nervous system in Parkinson's disease. Eur Neurol 38(Suppl 2):2–7
96. Wakamatsu M, Ishii A, Ukai Y, Sakagami J, Iwata S, Ono M et al (2007) Accumulation of phosphorylated alpha-synuclein in dopaminergic neurons of transgenic mice that express human alpha-synuclein. J Neurosci Res 85(8):1819–1825. https://doi.org/10.1002/jnr.21310
97. Weinshenker D (2018) Long road to ruin: noradrenergic dysfunction in neurodegenerative disease. Trends Neurosci. https://doi.org/10.1016/j.tins.2018.01.010
98. Yamada M, Iwatsubo T, Mizuno Y, Mochizuki H (2004) Overexpression of alpha-synuclein in rat substantia nigra results in loss of dopaminergic neurons, phosphorylation of alpha-synuclein and activation of caspase-9: resemblance to pathogenetic changes in Parkinson's disease. J Neurochem 91(2):451–461. https://doi.org/10.1111/j.1471-4159.2004.02728.x
99. Zarow C, Lyness SA, Mortimer JA, Chui HC (2003) Neuronal loss is greater in the locus coeruleus than nucleus basalis and substantia nigra in Alzheimer and Parkinson diseases. Arch Neurol 60(3):337–341
100. Zhang W, Wang T, Pei Z, Miller DS, Wu X, Block ML et al (2005) Aggregated alpha-synuclein activates microglia: a process leading to disease progression in Parkinson's disease. FASEB J 19(6):533–542. https://doi.org/10.1096/fj.04-2751com

D409H GBA1 mutation accelerates the progression of pathology in A53T α-synuclein transgenic mouse model

Donghoon Kim[1,2], Heehong Hwang[1], Seulah Choi[1], Sang Ho Kwon[1], Suhyun Lee[1], Jae Hong Park[1], SangMin Kim[1] and Han Seok Ko[1,2,3,4*]

Abstract

Heterozygous mutations in glucocerebrosidase 1 (*GBA1*) are a major genetic risk factor for Parkinson's disease and Dementia with Lewy bodies. Mutations in *GBA1* leads to GBA1 enzyme deficiency, and GBA1-associated parkinsonism has an earlier age of onset and more progressive parkinsonism. To investigate a potential influence of GBA1 deficiency caused by mutations in *GBA1* on the disease progression of PD, GBA1 mice carrying D409H knock-in mutation were crossbred with the human A53T (hA53T) α-synuclein transgenic mice. Here, we show that GBA1 enzyme activity plays a significant role in the hA53T α-synuclein induced α-synucleinopathy. The expression of D409H GBA1 markedly shortens the lifespan of hA53T α-synuclein transgenic mice. Moreover, D409H GBA1 expression exacerbates the formation of insoluble aggregates of α-synuclein, glial activation, neuronal degeneration, and motor abnormalities in the hA53T α-synuclein transgenic mice. Interestingly, the expression of D409H GBA1 results in the loss of dopaminergic neurons in the substantia nigra pars compacta of hA53T transgenic mice. Taken together, these results indicate that GBA1 deficiency due to D409H mutation affects the disease onset and course in hA53T α-synuclein transgenic mice. Therefore, strategies aimed to maintain GBA1 enzyme activity could be employed to develop an effective novel therapy for GBA1 linked-PD and related α-synucleinopathies.

Keywords: Parkinson's disease, Gaucher's disease, Glucocerebrosidase 1, D409H GBA1 mutation, α-synuclein

Introduction

Parkinson's Disease (PD) is a neurodegenerative disorder that affects approximately 1-2% of the elderly population [33]. Common characteristics of PD include the selective loss of dopaminergic neurons and the formation of Lewy bodies (LBs) and Lewy neurites (LNs) in surviving neurons in the substantia nigra pars compacta (SNpc) and locus coeruleus (LC), which eventually result in motor impairment [39]. Many pathologically sequestered protein aggregates are found in LBs in which α-synuclein is a dominating component [43]. Despite the remaining mystery of its exact function of α-synuclein, it has been known to foster neurodegeneration in several diseases such as PD, Dementia with Lewy Bodies (DLBs) and multiple system atrophy (MSA) [13].

Lysosomal glucocerebrosidase 1 (GBA1) enzyme catalyzes the breakdown of glycosylceramide into ceramide and glucose [18]. Homozygous mutations in *GBA1* cause a lysosomal storage disorder, Gaucher disease, whereas heterozygous mutations in *GBA1* are implicated in PD and DLB [9, 12, 42]. Mutations in *GBA1* lead to GBA1 enzyme deficiency and result in α-synuclein accumulation [27, 41]. Clinical pathology of PD, in which *GBA1* mutations are present, displayed the presence of a greater number of LBs and LNs [4, 25]. Recent studies have revealed that GBA1 enzyme activity and the steady-state level of wild type GBA1 protein are both reduced in the postmortem of PD patients with and without *GBA1* mutations [1, 2, 11, 31, 36], indicating the pivotal role of GBA1 on the development of sporadic PD.

To date, the relationship between Gaucher disease and α-synucleinopathies such as PD, DLBs, and MSA has

* Correspondence: hko3@jhmi.edu
[1]Neuroregeneration and Stem Cell Programs, Institute for Cell Engineering, The Johns Hopkins University School of Medicine, Baltimore, MD 21205, USA
[2]Department of Neurology, The Johns Hopkins University School of Medicine, Baltimore, MD 21205, USA
Full list of author information is available at the end of the article

been unraveled to some extent such that PD and LBDs patients with *GBA1* mutations typically show an earlier onset of the diseases and more severe symptoms than control group [32]. In addition, the early-onset PD was identified in the patients with low GBA1 enzyme activity through an imaging study [21]. Several studies attempted to define the effect of GBA1 deficiency on α-synuclein accumulation, turn over and its consequent pathology in vivo [8, 10, 30, 37, 44]. Although the studies have partially relationship among GBA1, α-synuclein, and PD, the animal models fail to represent GBA1-associated Parkinsonism, lacking an earlier age of PD onset and dopaminergic neurodegeneration. To investigate the linkage between GBA1 deficiency and PD, we crossbred GBA1 mice harboring D409H knock-in mutation with human A53T α-synuclein transgenic (Tg) mice. These mice have exhibited severe motor impairments and neuropathology accompanying typical alpha-synuclein pathology including serine 129 phosphorylation, the formation of alpha-synuclein fibrils and truncated alpha-synuclein, as well as biochemical defects including mitochondrial defects and endoplasmic reticulum stress, but there are no obvious neuropathological changes in the SNpc region [5, 6, 19, 24]. Using these mice, we assessed the effects of D409H GBA1 mutation on the major phenotypes such as neurodegeneration, accumulation of α-synuclein aggregates, endoplasmic reticulum (ER) stress, and neuroinflammation as well as shortened lifespan were all observed in the A53T α-synuclein Tg mice with the disease onset. Notably, the expression of D409H GBA1 mutation in the A53T α-synuclein Tg mice accelerated the PD progression.

Materials and methods

Animals

All experimental procedures were followed according to the guidelines of Laboratory Animal Manual of the National Institute of Health Guide to the Care and Use of Animals, which were approved by the Johns Hopkins Medical Institute Animal Care and Use Committee. GBA1 D409H knock-in (KI) mice were kindly provided by Dr. Gregory A. Grabowski [45] and human alpha-Syn (A53T) transgenic mice were purchased at the Jackson Lab (Stock#: 006823). The mice were back-crossed with C57BL/6 mice (Jackson Lab), and human A53T α-synuclein Tg mice with D409H GBA1 knock-in mice were generated for the present study.

Stereological assessment

For stereological assessment [47], mice were perfused with PBS followed by 4% paraformaldehyde. After post-fixed with 4% paraformaldehyde for 12 h, the tissue samples were cryoprotected with 30% sucrose, and processed for immunohistochemistry. 50 μm coronal sections were cut throughout the brain including substantia nigra and every 4th section was used for analysis. The rabbit polyclonal anti-TH (1:1000; Novus) was incubated in blocking solution. The signals were visualized using DAB kit (Vector Laboratories) followed by incubation with biotinylated secondary antibodies and streptavidin-conjugated horseradish peroxidase (HRP) (Vectastain ABC kit, Vector Laboratories). The stained tissue sections were mounted onto slides and counterstained with thionin for Nissl substance. The total number of TH-, and Nissl-positive neurons in the SNpc was counted using Optical Fractionator probe of Stereo Investigator software (MicroBrightfield).

Immunostaining

α-synuclein pathology in the brainstem and the SNpc region were visualized by staining with anti-pS^{129} antibody (1:1000; Abcam). The semi-quantitative grading of p-α-Syn pathology of the SNpc was quantified as previously described [16] with minor modification. The samples were graded using a 0-3 semi-quantitative density scale.

Microglia and astrocyte were stained with anti-Iba-1 (1:1000; Wako) or anti-GFAP (1:2000; Dako), antibodies followed by incubation with biotin-conjugated anti-rabbit antibody and ABC reagents (Vector Laboratories). Then, sections were developed using SigmaFast DAB Peroxidase Substrate (Sigma-Aldrich, St. Louis, MO, USA). The number of microglia and densities of astrocyte in the SNpc region were measured using ImageJ software. The GlcCer-positive signals were stained with anti-GlcCer antibody (1:500, Glycobiotech), followed by incubation with CY3-conjugated anti-donkey secondary antibody. The fluorescent images were acquired through a Zeiss confocal microscope (LSM 710, Zeiss Confocal).

Western blotting

The ventral midbrain tissues were dissected and prepared in lysis buffer that consist of 10 mM Tris-HCL, 150 mM NaCl, 5 mM EDTA, 0.5% Nonidet P-40, 10 mM Na-β-glycerophosphate, Phosphate inhibitor mixture I and II (Sigma-Aldrich, St. Louis, MO, USA), and complete protease inhibitor mixture (Roche) at pH 7.4. Then the tissues were homogenized using a Diax 900 homogenizer (Sigma-Aldrich, St. Louis, MO, USA). After homogenization, samples were centrifuged at 12000 × g for 20 min, supernatants were collected, and protein levels of each supernatant were quantified. Electrophoresis on 8-16% gradient SDS-PAGE was performed in order to resolve the 20 μg of proteins from the ventral midbrain tissues. The proteins were then transferred to nitrocellulose membranes. The membranes were blocked with blocking solution (Tris-buffered saline containing 5% non-fat dry milk and 0.1% Tween-20) for 1 h and incubated at

4 °C overnight with anti-α-synuclein (1:1000; Sigma S5566), anti-α-synuclein (1:1000; BD Biosciences), or anti-grp78 (1:500; Santa Cruz; sc-1050) antibodies, followed by HRP-conjugated secondary antibody (1:5000; GE Healthcare) for 1 h at RT. Finally, the membranes were re-probed with HRP-conjugated β-actin antibody (1:50,000; Sigma-Aldrich, St. Louis, MO, USA) after the blots were stripped.

GBA1 enzyme (GCase) activity assay

The GCase activity assay has been performed as previously described [3, 27]. Mouse ventral midbrain tissues were homogenized in the buffer containing 0.25 M sucrose, 10 mM HEPES (pH 7.4) and 0.1 M EDTA, centrifuged at 6800 × g, 4 °C, for 5 min, and the supernatant was collected. The supernatant was centrifuged at 17,000 × g for 10 min, and the pellet enriched with lysosomes was collected in 50 μl of activity assay buffer 0.25% Triton X-100 (Sigma-Aldrich), 0.25% Taurocholic acid (Sigma-Aldrich), 1 mM EDTA, in citrate/phosphate buffer, pH 5.4. The GCase activity was measured by adding 50 μl of 1% BSA, adding 1 mM 4-Methylumbelliferyl β-glucophyranoside (4-MU; M3633, Sigma-Aldrich) and/or 10 mM conduritol B epoxide (CBE, Sigma-Aldrich). The samples were incubated for 40 min at 37 °C, followed by the addition of 50 μl (equi-volume) of 1 M glycine at pH of 12.5 to terminate the reaction. Sample volume of 100 μL per well was prepared on 96 well plate (Nunc, # 136101). The fluorescence was measured via a Perkin Elmer plate reader (ex = 355 nm, em = 460 nm, 0.1 s). GCasel activity was obtained by subtracting the GCase activity in presence of CBE from the total GCase activity of each sample. 95-97% of GCase activity was reduced by CBE treatment.

Dot-blot assay

Samples were loaded onto the pre-wetted nitrocellulose membrane using Bio-Dot microfiltration apparatus (Bio-rad). After washing each sample with tris-buffered saline, samples were blocked with 5% non-fat dry milk in tris-buffered saline containing 0.1% tween-20. Membranes were incubated with anti-α-synuclein filament antibody (1:1000; Abcam) or GlcCer antibody (1:500, Glycobiotech) at 4 °C overnight, followed by HRP-conjugated rabbit secondary antibody (GE Healthcare) for 1 h at RT.

Behavioral test

For the pole test [47], the mice were trained for two consecutive days before the actual test. Each training session consisted of three test trials. Animals were placed on the top of the pole (75 cm of metal rod at diameter of 9 mm) facing the head up direction. The time taken to turn and total time taken to reach the base of the pole were recorded. The maximum cutoff time to stop was 120 s. For the rotarod test [23], the mice were trained for three consecutive days (four 5-min trials, 5-min apart) to acclimate them to the rotarod apparatus. During the test period, mice were placed on the rotarod with increasing speed, from 4 rpm to 40 rpm in 300 s. The latency to fall off was recorded under blind condition to different groups.

Statistical analysis

Data were presented as mean ± SEM with at least 3 independent experiments. Representative morphological images were taken out of at least 3 experiments with parallel results. An unpaired two-tailed Student's test or an ANOVA test followed by Bonferroni post hoc analysis was conducted to assess the statistical significance. Assessments with $p < 0.05$ were considered significant.

Results

GBA1 enzyme deficiency caused by GBA1 D409H mutation increases the levels of α-synuclein

To test our hypothesis that decreased GBA1 enzyme activity due to mutation in GBA1 affects neurodegeneration in the hA53T α-synuclein transgenic (Tg) mouse model of PD, the GBA1$^{D409H/D409H}$ mutant mice [45] were crossbred with the hA53T α-synuclein (α-Syn) Tg mice (Fig. 1). GBA1 expression level was reduced to 70% in the ventral midbrain tissues of the GBA1$^{+/D409H}$ mice and to 55% in the ventral midbrain tissues of the GBA1$^{D409H/D409H}$ mice when compared to the wild type mice. GBA1 expression was further reduced to 48% in the hA53T α-Syn; GBA1$^{+/D409H}$ and to 42% in the hA53T α-Syn; GBA1$^{D409H/D409H}$ mice (Fig. 2a and b). GBA1 enzyme activity was reduced to 71% in the brain tissues of the GBA1$^{+/D409H}$ mice and to 39% in the ventral midbrain tissues of the GBA1$^{D409H/D409H}$ mice when compared to the wild type mice. GBA1 enzyme activity was further reduced to 54% in the hA53T α-Syn;GBA1$^{+/D409H}$ and to 25% in the hA53T α-Syn;GBA1$^{D409H/D409H}$ mice (Fig. 2c). Glucosylceramide (GlcCer), a substrate of GBA1, was accumulated by 3.4 folds and 6.9 folds in the hA53T α-Syn;GBA1$^{+/D409H}$ and the hA53T α-Syn;GBA1$^{D409H/D409H}$ mice, respectively (Fig. 2d and e). Similar result was observed in the SN tissues as assessed by GlcCer immunofluorescence staining (Fig. 2f). The levels of overexpressed hA53T α-synuclein were increased by 1.8 folds in the hA53T α-Syn;GBA1$^{+/D409H}$ and by 2.5 folds in the hA53T α-Syn;GBA1$^{D409H/D409H}$ mice at 6 months of age (Fig. 2g and h). The levels of total α-synuclein expression (endogenous mouse α-synuclein and overexpressed hA53T α-synuclein) were increased by 6.6 folds in the hA53T α-Syn;GBA1$^{+/D409H}$ and by 8.3 folds in the hA53T α-Syn;GBA1$^{D409H/D409H}$ mice at 6 months of age compared

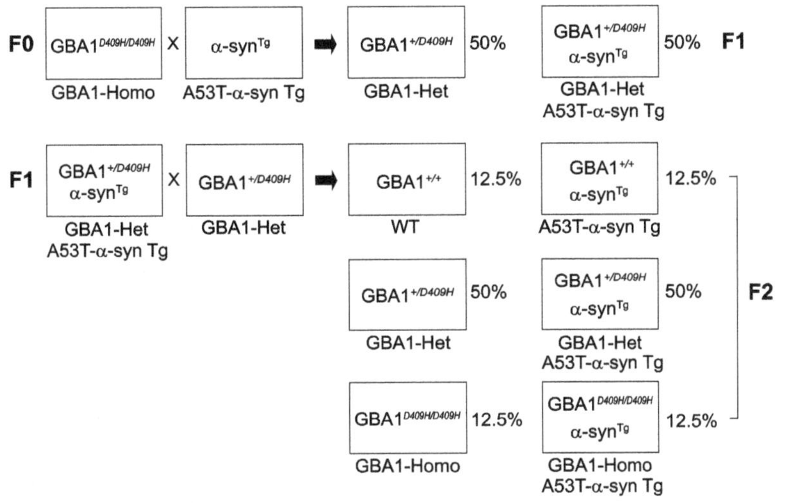

Fig. 1 Breeding strategy. To test our hypothesis that decreased GBA1 enzyme activity affects neurodegeneration in human A53T α-synuclein mouse model of PD, the $GBA1^{D409H/D409H}$ knock-in mice were crossbred with the hA53T α-synuclein mice

with non-Tg mice. Additionally, we found that the levels of endogenous mouse α-synuclein are increased in the dependent manner of GBA1 enzyme activity in GBA1 mutant mice (Fig. 2i). Thus, the steady-state levels of both endogenous α-synuclein and hA53T α-synuclein are dependent on the enzyme activity of GBA1 resulting from D409H mutation.

D409H GBA1 expression shortens lifespan and leads to dopaminergic degeneration in hA53T α-synuclein Tg mice

The hA53T mutant α-synuclein Tg mice develop adult-onset phenotypes with rapidly progressive motor impairment that eventually leads to death [19]. To examine whether D409H GBA1 expression bearing decreased enzyme activity affects the lifespan of hA53T α-synuclein Tg mice, littermates with the following genotypes were separated and aged: hA53T α-Syn, hA53T α-Syn;$GBA1^{+/D409H}$, hA53T α-Syn;$GBA1^{D409H/D409H}$, and their survival was monitored (Fig. 3a). The hA53T α-synuclein Tg mice lived an average of 10.8 months, as previously described [7]. The hA53T α-Syn;$GBA1^{+/D409H}$ lived an average of 9.7 months and the hA53T α-Syn;$GBA1^{D409H/D409H}$ lived an average of 8.6 months, indicating that the hA53T α-Syn;$GBA1^{D409H/D409H}$ significantly shortens lifespan of the hA53T α-synuclein Tg mice by 2.2 months. Therefore, decreased enzyme activity due to D409H GBA1 expression has a boosting impact that expedites the onset and progression of the lethal phenotype induced by α-synuclein pathologies in the hA53T α-synuclein Tg mice.

To determine whether the reduced GBA1 enzyme activity induces the loss of dopaminergic neurons in the hA53T α-synuclein mice, the number of TH positive neurons in the SNpc was counted via an unbiased stereological analysis of the genotypes at 6 months of age (Fig. 3b and c). As previously described, at 6 months of age when the mice are asymptomatic, there was no obvious dopaminergic neurodegeneration in the hA53T α-synuclein Tg mice. In contrast, there was an approximately 24% loss of dopaminergic neurons in the SNpc of the hA53T α-Syn;$GBA1^{+/D409H}$. Furthermore, there was 43% neuronal loss in the SNpc of the hA53T α-Syn;$GBA1^{D409H/D409H}$ mutant mice.

D409H GBA1 expression leads to reduction of the dopaminergic fiber density and alters behavioral deficits in the A53T α-synuclein Tg mouse models

Since D409H GBA1 expression leads to dopaminergic neurodegeneration in the SNpc, next, tyrosine hydroxylase (TH)-immunopositive fiber density in the striatum was assessed (Fig. 4a). At 6 months of age when the mice were asymptomatic, there was no obvious dopaminergic terminal loss in the hA53T α-synuclein mice. However, there was approximately 32% TH fibers were lost in the striatum of the hA53T α-syn;$GBA1^{+/D409H}$ and 58% in the striatum of the hA53T α-Syn;$GBA1^{D409H/D409H}$ compared to the control group (Fig. 4b).

To determine whether D409H GBA1 expression leading to decreased GBA1 enzyme activity leads to the abnormal behavior in the A53T α-synuclein, we performed a pole test, and rotarod analysis using a cohort of 6 months of age of different genotypes (Fig. 4c and d). At 6 months of age, when the hA53T α-synuclein mice were asymptomatic, there was no

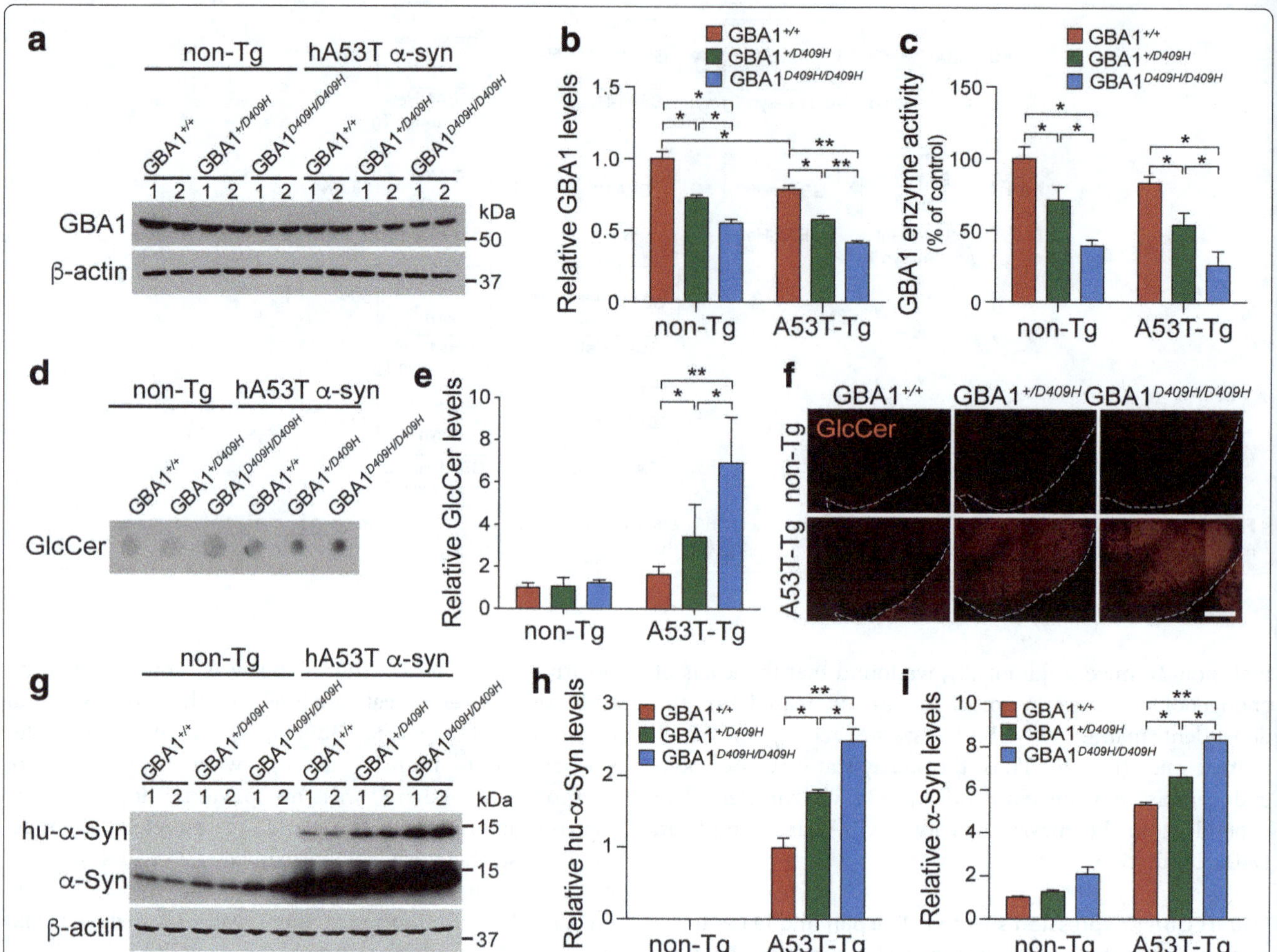

Fig. 2 The levels of α-synuclein are dependent on GBA1 enzyme activity. **a** and **b,** The expression levels of GBA1 were quantified in the ventral midbrain of the indicated genotypes at 6 months of age. **c,** GBA1 enzyme activity assay was conducted in the ventral midbrain of the indicated genotypes at 6 months of age. **d,** Dot blot shows relative GlcCer levels in the ventral midbrain of the indicated genotypes at 6 months of age. **e,** The relative levels of GlcCer were quantified. **f,** Representative images of GlcCer by immunostaining in the SN of the indicated genoypes at 6 months of age. The scale bar is 200 μm. **g,** Steady-state levels of human and mouse α-synuclein were monitored in the ventral midbrain of the indicated genotypes via Western blot analysis at 6 months of age. **h** and **i,** The expression levels of human and mouse α-synuclein were quantified. DATA are expressed as mean ± SEM (*n* = 6 for the each group)

significant behavioral impairment on the rotarod test. Average latency to fall in the accelerating rotarod was reduced in the hA53T α-Syn;GBA1$^{+/D409H}$. The reduction in latency times was greater in the hA53T α-Syn;GBA1$^{D409H/D409H}$ mice at the 6 months of age (Fig. 4c). We also conducted the pole test since it is a useful method for evaluating the mouse movement disorder caused by striatal dopamine depletion [26]. The pole test revealed that there was a moderate increase in the time to reach to the base of the pole in the hA53T α-Syn;GBA1$^{+/D409H}$ and a significantly greater increase in the hA53T α-Syn;GBA1$^{D409H/D409H}$ at 6 months of age (Fig. 4d). At 6 months of age, however, there was no significant difference in body weight (Fig. 4e).

D409H GBA1 expression accelerates the accumulation of insoluble α-synuclein species in the brainstem and SNpc of A53T α-synuclein Tg mice

As the accumulation of insoluble high molecular weight species of α-synuclein is a prominent indicator of pathology in the A53T α-synuclein mice [19], it was assessed via various techniques such as immunohistochemistry, dot blot, and immunoblot analysis (Fig. 5). Immunohistochemistry was conducted at 6 months of age when the mice were asymptomatic. At this time point, there was no obvious accumulation of α-synuclein phosphorylated at serine 129, which is closely associated with α-synuclein aggregation, in the SNpc and brainstem of the hA53T α-Syn mice. In contrast, immunohistochemistry revealed that some accumulation of α-synuclein phosphorylated at serine 129 in the

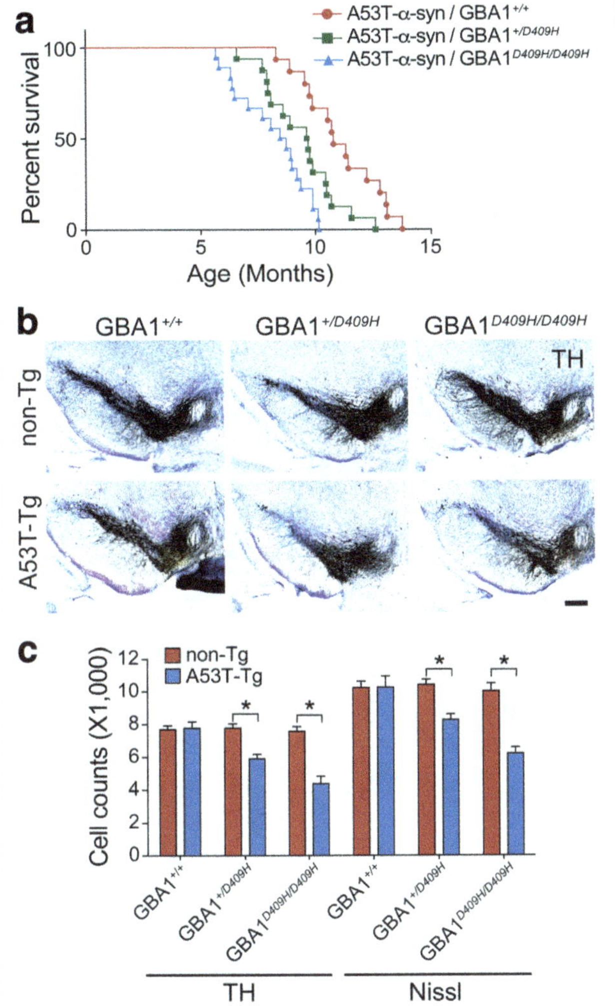

Fig. 3 D409H GBA1 expression shortens lifespan and leads to dopaminergic degeneration in the hA53T α-synuclein transgenic mice. **a,** Survival was monitored from littermates with the following genotypes: hA53Ta-Syn/GBA1$^{+/+}$ (n = 15), hA53T α-Syn/GBA1$^{+/D409H}$(n = 16), hA53T α-Syn/GBA1$^{D409H/D409H}$ (n = 18) mice. GBA1 mutation induces the lethal phenotype and TH-positive neuronal loss in the SNpc of A53T mutant α-synuclein transgenic mice. **b** and **c,** The number of TH-positive neurons in the SNpc was counted using stereological analysis with the indicated genotypes at 6 months of age. The scale bar is 200 μm. DATA are expressed as mean ± SEM (n = 6 for the each group)

brainstem and SNpc of the hA53T α-Syn;GBA1$^{+/D409H}$ and significant accumulation in the brainstem and SNpc of the hA53T α-Syn;GBA1$^{D409H/D409H}$ at 6 months of age (Fig. 5a, b, and c). None of the aggregates was detected in the brainstem and SNpc of non-Tg mice. Dot blot (Fig. 5d, and e) and immunoblot analysis (Fig. 5f and g) also demonstrated that the detergent-insoluble high molecular weight species of α-synuclein accumulated in the ventral midbrain of the hA53T α-Syn;GBA1$^{+/D409H}$ and the accumulation was significantly increased in the ventral midbrain of the hA53T α-Syn;GBA1$^{D409H/D409H}$ at 6 months of age (Fig. 5d, e, f, and g).

D409H GBA1 expression shows early neuroinflammation in the A53T α-synuclein Tg mice

At 6 months of age there was no significant accumulation of Iba-1 and GFAP in the SNpc of A53T α-synuclein mice. For microglia activation, characterized by the increased expression of Iba-1, serves as an indirect indicator of neuronal abnormality in the A53T α-synuclein Tg mice. Thus, the enhanced expression of Iba1 was determined by immunohistochemistry. There was an increased Iba-1 immunoreactivity in the SNpc of hA53T α-Syn;GBA1$^{+/D409H}$. The immunoreactivity was dramatically increased in the SNpc of the hA53T α-Syn; GBA1$^{D409H/D409H}$ at 6 months of age (Fig. 6a and b). As the accumulation of glial fibrillary acidic protein (GFAP) is a prominent pathological indicator in the A53T α-synuclein Tg mice, its accumulation was also assessed via immunohistochemistry. There was an increased GFAP immunoreactivity in the SNpc of hA53T α-Syn; GBA1$^{+/D409H}$. The accumulation was further increased in the SNpc of the hA53T α-Syn;GBA1$^{D409H/D409H}$ at 6 months of age (Fig. 6c and d).

D409H GBA1 expression triggers ER stress early in the A53T α-synuclein Tg mice

In symptomatic A53T α-synuclein Tg mice there was an accumulation of indicators of ER stress in a number of brain regions, including the brainstem and spinal cord [5]. 78 kDa glucose-regulated protein (grp78/BiP), an indicator of ER stress, was analyzed via immunohistochemisty and Immunoblot analysis using grp78 antibody (Fig. 7). Strikingly, immunohistochemistry demonstrated that there was a moderate increase of grp78 protein level in the SNpc tissues of the hA53T α-Syn;GBA1$^{+/D409H}$ and the upregulation of grp78 was significantly increased in the SNpc tissues of the hA53T α-Syn;GBA1$^{D409H/D409H}$ at 6 months of age (Fig. 7a and c). Immunoblot analysis also demonstrated that the grp78 protein accumulated in the ventral midbrain of the hA53T α-Syn;GBA1$^{+/D409H}$ and the accumulation was further promoted in the ventral midbrain of the hA53T α-Syn;GBA1$^{D409H/D409H}$ at 6 months of age (Fig. 7c and d).

Discussion

The hypothesis that GBA1 could affect α-synuclein degradation and pathology has been tested in several animal models [8, 10, 30, 37, 44]. These models have allowed us to elucidate the relationship among GBA1, α-synuclein, and PD. However, these animal models do not fully represent the clinical observations seen in the GBA1-associated Parkinsonism such as earlier PD onset and DA neuronal loss. To gain further insights into the mechanisms by which *GBA1* mutations increase the risk for PD and lead to the development of GBA1-assiciated parkinsonism, we crossbred GBA1 mice carrying D409H

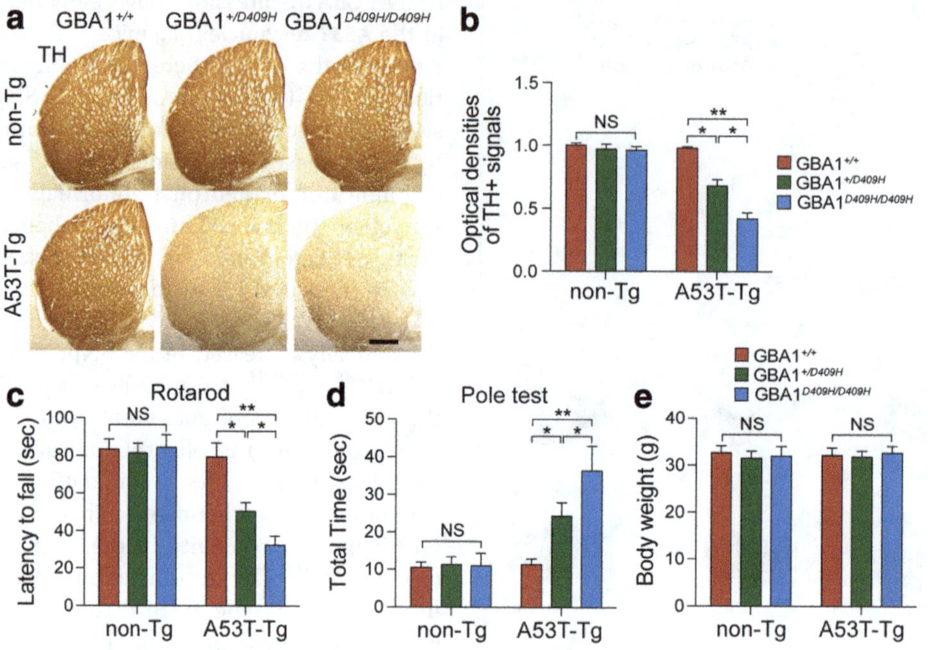

Fig. 4 D409H GBA1 expression promotes reduction of dopaminergic fiber densities and motor deficit in the striatum of hA53T α-synuclein transgenic mice. **a,** The striatal TH-immunopositive fiber density was assessed in the striatum of the indicated genotypes at 6 months of age ($n = 6$ per each group). The scale bar is 250 μm. **b,** The optical densities of TH positive signals were quantified. **c** and **d**, Rotarod and Pole test were assessed at 6 months of age with the indicated genotypes ($n = 7$ per each group). e, the body weight of mice were measured with the indicated genotypes ($n = 15$ per each group). DATA are expressed as mean ± SEM

knock-in mutation with human A53T α-synuclein Tg mice exhibiting neurological abnormalities, accumulation of α-synuclein aggregates, increased ER stress, neuroinflammation, and shortened lifespan [5, 19]. Using this mouse model, we assessed the impact of D409H GBA1 mutation on the major phenotypes of the A53T α-synuclein Tg mice with disease onset and further examined the cardinal features seen in the GBA1-associated Parkinsonism through biochemical and immunohistochemical analyses. Importantly, our findings reveal that the expression of D409H GBA1 mutation resulted in the loss of DA neurons, accelerates disease onset, exacerbates neuroinflammation and ER stress more extensively than the degree seen in the hA53T α-synuclein Tg mice.

It has been reported that mutations in *GBA1* result in the production of misfolded GBA1, increased GBA1 ubiquitination, and premature degradation leading to quantitative loss in the protein levels [22, 46]. We found the reduction of GBA1 protein expression and GBA1 enzyme activity in the brains of $GBA1^{+/D409H}$ and $GBA1^{D409H/D409H}$, which is similar to previous findings that GBA1 deficiency due to expression of L444P mutation or heterozygous *GBA1*-null mutations results in GBA1 enzyme activity deficiency [30]. Importantly, there was even lower GBA1 enzyme activity in the brains of hA53T α-Syn;$GBA1^{+/D409H}$ and hA53T α-Syn;$GBA1^{D409H/D409H}$, which differs from the earlier finding that heterozygous *GBA1*-null mutations in the A53T α-synuclein Tg mice does not lead to GBA1 enzyme deficiency [44]. Although the reason for this discrepancy is unclear, it is conceivable that the GBA1 enzyme deficiency due to D409H mutation may affects the disease onset in A53T α-synuclein Tg mice differently from heterozygous GBA1-null mutations. For instance, the buildup of the misfolded GBA1 D409H mutant protein [29] and α-synuclein aggregates trigger ER stress [5], which would form a positive feedback loop to further impair GBA1 enzyme activity and consequently contribute to α-synuclein pathology and loss of DA neurons in the model. Since it is known that GBA1 enzyme activity was lowest in the SN of PD patients [1, 2, 11, 31], a further investigation will be required to determine GBA1 enzyme activity in different brain regions in this mouse model. In addition, it is possible that GBA1 D409H mutation may affect the lysosomal dysfunction in hA53T α-synuclein Tg, thereby hampering the autophagy/lysosomal degradation of pathological α-synuclein [34]. Future study will be required to test this possibility in our animal model.

In our model, the relationship between GBA1 enzyme activity and α-synuclein accumulation revealed that

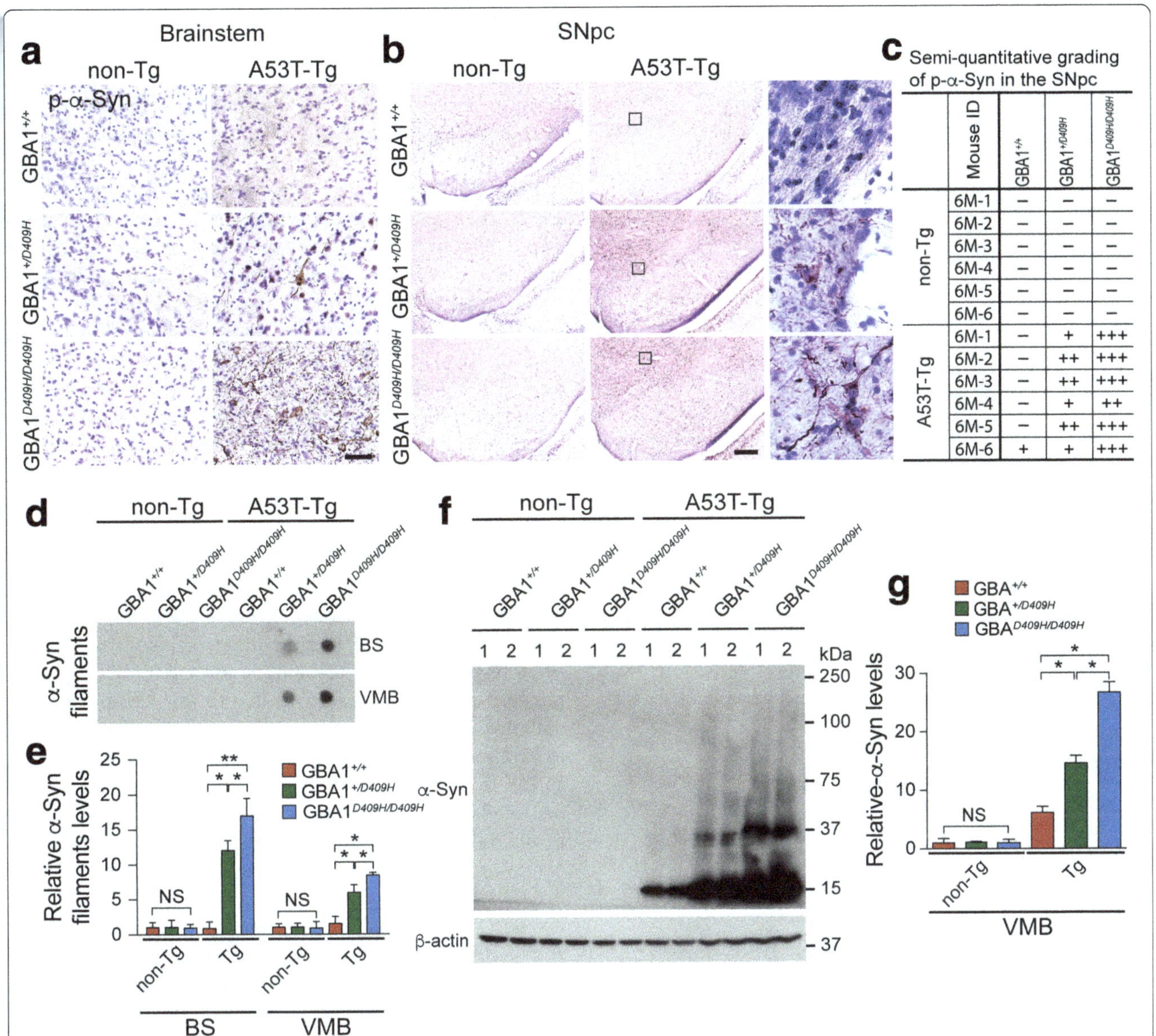

Fig. 5 D409H GBA1 expression leads to the accumulation of pathologic α-synuclein aggregates in the brainstem and SNpc of A53T α-synuclein transgenic mice. **a,** Representative images of p-α-Syn positive signals in the brainstem . Immunohistochemistry with phosphor-S^{129} α-synuclein (p-α-Syn) antibody was conducted in the lateral vestibular nucleus of the brainstem of the indicated genotypes at 6 months of age. The scale bar represents 50 μm. **b,** Representative images of p-α-Syn signals in the SNpc of the indicated genotypes at 6 months of age at low-magnification and high-magnification. The scale bar is 200 μm. **c,** Semi-quantitative grading of p-α-Syn pathology in the indicated genotypes. **d** and **e,** Dot-blot analysis of brainstem (BS) and ventral midbrain (VMB) of bigenic mice ($n = 3$) with α-synuclein filament antibody was performed and quantified. **f** and **g,** Accumulation of high molecular weight species of α-synuclein in the ventral midbrain was assessed in the VMB. The ventral midbrain lysates were immunoblotted with α-Syn antibody. The high molecular weight species were quantified

GBA1 deficiency due to D409H mutation was associated with the increased levels of human and mouse α-synulcein proteins as well as the enhanced levels of high molecular weight α-synuclein aggregates in the ventral midbrain regions. Consistent with previous findings, our observations confirm that decreased GBA1 enzyme activity due to *GBA1* mutations or null leads to increased α-synuclein levels in other models [8, 10, 30] and PD postmortem brains [11, 31]. Since the levels of α-synuclein are greater in the brain of hA53T α-Syn;GBA1$^{D409H/D409H}$ compared to hA53T α-Syn; GBA1$^{+/D409H}$, the accumulation of α-synuclein is dependent on the levels of GBA1 enzyme activity. On the other hand, our study revealed that phosphoserine 129 (pSer) α-synuclein immunoreactivity and high molecular weight α-synuclein species were detected in

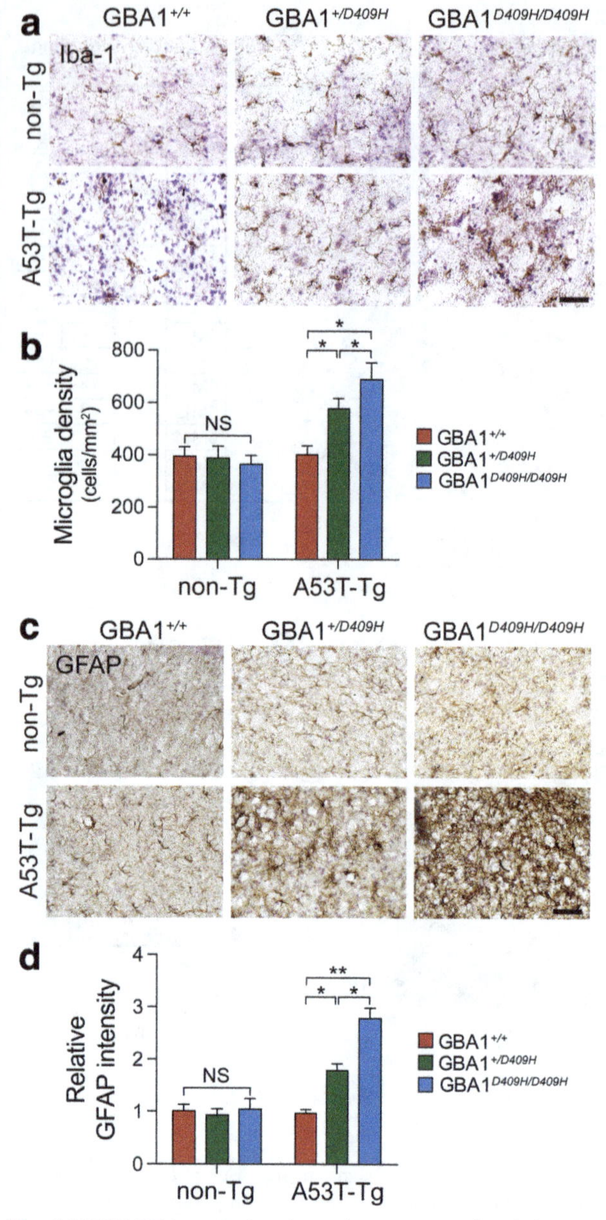

Fig. 6 D409H GBA1 expression shows the activation of pathology-associated microglia and astrocyte activation in the SNpc of A53T α-synuclein transgenic mice. **a,** Iba-1 immunoreactive microglia were observed in the SNpc region of the indicated genotypes at 6 months of age. The scale bar is 50 μm. **b,** The number of microglia was counted. **c,** GFAP immunoreactive astrocytes were observed in the SNpc region of the indicated genotypes at 6 months of age. The scale bar is 50 μm. **d,** The signals were measured using ImageJ

the ventral midbrain of hA53T α-Syn;GBA1$^{+/D409H}$ and hA53T α-Syn;GBA1$^{D409H/D409H}$ mice at 6 months of age. Moreover, intensities of both pSer α-synuclein immunoreactivity and high molecular weight α-synuclein species were correlated with the enzyme activity levels of GBA1 in the hA53T α-Syn;GBA1$^{+/D409H}$ and hA53T α-Syn;GBA1$^{D409H/D409H}$ mice. However, the pSer immunoreactivity and high molecular weight α-synuclein species were not present in the ventral midbrain of the hA53T α-Syn Tg mice at 6 months of age. Although the underlying mechanism of how D409H expression results in increased pathologic α-synuclein aggregates at the early time point is not clear, it is likely that additional α-synuclein accumulation triggered by GBA1 deficiency due to D409H expression pushes forward the levels of α-synuclein protein to reach quickly the threshold required for pathologic α-synuclein aggregates in the model at 6 months of age, eliciting overt DA neurodegeneration loss in the SNpc and PD related motor deficits in the same model. Based on our current observations, the hA53T α-Syn Tg mouse model may provide a valuable resource to uncover mechanisms of how PD-associated gene mutations can impact PD pathogenesis.

Importantly, we found the loss of nigrostriatal DA neurons in the SNpc of the hA53T α-Syn;GBA1$^{+/D409H}$ and hA53T α-Syn;GBA1$^{D409H/D409H}$, which were not detected in the A53T α-synuclein Tg mice, GBA1$^{+/D409H}$, and GBA1$^{D409H/D409H}$ at 6 months of age. This result has not been reported in the previous studies [10, 37, 44]. One possible explanation for this is due to the accumulation of pathologic α-synuclein aggregates, which may be sufficient to lead to the loss of nigrostriatal DA neurons in the SNpc at the time point. Another explanation might be behind neuroinflammation that contributes to neurodegeneration in neurodegenerative disorders including PD [20, 35, 38]. Neuroinflammation was present in the SNpc of hA53T α-Syn;GBA1$^{+/D409H}$ and hA53T α-Syn;GBA1$^{D409H/D409H}$, but not observed in A53T α-synuclein Tg mice, GBA1$^{+/D409H}$, and GBA1$^{D409H/D409H}$ at 6 months of age. The last explanation for this might be ER stress that contributes to neurodegeneration in neurodegenerative disorders including PD [14, 15, 28]. We also observed significantly changed levels of ER stress in the SNpc of hA53T α-Syn; GBA1$^{+/D409H}$ and hA53T α-Syn;GBA1$^{D409H/D409H}$ at 6 month of age, which were not detected in A53T α-synuclein Tg mice, GBA1$^{+/D409H}$, and GBA1$^{D409H/D409H}$ at the time point.

Although the penetrance of D409H GBA1 mutation is relatively lower than other mutations such as N370S and L444P GBA1 mutations [40], our current findings suggest that GBA1 deficiency due to D409H GBA1 mutation alone is not sufficient to cause PD but additional factors, such as environmental factors or increased levels of α-synuclein could increase the penetrance through rendering the levels of α-synuclein accumulation close to the threshold required for α-synuclein aggregation. Our previous finding that GBA1 deficiency due to L444P GBA1 heterozygous mutation renders DA neurons more susceptible to MPTP intoxication [47] further

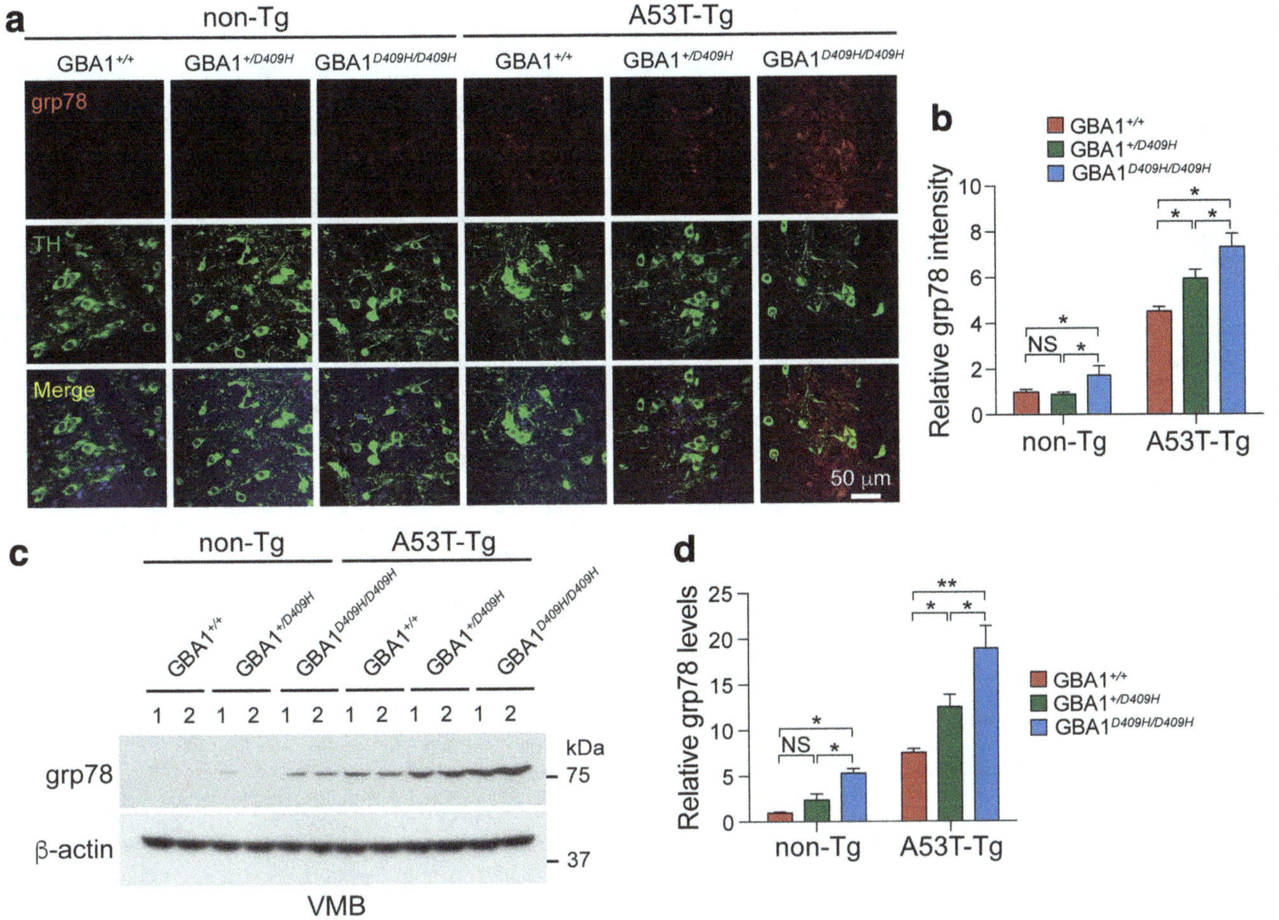

Fig. 7 D409H GBA1 expression shows early induction of ER chaperone grp78 in the A53T α-synuclein transgenic mice. **a,** Accumulation of grp78, an indicator of ER stress, was analyzed via immunostaining with grp78 and TH antibodies in the SNpc of indicated genotypes at 6 months of age. The scale bar is 50 μm. **b,** The fluorescence levels of grp78 were analyzed using Image J and compared to non-Tg ($n = 3$). **c** and **d,** Accumulation of grp78 was analyzed via Western blot analysis with grp78 antibody in the ventral midbrain of the indicated genotypes. The grp78 levels were measured using ImageJ

supports this hypothesis. Our study does not provide a detailed explanation on how D409H GBA1mutation contributes to severe neurodegeneration with the loss of DA neurons in the A53T α-synuclein Tg mice. Further studies need to be undertaken to account for the DA neurodegeneration. Also, it would be interesting to study how the regulation of formation of α-synuclein tetramers and other related multimers as well as the changes in the status of glycosphingolipids (GSLs) in the model is regulated [17].

Conclusions

In conclusion, our results indicate that GBA1 deficiency due to D409H GBA1 mutation that contributes to α-synuclein accumulation exacerbates neuronal vulnerability in neurodegenerative processes triggered by A53T α-synuclein expression in vivo. The model that recapitulates the cardinal PD phenotypes including loss of DA neurons, LB pathology, and motor deficits can be a useful tool to study in depth the possible mechanisms underlying neurodegeneration due to *GBA1* mutations and to test the efficacy of potential treatment against GBA1-associated PD and Dementia with Lewy bodies (DLB).

Acknowledgements

The authors acknowledge the joint participation by the Adrienne Helis Malvin Medical Research Foundation and the Diana Helis Henry Medical Research Foundation through its direct engagement in the continuous active conduct of medical research in conjunction with The Johns Hopkins Hospital and the Johns Hopkins University School of Medicine and the Foundation's Parkinson's Disease Program M-2014, H-1, H-2013.

Funding

This work was supported by grants from the NIH/NINDS NS38377 Morris K. Udall Parkinson's Disease Research Center and NIH/NINDS NS082205 and R21NS098006 and the Maryland Stem Cell Research Foundation 2012-MSCRFE-0059.

Authors' contributions

DK and HSK designed research; DK, HH, SC, SHK, SL, JHP and S K performed research; DK analyzed data; DK and HSK wrote the paper. All authors read and approved the final manuscript.

Competing interests

The authors declare that they have no competing interests.

Author details

[1]Neuroregeneration and Stem Cell Programs, Institute for Cell Engineering, The Johns Hopkins University School of Medicine, Baltimore, MD 21205, USA. [2]Department of Neurology, The Johns Hopkins University School of Medicine, Baltimore, MD 21205, USA. [3]Diana Helis Henry Medical Research Foundation, New Orleans, Louisiana 70130, USA. [4]Adrienne Helis Malvin Medical Research Foundation, New Orleans, Louisiana 70130, USA.

References

1. Alcalay RN, Levy OA, Waters CC, Fahn S, Ford B, Kuo SH, Mazzoni P, Pauciulo MW, Nichols WC, Gan-Or Z et al (2015) Glucocerebrosidase activity in Parkinson's disease with and without GBA mutations. Brain 138:2648–2658. https://doi.org/10.1093/brain/awv179
2. Chiasserini D, Paciotti S, Eusebi P, Persichetti E, Tasegian A, Kurzawa-Akanbi M, Chinnery PF, Morris CM, Calabresi P, Parnetti L et al (2015) Selective loss of glucocerebrosidase activity in sporadic Parkinson's disease and dementia with Lewy bodies. Mol Neurodegener 10:15. https://doi.org/10.1186/s13024-015-0010-2
3. Choi S, Kim D, Kam TI, Yun S, Kim S, Park H, Hwang H, Pletnikova O, Troncoso JC, Dawson VL et al (2015) Lysosomal enzyme Glucocerebrosidase protects against Abeta1-42 oligomer-induced neurotoxicity. PLoS One 10: e0143854. https://doi.org/10.1371/journal.pone.0143854
4. Clark LN, Kartsaklis LA, Wolf Gilbert R, Dorado B, Ross BM, Kisselev S, Verbitsky M, Mejia-Santana H, Cote LJ, Andrews H et al (2009) Association of glucocerebrosidase mutations with dementia with lewy bodies. Arch Neurol 66:578–583. https://doi.org/10.1001/archneurol.2009.54
5. Colla E, Coune P, Liu Y, Pletnikova O, Troncoso JC, Iwatsubo T, Schneider BL, Lee MK (2012) Endoplasmic reticulum stress is important for the manifestations of alpha-synucleinopathy in vivo. J Neurosci 32:3306–3320. https://doi.org/10.1523/JNEUROSCI.5367-11.2012
6. Colla E, Jensen PH, Pletnikova O, Troncoso JC, Glabe C, Lee MK (2012) Accumulation of toxic alpha-synuclein oligomer within endoplasmic reticulum occurs in alpha-synucleinopathy in vivo. J Neurosci 32:3301–3305. https://doi.org/10.1523/JNEUROSCI.5368-11.2012
7. Daher JP, Pletnikova O, Biskup S, Musso A, Gellhaar S, Galter D, Troncoso JC, Lee MK, Dawson TM, Dawson VL et al (2012) Neurodegenerative phenotypes in an A53T alpha-synuclein transgenic mouse model are independent of LRRK2. Hum Mol Genet 21:2420–2431. https://doi.org/10.1093/hmg/dds057
8. Davis MY, Trinh K, Thomas RE, Yu S, Germanos AA, Whitley BN, Sardi SP, Montine TJ, Pallanck LJ (2016) Glucocerebrosidase deficiency in Drosophila results in alpha-Synuclein-independent protein aggregation and neurodegeneration. PLoS Genet 12:e1005944. https://doi.org/10.1371/journal.pgen.1005944
9. DePaolo J, Goker-Alpan O, Samaddar T, Lopez G, Sidransky E (2009) The association between mutations in the lysosomal protein glucocerebrosidase and parkinsonism. Mov Disord 24:1571–1578. https://doi.org/10.1002/mds.22538
10. Fishbein I, Kuo YM, Giasson BI, Nussbaum RL (2014) Augmentation of phenotype in a transgenic Parkinson mouse heterozygous for a Gaucher mutation. Brain 137:3235–3247. https://doi.org/10.1093/brain/awu291
11. Gegg ME, Burke D, Heales SJ, Cooper JM, Hardy J, Wood NW, Schapira AH (2012) Glucocerebrosidase deficiency in substantia nigra of parkinson disease brains. Ann Neurol 72:455–463. https://doi.org/10.1002/ana.23614
12. Gegg ME, Schapira AHV (2018) The role of glucocerebrosidase in Parkinson disease pathogenesis. FEBS J. https://doi.org/10.1111/febs.14393
13. Goedert M (2001) Alpha-synuclein and neurodegenerative diseases. Nat Rev Neurosci 2:492–501. https://doi.org/10.1038/35081564
14. Hetz C, Mollereau B (2014) Disturbance of endoplasmic reticulum proteostasis in neurodegenerative diseases. Nat Rev Neurosci 15:233–249. https://doi.org/10.1038/nrn3689
15. Hetz C, Saxena S (2017) ER stress and the unfolded protein response in neurodegeneration. Nat Rev Neurol 13:477–491. https://doi.org/10.1038/nrneurol.2017.99
16. Kim C, Lv G, Lee JS, Jung BC, Masuda-Suzukake M, Hong CS, Valera E, Lee HJ, Paik SR, Hasegawa M et al (2016) Exposure to bacterial endotoxin generates a distinct strain of alpha-synuclein fibril. Sci Rep 6:30891. https://doi.org/10.1038/srep30891
17. Kim S, Yun SP, Lee S, Umanah GE, Bandaru VVR, Yin X, Rhee P, Karuppagounder SS, Kwon SH, Lee H et al (2018) GBA1 deficiency negatively affects physiological alpha-synuclein tetramers and related multimers. Proc Natl Acad Sci U S A 115:798–803. https://doi.org/10.1073/pnas.1700465115
18. Kitatani K, Sheldon K, Rajagopalan V, Anelli V, Jenkins RW, Sun Y, Grabowski GA, Obeid LM, Hannun YA (2009) Involvement of acid beta-glucosidase 1 in the salvage pathway of ceramide formation. J Biol Chem 284:12972–12978. https://doi.org/10.1074/jbc.M802790200
19. Lee MK, Stirling W, Xu Y, Xu X, Qui D, Mandir AS, Dawson TM, Copeland NG, Jenkins NA, Price DL (2002) Human alpha-synuclein-harboring familial Parkinson's disease-linked ala-53 -> Thr mutation causes neurodegenerative disease with alpha-synuclein aggregation in transgenic mice. Proc Natl Acad Sci U S A 99:8968–8973. https://doi.org/10.1073/pnas.132197599
20. Liddelow SA, Guttenplan KA, Clarke LE, Bennett FC, Bohlen CJ, Schirmer L, Bennett ML, Munch AE, Chung WS, Peterson TC et al (2017) Neurotoxic reactive astrocytes are induced by activated microglia. Nature 541:481–487. https://doi.org/10.1038/nature21029
21. Lopez G, Sidransky E (2013) Predicting parkinsonism: new opportunities from Gaucher disease. Mol Genet Metab 109:235–236. https://doi.org/10.1016/j.ymgme.2013.04.012
22. Lu J, Chiang J, Iyer RR, Thompson E, Kaneski CR, Xu DS, Yang C, Chen M, Hodes RJ, Lonser RR et al (2010) Decreased glucocerebrosidase activity in Gaucher disease parallels quantitative enzyme loss due to abnormal interaction with TCP1 and c-Cbl. Proc Natl Acad Sci U S A 107:21665–21670. https://doi.org/10.1073/pnas.1014376107
23. Luk KC, Kehm V, Carroll J, Zhang B, O'Brien P, Trojanowski JQ, Lee VM (2012) Pathological alpha-synuclein transmission initiates Parkinson-like neurodegeneration in nontransgenic mice. Science 338:949–953. https://doi.org/10.1126/science.1227157
24. Martin LJ, Pan Y, Price AC, Sterling W, Copeland NG, Jenkins NA, Price DL, Lee MK (2006) Parkinson's disease alpha-synuclein transgenic mice develop neuronal mitochondrial degeneration and cell death. J Neurosci 26:41–50. https://doi.org/10.1523/JNEUROSCI.4308-05.2006
25. Mata IF, Samii A, Schneer SH, Roberts JW, Griffith A, Leis BC, Schellenberg GD, Sidransky E, Bird TD, Leverenz JB et al (2008) Glucocerebrosidase gene mutations: a risk factor for Lewy body disorders. Arch Neurol 65:379–382. https://doi.org/10.1001/archneurol.2007.68
26. Matsuura K, Kabuto H, Makino H, Ogawa N (1997) Pole test is a useful method for evaluating the mouse movement disorder caused by striatal dopamine depletion. J Neurosci Methods 73:45–48
27. Mazzulli JR, Xu YH, Sun Y, Knight AL, McLean PJ, Caldwell GA, Sidransky E, Grabowski GA, Krainc D (2011) Gaucher disease glucocerebrosidase and alpha-synuclein form a bidirectional pathogenic loop in synucleinopathies. Cell 146:37–52. https://doi.org/10.1016/j.cell.2011.06.001
28. Mercado G, Castillo V, Soto P, Sidhu A (2016) ER stress and Parkinson's disease: pathological inputs that converge into the secretory pathway. Brain Res 1648:626–632. https://doi.org/10.1016/j.brainres.2016.04.042
29. Migdalska-Richards A, Schapira AH (2016) The relationship between glucocerebrosidase mutations and Parkinson disease. J Neurochem 139(Suppl 1):77–90. https://doi.org/10.1111/jnc.13385
30. Migdalska-Richards A, Wegrzynowicz M, Rusconi R, Deangeli G, Di Monte DA, Spillantini MG, Schapira AHV (2017) The L444P Gba1 mutation enhances alpha-synuclein induced loss of nigral dopaminergic neurons in mice. Brain 140:2706–2721. https://doi.org/10.1093/brain/awx221
31. Murphy KE, Gysbers AM, Abbott SK, Tayebi N, Kim WS, Sidransky E, Cooper A, Garner B, Halliday GM (2014) Reduced glucocerebrosidase is associated with increased alpha-synuclein in sporadic Parkinson's disease. Brain 137: 834–848. https://doi.org/10.1093/brain/awt367
32. Nalls MA, Duran R, Lopez G, Kurzawa-Akanbi M, McKeith IG, Chinnery PF, Morris CM, Theuns J, Crosiers D, Cras P et al (2013) A multicenter study of glucocerebrosidase mutations in dementia with Lewy bodies. JAMA Neurol 70:727–735. https://doi.org/10.1001/jamaneurol.2013.1925

33. Nussbaum RL (2003) Alzheimer's disease and Parkinson's disease (vol 348, pg 1356, 2003). New Engl J Med 348:2588–2588
34. Pitcairn C, Wani WY, Mazzulli JR (2018) Dysregulation of the autophagic-lysosomal pathway in Gaucher and Parkinson's disease. Neurobiol Dis. https://doi.org/10.1016/j.nbd.2018.03.008
35. Poewe W, Seppi K, Tanner CM, Halliday GM, Brundin P, Volkmann J, Schrag AE, Lang AE (2017) Parkinson disease. Nat Rev Dis Primers 3:17013. https://doi.org/10.1038/nrdp.2017.13
36. Rocha EM, Smith GA, Park E, Cao H, Brown E, Hallett P, Isacson O (2015) Progressive decline of glucocerebrosidase in aging and Parkinson's disease. Ann Clin Transl Neurol 2:433–438. https://doi.org/10.1002/acn3.177
37. Rockenstein E, Clarke J, Viel C, Panarello N, Treleaven CM, Kim C, Spencer B, Adame A, Park H, Dodge JC et al (2016) Glucocerebrosidase modulates cognitive and motor activities in murine models of Parkinson's disease. Hum Mol Genet 25:2645–2660. https://doi.org/10.1093/hmg/ddw124
38. Salter MW, Stevens B (2017) Microglia emerge as central players in brain disease. Nat Med 23:1018–1027. https://doi.org/10.1038/nm.4397
39. Savitt JM, Dawson VL, Dawson TM (2006) Diagnosis and treatment of Parkinson disease: molecules to medicine. J Clin Invest 116:1744–1754. https://doi.org/10.1172/JCI29178
40. Schapira AH (2015) Glucocerebrosidase and Parkinson disease: recent advances. Mol Cell Neurosci 66:37–42. https://doi.org/10.1016/j.mcn.2015.03.013
41. Schondorf DC, Aureli M, McAllister FE, Hindley CJ, Mayer F, Schmid B, Sardi SP, Valsecchi M, Hoffmann S, Schwarz LK et al (2014) iPSC-derived neurons from GBA1-associated Parkinson's disease patients show autophagic defects and impaired calcium homeostasis. Nat Commun 5:4028. https://doi.org/10.1038/ncomms5028
42. Sidransky E, Lopez G (2012) The link between the GBA gene and parkinsonism. Lancet Neurol 11:986–998. https://doi.org/10.1016/S1474-4422(12)70190-4
43. Spillantini MG, Schmidt ML, Lee VM, Trojanowski JQ, Jakes R, Goedert M (1997) Alpha-synuclein in Lewy bodies. Nature 388:839–840. https://doi.org/10.1038/42166
44. Tayebi N, Parisiadou L, Berhe B, Gonzalez AN, Serra-Vinardell J, Tamargo RJ, Maniwang E, Sorrentino Z, Fujiwara H, Grey RJ et al (2017) Glucocerebrosidase haploinsufficiency in A53T alpha-synuclein mice impacts disease onset and course. Mol Genet Metab 122:198–208. https://doi.org/10.1016/j.ymgme.2017.11.001
45. Xu YH, Quinn B, Witte D, Grabowski GA (2003) Viable mouse models of acid beta-glucosidase deficiency: the defect in Gaucher disease. Am J Pathol 163:2093–2101
46. Yang C, Wang H, Zhu D, Hong CS, Dmitriev P, Zhang C, Li Y, Ikejiri B, Brady RO, Zhuang Z (2015) Mutant glucocerebrosidase in Gaucher disease recruits Hsp27 to the Hsp90 chaperone complex for proteasomal degradation. Proc Natl Acad Sci U S A 112:1137–1142. https://doi.org/10.1073/pnas.1424288112
47. Yun SP, Kim D, Kim S, Kim S, Karuppagounder SS, Kwon SH, Lee S, Kam TI, Lee S, Ham S et al (2018) Alpha-Synuclein accumulation and GBA deficiency due to L444P GBA mutation contributes to MPTP-induced parkinsonism. Mol Neurodegener 13:1. https://doi.org/10.1186/s13024-017-0233-5

13

TDP-43 pathology in anterior temporal pole cortex in aging and Alzheimer's disease

Sukriti Nag[1,2*], Lei Yu[1,3], Patricia A. Boyle[1,4], Sue E. Leurgans[1,3], David A. Bennett[1,3] and Julie A. Schneider[1,2,3]

Abstract

TDP-43 pathology was investigated in the anterior temporal pole cortex (ATPC) and orbital frontal cortex (OFC), regions often degenerated in frontotemporal lobar degenerations (FTLD), in aging and Alzheimer's disease (AD). Diagnosis of dementia in the 1160 autopsied participants from 3 studies of community-dwelling elders was based on clinical evaluation and cognitive performance tests which were used to create summary measures of the five cognitive domains. Neuronal and glial TDP-43 cytoplasmic inclusions were quantitated in 8 brain regions by immunohistochemistry, and used in ANOVA and regression analyses. TDP-43 pathology was present in 547 (49.4%) participants in whom ATPC (41.9%) was the most frequently involved neocortical region and in 15.5% of these cases, ATPC was the only neocortical area with TDP-43 pathology suggesting not only that ATPC is involved early by TDP-43 but that ATPC may represent an intermediate stage between mesial temporal lobe involvement by TDP-43 and the last stage with involvement of other neocortical areas. To better study this intermediary neocortical stage, and to integrate with other staging schemes, our previous 3 stage distribution of TDP-43 pathology was revised to a 5 stage distribution scheme with stage 1 showing involvement of the amygdala only; stage 2 showed extension to hippocampus and/or entorhinal cortex; stage 3 showed extension to the ATPC; stage 4 – showed extension to the midtemporal cortex and/or OFC and finally in stage 5, there was extension to the midfrontal cortex. Clinically, cases in stages 2 to 5 had impaired episodic memory, however, stage 3 was distinct from stage 2 since stage 3 cases had significantly increased odds of dementia. The proportion of cases with hippocampal sclerosis increased progressively across the stages with stage 5 showing the largest proportion of hippocampal sclerosis cases. Stage 5 cases differed from other stages by having impairment of semantic memory and perceptual speed, in addition to episodic memory impairment. These data suggest that of the regions studied, TDP-43 pathology in the ATPC is an important early neocortical stage of TDP-43 progression in aging and AD while extension of TDP-43 pathology to the midfrontal cortex is a late stage associated with more severe and global cognitive impairment.

Keywords: Alzheimer's disease, Anterior temporal pole, Dementia, Episodic memory, Hippocampal sclerosis, Orbital frontal cortex, Semantic memory, TDP-43

Introduction

The transactive response DNA-binding protein 43 (TDP-43) was first localized in brains of cases with frontotemporal lobar degeneration (FTLD) and amyotrophic lateral sclerosis (ALS) [1, 20]. Subsequent studies localized this protein in Alzheimer's disease (AD) [8, 24] and other neurodegenerative diseases such as age-related hippocampal sclerosis [14, 18], Lewy body (LB) diseases [11, 16] and chronic traumatic encephalopathy [12]. TDP-43 protein was also reported in the aging brain in the absence of a pathological diagnosis of AD [11, 15, 24] and in cognitively normal Asians [17]. The TDP-43 protein deposition was in the form of intranuclear or intracytoplasmic inclusions in neurons and glia, as well as dystrophic neurites in the affected regions; findings collectively referred to as TDP-43 pathology.

Few studies have investigated the regional distribution of TDP-43 pathology in the brain. In the behavioral variant FTLD, 4 patterns of TDP-43 distribution were reported [5] with early involvement of the orbital and inferior frontal gyri and anteromedial temporal structures to widespread

* Correspondence: Sukriti_Nag@rush.edu
[1]Rush Alzheimer Disease Center, Rush University Medical Center, Suite 1000, 1750 W Harrison Street, Chicago, IL 60612, USA
[2]Departments of Pathology (Neuropathology), Rush University Medical Center, Chicago, IL, USA
Full list of author information is available at the end of the article

cortical TDP-43 pathology, depending on the specific pattern. By contrast, TDP-43 distribution in AD was reported to follow 6 stages with medial temporal structures (stages 1-3) being affected early followed by ventral striatum, insular and inferior temporal cortices (stage 4), the brainstem (Stage 5) and finally basal ganglia and midfrontal cortex (stage 6) [8]. Our previous studies in a cohort of older community dwelling persons without FTLD, reported 3 stages of regional TDP-43 distribution regardless of presence or absence of AD [14, 15, 26]. In stage 1, TDP-43 was localized to the amygdala, in stage 2 there was extension of TDP-43 pathology to the hippocampus and/or entorhinal cortex while in stage 3 there was further extension to neocortical areas such as the midtemporal or midfrontal cortices.

TDP-43 pathology is considered central to the pathogenesis of FTLD/ALS whereas its role in other neurodegenerative diseases is less clear. Given the propensity for TDP-43 pathology to affect the anterior and/or orbital frontal cortex (OFC) and temporal lobe structures with prominent neurodegeneration in FTLD-TDP, the hypothesis that TDP-43 pathology may also preferentially involve the anterior temporal pole cortex (ATPC) and OFC in aging and AD was tested. ATPC is the most rostral neocortical area of the superior and middle temporal gyri and is highly interconnected with the amygdala and the OFC.

Our results show that the ATPC, but not the OFC, appears to be a prominent and early neocortical site of involvement in TDP-43 pathology associated with aging and AD and that this stage is related to dementia. To better study this early neocortical stage, and to integrate with other staging schemes, we propose a new 5 stage system of TDP-43 distribution that includes TDP-43 in ATPC. The association of all 5 stages of TDP-43 pathology with dementia, memory, and other cognitive domains was studied in participants of 3 longitudinal studies of aging and dementia: the Rush Memory and Aging Project (MAP), the Religious Orders Study (ROS) and the Minority Aging Research Project (MARS).

Materials and methods

Participants and clinical evaluation

Autopsied participants ($n = 1160$) were from 3 longitudinal clinical-pathologic cohort studies of aging and dementia, Rush MAP ($n = 636$), ROS ($n = 501$) and MARS ($n = 23$), each approved by the Institutional Review Board of Rush University Medical Center. All data collections (antemortem and postmortem) were similar in these studies allowing combined analyses of the cohorts. A signed, informed consent was obtained from each participant for an annual clinical evaluation and for brain donation. Fifteen cases having a pathologic diagnosis of FTLD in accordance with previous FTLD classifications [6, 10], were excluded from the study and are not included in the total number mentioned above. These excluded cases were diagnosed as having corticobasal degeneration, Pick's disease, progressive supranuclear palsy, and FTLD-TDP. Thirty-four cases with missing tissue from any of the mandatory regions of interest were also excluded from the study. 18 cases having skipped areas (see below) were also excluded leaving 1108 cases available for statistical analyses. All 1108 cases had TDP-43 pathology data available from the amygdala since previous studies [8, 14] demonstrate that TDP-43 pathology in aging and AD appears to start and then spread from the amygdala.

Uniform clinical evaluation at baseline and annually thereafter included a standardized battery of 19 cognitive performance tests as described previously [3, 25]. The Mini-Mental State Examination (MMSE) and Complex Ideational Material were used for descriptive purposes or diagnostic classification, respectively. The remaining 17 tests assessed function of five cognitive domains including episodic, semantic, and working memory, perceptual speed and visuospatial ability. In order to reduce ceiling and floor artifacts as well as random variability, composite measures were obtained by converting the raw scores of the individual tests to z scores using the baseline mean and standard deviation (SD) of all participants and then averaging results for each domain of cognitive function [25].

Dementia and probable AD were diagnosed using criteria of the joint working group of the National Institute of Neurological and Communicative Disorders and Stroke and the AD and Related Disorders Association [13]. Dementia status proximate-to-death was assigned by a Board-certified neurologist after review of all clinical information.

Pathological analyses

The average post-mortem interval was 9.3 h (SD 8.3). Brains were fixed with 4% paraformaldehyde in 0.1 M phosphate buffer. Blocks were dissected from 11 brain regions which included the following cortices: midfrontal (Brodmann9/46), midtemporal (Brodmann 21), inferior parietal (Brodmann 39/40), occipital (Brodmann17), anterior cingulate (Brodmann 24) and entorhinal (Brodmann 28) with amygdala. Blocks were also taken of the mid-hippocampus, basal ganglia at the level of the anterior commissure, anterior thalamus, midbrain at the level of the exiting 3rd nerve fibers and the cerebellum which included the dentate nucleus. Blocks were processed using standard techniques and paraffin-embedded sections (6 μm) stained with hematoxylin-eosin were used to detect microinfarcts and arteriolosclerosis as described below and hippocampal sclerosis (HS). The latter was evaluated unilaterally in a coronal section of the midhippocampus at the level of the lateral geniculate body, and graded as absent or present based on severe neuronal loss and gliosis in CA1 and/or subiculum or other sectors.

TDP-43 pathology

TDP-43 protein was localized in four brain regions (amygdala, entorhinal cortex, hippocampus CA1 and subiculum and the dentate nucleus) and four neocortical areas (ATPC, midtemporal cortex, OFC and midfrontal cortex) having the Brodmann designation of 38, 21, 11 and 9/46 respectively (Fig. 1a-g). A phosphorylated monoclonal TAR5P-1D3 (pS409/410; 1:100, Ascenion, Munich, Germany) TDP-43 antibody [19] was used. A semiquantitative estimate of TDP-43 cytoplasmic inclusions in neurons and glia was obtained at 200 X, in a 0.25 mm^2 area of greatest density using a 6-point scale (none, sparse [1-2 inclusions], sparse to moderate [3-5 inclusions], moderate [6-12 inclusions], moderate to frequent [13-19 inclusions], and frequent [20 or more inclusions]) (Fig. 2a-d). In analyses, a dichotomous variable was used to define presence of TDP-43 pathology in each region.

AD pathology

The National Institute on Aging-Reagan criteria [7] were used with intermediate and high likelihood cases

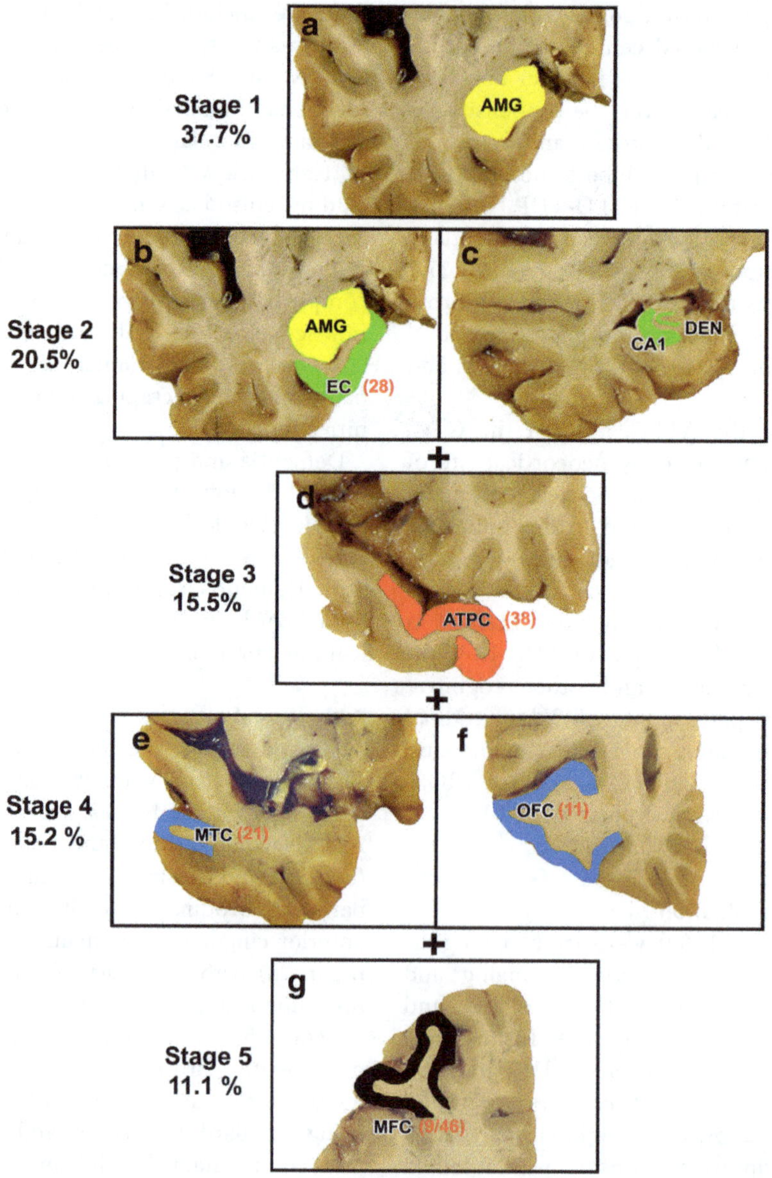

Fig. 1 (**a-g**) The regional distribution of TDP-43 inclusions and percentage of cases showing TDP-43 inclusions in stages 1-5 are shown (**a-g**). This is a cumulative staging system such that any stage from 2 to 5 is considered to be positive if the previous stages are positive. The Brodmann designation of the cortices is shown in parentheses. AMG = amygdala, EC = entorhinal cortex, CA1 = CA1 sector of the hippocampus, DEN = dentate gyrus, ATPC = anterior temporal pole cortex, MTC = midtemporal cortex, OFC = orbital frontal cortex and MFC = midfrontal cortex

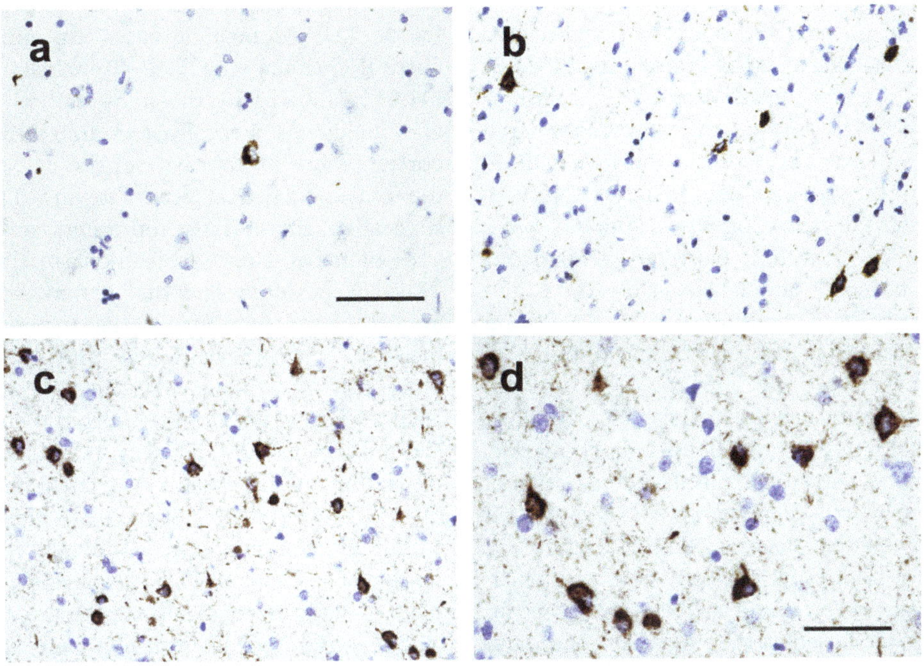

Fig. 2 TDP-43 inclusions in neuronal cytoplasm and neurites in the ATPC are shown (a-d). Representative areas of the ATPC show sparse (**a**), moderate (**b**) and frequent (**c**) intracytoplasmic neuronal TDP-43 inclusions and neurite immunostaining. The areas depicted (**a-c**) are smaller than the 0.25 mm^2 counting frame used to quantitate the inclusions. (**d**) Cytoplasmic TDP-43 in neurons and prominent neurite staining are shown in high magnification. Scale bar = 25 μm (**a-c**) and 50 μm (**d**)

indicating a pathologic diagnosis of AD. Modified Bielschowsky silver stain was used to quantitate neuritic and diffuse plaques and neurofibrillary tangles in 5 brain regions (midfrontal, midtemporal, inferior parietal and entorhinal cortices and hippocampus), having the highest density of these structures, as described previously [23]. The raw count for each of the three pathologies within each region was divided by the SD of each marker and values were averaged across the regions to obtain a summary score for each subject. The summary scores of these three AD markers were then averaged to yield the global measure of AD pathology for each subject, which was used in analyses.

Infarcts

The age, volume and anatomic location of all macroscopic infarcts and the age and location of microscopic infarcts were documented. Only chronic macro and microinfarcts were included in the analyses as dichotomous variables.

Vascular diseases

Atherosclerosis was assessed in basal cerebral arteries while arteriolosclerosis was assessed in the basal ganglia and both vessel pathologies were graded using a semi-quantitative scale from 0 (none) to 6 (severe) as described previously [22]. Cerebral amyloid angiopathy (CAA) was assessed in meningeal and intracortical vessels in four cortical sections (midfrontal, midtemporal, inferior parietal and occipital) immunostained for β-amyloid and graded as described previously [27].

Lewy bodies

These were assessed in 6 regions (midfrontal, midtemporal, entorhinal and cingulate cortices, amygdala and substantia nigra) as described previously [25] and recorded and analyzed as a dichotomous variable.

Where pertinent, immunohistochemistry was done for anti-phospho-PHF tau pSer202/Thr205 (1:3000, Thermo Fisher Scientific, Waltham, MA) and 'fused in sarcoma' (FUS) protein (1:1000, Sigma Aldrich Corp, St. Louis, MO) to exclude FTLD cases. All immunohistochemistry was done using a Leica-Bond Max autostainer (Leica Microsystems, New Buffalo, IL). Antigen retrieval was done using heat-induced epitope retrieval (HIER) solution 1 (citrate-base) (Leica Microsystems) for 10 min for α-synuclein, and 30 min for FUS and HIER solution 2 (EDTA-base) (Leica Microsystems) for 20 min for phosphorylated TDP-43. Sections were pretreated with formic acid prior to immunostaining for β-amyloid. In case of α-synuclein the Bond polymer alkaline phosphatase red detection kit was used while for the other antibodies the Bond Polymer Refine Detection Kit was used which produced a brown reaction product.

Statistical analyses

Demographics, clinical characteristics and age-related pathologies including macro and microinfarcts, HS, LBs and AD pathologies and vascular pathologies (arteriolosclerosis, atherosclerosis, and CAA), were compared between subjects without and those in the five TDP-43 stages using χ^2 or the analysis of variance (ANOVA). Age, education, MMSE and cognitive domains were further compared by post hoc pairwise comparisons between TDP-43 stages 2 and 3, stages 3 and 4 and stages 4 and 5 cases with application of a Bonferroni Correction ($\alpha = 0.05/3$) to adjust for multiple testing.

Multivariable linear regression analyses were used to determine the association of the 5 TDP-43 pathology stages with the outcome measures of episodic, semantic, and working memory, perceptual speed and visuospatial skills. Multivariable logistic regression analyses evaluated the association of the five stages of TDP-43 pathology with dementia as a binary outcome. In both multivariable linear and logistic regression analyses, Stage 0 (no TDP-43 pathology) was used as the reference group and all models controlled for age, sex, education and the age-related pathologies listed above. All analyses were carried out using SAS software, (SAS Institute Inc. SAS/STAT 14.1 User's Guide, Cary, NC). Model assumptions were examined graphically and analytically and were adequately met. A nominal threshold of $p < 0.05$ was used for statistical significance throughout except for the post hoc pairwise comparisons mentioned above.

Results

TDP-43 neuronal and glial inclusions were present in 547 of 1108 (49.4%) participants. TDP-43 cytoplasmic inclusions in entorhinal and neocortical regions tended to be more frequent in the second layer than in deeper cortical layers. Most inclusions were compact (Fig. 2d) while granular inclusions were less frequent.

TDP-43 in ATPC and OFC

In the TDP-43 positive cases, the most frequent neocortical area showing TDP-43 inclusions was the ATPC (41.9%) followed by the midtemporal cortex, the OFC and inclusions were least common in the midfrontal cortex (Table 1). In 15.5% of the 547 cases, ATPC was the only neocortical area showing TDP-43 pathology suggesting that ATPC represents one of the earliest sites of neocortical involvement in the progression of TDP-43 pathology and that it may represent an intermediate stage between mesial temporal lobe involvement by TDP-43 pathology and the last stage with more extensive neocortical involvement. Extension of TDP-43 pathology to the midfrontal cortex (see below), had a distinct pathological and clinical profile justifying separation of these cases into an additional stage. We therefore revised our 3 stage distribution of TDP-43 pathology to include two additional stages. Our new 5 stage distribution of TDP-43 pathology was as follows: stage 1 – localized to amygdala; stage 2 –extension to hippocampus and/or entorhinal cortex; stage 3 – extension to the ATPC, stage 4 – extension to other neocortical areas such as midtemporal or OFC and finally in stage 5 there was extension to the midfrontal cortex (Fig. 1a-g). Stages 2 and 4 were considered to be positive if any of the new regions included in these stages showed TDP-43 pathology.

All participants having TDP-43 pathology ($n = 547$), showed inclusions in the amygdala and in 206 of the 547 cases (37.7%), the inclusions were confined to the amygdala (stage 1) (Fig. 1a, Table 1). Extension of TDP-43 to the entorhinal cortex or CA1 sector of the hippocampus or dentate neurons was observed in 112 of the 547 (20.5%) cases (stage 2). Further extension of TDP-43 to the ATPC (stage 3) was observed in 85 of the 547 (15.5%) cases while additional extension to midtemporal or OFC (stage 4) was observed in 83 of the 547 (15.2%) cases and extension to the midfrontal

Table 1 Frequency of TDP-43 pathology in brain regions by stage in 547 participants

Regions	TDP-43 stages					Total
	1	2	3	4	5	TDP-43 positive cases by brain regions n, %
	n = 206	*n* = 112	*n* = 85	*n* = 83	*n* = 61	
	37.7%	20.5%	15.5%	15.2%	11.1%	
Amygdala	206	112	85	83	61	547, *100*
Entorhinal Cortex	0	92	83	82	60	317, *58.0*
Hippocampus, CA1	0	84	74	82	59	299, *54.7*
Hippocampus, dentate gyrus	0	60	59	76	59	244, *44.6*
Anterior temporal pole cortex	0	0	85	83	61	229, *41.9*
Midtemporal cortex	0	0	0	70	57	127, *23.2*
Orbital frontal cortex	0	0	0	32	57	89, *16.3*
Midfrontal cortex	0	0	0	0	61	61, *11.1*

cortex (stage 5) was observed in 61 of the 547 (11. 1%) cases. In both stage 4 and 5 cases the number of TDP-43 inclusions in ATPC was greater than observed in stage 3 cases (Fig. 3). Stage 4 or 5 cases did not show significant microvacuolation or obvious neurodegeneration of the frontal and/or midtemporal cortices that characterize FTLD cases. Nine cases in stage 5, having no dementia (Table 2) did not have AD but other pathologies such as HS ($n = 4$), a combination of HS and LB disease (n = 4) and 1 case had a chronic macroinfarct in the caudate. Phospho-PHF-tau and FUS immunostaining done in these cases was negative excluding a diagnosis of FTLD.

18 of the 1160 (1.5%) cases failed to show the proposed regional progression of TDP-43 pathology due to one skipped stage despite examination of an additional section of the regions without identified TDP-43 pathology. Of the 18 cases, eight showed no TDP-43 pathology in the amygdala which showed no degenerative changes on microscopy. In 5 cases the hippocampus/entorhinal cortex was skipped, in another 3 cases the ATPC was skipped and in 2 cases the midtemporal cortex was skipped. The clinical diagnoses of these 18 cases were probable AD (6 cases), mild cognitive impairment (7 cases) and no cognitive impairment (5 cases). Fourteen of the 18 cases met criteria for pathologic AD while the remaining 4 cases did not, however, numerous macroinfarcts/microinfarcts with significant tissue loss was present in these cases. These18 cases were not included in the statistical analyses.

TDP-43 stages and age-related pathologies

Overall, the frequency of a pathologic diagnosis of AD was higher in those having TDP-43 pathology (73.5%) as compared to those negative for TDP-43 (56.2%). The proportion of cases with a pathologic diagnosis of AD increased across the TDP-43 stages to 80% in Stage 3 and 85% in each of stages 4 or 5 (Table 2). Bivariate analyses showed that HS frequency was 10-fold higher in cases having TDP-43 pathology as compared to those without TDP-43 pathology. In addition, a progressive increase in percentage of HS was noted across the TDP-43 stages with a nine-fold increase in HS frequency in stage 3 cases and a 35-fold increase in stage 5 cases. Lewy body disease was significantly higher in those with TDP-43 pathology as compared to those having no TDP-43 with a 2-fold increase in frequency in the stage 5 cases as compared with those without TDP-43 pathology. The frequencies of other age-related pathologies including macro and microinfarcts, and vessel pathologies such as arteriolosclerosis, atherosclerosis, and CAA did not differ by TDP-43 pathology.

Clinical findings in TDP-43 stages

The demographic and clinical data for participants in each of the 5 TDP-43 stages are shown in Table 2. Overall, age was significantly higher in cases with TDP-43 pathology as compared to those without TDP-43 pathology ($p < 0.001$). Post hoc pairwise comparisons between the age of stage 2 and 3 cases, stage 3 and 4 cases and stage 4 and 5 cases showed no statistical difference

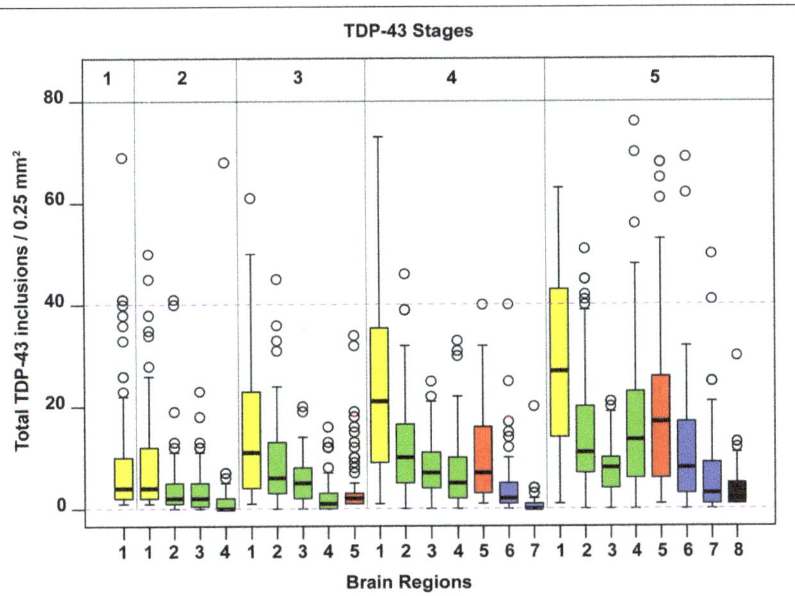

Fig. 3 Box plots showing the total number of TDP-43 inclusions per 0.25 mm^2 area in the eight brain regions by stage. The numbers on the x axis denote the brain regions which are designated as 1: amygdala, 2: entorhinal cortex, 3:CA1 sector of the hippocampus, 4: dentate neurons of the hippocampus, 5: anterior temporal pole cortex, 6: midtemporal cortex, 7: orbital frontal cortex, 8: midfrontal cortex. There is progressive increase of inclusions in the amygdala by stage. Inclusions in all regions including the ATPC are maximal in stage 5

Table 2 Clinical pathologic characteristics of 1108 participants by TDP-43 stages

Characteristics	TDP-43 Stages						*p*-value
	Stage 0 *n* = *561*	Stage 1 *n* = *206*	Stage 2 *n* = *112*	Stage 3 *n* = *85*	Stage 4 *n* = *83*	Stage 5 *n* = *61*	
Age at death, y, mean (SD)	87.7 (6.9)	89.6 (6.6)	91.5 (6.1)	92.0 (5.6)	92.1 (5.3)	90.3 (5.3)	< 0.001*
Female, n (%)	370 (66.0)	144 (69.9)	79 (70.5)	67 (78.8)	67 (80.7)	41 (67.2)	0.036
Education, mean (SD),	16.1 (3.9)	16.2 (3.6)	16.1 (3.6)	15.7 (3.5)	15.5 (3.4)	15.8 (3.3)	0.705*
Clinical characteristics, n (%)							
No Dementia	376 (67.4)	130 (63.1)	55 (49.1)	30 (35.3)	27 (32.9)	9 (14.8)	< 0.001
Dementia	182 (32.6)	76 (36.9)	57 (50.9)	55 (64.7)	55 (67.1)	52 (85.3)	
Cognitive function tests proximate to death, mean (SD)							
MMSE score	22.8 (8.2)	21.5 (8.6)	19.0 (9.8)	18.3 (9.5)	15.6 (9.2)	11.2 (10.5)	< 0.001*
Episodic memory	−0.60 (1.3)	−0.71 (1.3)	−1.23 (1.4)	−1.38 (1.3)	−1.97 (1.2)	−2.19 (1.3)	< 0.001*
Semantic memory	−0.91 (1.5)	−1.05 (1.5)	−1.63 (1.9)	−1.51 (1.7)	−1.96 (1.7)	−2.80 (2.1)	< 0.001*
Working memory	−0.61 (1.1)	−0.65 (1.1)	− 0.95 (1.2)	−0.87 (1.0)	− 0.97 (1.0)	− 1.27 (1.3)	< 0.001*
Perceptual speed	− 1.03 (1.2)	− 1.08 (1.1)	− 1.42 (1.2)	−1.51 (1.1)	− 1.68 (1.1)	−2.10 (1.2)	< 0.001*
Visuospatial ability	− 0.42 (1.1)	−0.41 (1.2)	− 0.64 (1.2)	−0.68 (1.1)	− 0.91 (1.1)	− 1.05 (1.3)	< 0.001*
Pathologic characteristics, n (%)							
AD, NIA-Reagan	315 (56.2)	136 (66.0)	75 (67.0)	68 (80.0)	71 (85.5)	52 (85.3)	< 0.001
Hippocampal sclerosis	10 (1.8)	7 (3.4)	14 (12.5)	14 (16.5)	27 (32.5)	38 (62.3)	< 0.001
Macroinfarcts	196 (34.9)	77 (37.4)	38 (33.9)	29 (34.1)	37 (44.6)	21 (34.4)	0.724
Microinfarcts	158 (28.2)	61 (29.6)	36 (32.1)	21 (24.8)	26 (31.3)	23 (37.7)	0.678
Arteriolosclerosis	161 (28.9)	76 (37.1)	32 (28.6)	33 (38.8)	30 (36.1)	20 (29.5)	0.145
Atherosclerosis	174 (31.1)	71 (34.5)	37 (33.0)	27 (31.8)	28 (33.7)	20 (32.8)	0.966
Cerebral amyloid angiopathy	418 (75.2)	155 (75.6)	95 (84.8)	69 (81.2)	66 (79.5)	51 (83.6)	0.171
Lewy body disease	115 (21.1)	50 (24.9)	32 (29.4)	24 (29.6)	16 (20.5)	25 (40.0)	0.008

p-value derived from ANOVA* or chi-square

($p = 0.574$, $p = 0.945$ and $p = 0.104$ respectively). Frequency of females was slightly higher in those having TDP-43 pathology while education did not differ by TDP-43 status. Of the cases having no TDP-43 pathology, 67% had no dementia and the percentage of participants with no dementia decreased across the TDP-43 stages with only 15% showing no dementia in stage 5 (Table 2).

Relation of TDP-43 stages to dementia

The mean MMSE score, proximate to death was 22.8 (SD 8.2) in the group without TDP-43 pathology while the mean MMSE score was significantly lower in those having TDP-43 pathology being 18.5 (SD 9.8). The MMSE scores were progressively lower across TDP-43 stages 2 to 5 (Table 2). Post hoc pairwise comparisons between the mean MMSE scores of stages 2 and 3 and stages 3 and 4 cases showed no difference while comparison between stages 4 and 5 cases showed significantly lower ($p = 0.003$) MMSE scores in the stage 5 cases. Of the cases without TDP-43 pathology, one-third had dementia. The percentage frequency of dementia increased across the TDP-43 stages with 65% of stage 3, and 85% of stage 5 cases having dementia.

In logistic regression analyses, controlling for demographics and other age-related pathologies, higher odds of dementia were observed in TDP-43 stages 3 (odds ratio 2.68, confidence interval 1.51-4.75, $p < 0.001$), 4 (odds ratio 1.90, confidence interval 1.05-3.42, $p = 0.034$) and 5 cases (odds ratio 5.20, confidence interval 2.23-12. 1, $p < 0.001$) as compared to those without TDP-43 pathology (Table 3). Additional models with dementia as an outcome included interaction terms between the TDP-43 stages and AD, or LB disease or HS. These interaction terms were not significant suggesting that the association of the TDP-43 stages with dementia were not affected by the presence of these diseases.

TDP-43 stages and cognitive domains

Overall impairment of cognitive domains was greater in those with TDP-43 pathology as compared with those without TDP-43 pathology ($p < 0.001$). In those with TDP-43 pathology impairment of specific cognitive domains was varied by the TDP-43 stage (Table 2). The mean scores for the cognitive domains

Table 3 Relation of the five TDP-43 positive stages and age-related pathologies to dementia

Model terms	Relation to dementia	
	OR (95% CI)	*p*-value
TDP-43 stage 1[a]	0.91 (0.62,1.35)	0.645
TDP-43 stage 2[a]	1.38 (0.84, 2.24)	0.203
TDP-43 stage 3[a]	2.68 (1.51, 4.75)	< 0.001
TDP-43 stage 4[a]	1.90 (1.05, 3.42)	0.034
TDP-43 stage 5[a]	5.20 (2.23, 12.1)	< 0.001
AD Pathology	3.81 (2.93, 4.96)	< 0.001
Macroinfarcts	2.27 (1.66, 3.11)	< 0.001
Microinfarcts	1.26 (0.91,1.74)	0.167
Atherosclerosis	1.48 (1.07, 2.04)	0.019
Arteriolosclerosis	1.38 (1.00,1.90)	0.054
Lewy bodies	3.09 (2.20, 4.34)	< 0.001
Hippocampal sclerosis	3.48 (1.86, 6.49)	< 0.001

Estimated from multiple logistic regression models, adjusted for age at death, sex and education
[a]represents contrasts with TDP-43 stage 0

of episodic, semantic, working memory, perceptual speed and visuospatial ability were progressively lower across TDP-43 stages 2 through 5 with lowest values in stage 5 cases. Post hoc pairwise comparisons between stages 2 and 3 cases showed no difference in the values of the five cognitive domains. Comparison of stage 3 and 4 cases showed that episodic memory was more impaired ($p = 0.003$) in the stage 4 cases while impairment of semantic memory was greater ($p = 0.002$) in stage 5 cases as compared to stage 4 cases.

Using linear regression models which controlled for demographics, degenerative and vascular pathologies and infarcts, cases with TDP-43 stages 2 through 5 had a lower level of episodic memory as compared to those without TDP-43 pathology (Table 4). Only Stage 5 subjects showed additional impairment in semantic memory, and perceptual speed.

Discussion

This clinical-pathologic study of community-dwelling older subjects focuses on the pathological and clinical significance of detecting TDP-43 pathology in the ATPC, OFC and midfrontal cortex. Our results show that TDP-43 pathology in the ATPC, but not in the OFC, represents an early neocortical stage in the progression of TDP-43 pathology in aging and AD being intermediate between stage 2 (mesial temporal) and the later stages with more widespread neocortical TDP-43 distribution and that involvement of the ATPC is an important pathologic marker of the transition to dementia. While episodic memory is impaired in stages 2-5, significantly lower MMSE scores, impairment of semantic memory and perceptual speed only occurs when TDP-43 protein involves the midfrontal cortex.

Although the ATPC is known to be degenerated in FTLD [2, 9], and AD [2], there are no reports of TDP-43 protein localization in this region. Several studies of AD [8, 11] and elders without a pathological diagnosis of AD [15, 17] have documented the regional distribution of TDP-43 pathology which occurs in a stereotyped manner with involvement of amygdala and medial temporal structures before involvement of the neocortex. In the present study, the ATPC was the most frequently

Table 4 Relation of TDP-43 stages and age-related pathologies to cognitive outcomes

Model terms	Estimate (SE) *p*-value				
	Episodic Memory	Semantic Memory	Working Memory	Perceptual Speed	Visuospatial Abilities
TDP-43 stage 1[a]	0.05 (0.09) 0.591	0.06 (0.12) 0.592	0.08 (0.09) 0.374	0.10 (0.09) 0.273	0.12 (0.09) 0.174
TDP-43 stage 2[a]	−0.32 (0.12) 0.008	− 0.34 (0.15) 0.024	− 0.16 (0.11) 0.141	− 0..12 (0.12) 0.290	− 0.02 (0.11) 0.874
TDP-43 stage 3[a]	− 0.31 (0.14) 0.023	− 0.06 (0.17) 0.717	0.02 (0.13) 0.879	− 0.13 (0.13) 0.337	0.07 (0.13) 0.594
TDP-43 stage 4[a]	− 0.76 (0.15) < 0.001	− 0.34 (0.18) 0.064	−0.02 (0.13) 0.886	− 0.22 (0.14) 0.108	−0.08 (0.14) 0.574
TDP-43 stage 5[a]	−0.83 (0.18) < 0.001	− 0.97 (0.22) < 0.001	−0.24 (0.16) 0.142	− 0.61 (0.17) < 0.001	−0.20 (0.17) 0.254
AD pathology	−0.90 (0.06) < 0.001	− 0.96 (0.07) < 0.001	−0.55 (0.05) < 0.001	−0.54 (0.06) < 0.001	−0.40 (0.06) < 0.001
Macroinfarcts	−0.40 (0.08) < 0.001	−0.42 (0.10) < 0.001	−0.37 (0.07) < 0.001	−0.25 (0.07) < 0.001	−0.12 (0.07) 0.097
Microinfarcts	−0.08 (0.08) 0.288	−0.15 (0.10) 0.134	− 0.01 (0.07) 0.845	−0.14 (0.07) 0.053	− 0.01 (0.07) 0.905
Atherosclerosis	−0.14 (0.08) 0.078	− 0.10 (0.10) 0.321	−0.05 (0.07) 0.465	− 0.15 (0.07) 0.041	−0.14 (0.07) 0.063
Arteriolosclerosis	−0.23 (0.08) 0.003	−0.20 (0.10) 0.039	− 0.13 (0.07) 0.063	−0.19 (0.07) 0.011	− 0.12 (0.07) 0.107
Lewy body disease	−0.44 (0.08) < 0.001	− 0.79 (0.10) < 0.001	−0.42 (0.07) < 0.001	− 0.42 (0.08) < 0.001	−0.28 (0.08) < 0.001
Hippocampal sclerosis	−0.59 (0.14) < 0.001	− 0.66 (0.17) < 0.001	− 0.24 (0.12) 0.055	−0.21 (0.13) 0.100	− 0.34 (0.13) 0.009

Cognitive outcomes are estimated from separate linear regressions, all adjusted for age at death, sex, and education. Cell entries are estimate, standard error (SE), and probability value
[a]represent contrasts with TDP-43 stage 0

involved neocortical area while OFC involvement was less frequent, although somewhat greater than the midfrontal cortex. Since the ATPC is the most frequently involved neocortical area showing TDP-43 pathology, adding this region to TDP-43 staging protocols will detect more cases having a higher TDP-43 stage with early neocortical involvement. The late involvement of the OFC (stage 4), differentiates the present cases from the FTLD cases which show early involvement of this region [5]. Overall, it appears that TDP-43 pathology in aging is a temporal lobe predominant neurodegenerative disorder with early involvement of the mesial and anterior temporal lobe structures and later involvement of frontal cortex. In 11% of cases there was extension of TDP-43 pathology to the midfrontal cortex which represents the last stage of TDP-43 distribution. In this respect the present staging is similar to the 6 stage TDP-43 distribution scheme in AD in which midfrontal cortex was involved last [8]. However, the present TDP-43 staging is simplified since the last stage was reached by sectioning 8 regions instead of the 14 regions studied in the previous paper and with the present scheme, cases can be staged if for example the brainstem or subcortical regions are unavailable.

Eighteen of the 1160 cases (1.5%) failed to show the proposed regional progression of TDP-43 pathology due to one skipped stage. Since additional sections of these skipped regions were examined and significant neuronal loss was not detected, lack of TDP-43 pathology in these regions was ascribed to the biological variation of TDP-43 distribution. Skipped regions were also reported in other studies of TDP-43 staging [8, 17].

TDP-43 pathology in the ATPC was associated with a higher percentage of cases with pathologic AD and slightly higher percentage of cases with HS pathology compared to TDP-43 involvement limited to the hippocampus or entorhinal cortex (stage 2). These observations support the ATPC being an intermediate pathologic stage of age-related TDP-43 proteinopathy. The observation that the frequency of AD was significantly higher in cases as the TDP-43 stage increases beyond the amygdala was reported previously [11, 14]. Also, the frequency of HS in cases having TDP-43 pathology was 10 fold that observed in those without TDP-43 pathology. In addition, the percentage of HS was higher in the higher TDP-43 stages. Increased frequency of TDP-43 pathology in cases with HS [11, 14, 26] and increased frequency of HS in the higher TDP-43 stages [8, 14] has been noted previously. Frequencies of macro and microinfarcts and vascular diseases were not different in those without and those with TDP-43 pathology including those with involvement of the ATPC. As reported previously [11, 14, 15, 24], there was coexistence of TDP-43 pathology and LB disease, with a significant increase in LB disease in those having TDP-43 pathology as compared to those without TDP-43 pathology. The interrelationship between the TDP-43 pathology stages and these co-morbid pathologies require further study.

TDP-43 pathology stages 3 through 5 were associated with higher odds of dementia which was independent of coexisting pathologic diagnoses of AD, LB disease or HS, suggesting that the progression of TDP-43 from the mesial temporal lobe to the ATPC represents an important transition and likely marks the onset of more severe functional changes.

Impaired episodic memory, a significant finding in AD was present across all the TDP-43 stages except stage 1. The independent association of TDP-43 pathology with impaired episodic memory was also observed in our previous studies of mixed AD and non-AD cases [14, 26] and in community dwelling elders without a pathologic diagnosis of AD or FTLD [15]. Post hoc pairwise comparisons emphasized the differences in the cognitive profiles of stage 3, 4 and 5 cases with impairment of semantic memory occurring only in stage 5 cases. Linear regression did not show an association between stage 3 and 4 cases with semantic memory. Possibly impairment of this modality only occurs with more widespread TDP-43 pathology localization in the midfrontal cortex suggesting that degenerative/functional changes occur as the pathology accumulates. In addition, although ATPC and the midtemporal cortex are known to have a critical role in semantic representation and/or processing [21], the neuroanatomic model of semantic processing is more extensive than just temporal cortex with seven regions (angular, middle temporal, fusiform and parahippocampal, inferior frontal and posterior cingulate gyri, dorsomedial and ventromedial prefrontal cortices) being consistently engaged during functional magnetic resonance imaging and positron emission tomography of subjects [4].

Strengths of this study include detailed data on multiple neuropathologies on a large number of participants obtained in a blinded manner and the availability of detailed clinical data on diagnosis and neuropsychological testing of these participants performed proximate to death. These studies also have high follow-up and autopsy rates that provide internal validity of findings.

A perceived limitation could be the lack of TDP-43 data from the basal ganglia and brainstem. Although, the staging presented in this study is contracted as compared to a previous study of TDP-43 staging in AD [8], the highest stage in both studies shows involvement of the midfrontal cortex. Another potential limitation may be that only one hemisphere was sampled raising the possibility of misclassification. While over half the participants were derived from the community, many were from ROS and these participants likely had better dietary intake, access to health care and levels of education, all factors affecting cognitive risk. The number of minorities in this study is small therefore further studies will be required of minority cohorts.

Conclusions

Pathological and clinical data justified expansion of our previous 3 stage TDP-43 pathology distribution scheme to a 5 stage distribution scheme. Of the neocortical areas studied, ATPC was the earliest neocortical region showing TDP-43 pathology therefore TDP-43 pathology involves the temporal cortex earlier than the frontal cortex. Cases with TDP-43 in the ATPC had significantly increased odds of dementia justifying separation of ATPC to a distinct stage. Impairment of episodic memory was present in stages 2 to 5 but impairment of semantic memory and perceptual speed was only observed when TDP-43 pathology spread from the temporal cortex to involve the midfrontal cortex.

Abbreviations

AD: Alzheimer's disease; ALS: Amyotrophic lateral sclerosis; ANOVA: Analysis of variance; ATPC: Anterior temporal pole cortex; CAA: Cerebral amyloid angiopathy; FTLD: Fronto-temporal lobar degeneration; HS: Hippocampal sclerosis; LB: Lewy body; MAP: Memory and Aging Project; MARS: Minority Aging Research Project; MMSE: Mini-mental state examination; OFC: Orbital frontal cortex; ROS: Religious Orders Study; SD: Standard deviation; TDP-43: Transactive response DNA-binding protein 43

Acknowledgements

We thank the participants of the Religious Orders Study, the Memory and Aging Project and the Minority Aging Research Project, and staff of the Rush Alzheimer's Disease Center including Er-Yun Chen and Wenqing Fan. We also thank M. Neumann and E. Kemmer for providing the phosphorylation specific TDP-43 1D3 antibody.

Funding

This study was supported by NIH National Institute on Aging (R01AG017917, P30AG010161, RF1AG022018, R01AG042210) and the Illinois Department of Public Health.

Authors' contributions

SN and JAS made substantial contributions to conception and design, acquisition of data, analysis and interpretation of data. SN drafted the manuscript and revised it following review of the initial manuscript by all authors. LY and SAL made substantial contributions to the design of the statistical analysis of the data. All authors have given final approval of the version to be published. SN and JAS are accountable for all aspects of the work and will ensure that questions related to the accuracy or integrity of any part of the work are appropriately investigated and resolved.

Competing interests

The authors declare that they have no competing interests.

Author details

[1]Rush Alzheimer Disease Center, Rush University Medical Center, Suite 1000, 1750 W Harrison Street, Chicago, IL 60612, USA. [2]Departments of Pathology (Neuropathology), Rush University Medical Center, Chicago, IL, USA. [3]Departments of Neurological Sciences, Rush University Medical Center, Chicago, IL, USA. [4]Departments of Behavioral Sciences, Rush University Medical Center, Chicago, IL, USA.

References

1. Arai T, Hasegawa M, Akiyama H, Ikeda K, Nonaka T, Mori H, Mann D, Tsuchiya K, Yoshida M, Hashizume Y, Oda T (2006) TDP-43 is a component of ubiquitin-positive tau-negative inclusions in frontotemporal lobar degeneration and amyotrophic lateral sclerosis. Biochem Biophys Res Commun 351:602–611
2. Arnold SE, Hyman BT, Van Hoesen GW (1994) Neuropathologic changes of the temporal pole in Alzheimer's disease and Pick's disease. Arch Neurol 51: 145–150
3. Bennett DA, Schneider JA, Aggarwal NT, Arvanitakis Z, Shah RC, Kelly JF, Fox JH, Cochran EJ, Arends D, Treinkman AD, Wilson RS (2006) Decision rules guiding the clinical diagnosis of Alzheimer's disease in two community-based cohort studies compared to standard practice in a clinic-based cohort study. Neuroepidemiology 27:169–176
4. Binder JR, Desai RH (2011) The neurobiology of semantic memory. Trends Cogn Sci 15:527–536
5. Brettschneider J, Del TK, Irwin DJ, Grossman M, Robinson JL, Toledo JB, Fang L, Van Deerlin VM, Ludolph AC, Lee VM, Braak H, Trojanowski JQ (2014) Sequential distribution of pTDP-43 pathology in behavioral variant frontotemporal dementia (bvFTD). Acta Neuropathol 127:423–439
6. Cairns NJ, Bigio EH, Mackenzie IR, Neumann M, Lee VM, Hatanpaa KJ, White CL III, Schneider JA, Grinberg LT, Halliday G, Duyckaerts C, Lowe JS, Holm IE, Tolnay M, Okamoto K, Yokoo H, Murayama S, Woulfe J, Munoz DG, Dickson DW, Ince PG, Trojanowski JQ, Mann DM (2007) Neuropathologic diagnostic and nosologic criteria for frontotemporal lobar degeneration: consensus of the consortium for frontotemporal lobar degeneration. Acta Neuropathol 114:5–22
7. Hyman BT, Trojanowski JQ (1997) Consensus recommendations for the postmortem diagnosis of Alzheimer disease from the National Institute on Aging and the Reagan institute working group on diagnostic criteria for the neuropathological assessment of Alzheimer disease. J Neuropathol Exp Neurol 56:1095–1097
8. Josephs KA, Murray ME, Whitwell JL, Tosakulwong N, Weigand SD, Petrucelli L, Liesinger AM, Petersen RC, Parisi JE, Dickson DW (2016) Updated TDP-43 in Alzheimer's disease staging scheme. Acta Neuropathol 131:571–585
9. Kril JJ, Halliday GM (2011) Pathological staging of frontotemporal lobar degeneration. J Mol Neurosci 45:379–383
10. Lashley T, Rohrer JD, Mead S, Revesz T (2015) Review: an update on clinical, genetic and pathological aspects of frontotemporal lobar degenerations. Neuropathol Appl Neurobiol 41:858–881
11. McAleese KE, Walker L, Erskine D, Thomas AJ, McKeith IG, Attems J (2017) TDP-43 pathology in Alzheimer's disease, dementia with Lewy bodies and ageing. Brain Pathol 27:472–479
12. McKee AC, Gavett BE, Stern RA, Nowinski CJ, Cantu RC, Kowall NW, Perl DP, Hedley-Whyte ET, Price B, Sullivan C, Morin P, Lee HS, Kubilus CA, Daneshvar DH, Wulff M, Budson AE (2010) TDP-43 proteinopathy and motor neuron disease in chronic traumatic encephalopathy. J Neuropathol Exp Neurol 69:918–929
13. McKhann G, Drachman D, Folstein M, Katzman R, Price D, Stadlan EM (1984) Clinical diagnosis of Alzheimer's disease: report of the NINCDS-ADRDA work group under the auspices of Department of Health and Human Services Task Force on Alzheimer's disease. Neurology 34:939–944
14. Nag S, Yu L, Capuano AW, Wilson RS, Leurgans SE, Bennett DA, Schneider JA (2015) Hippocampal sclerosis and TDP-43 pathology in aging and Alzheimer disease. Ann Neurol 77:942–952
15. Nag S, Yu L, Wilson RS, Chen EY, Bennett DA, Schneider JA (2017) TDP-43 pathology and memory impairment in elders without pathologic diagnoses of AD or FTLD. Neurology 88:653–660
16. Nakashima-Yasuda H, Uryu K, Robinson J, Xie SX, Hurtig H, Duda JE, Arnold SE, Siderowf A, Grossman M, Leverenz JB, Woltjer R, Lopez OL, Hamilton R, Tsuang DW, Galasko D, Masliah E, Kaye J, Clark CM, Montine TJ, Lee VM, Trojanowski JQ (2007) Co-morbidity of TDP-43 proteinopathy in Lewy body related diseases. Acta Neuropathol 114:221–229
17. Nascimento C, Suemoto CK, Rodriguez RD, Alho AT, Leite RP, Farfel JM, Pasqualucci CA, Jacob-Filho W, Grinberg LT (2016) Higher prevalence of TDP-43 Proteinopathy in cognitively normal Asians: a Clinicopathological study on a multiethnic sample. Brain Pathol 26:177–185
18. Nelson PT, Smith CD, Abner EL, Wilfred BJ, Wang WX, Neltner JH, Baker M, Fardo DW, Kryscio RJ, Scheff SW, Jicha GA, Jellinger KA, Van Eldik LJ, Schmitt FA (2013) Hippocampal sclerosis of aging, a prevalent and high-morbidity brain disease. Acta Neuropathol 126:161–177

19. Neumann M, Kwong LK, Lee EB, Kremmer E, Flatley A, Xu Y, Forman MS, Troost D, Kretzschmar HA, Trojanowski JQ, Lee VM (2009) Phosphorylation of S409/410 of TDP-43 is a consistent feature in all sporadic and familial forms of TDP-43 proteinopathies. Acta Neuropathol 117:137–149
20. Neumann M, Sampathu DM, Kwong LK, Truax AC, Micsenyi MC, Chou TT, Bruce J, Schuck T, Grossman M, Clark CM, McCluskey LF, Miller BL, Masliah E, Mackenzie IR, Feldman H, Feiden W, Kretzschmar HA, Trojanowski JQ, Lee VM (2006) Ubiquitinated TDP-43 in frontotemporal lobar degeneration and amyotrophic lateral sclerosis. Science 314:130–133
21. Patterson K, Nestor PJ, Rogers TT (2007) Where do you know what you know? The representation of semantic knowledge in the human brain. Nat Rev Neurosci 8:976–987
22. Schneider JA, Bienias JL, Wilson RS, Berry-Kravis E, Evans DA, Bennett DA (2005) The apolipoprotein E epsilon4 allele increases the odds of chronic cerebral infarction [corrected] detected at autopsy in older persons. Stroke 36:954–959
23. Schneider JA, Wilson RS, Bienias JL, Evans DA, Bennett DA (2004) Cerebral infarctions and the likelihood of dementia from Alzheimer disease pathology. Neurology 62:1148–1155
24. Uchino A, Takao M, Hatsuta H, Sumikura H, Nakano Y, Nogami A, Saito Y, Arai T, Nishiyama K, Murayama S (2015) Incidence and extent of TDP-43 accumulation in aging human brain. Acta Neuropathol Commun 3:35. https://doi.org/10.1186/s40478-015-0215-1
25. Wilson RS, Bennett DA, Bienias JL, Aggarwal NT, Mendes De Leon CF, Morris MC, Schneider JA, Evans DA (2002) Cognitive activity and incident AD in a population-based sample of older persons. Neurology 59:1910–1914
26. Wilson RS, Yu L, Trojanowski JQ, Chen EY, Boyle PA, Bennett DA, Schneider JA (2013) TDP-43 pathology, cognitive decline, and dementia in old age. JAMA Neurol 70:1418–1424
27. Yu L, Boyle PA, Nag S, Leurgans S, Buchman AS, Wilson RS, Arvanitakis Z, Farfel JM, De Jager PL, Bennett DA, Schneider JA (2015) APOE and cerebral amyloid angiopathy in community-dwelling older persons. Neurobiol Aging 36:2946–2953

14

Iatrogenic Creutzfeldt-Jakob disease with Amyloid-β pathology: an international study

Ignazio Cali[1,20*], Mark L. Cohen[1,4], Stéphane Haïk[5,6,7], Piero Parchi[8,9], Giorgio Giaccone[10], Steven J. Collins[11], Diane Kofskey[1,4], Han Wang[12], Catriona A. McLean[13,14], Jean-Philippe Brandel[5,6], Nicolas Privat[5], Véronique Sazdovitch[5,7], Charles Duyckaerts[5,7], Tetsuyuki Kitamoto[15], Ermias D. Belay[16], Ryan A. Maddox[16], Fabrizio Tagliavini[10], Maurizio Pocchiari[17], Ellen Leschek[18], Brian S. Appleby[2,3,4], Jiri G. Safar[1,2,4], Lawrence B. Schonberger[16] and Pierluigi Gambetti[1,19*]

Abstract

The presence of pathology related to the deposition of amyloid-β (Aβ) has been recently reported in iatrogenic Creutzfeldt-Jakob disease (iCJD) acquired from inoculation of growth hormone (GH) extracted from human cadaveric pituitary gland or use of cadaveric dura mater (DM) grafts.

To investigate this phenomenon further, a cohort of 27 iCJD cases – 21 with adequate number of histopathological sections – originating from Australia, France, Italy, and the Unites States, were examined by immunohistochemistry, amyloid staining, and Western blot analysis of the scrapie prion protein (PrP^{Sc}), and compared with age-group matched cases of sporadic CJD (sCJD), Alzheimer disease (AD) or free of neurodegenerative diseases (non-ND). Cases of iCJD and sCJD shared similar profiles of proteinase K-resistant PrP^{Sc} with the exception of iCJD harboring the "MMi" phenotype. Cerebral amyloid angiopathy (CAA), either associated with, or free of, Thioflavin S-positive amyloid core plaques (CP), was observed in 52% of 21 cases of iCJD, which comprised 37.5% and 61.5% of the cases of GH- and DM-iCJD, respectively. If only cases younger than 54 years were considered, Aβ pathology affected 41%, 2% and 0% of iCJD, sCJD and non-ND, respectively. Despite the patients' younger age CAA was more severe in iCJD than sCJD, while Aβ diffuse plaques, in absence of Aβ CP, populated one third of sCJD. Aβ pathology was by far most severe in AD. Tau pathology was scanty in iCJD and sCJD.

In conclusion, (i) despite the divergences in the use of cadaveric GH and DM products, our cases combined with previous studies showed remarkably similar iCJD and Aβ phenotypes indicating that the occurrence of Aβ pathology in iCJD is a widespread phenomenon, (ii) CAA emerges as the hallmark of the Aβ phenotype in iCJD since it is observed in nearly 90% of all iCJD with Aβ pathology reported to date including ours, and it is shared by GH- and DM-iCJD, (iii) although the contributions to Aβ pathology of other factors, including GH deficiency, cannot be discounted, our findings increase the mounting evidence that this pathology is acquired by a mechanism resembling that of prion diseases.

Keywords: Amyloid-β, Pathology, iCJD, Cerebral amyloid angiopathy, Thioflavin S

* Correspondence: ixc20@case.edu; pxg13@case.edu
[1]Departments of Pathology, Case Western Reserve University, School of Medicine, Cleveland, OH 44106, USA
Full list of author information is available at the end of the article

Introduction

The key pathogenic event of all prion diseases is the conversion of a normal or cellular prion protein (PrP^{C}) into a misfolded and disease-associated isoform commonly identified as scrapie prion protein (PrP^{Sc}) or prion. Newly converted PrP^{Sc} then propagates and accumulates preferentially in the central nervous system (CNS) typically accompanied by spongiform degeneration, gliosis and neuronal cell death. These pathogenetic features apply especially to Creutzfeldt-Jakob disease (CJD), by far the most common human prion disease. The pathogenic mechanism based on the conformational conversion of PrP^{C} into PrP^{Sc}, which then acts as a seed, can conceptually accommodate not only PrP^{Sc} accumulation and propagation in the affected subject, but also the potential transmission of the process from affected to non-affected subjects. Although the sporadic and inherited forms account for the majority of human prion diseases [24], less than 1% of the prion diseases is acquired from animals or humans via an infectious mechanism [7]. Within this group, iatrogenic CJD (iCJD) is of particular interest. More than 492 cases of iCJD have been reported worldwide [4]. Most cases have been associated with the administration of growth hormone (GH) extracted from cadaveric pituitary glands and the application of cadaveric dura mater (DM) grafts [7]. The existence of iCJD and experimental evidence have firmly established the infectious property of prion diseases [18, 26, 27].

The central pathogenic event in Alzheimer's disease (AD), the most common cause of dementia, is the deposition of amyloid β (Aβ), a truncated fragment of the amyloid precursor protein (*APP*), which leads to the formation of extracellular Aβ plaques [22, 30]. Deposition of highly phosphorylated, microtubule-associated tau protein (p-tau) also occurs [57] and, is believed to be a downstream event [33]. Most evidence indicates that deposition of Aβ and p-tau in the affected brain is stereotypical and hierarchical [5, 63]. More recently, it has been pointed out that Aβ and p-tau mimic several major characteristics of PrP^{Sc} including mechanisms of accumulation and propagation and formation of distinct Aβ and p-tau species that fulfill some of the characteristics of strains [16, 28, 56, 67, 68]. Like PrP^{Sc}, Aβ has been detected in tissues other than CNS parenchyma including dura mater and pituitary glands [35, 43]. Furthermore, Aβ and p-tau pathologies (but not fully developed AD) have been replicated following Aβ or p-tau intracerebral or peripheral inoculations to transgenic mice that express human *APP* harboring AD pathogenic mutations as well as wild type human *APP*, indicating that Aβ pathology is transmissible [11, 20, 47, 48, 70]. In contrast to prion diseases, there is no evidence that AD and/or tauopathy (e.g., frontotemporal lobar degeneration) transmit from human-to-human.

Five recent studies have independently reported the presence of significant Aβ pathology in 4 of 8, 18 of 33, and 1 of 24 cases of iCJD from the United Kingdom (UK) and France, linked to injections of cadaveric GH (GH-iCJD) [19, 37, 53], and in 5 of 7 Swiss and Austrian iCJD and 13 of 16 Japanese iCJD cases who had received DM grafts (DM-iCJD) [23, 31]. In the most severely affected cases, Aβ amorphous aggregates were also detected in the pituitary gland and DM [37, 43]. The concomitant presence of Aβ and PrP^{Sc} deposits resulting in mixed AD and CJD phenotypes has been reported [8, 25, 50, 65]. However, while the AD-CJD mixed phenotype has been observed in older CJD-affected individuals [29, 64], most of the 28 iCJD cases harboring significant Aβ pathology were under 55 years of age [19, 23, 37, 53]. A possible explanation for the higher prevalence of Aβ pathology at a relatively young age in iCJD-affected subjects is that both Aβ and PrP^{Sc} seeds are transmitted during the iatrogenic procedures and then accumulate and propagate concurrently. However, Ritchie and coworkers have also observed brain Aβ pathology in absence of PrP^{Sc} deposition in recipients of cadaveric GH [53]. This important finding strongly argues for human-to-human transmission of an Aβ-related condition independently from the PrP^{Sc} seeding process. Nonetheless, whether the neuroendocrine deficiency may favor the Aβ pathology in some cases is still unknown [21].

To further investigate the iatrogenic seeding of Aβ pathology, we examined whether this condition occurs not only with UK and French GH as previously described but with receipt of GH produced before 1977 in the United States (US) as well. All US GH-iCJD patients to date received GH made before 1977, when a GH purification procedure was adopted that reduced or eliminated prion contamination. We also wanted to further examine the phenotypes of the DM-iCJD linked to the use of the Lyodura® brand. Out of 27 cases of definite iCJD, we selected 21 which were suitable for detailed histopathological examination and were provided by national prion surveillance centers of Australia, France, Italy, and the US. Cases of sporadic CJD (sCJD), non-neurodegenerative disorders (non-ND), and AD were used as comparison groups. Two autopsied cases who underwent GH treatment but did not develop iCJD were also examined. We report that (i) over 50% of iCJD cases harbored significant Aβ pathology, which included cerebral amyloid angiopathy (CAA) in all cases; (ii) the prevalence of the Aβ-positive iCJD subset was significantly higher than that of Aβ-positive sCJD cases, which were on average 17 years older; (iii) p-tau pathology was present but did not distinguish Aβ-positive iCJD cases from the sCJD controls, and seemed to be age-related; (iv) the phenotypic characteristics of the Aβ pathology in iCJD were distinct from those of typical AD.

Materials and methods

Reagents and antibodies

Dulbecco's Phosphate Buffered Saline (DPBS), NaCl, Nonidet P-40, Sodium deoxycholate, Tris–HCl, Phenylmethanesulfonyl fluoride (PMSF), proteinase K (PK), Thioflavin S, and Kodak Biomax MR and XAR films were from Sigma-Aldrich (St. Louis, MO, USA). Tween 20, β–mercaptoethanol, Tris buffered saline (TBS), 2X Laemmli sample buffer, non-fat dry milk, 15% Criterion Tris–HCl polyacrylamide precast gels, 30% Acrylamide/Bis solution, tetramethylethylenediamine (TEMED), 10% sodium dodecyl sulfate (SDS) and ammonium persulphate (APS) were from Bio-Rad Laboratories (Hercules, CA, USA). Odyssey Blocking Buffer was from LI-COR Biosciences (Lincoln, NE, USA); polyvinylidene difluoride (PVDF) membrane (Immobilon-FL and Immobilon-P) was from EMD Millipore (Billerica, MA, USA). The primary antibodies (Abs) included the AT8 (to human phospho-tau residues Ser202 and Thr205) from Thermo Fisher Scientific Inc. (Waltham, MA, USA), 4G8 (to human Aβ residues 17–24), and 3F4 (to human PrP residues 106–110) [38, 71] from Richard Kascsak at the N.Y.S. Institute for Basic Research; 12B2 (to human PrP residues 89–93) [45] was from the Wageningen University & Research (Lelystad, Netherlands), whereas Tohoku-2 (to human PrP residues 97–103) [42] was kindly provided by Dr. Tetsuyuki Kitamoto. Secondary Abs were the sheep anti-mouse IgG from Life Sciences (Piscataway, NJ, USA), IRDye 800CW goat anti-mouse IgG (1 mg/ml) and IRDye 680RD goat anti-rabbit IgG (1 mg/ml) from LI-COR Biosciences (Lincoln, NE, USA). Reagents ECL and ECL plus were from GE Healthcare, Life Sciences (Piscataway, NJ, USA); Envision Flex Peroxidase Blocking Reagent, Envision Flex/HRP and Envision Flex DAB were from Dako (Dako North America Inc., Carpinteria, USA); the Vectashield mounting medium for fluorescence was from Vector Laboratories Inc. (Burlingame, CA, USA).

Patients

Brain tissue from 27 confirmed iCJD patients was collected in this study. Thirteen of these cases were associated with cadaveric GH extracted from pituitary glands, whereas the other 14 cases were associated with cadaveric DM graft (Table 1 and Additional file 1: Table S1). All GH-iCJD were from the US and were treated with GH under the US National Hormone and Pituitary Program and started their treatment between 1969 and 1974. Tissue from 12 of the 13 US GH-iCJD was obtained at autopsy and one at biopsy. Two DM-iCJD were US cases, but only one -a 26 years old man -had received the Lyodura® brand dura (B. Braun Melsungen AG, Melsungen, Germany) (DM_L-iCJD) whereas the other case -a 39 years old woman -had received the Tutoplast® brand dura (Pfrimmer-Viggo GmbH + Co, Erlangen, Germany) (DM_T-iCJD). An important difference between these brands of dural graft is that unlike Tutoplast, Lyodura brand dural grafts were intermingled with many other dural grafts during the manufacturing procedure, thereby increasing the risk of cross-contamination. Other DM-iCJD cases included 1) two cases from the Australian National CJD Registry (Melbourne, Australia), 2) six cases from the Réseau National de Référence de maladies de Creutzfeldt-Jakob and Centre National de Référence des agents transmissibles non conventionnels (Paris, France), and 3) four cases from the Istituto Superiore di Sanita' (Rome, Italy). With the exception of one French DM-iCJD case, for which the medical product Lyodura® brand could not be confirmed, all cases were DM_L-iCJD. The histopathology and/or clinical and molecular features have been published for two US DM-iCJD (cases 1 and 2, Table 1) [3, 10, 32], three US GH-iCJD (cases 6, 9 and 10, Table 1) [10], and one Australian DM_L-iCJD (case 17, Table 1) [58]. The five distinct comparison groups included 1) two US non-CJD patients who received the GH between years 1973–1977 (50 years) or between years 1977–1981 (46 years). The latter case may not have received any of the pre-1977 produced higher risk US GH material because 1977 was the transition year when a new purification procedure of GH extraction was started [1]; 2) 67 confirmed sCJD cases from Australia ($N = 4$), France ($N = 11$), Italy ($N = 8$) and US ($N = 44$) (Additional file 1: Tables S1 and S2); 3) 11 US autopsied cases of non-ND with age at death of 40 ± 12 years (range, 25–59 years) following diagnosis of blood cancer ($N = 3$; 25, 27 and 41 years), intracranial tumors ($N = 2$; 35 and 44 years), hemoglobin sickle cell disease (28 years), scrotal abscess and pulmonary embolus (31 years), type II diabetes mellitus (47 years), gastrointestinal hemorrhage (50 years), systemic lupus erythematosus (56 years), end stage renal disease and cardiac arrest (59 years); 4) seven US cases of AD with age at death of 64 ± 8 years, and disease duration of 75 ± 39 months [12]. Disease duration was not available in one AD case. All sporadic and iatrogenic CJD cases were classified according to Parchi and collaborators (1999). Since all Aβ-positive cases had multiple cortical sections not all of which were positive, we excluded from the study six Aβ-negative cases with only one section available.

All of the US iCJD and the two CJD-free recipients of GH were collected at the National Prion Disease Pathology Surveillance Center (NPDPSC) in Cleveland (OH) in collaboration with the National Institute of Diabetes, Digestive and Kidney Diseases, NIH, (Bethesda, MD) and Division of High Consequence Pathogens and Pathology, CDC, (Atlanta, GA) and Westat Agency (Rockville, MD). The AD and US sCJD controls were

Table 1 All examined cases of iCJD from countries of treatment with clinical, molecular and histopathological features

Case number	Iatrogenic exposure	Country	Sex	Age at death (years)	Disease duration (months)	Mean incubation period[a] (years)	Codon 129 genotype	PrP^{Sc} type	Histopath. phenotype	Two or more histological sections
1[b,c]	DM_L	United States	M	26	5	19	na	na	MM(MV)1	yes
2[d,e]	DM_T		F	39	4	6	MM	1	MM(MV)1	yes
3	GH		M	33	6	23	VV	na	VV2	yes
4	GH		M	39	17	24	MV	na	MV2K	yes
5	GH		M	39	7	27	MM	2	Atypical	yes
6[e]	GH		F	41	2	26	MM	1	MM(MV)1	yes
7	GH		M	43	26	23	MV	i+2	MV2K	yes
8	GH		M	44	18	32.5	MV	i+2	MV2K	yes
9[e]	GH		M	51	14	38	MM	i	MMi	yes
10[e]	GH		M	54	2	41.5	MM	1	MM(MV)1	yes
11	GH		M	23	19	10	na	na	MV2K or MMi	no
12	GH		M	34	18	23	na	na	MV2K or MMi	no
13	GH		M	37	3	21	na	na	MM(MV)1	no
14	GH		M	42	5	>28[f]	MM	na	Undetermined[g]	no
15[h]	GH		M	52	4	43	na	na	MM(MV)1	no
mean±SD[i]				41±8.5	11±8	28±9.5[j]				
16	DM_L	Australia	M	32	3.5	16.5	MV	na	MM(MV)1	yes
17[k]	DM_L		M	62	2	5	na	na	MM(MV)1	yes
mean±SD				47±21	3±1	11±8				
18	DM_L	France	M	25	8	8	MV	na	MM(MV)1	yes
19	DM_{Unk}		M	29	6	25	MV	1	MM(MV)1	yes
20	DM_L		M	42	5	6	VV	na	VV2	yes
21	DM_L		F	50	14	11	MM	na	MMi	yes
22	DM_L		F	62	4	4	VV	na	VV2	yes
23	DM_L		F	71	4	4	MV	na	MV2K	yes
mean±SD				46.5±18	7±4	10±8				
24	DM_L	Italy	F	23	27	21	VV	2	VV2	yes
25	DM_L		F	26	6	12	MM	na	MM(MV)1	no
26	DM_L		M	42	3.5	18	MM	1+2	MM1+2	yes
27	DM_L		M	75	3	18	VV	2	VV2	yes
mean±SD				41.5±24	10±11.5	17±4				

[a]The mean incubation period was measured from the mid-point of GH therapy or date of receipt of the dura graft to the clinical onset of the disease; [b][3]; [c]Numbers in bold indicate iCJD cases with Aβ-positive pathology; [d][32]; [e] [10]; [f]Unknown starting date for GH treatment (incubation period thought to be greater than 28 years); [g]Associated with severe spongiosis and gliosis; [h]Biopsy; [i]Mean±SD of the US iCJD cases does not include DM_L (case 1) and DM_T (case 2); [j]It does not include case 14; [k][58]; Histopath. histopathological, DM_{Unk} dura mater of an unknown (Unk) brand, *na* not available *SD* standard deviation

from the NPDPSC whereas the 11 non-ND cases were collected in the repository of the Department of Pathology at Case Western Reserve University. The neuropathological study was carried out either in our laboratory or in the laboratories of the participating countries. Neuropathology was reviewed by IC and MC. Western blot (WB) examination of iCJD cases was performed in our laboratory in Cleveland (cases 2, 6–10, 24, 26 and 27, Table 1), at University of California, San Francisco (UCSF) (case 5) as well as in France (case 19, Table 1) and Italy (cases 24, 26 and 27, Table 1).

Histology and immunohistochemistry

Formalin-fixed brain tissue was treated as previously described [9]. Briefly, sections were deparaffinized and rehydrated, immersed in 1X Tris buffered saline-Tween 20 (TBS-T), and endogenous peroxidase blocked after incubation with the Envision Flex Peroxidase Blocking Reagent for 10 minutes (min). Sections were washed, immersed in 1.5 mmol/L hydrochloric acid, microwaved for 15 min and probed with Abs 3F4 (1:1000), 4G8 (1:3000), and AT8 (1:200) for 1 hour (h). After washing and incubation with Envision Flex/HRP polymer for 30 min, sections were treated with Envision Flex DAB to show the immunostaining.

Thioflavin S staining

After deparaffinization, formalin-fixed sections were stained in Thioflavin S for 7 min, washed three times in 80% alcohol, dehydrated in ethanol, cleared in xylene, and cover slipped with Vectashield mounting medium for fluorescence. Sections were kept in the dark at 4 °C for 30 min before being viewed under the fluorescence microscope (Olympus IX71).

Evaluation of the histopathological changes associated with Alzheimer's disease and Prion disease

Histopathological evaluation was performed in 10 or more anatomical regions in most cases. Standard brain locations included the frontal, temporal, parietal, occipital and entorhinal cortices, hippocampus, striatum, thalamus, midbrain and cerebellar hemispheres and/or vermis. Histopathological evaluation included 1) Hematoxylin-eosin (HE) staining, to assess the presence of spongiform degeneration, gliosis, and amyloid Aβ cores; 2) Immunostaining with Abs 4G8, AT8 and 3F4 to Aβ, p-tau and PrP, respectively; 3) Staging of Aβ plaques using monoclonal Ab 4G8 and Thioflavin S, according to Thal et al. [63]. This method identifies five major stages or phases of Aβ plaques deposition affecting the neocortex, including frontal, temporal, parietal and occipital cortices (Phase 1), hippocampus and entorhinal cortex (Phase 2), striatum thalamus and midbrain (Phase 3–4), and cerebellum (Phase 5); 4) Description of the morphology of the Aβ plaques, including a) diffuse plaques, b) core plaques (CP) (i.e., a plaque with a dense core surrounded by a halo and a corona of lightly stained Aβ), c) neuritc plaques (i.e., a core plaque surrounded by p-tau dystrophic neurites); 5) Staging of Aβ CAA, according to previous procedures [61] with recognition of three major phases: CAA affecting the neocortex (Phase 1), hippocampus, entorhinal cortex, cerebellum and midbrain (Phase 2), striatum and thalamus (Phase 3); 6) Typing of CAA, identified as CAA type 1 or type 2 depending on the presence or absence of Aβ deposits in the cortical capillaries [60]. The criteria for the identification of CAA type 1 were i) diameter of the vessels ≤ 10 μm, and ii) deposition of Aβ in the outer basement membrane; 7) Severity of CAA, based on a modified protocol by Vonsattel and coworkers that uses 4G8-stained sections (with the addition of Thioflavin S in some cases) instead of Congo red [66]; 8) Brain distribution of neurofibrillary tangles (NFT) and neocortical distribution of dystrophic neurites (DN); 9) Severity of NFT and DN expressed as NFT or DN density in one microscopic field (area: 1.3×1.0 mm^2, using a 10X objective) harboring the highest density of NFT or DNs in one or more brain regions; severity was scored as mild (≤ 10 NFT or DN), moderate (> 10 to < 30 NFT or DN) and severe (≥ 30 NFT or DN); 10) Automated image acquisition and morphometric analysis to assess density (expressed as the percentage of the area of the cerebral cortex occupied by plaques) and size (diameter) of Thioflavin S-positive Aβ core plaques as well as size (perimeter) of the blood vessel; 11) Semiquantitative analysis of the percentage of 4G8-positive Aβ deposits along the wall of blood vessels; and 12) Double immunostaining with 4G8 and 3F4 to rule out the co-localization of PrP and Aβ [25].

Image acquisition and statistical analysis

Image acquisition was carried out with a Leica DFC 425 digital camera mounted on a Leica DM 2000 microscope. Images were analyzed by the software Image-Pro Plus 7.0 (Media Cybernetics, Inc.). Cumulative survival curves were generated by the Kaplan–Meier analysis. Statistical significance between the survival curves of the individual groups were determined by the log rank (Mantel-Cox) test. When comparing different patient groups, *P*-values were calculated with Chi-square test, Fisher's exact test, Student's t-test (two-tailed). All the statistical analyses were performed using GraphPad Prism 6.0.

Preparation of brain homogenates, proteinase K digestion and Western blot analysis

10% (wt/vol) brain homogenates (BH) prepared in 1X LB100 buffer (100 mM NaCl, 0.5% Nonidet P-40, 0.5% sodium deoxycholate, 10 mM EDTA, 100 mM Tris–HCl, pH 6.9 at 37 °C), were centrifuged at 1000 x g for 5 min at 4 °C, pellets discarded and supernatants (S1) collected. S1 aliquots were incubated with 100 U/ml PK at 37 °C for 1 h [PK specific activity was 48 U/mg at 37 °C, with 1 U/ml equal to 20.8 μg/ml PK]. The enzymatic digestion was stopped with PMSF (3 mM final concentration). Each sample was diluted with an equal volume of 2X Laemmli sample buffer (6% SDS, 20% glycerol, 4 mM EDTA, 5% β –mercaptoethanol, 125 mM Tris–HCl, pH 6.8) and denatured at 100 °C for 10 min. Proteins were separated on 15% Criterion™ Tris–HCl Precast Gels (W x L: 13.3 cm × 8.7 cm) at 120 Volts (V) for 20 min followed by 150 V for 1 h 45 min, or using 15% Tris–HCl SDS–polyacrylamide gels (W x L: 20 cm × 20 cm) at 25 mA/gel for 1 h 45 min followed by 35 mA/gel for 6 h 30 min (Bio-Rad PROTEAN® II xi cell system). For near-infrared WB analysis, proteins were blotted onto the Immobilon-FL PVDF membrane for 2 h, blocked with the Blocking Buffer Odyssey for 45 min and incubated with Abs 3F4 (1:20,000), 12B2 (200 ng/ml) or Tohoku-2 (1:10,000) for 2 h. Membranes were then washed with 1X DPBS containing 0.1% of Tween 20 (1X DPBS-T) and incubated with Abs IRDye 800CW goat anti-mouse IgG (1:15,000) or IRDye 680RD goat anti-rabbit IgG (1:15,000) for 1 h. After washing in 1X DPBS-T, membranes were developed with the Odyssey infrared imaging system (LI-COR Biosciences) as described by the manufacturer. For chemiluminescence, proteins were blotted onto the Immobilon-P PVDF membrane, blocked with 5% non-fat dry milk in 0.1% Tween 20-1X TBS (blocking buffer), and incubated with primary Abs and horseradish peroxidase-conjugated goat anti-mouse secondary Ab (1:3000). Membranes were developed by the enhanced chemiluminesce reaction using ECL and ECL plus reagents, and signal captured on MR and XAR films.

Clinical evaluation

Medical records were reviewed by a clinician (BSA) and data were collected on demographics (age at death, gender, and race/ethnicity). Disease onset was defined as the time at which the first persistent and consistent symptom of prion disease was observed. Data on family history of dementia as well as past medical and surgical history were also collected. The mean incubation period in iCJD was measured from the mid-point of GH therapy or date of receipt of the DM graft to the clinical onset of the disease.

Genetic analysis

DNA was extracted from frozen brain tissues and *APP*, presenilin 1 (*PSEN1*), presenilin 2 (*PSEN2*), and *PRNP* gene analysis was performed as previously described using Illumina and Sanger Sequencing for exons 4 and 5 in *PSEN1* [12]. Sequencing analysis was performed using Mutation Surveyor Version 4.0.7 (Softgenetics, State College, PA). Genotyping of Apolipoprotein E (*ApoE*) single-nucleotide polymorphisms was performed by Sanger sequencing (Center for Human Genetics, Cleveland, OH).

Results

Demographics, molecular features and histopathological phenotype of iCJD and controls including sCJD

We examined 27 cases of iCJD linked to cadaveric DM graft ($N = 14$) or GH ($N = 13$), who received the iatrogenic treatment in Australia, France, Italy and the US (Table 1). Sixty-seven cases of sCJD obtained from the same countries as the iCJD cases were used as controls (Additional file 1: Table S2). The sCJD case population was selected to be as similar to the age of the iCJD case population as possible. As expected, the iCJD cases had a higher percentage of premorbid neurological conditions (including intracranial tumors and head trauma) and neurosurgery given that these conditions often led to treatment with GH and/or DM grafts. No statistical correlations were found when intracranial tumor or head trauma were tested against either Aβ or tau pathologies in the iCJD and sCJD populations (Additional file 1: Table S3). Both iCJD and sCJD cohorts were compared to a seven case group with typical AD (Tables 2 and 3, and Additional file 2: Table S6). The iCJD cases were stratified by country of origin, age at death, disease durations and incubation period (Table 1). The data stratified according to diagnosis, i.e. all-iCJD, GH-iCJD, DM-iCJD and sCJD, as well as according to the age at death, i.e. ≤ 54 years ("young") and > 54 years ("old") are shown in Additional file 1: Table S1 and Additional file 3: Figure S1. For all the cases combined, the three iCJD diagnostic groups revealed no significant difference in mean age at death, disease duration and median survival, while the incubation period was significantly shorter in DM-iCJD than in GH-iCJD ($P < 0.0001$) (Additional file 1: Table S1 and Additional file 3: Figure S1). Separation of cases into young and old subsets underscored the younger age of the GH-iCJD cases, which exclusively populated the young group, and the wide age range of DM-iCJD (Additional file 1: Table S1). In the young group, the incubation period again was significantly shorter in DM-iCJD than GH-iCJD ($P < 0.002$). Overall, disease duration and incubation period were significantly shorter in the older group ($P < 0.0008$ and $P < 0.03$, respectively) (Additional file 1: Table S1). The sCJD control population was 8 years older at death than the iCJD population while disease duration was comparable in the two conditions. Sporadic CJD young cases had a mean age at death comparable to that of GH-iCJD while disease duration in old cases matched that of DM-iCJD (Additional file 1: Table S1).

Table 2 Staging and amyloid presence in Aβ CP from iCJD associated with Aβ pathology along with cases of sCJD and AD used as controls

Case number	Age (y)	Disease durat. (mo)	Codon 129 genotype	PrP^{Sc} type	Phase 1		Phase 2		Phase 3-4		Phase 5	
					Neocortex	Thiofl	Hippoc.	Thiofl	Subcortical	Thiofl	Cerebellum	Thiofl
iCJD												
1 (1)[a]	26	5	na	na	+++[b,c]	+[d]	++	-	+[e]	-	+	-
2 (19)	29	6	MV	1	+++[f]	+	+	+	-	nt	-	nt
3 (8)	44	18	MV	i+2	++++	+	++	-	+++	-	-	-
4 (9)	51	14	MM	i	-	-	-	-	-	nt	+	+
5 (17)	62	2	na	na	++++	+[g]	na	na	na	na	-	-
mean±SD	42±15	9±7			78%[h]		62.5%		40%		40%	
sCJD												
1 (57)[i]	63	3	MV	1	+++[f]	+	++	+	++	nt	-	nt
2 (59)	71	9	MV	2	+[f]	+	-	-	-	nt	-	nt
3 (65)	71	10	VV	2	+	+	-	nt	-	nt	-	nt
4 (67)	79	6	VV	2	+++	+	-	nt	-	nt	-	nt
mean±SD	71±6.5	7±3			57%		25%		17%		0%	
P value[j]					NS		NS		NS		NS	
AD												
1	56	60	na	na	++++	+	++	+	+++	+	+	+
2	56	60	na	na	++++	+	++	+	+++	+	+	+
3	59	na	na	na	++++	+	++	+	+++	+	+	+
4	60	130	na	na	++++	+	++	+	+++	+	+	-
5	70	66	na	na	++++	+	++	+	+++	+	+	+
6	72	111	na	na	++++	+	++	+	+++	-	+	+
7	74	22	na	na	++++	+	++	+	+++	+	+	+
mean±SD	64±8	75±39			100%		100%		100%		100%	
P value[k]					< 0.02		< 0.04		< 0.0004		< 0.05	

Phases 1 to 5 refer to Aβ plaques deposition in various brain regions reflecting disease progression according to Thal et al [63]; [a,i]Numbers in parenthesis in the first column refer to numerals used in [a]Table 1 and [i]Additional file 1: Table S2; [b]Minus and plus signs indicate absence (-) or presence (+) of Aβ pathology affecting one (+), two (++), three (+++) or four (++++) of the brain regions that characterize each phase; Phase 1: frontal, temporal, parietal and occipital cortical regions; Phase 2: hippocampus and entorhinal cortex; Phase 3-4: striatum, thalamus and midbrain; Phase 5: cerebellum; [c,e]Refers to one iCJD with one or two missing sections from the [c]neocortex or [e]subcortical regions; [d]The (+) sign under Thiofl (Thioflavin S) indicates presence of amyloid plaques in at least one brain region; the (-) sign indicates that all regions tested had Thioflavin S negative staining; [f]Refers to one iCJD and two sCJD cases with missing parietal cortex; [g]Positive staining with Congo red [58]; [h]Percentage of brain regions with CP; [j,k]Fisher's exact test comparing iCJD to [j]sCJD or [k]AD; *Hippoc.* hippocampal formation (hippocampus and entorhinal cortex), *y* years, *durat.* duration, *mo* months, *na* not available, *nt* not tested, *NS* not significant, *SD* standard deviation

With regard to the molecular features, the percent distribution of the three genotypes (MM, MV, VV) at codon 129 of the PrP gene in the iCJD population (MM 43%, MV 33%, VV 24%) significantly differed from that of the sCJD controls (MM 65%, MV 18%, VV 17%) as well as those reported for unselected sCJD populations (MM 71%, MV 12%, VV 17%) [15] pointing to an increased relative prevalence of the MV and VV genotypes at the expense of the MM genotype in our iCJD cohort (Fig. 1). The iCJD genotype distribution also differed from those of Western European, Australian and the North American general populations (MM 37%, MV 51%, VV 12%) [14]. Keeping in mind the limited number of cases for some of these analyses, 129 genotype distribution also diverged in the GH-iCJD and DM-iCJD subsets: while the relative representation of the MV genotype was increased in both subsets, the DM-iCJD showed a three times higher representation of the VV genotype (33% vs. 11%) (Fig. 1). Analyses of the PK-resistant PrP^{Sc} ($resPrP^{Sc}$) type distribution showed that in iCJD the combined representation of types 2 (with unglycosylated $resPrP^{Sc}$ of ~19 kDa), "intermediate" (i; ~20 kDa), i + 2 (~20 + 19 kDa), and 1 + 2 (~21 + 19 kDa) (63%) was much higher than the representation of combined type 2 and i + 2 (28%) in sCJD unselected populations [15, 49], as well as in our sCJD controls, a finding consistent with the combined prevalence of the MV and VV genotypes which often are paired with type 2 and i + 2 (Fig. 1). Next, we compared phenotypic characteristics, such as disease duration and histopathological features in age-

Table 3 Staging of Aβ CAA in iCJD and control cases of sCJD and AD

Case number	Age (y)	Disease duration (mo)	Codon 129 genotype	PrP^{Sc} type	Phase 1		Phase 2					Phase 3		Vstl.[a] score	CAA[b] type
					Neocortex	Thiofl	Hippoc.	Thiofl	Crbl	Thiofl	Midb.	Subcort.	Thiofl		
iCJD															
1 (1)[c]	26	5	na	na	+++[d,e]	+[f]	++	+	+	+	na	-[e]	-	3	1
2 (19)	29	6	MV	1	+++[g]	+	+	+	+	nt	+	+	nt	2	2
3 (16)	32	3.5	MV	na	+[h]	na	-	na	-	na	-	-	na	1	2
4 (8)	44	18	MV	i+2	++++	+	++	-	+	+	-	-	-	3	2
5 (21)	50	14	MM	na	+++[g]	+	-	nt	-	nt	+	+	nt	1	2
6 (9)	51	14	MM	i	++	+	-	-	+	+	-	-	-	2	2
7 (10)	54	2	MM	1	+	+	-	-	-	-	-	-	nt	1	2
8 (17)	62	2	na	na	++++	+[i]	na	na	+	+[i]	na	na	na	na	na
9 (22)	62	4	VV	na	++[g]	-	-	nt	+	-	+	+	nt	1	2
10 (23)	71	4	MV	na	-	nt	+	-	+	-	-	-	nt	1	2
11 (27)	75	3	VV	2	++++	-	+	-	+	-	-	-	nt	1	2
mean±SD	50.5±17	7±6			69%[j]		35%		73%		33%	16%			
sCJD															
1 (55)[k]	49	4	MM	1	+[g]	-	-	-	-	nt	-	-	nt	1	2
2 (56)	63	4	MM	1	+[g]	-	++	-	+	-	+	++	nt	1	2
3 (57)	63	3	MV	1	-	-	-	-	+	nt	-	+	nt	1	2
4 (44)	64	1	MM	1	++	+	-	-	-	nt	-	-	-	1	2
5 (58)	71	8	VV	2	+++[g]	-	++	-	+	-	-	-	nt	1	2
6 (66)	74	4.5	VV	2	+	-	-	nt	-	nt	-	-	nt	1	2
mean±SD	64±9	4±2			38%		33%		50%		17%	25%			
P value[l]					< 0.03		NS		NS		NS	NS		= 0.05*	NS*
AD															
1	56	60	na	na	++++	+	-	-	+	+	+	+	-	2	2
2	56	60	na	na	++++	+	-	-	+	+	-	-	-	3	2
3	59	na	na	na	++++	-	-	-	+	+	-	-	-	3	2
4	60	130	na	na	++++	-	-[n]	-	+	-	-	+	+	2	2
5	70	66	na	na	++++	+	+	-	+	+	-	-	-	2	2
6	72	111	na	na	++++	+	+	+	+	+	+	+	+	3	1
7	74	22	na	na	+++	-	-	-	+	+	-	+	-	3	2
mean±SD	64±8	75±39			96%		15%		100%		29%	29%			
P value[m]					< 0.006		NS		NS		NS	NS		< 0.02*	NS*

Phases 1 to 3 refer to Aβ CAA deposition in various brain regions, reflecting disease progression according to Thal et al [61]; [a]Vonsattel (Vstl) 0-3 score of Aβ CAA severity to the highest score in one or more brain locations [66]; [b]Presence (type 1) or absence (type 2) of Aβ deposits in the cortical capillaries [60]; [c,k]Numbers in parenthesis in the first column refer to numerals used in [c]Table 1 and [k]Additional file 1: Table S2; [d]Minus and plus signs indicate absence (-) or presence (+) of Aβ CAA affecting one (+), two (++), three (+++) or four (++++) brain regions in each phase; Phase 1: frontal, temporal, parietal and occipital cortical regions; Phase 2: hippocampus, entorhinal cortex, cerebellum and midbrain; Phase 3: striatum, thalamus; [e]Refers to one iCJD patient with one missing section from neocortex and subcortical regions; [f]The (+) sign under Thiofl (Thioflavin S) indicates presence of positive staining of at least one brain region; the (-) sign indicates that all regions examined had Thioflavin S negative staining; [g]Refers to 3 iCJD and 3 sCJD cases with missing parietal cortex; [h]Refers to one iCJD with missing frontal cortex; [i]Positive staining with Congo red [58]; [j]Percentage of brain regions with Aβ CAA; [l,m]Fisher's exact test comparing iCJD to [l]sCJD or [m]AD; [n]Refers to one AD patient with missing entorhinal cortex; *y* years, *mo* months *Hippoc.* hippocampal formation (hippocampus and entorhinal cortex), *Crbl* cerebellum, *Midb.* midbrain, *Subcort.* subcortical regions (striatum and thalamus), *na* not available, *nt* not tested, *NS* not significant, *SD* standard deviation; *Student's t-test

group matched cases of iCJD and sCJD controls which shared both 129 genotype and PrP^{Sc} type. Iatrogenic CJD with genotypes 129MM coupled with PrP^{Sc} type 1 (iCJDMM1), the only subset with a significant number of age-group matched cases, showed shorter mean disease duration than sCJDMM1 (2.7 vs. 5.6 months; $P > 0.05$). As for the histopathological features, when histopathological phenotypes associated with the same pairing of the 129 genotype and $resPrP^{Sc}$ type were compared, all iCJD phenotypes were found to match

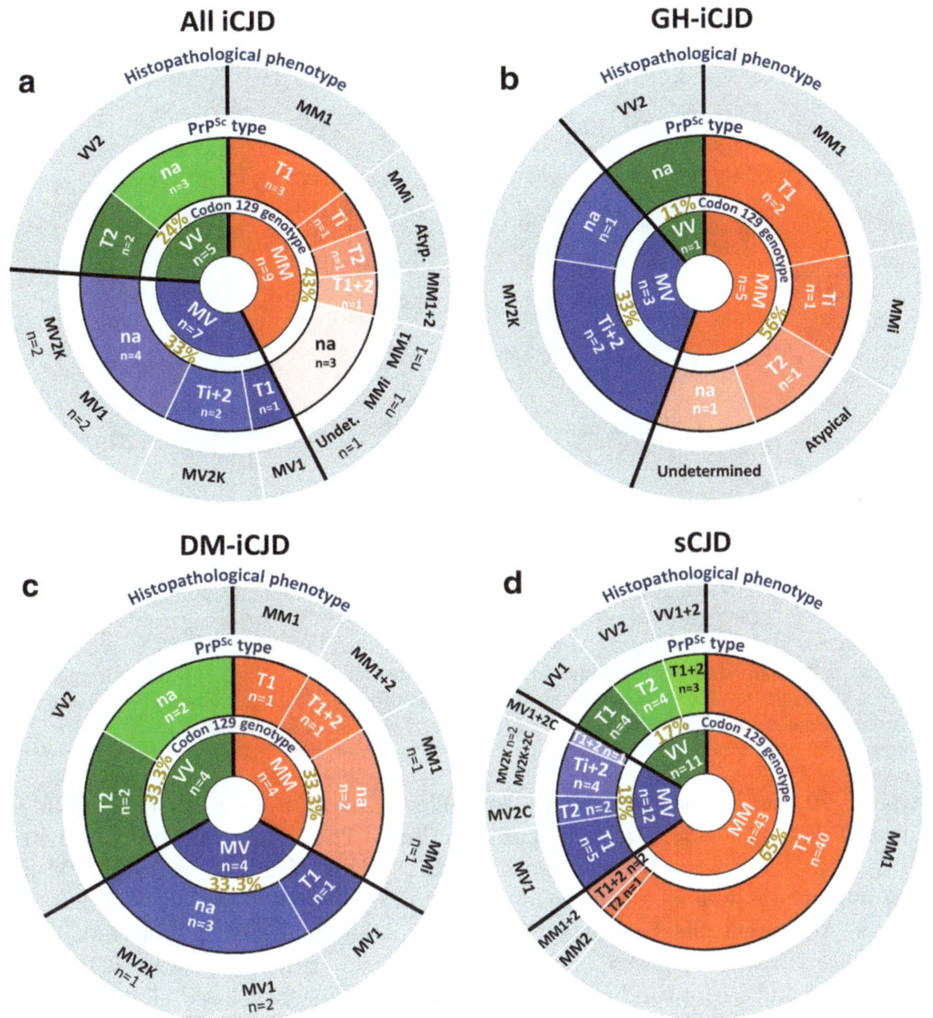

Fig. 1 Ring doughnut charts visualizing distributions of codon 129 genotypes, resPrP^{Sc} types and disease phenotypes among iCJD and sCJD cases examined. **a** whole iCJD cohort; inner circle: percent distribution of codon 129 genotype (MM, MV, VV); intermediate circle: distribution of resPrP^{Sc} types (T1, T2, Ti, Ti ± 2, T1 + 2); outer circle: distribution of histopathological phenotype. **b** GH-iCJD, legend as **a**; **c** DM-iCJD, legend as **a**; **d** sCJD. T1: type 1; Ti: type intermediate; T2: type 2; Ti + 2: type i + 2; T1 + 2: type 1 + 2; n: number of cases; na: not available; Atyp.: atypical; Undet.: undetermined. Percentages refer to the distribution of codon 129 genotype

the phenotypes of the corresponding sCJD, except for three cases. Two of these cases (GH-iCJD case 9 and DM-iCJD case 21), both harboring the 129MM genotype, had a phenotype characterized by the presence of kuru plaques resembling sCJDMV2K phenotype, which is typically not seen in sCJDMM associated either type 1 or 2 (Table 1). However, both these cases matched the previously described iCJDMMi phenotype [10, 39–41, 54]. The phenotype of the third case (GH-iCJD, case 5), which was associated with the 129MM genotype and resPrP^{Sc} type 2, differed in several features from typical phenotype of sCJDMM2. While spongiform degeneration type mimicked that of sCJDMM2, it was limited to the first cortical layers, rather than being widespread in the cerebral cortex, and it was accompanied by severe neuronal loss and astrogliosis while kuru plaques were lacking; furthermore, PrP immunostaining was punctate rather than forming coarse granular deposits (Additional file 4: Figure S2).

Western blot profiles of the resPrP^{Sc} in iCJD and matching sCJD controls

The profiles of resPrP^{Sc} from 10 iCJD suitable cases (2, 6–10, 19, 24, 26 and 27, Table 1) were compared with those of sCJD cases harboring the same 129 genotype and resPrP^{Sc} type (Fig. 2). This comparative study revealed that resPrP^{Sc} profiles from nine of the 10 iCJD cases matched those of the corresponding sCJD subtypes (Fig. 2). Thus, probing with 3F4, all CJDVV2 cases showed an unglycosylated resPrP^{Sc} fragment of ~19 kDa, which typically identifies type 2, whereas CJDMVi + 2

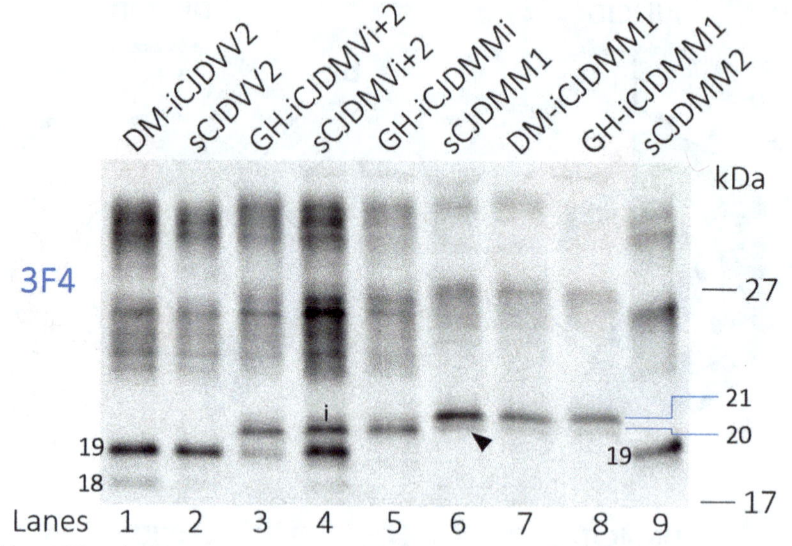

Fig. 2 WB profile of resPrP^{Sc} from iCJD and sCJD controls using high resolution gel electrophoresis. BHs from the frontal cortex (lanes 8 and 9) and cerebellum (lanes 1–7) treated with 100 U/ml PK (~2000 μg/ml) were probed with 3F4. PrP bands were resolved in a 15% Tris–HCl, 20 cm-long gel, and visualized with the near-infrared LI-COR system. The resPrP^{Sc} profiles from iCJD (lanes 1, 3, 5, 7 and 8) and matching sCJD subtypes (lanes 2, 4 and 6) are similar as shown by the co-migration of the unglycosylated resPrP^{Sc} type 2 (19) (lanes 1–4) and type 1 (21) (lanes 6–8). The different thickness of the type 2 (19) band is within the variability range for this subtype. The unglycosylated resPrP^{Sc} band of ~20 kDa, also identified as type i (i), is visible in GH-iCJDMVi + 2 (lane 3), sCJDMVi + 2 (lane 4) and GH-iCJDMMi case (lane 5); a thin band of ~20 kDa (arrowhead) is also present in CJDMM1. An ~18 kDa fragment (18) is also present in CJDVV2 and CJDMVi + 2

cases showed the type i ~20 kDa fragment in addition to the unglycosylated resPrP^{Sc} of ~19 kDa. In both iCJDMM1 and sCJDMM1, resPrP^{Sc} was characterized by the type 1 (~21 kDa) fragment as well as a faint band of ~20 kDa (Fig. 2 and Additional file 5: Figure S3). Conversely, iCJDMMi (case 9, Table 1) showed a prominent fragment matching type i and a faint band of ~21 kDa possibly representing type 1 (Fig. 2 and Additional file 5: Figure S3). These findings confirm the presence of type i in iCJDMMi and CJDMVi + 2 [39, 54], and indicate that in small amounts, a ~20 kDa fragment matching type i in mobility may be present also in iCJDMM1 and sCJDMM1 while type 1 may be present in iCJDMMi (Fig. 2 and Additional file 5: Figure S3). Tissue was not available for a detailed profile determination of resPrP^{Sc} from iCJDMM case 5 (Table 1), but it was reported to be matching resPrP^{Sc} type 2.

Aβ in iCJD, sCJD, prion disease free GH recipients and non-ND: Prevalence, clinical molecular and phenotype features

The presence of Aβ pathology was searched for in all of the 27 iCJD and 67 sCJD cases. Cases were considered positive when at least one Aβ CP containing amyloid (Thioflavin S or Congo red positive) and/or one blood vessel harboring Aβ deposits consistent with CAA were identified in at least one histology section of a minimum of two (Table 1, Fig. 3 and Materials and Methods). Eleven of 21 iCJD cases (52%) fulfilled these selection criteria. They comprised three of the eight cases of GH-iCJD, eight of the 13 cases of DM-iCJD including the two cases of iCJDMMi (cases 9 and 21 of Table 1, Fig. 4 and Additional file 2: Table S4). Despite the relatively small size of the Aβ-positive iCJD subset, a trend could be detected when basic clinical and molecular features as well as the histopathological phenotypes were comparatively analyzed in Aβ-affected and -unaffected groups and their subsets. Subjects harboring Aβ pathology were older in each iCJD subset. Age differentials varied from ~14 to 17 years, while the incubation period was ~13 years longer in Aβ-positive GH-iCJD cases (Fig. 5). Regarding the 129 genotype, the prevalence of the MV and VV genotypes over the MM genotype observed in all iCJD cohort was slightly increased in Aβ-positive iCJD cases (57% vs. 66%) ($P > 0.05$) (Figs. 1 and 5). Furthermore, histopathological phenotypes were similarly distributed in the two iCJD groups. In Aβ-positive iCJD cases (8, 9, 10 and 27 of Table 1) with available frozen tissue the Illumina and Sanger sequencing of *APP*, *PSEN1*, and *PSEN2* genes identified no novel rare variants nor known mutations. Furthermore, *ApoE* genotyping available in Aβ-positive iCJD (8, 9, 10 and 27 of Table 1) and sCJD (65, 66 and 67 of Additional file 1: Table S2) cases underlined the lack of *ApoE-ε4/4*, and the presence of *ApoE-ε3/3* in all CJD cases with the exception of one iCJD (case 8) that had genotype *ApoE-ε2/3*.

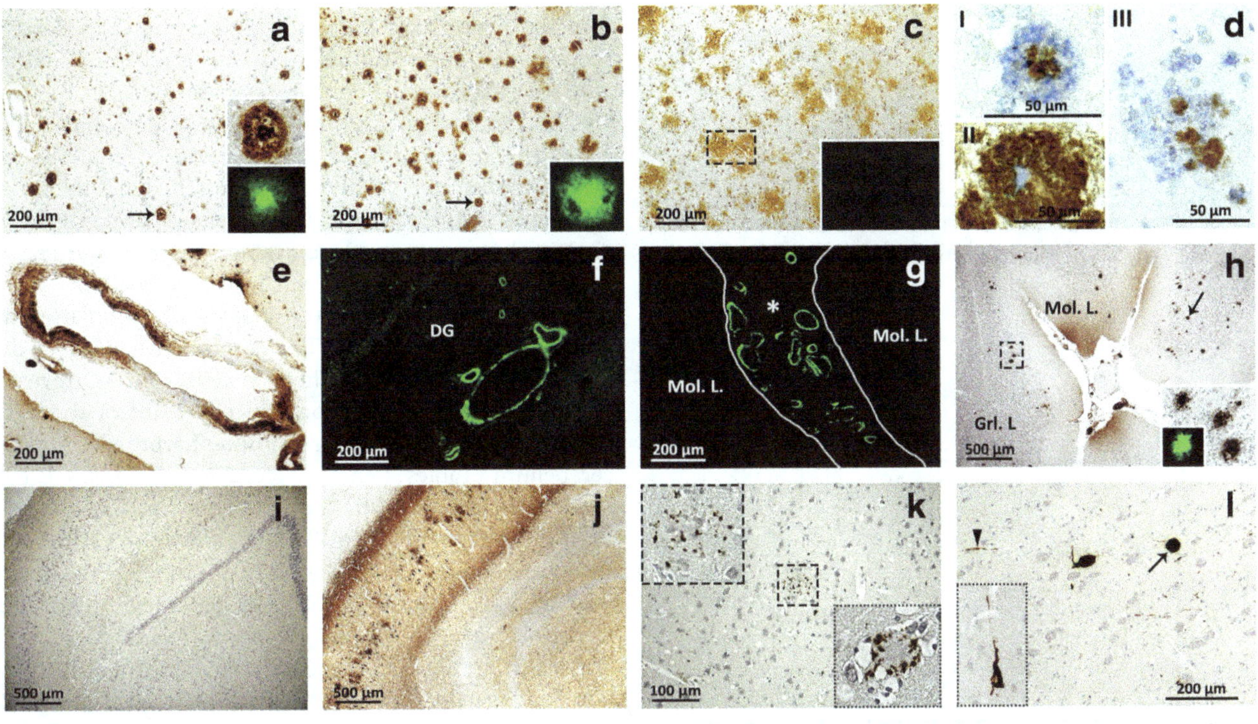

Fig. 3 Aβ and tau pathology of iCJD, sCJD and AD. **a** and **b** typical Aβ CP (arrows) from the frontal cortex of iCJD (**a**) and AD (**b**); inset **a**: Aβ CP at higher magnification immunoprobed for Aβ (top) or stained with Thioflavin S (bottom); inset **b**: Thioflavin S-positive Aβ CP. **c** diffuse plaques from the frontal cortex of a case of sCJD; inset: Thioflavin S-negative staining of plaques (dashed rectangle). **d** co-localization of Aβ (cyan dye) and PrP (brown dye) immunoreactivity in the same plaque from cerebral (I and III) and cerebellar (II) cortices of iCJD. I: plaque exhibiting a PrP-positive core surrounded by an Aβ immunoreactive crown; II-III: plaques showing either the immunostaining opposite to that of I, with Aβ-positive core and a PrP immunoreactive crown (II), or random distribution of PrP- and Aβ-reactive aggregates (III). **e-g** Aβ deposits (**e**) and Thioflavin S-positive staining (**f** and **g**) of vessels in frontal cortex (**e**), hippocampus (**f**) and cerebellum (**g**) in iCJD; **f**: DG, Dentate gyrus; **g**: asterisk, Aβ CAA in the subarachnoid space between two cerebellar folia. **h** Aβ CP predominantly affecting the granular layer (Grl. L) and Purkinje layer of the cerebellum in iCJD (case 9, Table 1); arrow indicates Aβ CP; large and small insets: enlargements of Aβ CP identified by the dashed rectangle in the main figure and a Thioflavin S-positive Aβ CP, respectively. **i-j** hippocampus free of tau pathology in iCJD (**i**) but severely affected in AD (**j**). **k** Tau-positive DN associated with an Aβ CP in frontal cortex of iCJD (case 8, Table 1) (dashed square); top inset: enlargement of tau reactive DN identified in dashed square; bottom inset: DN associated with a PrP kuru plaque in iCJD (occipital cortex, case 9, Table 1). **l** globose NFT (arrow) and neuropil threads (arrowhead) in the nucleus basalis of Meynert of iCJD (case 6, Table 1); inset: flame-shaped NFT in the temporal neocortex of the same iCJD case. Abs: 3F4 (**d**), 4G8 (**a-e**, **h**) and AT8 (**i-l**) to PrP, Aβ and phosphorylated tau, respectively; Thioflavin S to Aβ (**a-c**, **f-h**)

No Aβ pathology was detected in the two GH recipients, 46 and 50 years old, free of prion disease. However, the 50-year old case may not have received the higher risk US GH produced prior 1977.

Similar Aβ pathology was also present in nine of the 67 (13%) sCJD controls (Fig. 4 and Additional file 2: Table S4). The Aβ-positive cases were on average 20 years older than the negative cases ($P < 0.0001$) and had about half the disease duration (5.5 vs. 10.4 months) ($P = 0.029$). As for 129 genotype and PrP^{Sc} type, Aβ-positive sCJD showed a higher relative representation of the MV and VV genotypes and PrP^{Sc} type 2 than the negative cases, a trend resembling that of iCJD. However, contrary to iCJD, the MV2K phenotype was not observed but the VV2 phenotype was better represented in sCJD Aβ-positive cases. Aβ pathology was also searched for in 11 non-ND cases (age 40 ± 12 years, range 25–59 years). The two oldest cases (56- and 59-year-old) were Aβ-positive harboring CP one and CAA the other (Fig. 4).

Aβ in iCJD, sCJD and AD: Histopathological phenotype, severity and staging

All Aβ-positive iCJD cases harbored CAA. However, in about half of these subjects, CAA was accompanied by CP (CAA + CP) consistent with the presence of two phenotypes: CAA alone and CAA + CP (Additional file 2: Table S4). The mean age of the subjects harboring CAA + CP was about 15 years younger than that of the subjects with CAA alone (Tables 2 and 3). Although not statistically significant, this finding suggests that CP presence is not age-related, but more consistent with the existence of two phenotypes. In the sCJD cohort, the presence of CP alone was observed in three of the nine Aβ-positive cases along with five cases

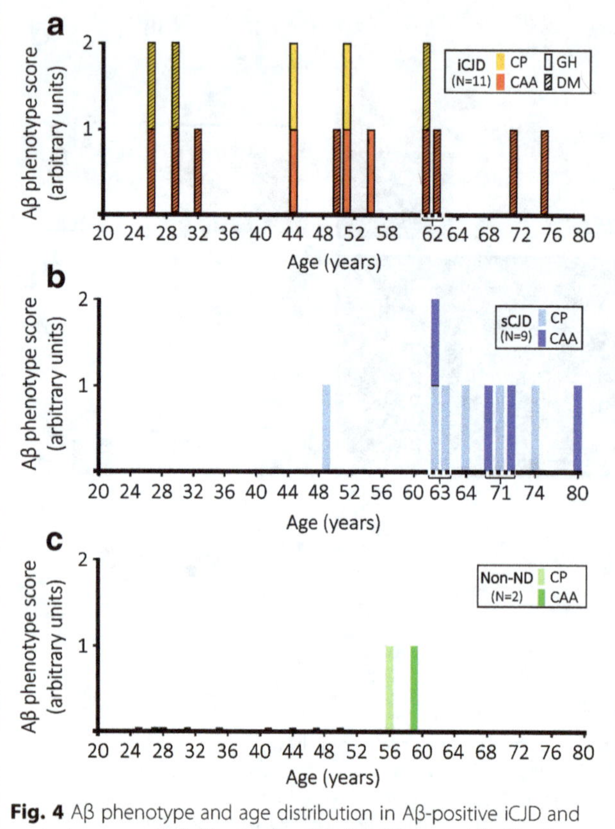

Fig. 4 Aβ phenotype and age distribution in Aβ-positive iCJD and control cases. **a**: iCJD ($N = 11$); **b**: sCJD ($N = 9$); **c**: non-ND ($N = 2$). Scores for the Aβ phenotype is relative to the presence of either Aβ CP or CAA (score 1), or combinations of both (score 2). Brackets below dotted line in the X-axis underline cases of the same age; GH: growth hormone; DM: dura mater

harboring CAA and one CAA + CP (Additional file 2: Table S4). Contrary to iCJD, sCJD cases harboring CP were older than those CP-free (71 vs. 64 years), possibly pointing to a relation to aging. Subpial Aβ deposition was observed in two DM- and one GH-iCJD young cases (≤ 54 years; cases 1, 8 and 16, Table 1) and in two old sCJD (> 54 years; cases 65 and 67, Additional file 1: Table S2).

As for the structural characteristics, most of the iCJD CP appeared to contain only Aβ as the only or dominant component since they reacted exclusively with Abs to Aβ; occasionally, however, they definitely also contained PrP either displaying an Aβ immunoreactive core with PrP reactive crown or the reverse or random mixtures of Aβ and PrP (Fig. 3). No significant difference was detected in the presence and brain distribution of Aβ diffuse (Thioflavin S-negative) plaques between iCJD ($N = 4$) and sCJD ($N = 21$) age-matched cases (Fig. 3 and Additional file 2: Table S5).

Staging of the Aβ pathology, a measure of disease progression, was carried out in 10 Aβ-positive cases of iCJD (Tables 2 and 3). Both CAA occurring alone and CAA + CP had a widespread distribution reaching at least phase 2 in the majority of the cases (82%). The CAA severity score (0–3) ranged from 1 to 3 with a mean of 1.6, and with the exception of one case (case 1, Table 3) CAA was of type 2 (capillaries unaffected) (Table 3 and Fig. 6). As expected according to the selection criteria, amyloid was demonstrated in the CP of all five CP-harboring cases, and in the vascular Aβ deposits of seven of the 10 (70%) CAA cases examined (Tables 2 and 3, and Fig. 3). In two cases, CP were present in the cerebellum (exclusively or along with other regions) mostly populating the granule cell layer (Fig. 3). The comparative study of disease staging in iCJD with those in sCJD and AD revealed that in the sCJD cohort, only in one third of the cases Aβ pathology reached phase 2; none harbored CP in the cerebellum (Tables 2 and 3). The CAA score was 1, 62% lower than that in iCJD, but the type was exclusively 2 as in most cases of iCJD (Table 3). Amyloid was demonstrated in one of six (17%) of the CAA-affected sCJD cases. Contrary to sCJD, Aβ pathology in AD surpassed in severity the Aβ pathology observed in iCJD (Tables 2 and 3). This especially applied to CP distribution that reached phase 5 in all cases, a level of disease progression reached only by half of the cases in iCJD. Furthermore, amyloid-positive CAA was observed in all cases. As for CAA, although the difference in distribution was less striking, the mean CAA score was 2.57, about 1.6 times greater than in iCJD, but CAA was almost exclusively type 2, as in iCJD.

Morphometric characteristics of amyloid-positive CP and of blood vessels carrying Aβ deposits in CAA were compared in iCJD and AD (Additional file 6: Figure S4 and Additional file 7: Figure S5). In iCJD cerebral cortex, the CP burden was over 4 times lower ($P < 0.004$) and CP about 17% smaller than in AD ($P < 0.0001$). A small population of large CP in AD were not detected in the iCJD cohort (Additional file 6: Figure S4). In iCJD CAA-affected vessels the Aβ deposits occupied a relatively larger portion of the vessel wall than in AD ($P < 0.0001$) (Additional file 7: Figure S5).

Tau pathology in iCJD, sCJD and AD: Lesion type, prevalence, staging and severity

NFT and DN, two prototypical lesions of tau pathology associated with typical AD, were found in 48% and 14%, respectively, of all iCJD cases (Additional file 2: Table S4). The NFT were found regardless of the presence of Aβ pathology while the DN were present in 3 cases, all harboring CP (Figs. 3 and 5). Although the NFT-positive iCJD subset was 8 years older than the NFT-free, the difference was not significant. Furthermore, the NFT prevalence in the entire iCJD cohort did not seem to change significantly as a function of age also when young (≤ 54 years) and old (> 54 years) NFT-positive iCJD subsets were assessed (47%

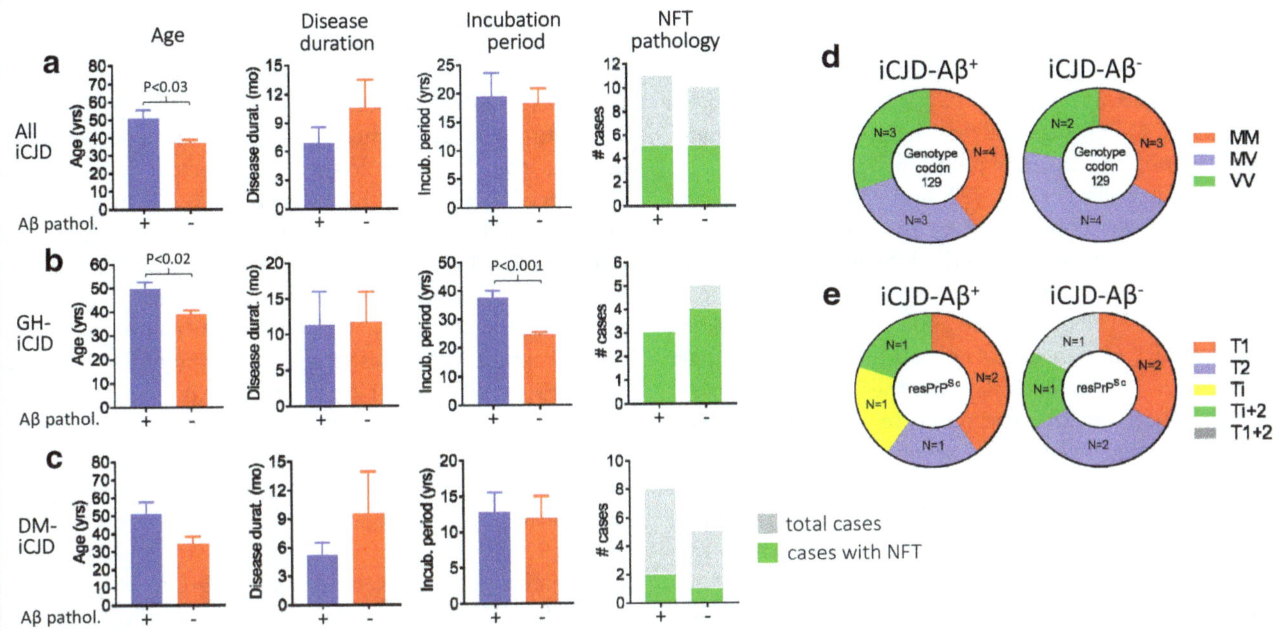

Fig. 5 Graphic representation of demographic data, NFT pathology, codon 129 genotype and resPrP^{Sc} type in iCJD with (+) and without (–) Aβ pathology. **a-c** age, disease duration, incubation period, and NFT pathology relative to All iCJD (**a**), GH-iCJD (**b**) and DM-iCJD (**c**); yrs.: years; mo: months. **d** and **e** ring doughnut charts visualizing genotype frequency at codon 129 (**d**) and resPrP^{Sc} type distribution (**e**) in iCJD with (iCJD-Aβ$^+$) and without (iCJD-Aβ$^-$) Aβ pathology; M: methionine; V: valine; T1: type 1; T2: type 2; Ti: type intermediate; Ti + 2: types intermediate +2; T1 + 2: types 1 + 2

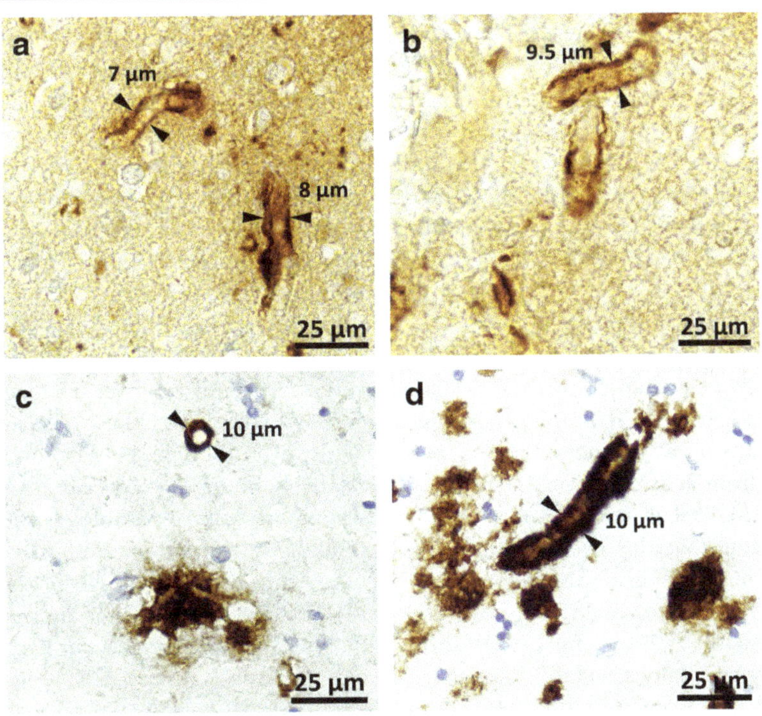

Fig. 6 Type 1 or capillary CAA in one iCJD (**a** and **b**) and one AD (**c** and **d**). **a-d** Aβ deposits along the basement membrane of capillaries in the parahippocampal gyrus (**a**), molecular layer of the cerebellum (**b**) and hippocampus (**c** and **d**). The mean diameter of capillaries in longitudinal sections resulted from three (**a** and **b**) and six (**d**) measurements along the capillary whereas the diameter of the capillary in cross-section in **c** is the mean diameter calculated by the software (Image-Pro Plus)

vs. 50%). In the Aβ-positive iCJD subset, NFT and DN were found in 5/11 and 3/11 cases, respectively. The similar NFT prevalence in the Aβ-positive iCJD population when compared with that of the general iCJD population (45.5% vs. 48%) [23] suggests that the presence of Aβ pathology does not influence the prevalence of NFT.

In sCJD, prevalences of NFT and DN were 53% and 1.5% respectively, comparable to the 48% prevalence of NFT in the iCJD cohort, while the DN prevalence in sCJD compared to iCJD was much lower (Additional file 2: Table S4). The NFT prevalence appeared to be age-related given the NFT presence in 41% and 80% of the younger and older cases, respectively, and the ~ 9.5 years older age of the NFT-positive compared to the negative cases ($P < 0.0006$). Distribution and severity of NFT also were comparable to those of the corresponding iCJD cohort and so was the age relation (Additional file 2: Table S6). Much higher burdens of both NFT and DN with no evidence of age effect were observed in all AD cases. However, brain distribution was comparable to that of iCJD.

Discussion

We report on 21 cases of iCJD including GH-iCJD and DM-iCJD subsets collected in Australia, France, Italy and the US, 11 (52%) of which harbored significant Aβ pathology. Despite the diversity of their geographic origin, our iCJD cases were remarkably similar concerning the 129 genotype and CJD histopathological phenotype distributions, and the features of the associated Aβ pathology.

For DM-iCJD, the similarities may reflect the use of the same Lyodura product in all these countries. In contrast, the cases of GH-iCJD were all from the US and can only be compared with the similar cohorts studied in the UK and France, where methods of GH production differed from those in the US (SH and JPB, personal communication).

Genotype and phenotype distribution in our iCJD cohort showed a relatively high prevalence of MV and VV over MM codon 129 genotypes when compared to sCJD as also observed in previous studies [54, 55]. Furthermore, we observed two iCJD with the MMi phenotype that has been shown to originate from adaptation of sCJDVV2 or sCJDMV2K to the 129MM background of the recipient [39, 42, 54, 59]. The finding that this event, initially described in Japanese DM-iCJD, is also observed in our international iCJD cohort as well as the UK cohort, and thus is widespread, suggests that 129VV and 129MV individuals may have been preferentially selected as donors in several countries. Alternatively, subjects with 129MV and 129VV genotypes might be more susceptible to acquire CJD than the carriers of the 129MM genotype, in whom the sCJDMM1 phenotype might be difficult to reproduce requiring strain adaptation [13, 46, 69]. The ~2 times longer incubation period in GH-iCJD than DM-iCJD cases resembles the longer incubation period associated with the peripheral (e.g., in the peritoneal cavity) vs. central (e.g., intracerebral) inoculations of prions or Aβ seeds in Tg mouse models for these proteinopathies [20, 36]. Concerning the Aβ pathology, iCJD-affected subjects had CAA accompanied by parenchymal Aβ CP in five cases and subpial deposits in three. The Aβ-positive iCJD subset also had a relatively young age (mean 50.5 years, range 26–75 years) along with the relative severity and widespread distribution of CAA [66]. Furthermore, with only one exception, CAA was type 2, i.e. did not affect cerebral capillaries unlike type 1 [66]. Since CAA type 1 has been directly associated with AD severity, including tau pathology, age, and with *ApoE-ε4* allele frequency, the predominance of type 2 CAA in iCJD is not surprising given the relatively younger age and short duration of this condition [52, 62].

Aβ pathology was examined in age-group matched cohorts of sCJD and of non-ND used as controls to rule out the possibility that Aβ deposition in iCJD was either related to aging or resulted from the concomitant aggregation of prion or prion-like proteins by a cross-seeding mechanism. Furthermore, type and severity of the iCJD Aβ pathology was compared with that of AD. The 13% prevalence of Aβ pathology in the sCJD cohort (mean age 50 years, range 24–79 years) was 4 times lower than that in iCJD (52%) even though the Aβ-positive sCJD subset was 17 years older. In the non-ND cohort (age 40 ± 12 years, range 25–59 years), the 2 (18%) Aβ-positive cases were 56 and 59 years of age and the oldest of this cohort. When all Aβ-positive subsets were considered in the 20–54 years range, the prevalence of Aβ pathology in iCJD, sCJD and non-ND populations was 41%, 2% and 0%, respectively. Furthermore, the Aβ pathology in iCJD cases was more severe than sCJD, and showed a significantly more widespread CP and CAA distribution and a trend toward a significantly higher CAA severity score. On the contrary, Aβ pathology in AD was dramatically more severe than in Aβ-positive iCJD with regard to number, size and distribution of CP as well as of CAA in neocortical regions, even though the AD cohort used as control had a relatively young age (64 ± 8 years). These features clearly distinguish the Aβ pathology of iCJD from typical AD. Although we cannot rule out that the Aβ pathology might have evolved toward an AD phenotype had the Aβ positive iCJD patients lived longer and not died of CJD this possibility is unlikely since no significant differences were found between the UK GH-iCJD and hGH recipients free of CJD. Even though we used a different criterion for Aβ plaque selection, our findings on Aβ pathology do not significantly differ from those reported in five previous studies [19, 23, 31, 37, 53], which collectively examined 95 cases of iCJD, including 67 GH-iCJD and 28 DM-iCJD.

However, the 54% prevalence of the Aβ pathology in UK GH-iCJD is higher than the 37.5% we observed. Similarly, the 18 year mean incubation period of UK GH-iCJD is significantly shorter than that of US cases (28 years) ($P <$ 0.004). These differences may relate to the relatively high prevalence of UK GH-iCJD cases (~4.2%) compared to the 1.2% prevalence among US recipients of pre-1977 produced human GH (hGH) as well as to variations in selecting pituitary donors and in protocols of GH purification [2, 4, 7, 54]. Regardless of the causes, the higher prevalence of the Aβ pathology, the significantly lower mean incubation period and the more than a decade younger age differential of UK Aβ-positive GH-iCJD cases, suggest that GH used in UK had a higher infectious dose not only of PrP^{Sc} but also of Aβ seeds. Remarkably, despite these differences, the Aβ phenotype in US and UK was similarly characterized by CAA alone or co-existing with CP. The small subset of Aβ-positive GH-iCJD cases harboring parenchymal Aβ deposits reported by Ritchie and co-workers (2017a) presumably included diffuse plaques, which may also account for the higher prevalence of positive Aβ pathology in UK GH-iCJD. Furthermore, CAA reached similar severity scores in US (1.6) and UK (2) and type 2 CAA markedly predominated in both countries [37, 53]. The very low prevalence of the Aβ pathology (4%) in French GH-iCJD cases compared to the US and UK GH-iCJD cases has been explained possibly by the few years shorter incubation period in French GH-iCJD and to differences in GH preparations [19]. The prevalence of the Aβ pathology in DM-iCJD reported here (61.5%) is similar to that of the previous studies combined (69%) but differs from the 81% prevalence reported by Hamaguchi et al. (2016). This difference may depend on the older age of the Japanese cohort compared to those examined by us and Frontzek et al. (2016) (10 and 16 years, respectively). The co-occurrence of CAA and Aβ parenchymal deposits was observed in all the cases of Frontzek and co-workers (2016) but in only half of ours (CAA occurred alone in the others). This discrepancy along with the aforementioned discrepancy of UK GH-iCJD cases are likely due to our different criteria of Aβ plaque validation. Unlike the five previous studies that also accepted diffuse plaques, we validated only CP (i.e. Aβ plaques that contained amyloid) to better distinguish Aβ pathology associated with iCJD from that related to aging [19, 23, 31, 37, 53]. The exclusion of the plaque amyloid requirement would have increased the the Aβ-positive iCJD cases from 11 to 13 and increased by 9 the number of Aβ-positive sCJD cases (Additional file 2: Table S5 and data not shown). The CP requirement in the Aβ pathology of iCJD might establish a qualitative difference in the Aβ phenotype between iCJD and sCJD in younger populations. Nonetheless, this and previous studies show that CAA, with or without CP, is the distinctive histopathological phenotype of Aβ deposition in iCJD [19, 23, 31, 37, 53]. Our study taking advantage of the direct comparison, also shows that the Aβ phenotype is similar in GH- and DM-iCJD.

Because tau pathology is considered a consistent but secondary feature of AD, we also searched for the presence of the two most common tau related lesions, NFT and DN [33, 34, 57]. NFT were present in Aβ-negative and Aβ-positive iCJD, as well as in sCJD controls with similar prevalences (45–53%), and they were age-related. Occurrence of NFT in absence of Aβ plaques was previously shown in sCJD and was considered as "primary age-related tauopathy" in the elderly [17, 44, 51]. Overall, the NFT prevalence in cases with less than 52 years were similar in iCJD (44%) and sCJD (40%) cases, and did not differ from that reported in a large population of unselected individuals of similar age (41%) [6]. Neocortical DN were observed in only three iCJD cases and one case of sCJD where they were occasionally associated with CP, as previously reported [53]. In contrast, NFT and DN were consistently present in the AD cohort. These findings indicate that tau pathology is (i) a non-obligatory component of iCJD Aβ phenotype, (ii) likely develops independently from the Aβ pathology in iCJD, and (iii) further distinguishes iCJD Aβ pathology from AD.

Further important questions raised by our and previous studies are the origin of Aβ seeding, how Aβ seed reaches the brain, and whether Aβ-seeded diseases are contagious.

In hGH recipients, Ritchie and colleagues [53] convincingly showed that Aβ deposition occurs in the absence of prion pathology and the phenotype associated with the Aβ deposition remains similar to that of Aβ-positive iCJD cases, suggesting that Aβ deposition is a primary co-pathology in GH-iCJD and that Aβ and PrP^{Sc} seeding processes occur independently.

Although we occasionally have observed Aβ-PrP mixed plaques supporting the possibility of co-seeding, the brunt of the two pathologies were anatomically segregated: Aβ deposition affected mostly vessel walls while PrP^{Sc} affected exclusively the brain parenchyma. Moreover, the fact that Aβ-positive iCJD is associated with different CJD subtypes argues against cross-seeding of Aβ by a specific prion strain. Additional support to the independent seeding of Aβ in DM-iCJD comes from two other observations. First, Aβ deposits occurred in the dura graft but not in the patient's original dura [43], secondly, the distribution of Aβ deposits is consistent with the propagation through the brain of Aβ pathology originating from the dura graft while the distribution of PrP^{Sc} pathology is uniform [31, 43]. These findings point to the dura graft as the source of the Aβ seed and to a different tempo of Aβ and PrP^{Sc} propagation further strengthening the notion that in iCJD PrP^{Sc} and Aβ are independent pathologies. In GH-iCJD, the Aβ seed is likely to propagate from the site of cutaneous injection to the brain. Experimental data have definitely provided the proof of principle that human Aβ seed may reach the brain causing Aβ amyloidosis following systemic inoculation [20]. Remarkably, a predominantly vascular distribution of the Aβ deposits consistent with Aβ-CAA was noted in these experiments [20].

Conclusions

Although our and previous studies do not rule out important roles for other factors contributing to Aβ pathology in iCJD such as hGH deficiency or the DM-associated neurosurgical procedures, they point to human-to-human transmission of Aβ with mechanisms similar to those of PrP^{Sc} [19, 23, 31, 37, 53].

Additional files

Additional file 1: Table S1. Age, disease duration and incubation period in iCJD and sCJD divided into three groups according to age at death. **Table S2.** Demographic data and molecular subtypes of 67 sCJD cases from the countries providing iCJD cases used as age-group matched controls in assessing prevalence of Aβ and tau pathologies. **Table S3.** Demographic and medical data on iCJD and sCJD used as controls. (DOCX 37 kb)

Additional file 2: Table S4. Prevalence of Aβ and tau pathologies in iCJD and sCJD used as controls. **Table S5.** Aβ diffuse plaque staging in cases of iCJD and sCJD not associated with Aβ CP pathology. **Table S6.** Brain distribution and severity of NFT and DN in iCJD and control cases of sCJD and AD. (DOCX 49 kb)

Additional file 3: Figure S1. Kaplan–Meier estimates of iCJD and sCJD controls. **A:** survival graphs representing whole iCJD cohort and its GH- and DM-iCJD subsets as well as sCJD cases. **B**: survival graphs of 21 iCJD and all sCJD divided into two groups according to age: 54 years or younger (≤54y), and older than 54 years (> 54y). Median survivals are indicated on the X-axis in **A** and **B** (arrowheads). Significant differences in median survivals, determined by the log rank (Mantel-Cox), were found between GH-iCJD and sCJD (P=0.0017) (**A**) or DM-iCJD ≤ 54y and sCJD ≤ 54y (P=0.0027) (**B**). (PDF 2348 kb)

Additional file 4: Figure S2. Histopathology of an atypical US iCJD (case 5, Table 1). **A-C**: HE staining. **D** and **E**: PrP immunohistochemistry. **A**: spongiform degeneration (SD) with large and confluent vacuoles typical of the sCJDMM2 subtype, but limited to layer II of the frontal cortex, and severe neuronal loss and gliosis affecting all layers. **B**: high magnification of the area highlighted in **A** showing SD with large vacuoles. **C**: severe loss of granule cells and gliosis of the cerebellum; Grl. L: granular layer; Mol. L: molecular layer. **D** and **E**: diffuse or "synaptic" PrP immunostaining in the frontal cortex (**D**), and molecular and granular layers of the cerebellum (**E**); **A-C**: HE staining. **D** and **E**: PrP immunohistochemistry with Ab 3F4. (PDF 30981 kb)

Additional file 5: Figure S3. WB profile of $resPrP^{Sc}$ from iCJD and sCJD controls using different WB systems for PrP detection. BHs from the frontal cortex (lanes 8-10) and cerebellum (lanes 1-7) treated with 100 U/ml PK (~2000 μg/ml) were probed with indicated Abs. PrP bands were resolved in 15% Tris-HCl, 8.7 cm-long (**A-C** and **E**) and 20 cm-long (**D**) gels, and visualized with near-infrared LI-COR system (**A-D** and **E(i)**) or chemiluminescence (**E(ii)** and **E(iii)**). **A**: profiles of $resPrP^{Sc}$ from CJD obtained with an 8.7 cm-long gel are similar to those obtained with the 20 cm-long gels in Fig. 2. The unglycosylated $resPrP^{Sc}$ ~21 kDa of type 1 (21), ~20 kDa of type i (i), ~19 kDa of type 2 (2) and ~18 kDa (18) are indicated. **B**: the ~20 kDa of type i (i) and ~21 kDa of type 1 (21) (lanes 3-8), but not the ~19 kDa band of type 2, immunoreact with Ab 12B2. Profile of $resPrP^{Sc}$ from iCJDMMi (lane 5) is indistinguishable from that of CJDMVi+2 (lanes 3 and 4), but differs from those of iCJDMM1 and sCJDMM1 (lanes 6-8), as the ~21 kDa band predominates in these three conditions. **C**: only ~19 kDa (type 2), but not ~21 kDa (type 1) and ~20 kDa (type i) immunoreacted with Tohoku-2 (To-2). An ~18 kDa (18) band in CJDVV2 and CJDMVi+2, and an unidentified lower size fragment (large arrow) in all cases harboring type 2 were also detected. A non-specific band (indicated by three asterisks) was present in all tested samples. **D**: high resolution gel electrophoresis in 20-cm long gel revealing ~21 kDa (21) and the ~20 kDa band (i and arrowhead). **E(i)**: enhanced image of dashed area in **A** showing the bands ~21 kDa (21), ~20 kDa (i and arrowhead), and ~19 kDa (19; lane 4). The detection of the $resPrP^{Sc}$ ~20 kDa band in addition to the prominent ~21 kDa fragment in CJDMM1 is most likely due to our use of a high resolution electrophoretic systems. **E(ii)**: profiles of unglycosylated $resPrP^{Sc}$ from the same cases in **E(i)** visualized on film by chemiluminescence. Note that the three CJDMM1 (lanes 6-8) show only ~21 kDa bands. **E(iii)**: the ~20 kDa and ~21 kDa bands visible in **B** (lanes 3-5) resolve as a single band of ~21 kDa (lanes 4 and 5) when visualized on film by chemiluminescence. (PDF 6122 kb)

Additional file 6: Figure S4. Quantitative estimates of Thioflavin S-positive Aβ CP affecting the cerebral cortex in subjects with iCJD and sporadic AD (sAD). **A**: the density of Aβ CP, expressed as the percentage of cerebral cortex area occupied, was 5 times greater in subjects with sAD than in iCJD. **B**: size of Aβ CP (N=500), expressed as diameter, was greater in patients with sAD than in those with iCJD. **C** and **D**: representative microscopic fields showing fewer and smaller CP (arrows) in iCJD (**C**) than sAD (**D**) where cluster of very large CP (dashed square) could be detected. Bar graphs are expressed as mean ± standard error of the mean (SEM) in **A** or as mean ± standard deviation in **B**. Student's t-test (two-tailed). (PDF 3338 kb)

Additional file 7: Figure S5. Size of blood vessels examined and semiquantitative evaluation of the percentage of the vessel wall perimeters occupied by Aβ deposits in subjects with iCJD and sporadic AD (sAD). **A**: scatter plot showing the similar sizes of the blood vessels from the subarachnoid spaces of frontal, occipital and cerebellar regions examined for the semiquantitative determinations made in **B**; size of individual vessels is measured as perimeter. **B**: the percentage of the blood vessel wall occupied by Aβ was significantly greater in iCJD than sAD. Bar graphs are expressed as mean±SEM. Student's t-test (two-tailed). (PDF 228 kb)

Abbreviations

Aβ: amyloid β; AD: Alzheimer's disease; *APP*: amyloid precursor protein; *PSEN1*: presenilin 1; *PSEN2*: presenilin 2; *ApoE*: Apolipoprotein E; Ab: antibody; GH: growth hormone; hGH: human GH; DM: dura mater; DM_L: Lyodura® brand DM; DM_T: Tutoplast® brand DM; CJD: Creutzfeldt-Jakob disease; sCJD: sporadic CJD; iCJD: iatrogenic CJD; GH-iCJD: GH-associated iCJD; DM-iCJD: DM-associated iCJD; p-tau: highly phosphorylated tau; PrP^C: normal or cellular prion protein (PrP); PrP^{Sc}: scrapie PrP; $resPrP^{Sc}$: proteinase K-resistant PrP^{Sc}; PK: proteinase K; BH: brain homogenate; WB: Western blot; M: methionine; V: valine; T1: type 1; T2: type 2; T1+2: type 1+2; Ti: type intermediate; Ti+2: type intermediate+2; CAA: cerebral amyloid angiopathy; CP: core plaques; NFT: neurofibrillary tangles; DN: dystrophic neurites; HE: hematoxylin-eosin; Non-ND: non-neurodegenerative disorders; NPDPSC: National Prion Disease Pathology Surveillance Center

Acknowledgements

We thank all the clinicians and administrative personnel for referring patients to the partecipating National Prion Diseases Surveillance Centers. We gratefully acknowledge Dr. Marta Couce, Alison Boyd, Dr. Christiane Stehmann, Dr. Colin L. Masters, Dr. Anna Ladogana, Yvonne Cohen, Dr. Laura Cracco, Dr. Wenquan Zou, Dr. Lan Zhou, James Metcalf, Miriam Warren, Katie Eppic, and Janis Blevins for their assistance and advices.

Funding

This work was supported by: CDC 000309CK14 to J.G. Safar; NIH P01AI106705, NIH 5R01NS083687 and Charles S. Britton Fund. to P. Gambetti; The Réseau National de Référence de maladies de Creutzfeldt-Jakob and the "Centre National de Référence des agents transmissibles non conventionnels" (Paris,

France) are supported by Santé Publique France; Inserm 1127 has received funding from the program "Investissements 276 d'avenir" ANR-10-IAIHU-06; Italian Ministry of Health funding to F. Tagliavini; Stivison Fund for CJD Research to B.S. Appleby; The Australian National Creutzfeldt-Jakob Disease Registry is funded by the Commonwealth Department of Health and S. Collins is funded in part by a NHMRC Practitioner Fellowship (#APP1105784); Grant-in-Aid for Scientific Research on Innovative Areas (Brain Protein Aging and Dementia Control) from MEXT to T. Kitamoto.

Authors' contributions

IC contributed to study design, conducted the experiments, analyzed the data, generated the figures, wrote the manuscript; MLC, SH, PP, GG, SJC, CAM, JPB, EL, FT, MP, JGS acquired and analyzed demographic, clinical and/or pathological data, edited the manuscript; NP, VS, DK, HW acquired clinical and/or pathological data; TK, RAM, EDB, CD edited the manuscript; BSA analyzed and wrote the clinical data, edited the manuscript; LBS: initiated the collaboration, aquired demographic data and edited the manuscript; PG designed and supervised the study, analyzed the data, wrote the manuscript. All authors read and approved the final manuscript.

Competing interests

The authors declare that they have no competing interests.

Author details

[1]Departments of Pathology, Case Western Reserve University, School of Medicine, Cleveland, OH 44106, USA. [2]Departments of Neurology, Case Western Reserve University, School of Medicine, Cleveland, OH 44106, USA. [3]Departments of Psychiatry, Case Western Reserve University, School of Medicine, Cleveland, OH 44106, USA. [4]National Prion Disease Pathology Surveillance Center, Case Western Reserve University, School of Medicine, Cleveland, OH 44106, USA. [5]Inserm U1127, CNRS UMR 7225, Sorbonne Universités, UPMC Univ Paris VI UMR S 1127, Institut du Cerveau et de la Moelle épinière, Paris, France. [6]AP-HP, Cellule Nationale de Référence des maladies de Creutzfeldt-Jakob, Groupe Hospitalier Pitié-Salpêtrière, Paris, France. [7]AP-HP, Laboratoire de Neuropathologie R Escourolle, Groupe Hospitalier Pitié-Salpêtrière, Paris, France. [8]Department of Experimental, Diagnostic and Specialty Medicine, University of Bologna, Bologna, Italy. [9]IRCCS, Institute of Neurological Sciences, Bologna, Italy. [10]Fondazione IRCCS, Istituto Neurologico Carlo Besta, Milan, Italy. [11]Australian National Creutzfeldt-Jakob Disease Registry, Department of Medicine, and The Florey Institute of Neuroscience and Mental Health, The University of Melbourne, Parkville 3010, Australia. [12]Department of Neurology, University Hospitals Cleveland Medical Center, Cleveland, OH 44106, USA. [13]Department of Anatomical Pathology, Alfred Health, Melbourne 3181, Australia. [14]Victorian Brain Bank, the Florey institute of Neuroscience and Mental Health, The University of Melbourne, Parkville 3010, Australia. [15]Department of Neurological Science, Tohoku University Graduate School of Medicine, Sendai, Japan. [16]Division of High-Consequence Pathogens and Pathology, National Center for Emerging and Zoonotic Infectious Diseases, Centers for Disease Control and Prevention, Atlanta, GA, USA. [17]Department of Neurosciences, Istituto Superiore di Sanità, Rome, Italy. [18]National Institute of Diabetes and Digestive and Kidney Diseases, National Institutes of Health, Department of Health and Human Services, Bethesda, MD, USA. [19]Department of Pathology, 4th floor, room 419, Case Western Reserve University, 2085 Adelbert Road, Cleveland, OH 44106, USA. [20]Department of Pathology, 4th floor, room 402C, Case Western Reserve University, 2085 Adelbert Road, Cleveland, OH 44106, USA.

References

1. Abrams JY, Schonberger LB, Belay ED, Maddox RA, Leschek EW, Mills JL, Wysowski DK, Fradkin JE (2011) Lower risk of Creutzfeldt-Jakob disease in pituitary growth hormone recipients initiating treatment after 1977. J Clin Endocrinol Metab 96:E1666–E1669. https://doi.org/10.1210/jc.2011-1357
2. Belay ED, Schonberger LB (2005) The public health impact of prion diseases. Annu Rev Public Health 26:191–212. https://doi.org/10.1146/annurev.publhealth.26.021304.144536
3. Blossom DB, Maddox RA, Beavers SF, Church KA, Thoroughman DA, Schonberger LB, Belay ED (2007) A case of Creutzfeldt-Jakob disease associated with a dura mater graft in the United States. Infect Control Hosp Epidemiol 28:1396–1397. https://doi.org/10.1086/523862
4. Bonda DJ, Manjila S, Mehndiratta P, Khan F, Miller BR, Onwuzulike K, Puoti G, Cohen ML, Schonberger LB, Cali I (2016) Human prion diseases: surgical lessons learned from iatrogenic prion transmission. Neurosurg Focus 41:E10. https://doi.org/10.3171/2016.5.FOCUS15126
5. Braak H, Braak E (1995) Staging of Alzheimer's disease-related neurofibrillary changes. Neurobiol Aging 16:271–278 discussion 278–284
6. Braak H, Thal DR, Ghebremedhin E, Del Tredici K (2011) Stages of the pathologic process in Alzheimer disease: age categories from 1 to 100 years. J Neuropathol Exp Neurol 70:960–969. https://doi.org/10.1097/NEN.0b013e318232a379
7. Brown P, Brandel J-P, Sato T, Nakamura Y, MacKenzie J, Will RG, Ladogana A, Pocchiari M, Leschek EW, Schonberger LB (2012) Iatrogenic Creutzfeldt-Jakob disease, final assessment. Emerg Infect Dis 18:901–907. https://doi.org/10.3201/eid1806.120116
8. Bugiani O, Giaccone G, Verga L, Pollo B, Frangione B, Farlow MR, Tagliavini F, Ghetti B (1993) Beta PP participates in PrP-amyloid plaques of Gerstmann-Sträussler-Scheinker disease, Indiana kindred. J Neuropathol Exp Neurol 52:64–70
9. Cali I, Castellani R, Yuan J, Al-Shekhlee A, Cohen ML, Xiao X, Moleres FJ, Parchi P, Zou W-Q, Gambetti P (2006) Classification of sporadic Creutzfeldt-Jakob disease revisited. Brain J Neurol 129:2266–2277. https://doi.org/10.1093/brain/awl224
10. Cali I, Miller CJ, Parisi JE, Geschwind MD, Gambetti P, Schonberger LB (2015) Distinct pathological phenotypes of Creutzfeldt-Jakob disease in recipients of prion-contaminated growth hormone. Acta Neuropathol Commun 3:37. https://doi.org/10.1186/s40478-015-0214-2
11. Clavaguera F, Bolmont T, Crowther RA, Abramowski D, Frank S, Probst A, Fraser G, Stalder AK, Beibel M, Staufenbiel M, Jucker M, Goedert M, Tolnay M (2009) Transmission and spreading of tauopathy in transgenic mouse brain. Nat Cell Biol 11:909–913. https://doi.org/10.1038/ncb1901
12. Cohen ML, Kim C, Haldiman T, ElHag M, Mehndiratta P, Pichet T, Lissemore F, Shea M, Cohen Y, Chen W, Blevins J, Appleby BS, Surewicz K, Surewicz WK, Sajatovic M, Tatsuoka C, Zhang S, Mayo P, Butkiewicz M, Haines JL, Lerner AJ, Safar JG (2015) Rapidly progressive Alzheimer's disease features distinct structures of amyloid-β. Brain J Neurol 138:1009–1022. https://doi.org/10.1093/brain/awv006
13. Collinge J (2010) Medicine. Prion strain mutation and selection Science 328: 1111–1112. https://doi.org/10.1126/science.1190815
14. Collinge J, Palmer MS, Dryden AJ (1991) Genetic predisposition to iatrogenic Creutzfeldt-Jakob disease. Lancet Lond Engl 337:1441–1442
15. Collins SJ, Sanchez-Juan P, Masters CL, Klug GM, van Duijn C, Poleggi A, Pocchiari M, Almonti S, Cuadrado-Corrales N, de Pedro-Cuesta J, Budka H, Gelpi E, Glatzel M, Tolnay M, Hewer E, Zerr I, Heinemann U, Kretzschmar HA, Jansen GH, Olsen E, Mitrova E, Alpérovitch A, Brandel J-P, Mackenzie J, Murray K, Will RG (2006) Determinants of diagnostic investigation sensitivities across the clinical spectrum of sporadic Creutzfeldt-Jakob disease. Brain J Neurol 129:2278–2287. https://doi.org/10.1093/brain/awl159
16. Condello C, Stöhr J (2017) Aβ propagation and strains: implications for the phenotypic diversity in Alzheimer's disease. Neurobiol Dis. https://doi.org/10.1016/j.nbd.2017.03.014
17. Crary JF, Trojanowski JQ, Schneider JA, Abisambra JF, Abner EL, Alafuzoff I, Arnold SE, Attems J, Beach TG, Bigio EH, Cairns NJ, Dickson DW, Gearing M, Grinberg LT, Hof PR, Hyman BT, Jellinger K, Jicha GA, Kovacs GG, Knopman DS, Kofler J, Kukull WA, Mackenzie IR, Masliah E, McKee A, Montine TJ, Murray ME, Neltner JH, Santa-Maria I, Seeley WW, Serrano-Pozo A, Shelanski ML, Stein T, Takao M, Thal DR, Toledo JB, Troncoso JC, Vonsattel JP, White CL, Wisniewski T, Woltjer RL, Yamada M, Nelson PT (2014) Primary age-related tauopathy (PART): a common pathology associated with human aging. Acta Neuropathol (Berl) 128:755–766. https://doi.org/10.1007/s00401-014-1349-0
18. Duffy P, Wolf J, Collins G, DeVoe AG, Streeten B, Cowen D (1974) Letter: possible person-to-person transmission of Creutzfeldt-Jakob disease. N Engl J Med 290:692–693
19. Duyckaerts C, Sazdovitch V, Ando K, Seilhean D, Privat N, Yilmaz Z, Peckeu L, Amar E, Comoy E, Maceski A, Lehmann S, Brion J-P, Brandel J-P, Haïk S (2017) Neuropathology of iatrogenic Creutzfeldt-Jakob disease and immunoassay of French cadaver-sourced growth hormone batches suggest possible transmission of tauopathy and long incubation periods for the transmission of Abeta pathology. Acta Neuropathol (Berl). https://doi.org/10.1007/s00401-017-1791-x

20. Eisele YS, Obermüller U, Heilbronner G, Baumann F, Kaeser SA, Wolburg H, Walker LC, Staufenbiel M, Heikenwalder M, Jucker M (2010) Peripherally applied Abeta-containing inoculates induce cerebral beta-amyloidosis. Science 330:980–982. https://doi.org/10.1126/science.1194516
21. Feeney C, Scott GP, Cole JH, Sastre M, Goldstone AP, Leech R (2016) Seeds of neuroendocrine doubt. Nature 535:E1–E2. https://doi.org/10.1038/nature18602
22. Friedrich RP, Tepper K, Rönicke R, Soom M, Westermann M, Reymann K, Kaether C, Fändrich M (2010) Mechanism of amyloid plaque formation suggests an intracellular basis of Abeta pathogenicity. Proc Natl Acad Sci U S A 107:1942–1947. https://doi.org/10.1073/pnas.0904532106
23. Frontzek K, Lutz MI, Aguzzi A, Kovacs GG, Budka H (2016) Amyloid-β pathology and cerebral amyloid angiopathy are frequent in iatrogenic Creutzfeldt-Jakob disease after dural grafting. Swiss Med Wkly 146:w14287. https://doi.org/10.4414/smw.2016.14287
24. Gambetti P, Notari S (2013) Human sporadic Prion diseases. In: Gambetti P (ed) Zou W-Q. Prions and Diseases, Springer New York, pp 59–72
25. Ghoshal N, Cali I, Perrin RJ, Josephson SA, Sun N, Gambetti P, Morris JC (2009) Codistribution of amyloid beta plaques and spongiform degeneration in familial Creutzfeldt-Jakob disease with the E200K-129M haplotype. Arch Neurol 66:1240–1246. https://doi.org/10.1001/archneurol.2009.224
26. Gibbs CJ, Asher DM, Brown PW, Fradkin JE, Gajdusek DC (1993) Creutzfeldt-Jakob disease infectivity of growth hormone derived from human pituitary glands. N Engl J Med 328:358–359. https://doi.org/10.1056/NEJM199302043280520
27. Gibbs CJ, Asher DM, Kobrine A, Amyx HL, Sulima MP, Gajdusek DC (1994) Transmission of Creutzfeldt-Jakob disease to a chimpanzee by electrodes contaminated during neurosurgery. J Neurol Neurosurg Psychiatry 57:757–758
28. Goedert M, Masuda-Suzukake M, Falcon B (2017) Like prions: the propagation of aggregated tau and α-synuclein in neurodegeneration. Brain J Neurol 140:266–278. https://doi.org/10.1093/brain/aww230
29. Hainfellner JA, Wanschitz J, Jellinger K, Liberski PP, Gullotta F, Budka H (1998) Coexistence of Alzheimer-type neuropathology in Creutzfeldt-Jakob disease. Acta Neuropathol (Berl) 96:116–122
30. Hamaguchi T, Eisele YS, Varvel NH, Lamb BT, Walker LC, Jucker M (2012) The presence of Aβ seeds, and not age per se, is critical to the initiation of Aβ deposition in the brain. Acta Neuropathol (Berl) 123:31–37. https://doi.org/10.1007/s00401-011-0912-1
31. Hamaguchi T, Taniguchi Y, Sakai K, Kitamoto T, Takao M, Murayama S, Iwasaki Y, Yoshida M, Shimizu H, Kakita A, Takahashi H, Suzuki H, Naiki H, Sanjo N, Mizusawa H, Yamada M (2016) Significant association of cadaveric dura mater grafting with subpial Aβ deposition and meningeal amyloid angiopathy. Acta Neuropathol (Berl) 132:313–315. https://doi.org/10.1007/s00401-016-1588-3
32. Hannah EL, Belay ED, Gambetti P, Krause G, Parchi P, Capellari S, Hoffman RE, Schonberger LB (2001) Creutzfeldt-Jakob disease after receipt of a previously unimplicated brand of dura mater graft. Neurology 56:1080–1083
33. Hardy JA, Higgins GA (1992) Alzheimer's disease: the amyloid cascade hypothesis. Science 256:184–185
34. Hawkes CA, Carare RO, Weller RO (2014) Amyloid and tau in the brain in sporadic Alzheimer's disease: defining the chicken and the egg. Acta Neuropathol (Berl) 127:617–618. https://doi.org/10.1007/s00401-014-1243-9
35. Irwin DJ, Abrams JY, Schonberger LB, Leschek EW, Mills JL, Lee VM-Y, Trojanowski JQ (2013) Evaluation of potential infectivity of Alzheimer and Parkinson disease proteins in recipients of cadaver-derived human growth hormone. JAMA Neurol 70:462 468. https://doi.org/10.1001/jamaneurol.2013.1933
36. Jacquemot C, Cuche C, Dormont D, Lazarini F (2005) High incidence of scrapie induced by repeated injections of subinfectious prion doses. J Virol 79:8904–8908. https://doi.org/10.1128/JVI.79.14.8904-8908.2005
37. Jaunmuktane Z, Mead S, Ellis M, Wadsworth JDF, Nicoll AJ, Kenny J, Launchbury F, Linehan J, Richard-Loendt A, Walker AS, Rudge P, Collinge J, Brandner S (2015) Evidence for human transmission of amyloid-β pathology and cerebral amyloid angiopathy. Nature 525:247–250. https://doi.org/10.1038/nature15369
38. Kascsak RJ, Rubenstein R, Merz PA, Tonna-DeMasi M, Fersko R, Carp RI, Wisniewski HM, Diringer H (1987) Mouse polyclonal and monoclonal antibody to scrapie-associated fibril proteins. J Virol 61:3688–3693
39. Kobayashi A, Matsuura Y, Mohri S, Kitamoto T (2014) Distinct origins of dura mater graft-associated Creutzfeldt-Jakob disease: past and future problems. Acta Neuropathol Commun 2:32. https://doi.org/10.1186/2051-5960-2-32
40. Kobayashi A, Parchi P, Yamada M, Brown P, Saverioni D, Matsuura Y, Takeuchi A, Mohri S, Kitamoto T (2015) Transmission properties of atypical Creutzfeldt-Jakob disease: a clue to disease etiology? J Virol 89:3939–3946. https://doi.org/10.1128/JVI.03183-14
41. Kobayashi A, Parchi P, Yamada M, Mohri S, Kitamoto T (2016) Neuropathological and biochemical criteria to identify acquired Creutzfeldt-Jakob disease among presumed sporadic cases. Neuropathol Off J Jpn Soc Neuropathol 36:305–310. https://doi.org/10.1111/neup.12270
42. Kobayashi A, Sakuma N, Matsuura Y, Mohri S, Aguzzi A, Kitamoto T (2010) Experimental verification of a traceback phenomenon in prion infection. J Virol 84:3230–3238. https://doi.org/10.1128/JVI.02387-09
43. Kovacs GG, Lutz MI, Ricken G, Ströbel T, Höftberger R, Preusser M, Regelsberger G, Hönigschnabl S, Reiner A, Fischer P, Budka H, Hainfellner JA (2016) Dura mater is a potential source of Aβ seeds. Acta Neuropathol (Berl) 131:911–923. https://doi.org/10.1007/s00401-016-1565-x
44. Kovacs GG, Rahimi J, Ströbel T, Lutz MI, Regelsberger G, Streichenberger N, Perret-Liaudet A, Höftberger R, Liberski PP, Budka H, Sikorska B (2017) Tau pathology in Creutzfeldt-Jakob disease revisited. Brain Pathol Zurich Switz 27:332–344. https://doi.org/10.1111/bpa.12411
45. Langeveld JPM, Jacobs JG, Erkens JHF, Bossers A, van Zijderveld FG, van Keulen LJM (2006) Rapid and discriminatory diagnosis of scrapie and BSE in retro-pharyngeal lymph nodes of sheep. BMC Vet Res 2:19. https://doi.org/10.1186/1746-6148-2-19
46. Makarava N, Savtchenko R, Alexeeva I, Rohwer RG, Baskakov IV (2016) New molecular insight into mechanism of evolution of mammalian synthetic Prions. Am J Pathol 186:1006–1014. https://doi.org/10.1016/j.ajpath.2015.11.013
47. Meyer-Luehmann M, Coomaraswamy J, Bolmont T, Kaeser S, Schaefer C, Kilger E, Neuenschwander A, Abramowski D, Frey P, Jaton AL, Vigouret J-M, Paganetti P, Walsh DM, Mathews PM, Ghiso J, Staufenbiel M, Walker LC, Jucker M (2006) Exogenous induction of cerebral beta-amyloidogenesis is governed by agent and host. Science 313:1781–1784. https://doi.org/10.1126/science.1131864
48. Morales R, Duran-Aniotz C, Castilla J, Estrada LD, Soto C (2012) De novo induction of amyloid-β deposition in vivo. Mol Psychiatry 17:1347–1353. https://doi.org/10.1038/mp.2011.120
49. Parchi P, Giese A, Capellari S, Brown P, Schulz-Schaeffer W, Windl O, Zerr I, Budka H, Kopp N, Piccardo P, Poser S, Rojiani A, Streichemberger N, Julien J, Vital C, Ghetti B, Gambetti P, Kretzschmar H (1999) Classification of sporadic Creutzfeldt-Jakob disease based on molecular and phenotypic analysis of 300 subjects. Ann Neurol 46:224–233
50. Preusser M, Ströbel T, Gelpi E, Eiler M, Broessner G, Schmutzhard E, Budka H (2006) Alzheimer-type neuropathology in a 28 year old patient with iatrogenic Creutzfeldt-Jakob disease after dural grafting. J Neurol Neurosurg Psychiatry 77:413–416. https://doi.org/10.1136/jnnp.2005.070805
51. Reiniger L, Lukic A, Linehan J, Rudge P, Collinge J, Mead S, Brandner S (2011) Tau, prions and Aβ: the triad of neurodegeneration. Acta Neuropathol (Berl) 121:5–20. https://doi.org/10.1007/s00401-010-0691-0
52. Richard E, Carrano A, Hoozemans JJ, van Horssen J, van Haastert ES, Eurelings LS, de Vries HE, Thal DR, Eikelenboom P, van Gool WA, Rozemuller AJM (2010) Characteristics of dyshoric capillary cerebral amyloid angiopathy. J Neuropathol Exp Neurol 69:1158–1167. https://doi.org/10.1097/NEN.0b013e3181fab558
53. Ritchie DL, Adlard P, Peden AH, Lowrie S, Le Grice M, Burns K, Jackson RJ, Yull H, Keogh MJ, Wei W, Chinnery PF, Head MW, Ironside JW (2017) Amyloid-β accumulation in the CNS in human growth hormone recipients in the UK. Acta Neuropathol (Berl). https://doi.org/10.1007/s00401-017-1703-0
54. Ritchie DL, Barria MA, Peden AH, Yull HM, Kirkpatrick J, Adlard P, Ironside JW, Head MW (2017) UK iatrogenic Creutzfeldt-Jakob disease: investigating human prion transmission across genotypic barriers using human tissue-based and molecular approaches. Acta Neuropathol (Berl) 133:579–595. https://doi.org/10.1007/s00401-016-1638-x
55. Rudge P, Jaunmuktane Z, Adlard P, Bjurstrom N, Caine D, Lowe J, Norsworthy P, Hummerich H, Druyeh R, Wadsworth JDF, Brandner S, Hyare H, Mead S, Collinge J (2015) Iatrogenic CJD due to pituitary-derived growth hormone with genetically determined incubation times of up to 40 years. Brain J Neurol 138:3386–3399. https://doi.org/10.1093/brain/awv235
56. Russo C, Schettini G, Saido TC, Hulette C, Lippa C, Lannfelt L, Ghetti B, Gambetti P, Tabaton M, Teller JK (2000) Presenilin-1 mutations in Alzheimer's disease. Nature 405:531–532. https://doi.org/10.1038/35014735
57. Serrano-Pozo A, Frosch MP, Masliah E, Hyman BT (2011) Neuropathological

alterations in Alzheimer disease. Cold Spring Harb Perspect Med 1:a006189. https://doi.org/10.1101/cshperspect.a006189
58. Simpson DA, Masters CL, Ohlrich G, Purdie G, Stuart G, Tannenberg AE (1996) Iatrogenic Creutzfeldt-Jakob disease and its neurosurgical implications. J Clin Neurosci Off J Neurosurg Soc Australas 3:118–123
59. Takeuchi A, Kobayashi A, Parchi P, Yamada M, Morita M, Uno S, Kitamoto T (2016) Distinctive properties of plaque-type dura mater graft-associated Creutzfeldt-Jakob disease in cell-protein misfolding cyclic amplification. Lab Investig J Tech Methods Pathol 96:581–587. https://doi.org/10.1038/labinvest.2016.27
60. Thal DR, Ghebremedhin E, Rüb U, Yamaguchi H, Del Tredici K, Braak H (2002) Two types of sporadic cerebral amyloid angiopathy. J Neuropathol Exp Neurol 61:282–293
61. Thal DR, Griffin WST, de Vos RAI, Ghebremedhin E (2008) Cerebral amyloid angiopathy and its relationship to Alzheimer's disease. Acta Neuropathol (Berl) 115:599–609. https://doi.org/10.1007/s00401-008-0366-2
62. Thal DR, Papassotiropoulos A, Saido TC, Griffin WST, Mrak RE, Kölsch H, Del Tredici K, Attems J, Ghebremedhin E (2010) Capillary cerebral amyloid angiopathy identifies a distinct APOE epsilon4-associated subtype of sporadic Alzheimer's disease. Acta Neuropathol (Berl) 120:169–183. https://doi.org/10.1007/s00401-010-0707-9
63. Thal DR, Rüb U, Orantes M, Braak H (2002) Phases of a beta-deposition in the human brain and its relevance for the development of AD. Neurology 58:1791–1800
64. Tousseyn T, Bajsarowicz K, Sánchez H, Gheyara A, Oehler A, Geschwind M, DeArmond B, DeArmond SJ (2015) Prion disease induces Alzheimer disease-like Neuropathologic changes. J Neuropathol Exp Neurol 74:873–888. https://doi.org/10.1097/NEN.0000000000000228
65. Vital A, Canron M-H, Gil R, Hauw J-J, Vital C (2007) A sporadic case of Creutzfeldt-Jakob disease with beta-amyloid deposits and alpha-synuclein inclusions. Neuropathol Off J Jpn Soc Neuropathol 27:273–277
66. Vonsattel JP, Myers RH, Hedley-Whyte ET, Ropper AH, Bird ED, Richardson EP (1991) Cerebral amyloid angiopathy without and with cerebral hemorrhages: a comparative histological study. Ann Neurol 30:637–649. https://doi.org/10.1002/ana.410300503
67. Walker LC, Jucker M (2015) Neurodegenerative diseases: expanding the prion concept. Annu Rev Neurosci 38:87–103. https://doi.org/10.1146/annurev-neuro-071714-033828
68. Watts JC, Condello C, Stöhr J, Oehler A, Lee J, DeArmond SJ, Lannfelt L, Ingelsson M, Giles K, Prusiner SB (2014) Serial propagation of distinct strains of Aβ prions from Alzheimer's disease patients. Proc Natl Acad Sci U S A 111:10323–10328. https://doi.org/10.1073/pnas.1408900111
69. Weissmann C, Li J, Mahal SP, Browning S (2011) Prions on the move. EMBO Rep 12:1109–1117. https://doi.org/10.1038/embor.2011.192
70. Ye L, Fritschi SK, Schelle J, Obermüller U, Degenhardt K, Kaeser SA, Eisele YS, Walker LC, Baumann F, Staufenbiel M, Jucker M (2015) Persistence of Aβ seeds in APP null mouse brain. Nat Neurosci 18:1559–1561. https://doi.org/10.1038/nn.4117
71. Zou W-Q, Langeveld J, Xiao X, Chen S, McGeer PL, Yuan J, Payne MC, Kang H-E, McGeehan J, Sy M-S, Greenspan NS, Kaplan D, Wang G-X, Parchi P, Hoover E, Kneale G, Telling G, Surewicz WK, Kong Q, Guo J-P (2010) PrP conformational transitions alter species preference of a PrP-specific antibody. J Biol Chem 285: 13874–13884. https://doi.org/10.1074/jbc.M109.088831

Zidovudine ameliorates pathology in the mouse model of Duchenne muscular dystrophy via P2RX7 purinoceptor antagonism

Rasha Al-Khalidi[1,6†], Chiara Panicucci[1,2†], Paul Cox[1], Natalia Chira[1], Justyna Róg[3], Christopher N. J. Young[1,7], Rhiannon E. McGeehan[1], Kameshwari Ambati[4], Jayakrishna Ambati[4,5], Krzysztof Zabłocki[3], Elisabetta Gazzerro[2], Stephen Arkle[1], Claudio Bruno[2] and Dariusz C. Górecki[1*]

Abstract

Duchenne muscular dystrophy (DMD) is the most common inherited muscle disorder that causes severe disability and death of young men. This disease is characterized by progressive muscle degeneration aggravated by sterile inflammation and is also associated with cognitive impairment and low bone density. Given that no current treatment can improve the long-term outcome, approaches with a strong translational potential are urgently needed. Duchenne muscular dystrophy (DMD) alters P2RX7 signaling in both muscle and inflammatory cells and inhibition of this receptor resulted in a significant attenuation of muscle and non-muscle symptoms in DMD^{mdx} mouse model. As P2RX7 is an attractive target in a range of human diseases, specific antagonists have been developed. Yet, these will require lengthy safety testing in the pediatric population of Duchenne muscular dystrophy (DMD) patients. In contrast, Nucleoside Reverse Transcriptase Inhibitors (NRTIs) can act as P2RX7 antagonists and are drugs with an established safety record, including in children. We demonstrate here that AZT (Zidovudine) inhibits P2RX7 functions acting via the same allosteric site as other antagonists. Moreover, short-term AZT treatment at the peak of disease in DMD^{mdx} mice attenuated the phenotype without any detectable side effects. Recovery was evident in the key parameters such as reduced sarcolemma permeability confirmed by lower serum creatine kinase levels and IgG influx into myofibres, decreased inflammatory cell numbers and inflammation markers in leg and heart muscles of treated mice. Moreover, this short-term therapy had some positive impact on muscle strength in vivo and no detrimental effect on mitochondria, which is the main side-effect of Nucleoside Reverse Transcriptase Inhibitors (NRTIs). Given these results, we postulate that AZT could be quickly re-purposed for the treatment of this highly debilitating and lethal disease. This approach is not constrained by causative DMD mutations and may be effective in alleviating both muscle and non-muscle abnormalities.

Keywords: AZT, Duchenne muscular dystrophy, eATP, mdx, Purinergic receptors, P2RX7

* Correspondence: darek.gorecki@port.ac.uk
†Equal contributors
[1]Molecular Medicine Laboratory, School of Pharmacy and Biomedical Sciences, University of Portsmouth, Portsmouth, UK
Full list of author information is available at the end of the article

Introduction

Duchenne muscular dystrophy (DMD) is the most common inherited muscle disorder with X-linked inheritance. Affected boys suffer from a progressive muscle degeneration and weakness, which lead to loss of ambulation in early teens. Skeletal deformities, respiratory insufficiency and cardiomyopathy developing in the second decade of life are typical for this debilitating and still lethal disease. The pleiotropic effects of the mutant gene also include non-muscle symptoms: cognitive impairment and structurally weakened bones [3, 55]. DMD is caused by mutations in the DMD gene encoding a range of dystrophin proteins. The muscle isoform is a 427 kDa protein with a role in anchoring the dystrophin-associated protein complex (DAPC) in the muscle sarcolemma. Lack of dystrophin is attributed to plasma membrane destabilization, cell signaling impairment and myofibre necrosis, accompanied by chronic sterile inflammation, and finally leading to irreversible replacement of muscle with fibrotic and adipose tissues [52]. Most recent studies indicated that expression of specific dystrophin isoforms is also important for the proper functioning of myogenic cells [19, 72] and dystrophinopathy is also responsible for the cognitive impairment and bone weakness [3, 41, 55, 59].

Importantly, numerous studies demonstrated that chronic muscle inflammation plays a crucial role in DMD pathogenesis. Specifically, in the *mdx* mouse model of DMD, treatments inducing depletion of CD4, CD8, neutrophils or macrophages or of anti-cytokine therapies significantly improved the dystrophic phenotype [13, 20, 28, 45, 60]. The mechanism underlying the sterile inflammation in dystrophic muscle is not completely understood but damage-associated molecular patterns (DAMPs) released from damaged myofibres seem to be the key factor. ATP released into the extracellular space (eATP) is one of the most important DAMPs acting as a "danger signal" triggering inflammation via activation of the P2RX7 purinoceptors. This "danger receptor" belongs to a family of ATP-gated ion channels. However, unlike other P2RXs, it requires millimolar concentrations of eATP for full activation [30]. Such high eATP levels are only encountered in pathologies. P2RX7 triggers complex downstream signaling producing increased IL-1b levels and the NLRP3 inflammasome activation. Interestingly, P2RX7 expression and activation in inflammatory cells has been well documented [48] but recent studies also showed a significant up-regulation of this purinoceptor in muscle cells from the mouse model of DMD [8, 54, 73]. When exposed to eATP, dystrophic DMD^{mdx} myoblasts respond with increased cytosolic Ca^{2+} influx and IL-1b release, suggesting that skeletal muscle cells can actively participate in the inflammatory process through purinergic signaling [54]. Moreover, high eATP acting on P2RX7 activates both abnormal Ca^{2+} influx and large pore opening triggering a unique mechanism of autophagic cell death [75] and increased MMP-2 activation [74]. Treatment with apyrase, an ATP degrading enzyme, reduced intracellular Ca^{2+} levels in *mdx* fibers [2] and P2RX7 antagonists reduced the cell death and MMP-2 activity [74, 75], thus confirming that P2RX7 contributes to the deregulated homeostasis in dystrophic muscles.

Therefore, activation of P2RX7 pathways in DMD results in direct muscle cell damage and death as well as an enhanced inflammatory response worsening the muscle pathology in a mechanism akin to the involvement of P2RX7 in other inflammatory diseases [14, 17].

We have previously demonstrated the therapeutic impact of both genetic ablation and pharmacological blockade of P2RX7 in *mdx* mice in vivo. This included significant improvements in muscle morphology and strength but also a significant reduction of the inflammatory phenotype [24, 58] as well as amelioration of non-muscle symptoms [41, 58]. This wide range of improvements reflects the involvement of P2RX7 in multiple disease mechanisms. Therefore, P2RX7 blockade emerges as an attractive target for translational approaches. Numerous P2RX7 antagonists have been developed [9, 27, 37, 63] and some of these e.g. AZD9056 and CE-224,535, have been used in clinical trials in inflammatory diseases [21, 34, 62]. However, none of these compounds have been approved as medicines and none tested in children.

Importantly, Fowler et al., [22] demonstrated that the Nucleoside Reverse Transcriptase Inhibitor (NRTI) class of compounds, commonly used as anti-HIV drugs, can act as P2RX7 antagonists [22, 40]. These drugs, with established safety records, could be repurposed for the treatment of this lethal disease. However, the mode of action of NRTI at the receptor and their efficacy in the specific pathology such as DMD were unknown.

Here we used a molecular modelling approach to establish whether NRTIs act as classical P2RX7 antagonists. Furthermore, we tested Zidovudnine (Azidothymidine, AZT), one of the mainstay NRTI therapeutics in HIV prevention and treatment, for its anti-P2RX7 properties in dystrophic muscle cells in vitro and for its efficacy in alleviating the pathology in the mouse model of DMD in vivo. It is the consensus opinion of experts that the *mdx* mouse is currently the most appropriate pre-clinical model to test treatment efficacy for DMD (http://www.treat-nmd.eu/research/preclinical/dmd-sops/). We established that even a short-term treatment with AZT significantly reduced muscle inflammation and improved the dystrophic phenotype. Consequently, AZT, which has established pharmacological profile also in the pediatric population, is an ideal candidate for rapid re-purposing as a DMD therapeutic.

Materials and methods

Molecular modelling

Molecular docking of the NRTIs: AZT, 2-Me-AZT [44], d4T and me-d4T in the P2RX7 receptor was performed using the Molecular Operating Environment (MOE) program [42]. The crystal structure for the giant panda P2RX7 with the ligand A804598 bound (5U1V) was downloaded from the Protein Database [5]. Human and mouse P2RX7 peptide sequences from UniProt were aligned with the Giant panda (Additional file 1: Figure S1) to establish the sequence homology of the critically important regions. The Protonate3D tool was used to add hydrogen atoms to the protein and partial charges were calculated for the protein atoms. Ligand binding sites were generated using the MOE Alpha Site Finder tool, which generates hydrophobic and hydrophilic α-spheres that are clustered together to represent regions of empty space in the protein. Ligand molecules were constructed using the builder tool, partial charges were calculated and the ligand molecule was energy minimized using the MMFF94× (Merck Molecular Forcefield 94×) prior to commencing a docking run. The Docking module was used to dock the ligand into appropriate ligand binding sites using 'Triangle Matcher' placement methodology and 300 placement poses. The lowest energy 100 unique receptor-ligand complexes were identified and scored according to the London dG scoring function. They were then submitted to a final forcefield minimization step retaining 100 unique ligand receptor complexes. The docking score, S, was calculated using the Generalised Born Solvation model (GB/VI). This interaction is the non-bonded interaction energy (van der Waals, Coulomb and GB implicit solvent interaction energies) between the receptor and the ligand. The self-energies of both the receptor and the ligand are excluded. Energy minimization was carried out using the conjugate gradient method with a cutoff distance of 6 Å and a convergence criterion of 0.04 kJ/mol. The atoms of the receptor were held fixed during the calculations.

Animals

All animal experiments were performed in accordance with the Principles of Laboratory Animal Care (NIH publication No. 86–23, revised 1985) and approvals of the Institutional Ethical Review Board and the Home Office UK (70/7479). Our experimental designs exploit the ARRIVE guidelines [58] and the TREAT-NMD guidelines designed to standardize experimental protocols used as efficacy readouts to allow comparisons of parallel efforts. Starting at 4 weeks of age, *mdx* male mice (unbiased by gender) were treated by i.p. injection twice a day either for 2 or 4 weeks with 50 mg/kg body weight of AZT (Zidovudine; Z1900000) or for 2 weeks with 25 mg/kg body weight of 2-Me-AZT. Dosage was based on previous studies [12, 22, 40]. Age-matched control mice received the same volume of phosphate buffered saline (pH 7.4, filter-sterilized, Sigma Aldrich).

Following the treatment, mice were killed by carbon dioxide inhalation; serum, tibialis anterior (TA), gastrocnemii (GC), and heart muscles were collected for further evaluations. Investigators were blinded to the sample group allocation, where possible.

Cell culture

Dystrophic *mdx* myoblasts [75] were cultured as primary cells in KnockOut DMEM (Invitrogen) supplemented with 10% $^{v}/_{v}$ KSR (Knockout Serum Replacement, Invitrogen), 5% $^{v}/_{v}$ DHS (Donor Horse Serum, Sera Labs) and 2 mM L-glutamine.

The P2RX7 large pore assay

For dye uptake assays, cells cultured under conditions described above were washed and incubated in the large pore buffer (145 mM NaCl, 5 mM KCl, 1 mM $MgCl_2$ and 10 mM Na-HEPES, pH 7.4) containing 5 μM EtBr. Following addition of agonists with or without AZT or me-AZT, EtBr uptake was analyzed under LSM510 confocal microscope (Zeiss) with heated stage at 37 °C and a dipping objective, or using a POLARstar Optima plate reader (BMG Labtech). Each experiment was repeated at least 3 times.

Intracellular Ca2+ measurements

Myoblasts were cultured on glass coverslips in a 6-well plate (500,000 cells/well) for 48 h under conditions described above. Cells (70–80% confluent) were loaded with Fura-2 AM (Molecular Probes, Oregon) in culture medium for 15 min at 37 °C in a 95% O_2, 5% CO_2 atmosphere. After 2 brief washes in the assay buffer (130 mM NaCl, 5 mM KCl, 2 mM $CaCl_2$, 1 mM $MgCl_2$, 0.5 mM Na_2HPO_4, 1 mM pyruvate, 5 mM D-glucose, and 25 mM HEPES; pH 7.4), the coverslips were mounted in a cuvette and maintained in the assay buffer at room temperature in an RF5301PC spectrofluorimeter (Shimadzu). Fluorescence was recorded at 510 nm with excitation at 340/380 nm. At the end of each experiment the Fura 2 fluorescence was calibrated by addition of 13 μM ionomycin to determine maximal fluorescence ratio followed by addition of EGTA to complete removal of Ca^{2+}. Cytosolic Ca^{2+} concentration $[Ca^{2+}]c$ was calculated according to Grynkiewicz et al. [26]. The cells were treated with: 300 μM BzATP; 20 μM AZT and 20 μM me-AZT (applied 30 and 10 min prior to the addition of BzATP, respectively). Each experiment was repeated at least 4 times for AZT and 3 times for me-AZT.

Serum CK level measurement

The blood samples were collected, allowed to coagulate and centrifuged for 10 min at 2500 g. Immediately after centrifugation, the serum was isolated and stored at -20 °C. The creatine kinase (CK) levels were analyzed using the Creatine Kinase Activity Assay Kit (Mak116-1kt, Sigma-Aldrich), according to manufacturer's instructions.

Treadmill test

A five lane treadmill (Panlab/Harvard Apparatus) equipped with a darkened far-end area to encourage running, was used. AZT- and PBS-treated *mdx* mice were challenged on the treadmill twice (at the end of the second and the fourth week of treatment) for 30 min according to the protocol described by Radley-Crabb [51]. Briefly, groups of 4 mice were settled for 2 min on the treadmill with a stationary belt, then acclimatized for 2 min at a speed of 4 m/min, warmed up for 8 min at 8 m/min and finally exercised for 30 min at 12 m/min. The number of stops during the last 30 min and the total period spent running for each animal were measured.

Forelimb grip strength test

AZT- and PBS-treated *mdx* mice were also compared in the forelimb grip strength test (Force Gauce FG-5000A, Lutron Electronic) at the end of the second and the fourth week of treatment according to the SOP (ID) DMD_M.2.2.001. Briefly, each trial consisted of five repetitions with at least 1 min elapsing between each of the five determinations per animal; the grip strength value for each mouse was recorded as the average of the three best efforts and was then divided by the mouse body weight.

Histochemical analysis

Sections (10 μm) from frozen tibialis anterior and heart muscles isolated from 8 weeks old AZT- and PBS-treated *mdx* mice were cut on a cryostat. Sections were obtained from the middle third of the muscle, collected on poly-L-lysine (0.5 mg/ml) – coated glass slides and subsequently stained with H&E and/or acid phosphatase (AP). AP staining was used to quantify the inflammatory infiltrate areas, exploiting the properties of AP-rich inflammatory cells producing an azo dye when coupled with a naphthol-based buffer. For AP staining frozen muscle sections were kept at ambient temperature for 30′. Afterwards sections were incubated for 1 h at 37 °C with the incubating solution made as follow: substrate solution (naphtol AS-B1 phosphate 0.02 M in dimethylformamide), buffer solution (veronal acetate 0.15 M), sodium nitrite 4% (*w*/*v*) and pararosaniline solution (pararosaniline 0.12 M in 2 N HCl). Sections were then dehydrated in ascending alcohols (50%, 70%, 80%, 95% X2, 100% X2), cleared with xylene and mounted with Permount [4]. The AP-positive (red signal) areas were captured using an automated method through the Ariol system (Leica Biosystem) for an unbiased analysis and expressed as % of the total cross-sectional area.

Immunofluorescence

10 μm thick cryosections were fixed in a 4% $^{w}/_{v}$ paraformaldehyde solution in TBST for 15 min at 4 °C. The primary antibody incubation in TBST containing 10% $^{v}/_{v}$ serum was applied overnight at 4 °C and secondary antibody incubation in TBST and 2% $^{v}/_{v}$ serum containing Hoechst fluorescent nuclear counterstain was applied for 1 h at room temperature. Sections were mounted using Fluor Preserve Reagent (Merk Millipore) mounting medium.

The following antibodies were used: CD68—MCA1957GA rat monoclonal (AbD Serotec), dilution 1:500; collagen type-IV—AB769 goat polyclonal (Chemicon), dilution 1:500; Dystrophin- mouse monoclonal (D8043 SIGMA Sigma Aldrich), dilution 1:500; Ly6G—14–593 rat monoclonal (eBioscience), dilution 1:250; P2RX4 rabbit polyclonal (Alomone), dilution 1:500. Images were captured using a confocal microscope (LSM 710, Zeiss); the whole cross-section area from TA or GC was captured by non-overlapping 10× magnification images.

Muscle fiber size and central nucleation were visualized by collagen type-IV and Hoechst immunofluorescence staining. Individual microscope fields-of-view were montaged using ImageJ to present whole cross-sections through the muscle. Image analysis was performed on these composite images using Fiji, ImageJ, open-source software (NIH, US). A macro developed as described [58] was used to measure morphometric variables including the minimum Feret diameter, the total fiber number and the centrally nucleated fiber number per analyzed area.

For P2RX4, CD68 and Ly6G detection, the whole TA section was scanned with the confocal microscope at 10× magnification and quantification of immunofluorescent signals was performed with a semi-automated (unbiased) method using a thresholding macro in ImageJ and divided by the number of fields thus obtaining a number expressed in arbitrary units (AU), which indicates the mean fluorescence signal per unit area. The same method was applied to quantify IgG permeability into muscle fibers. Dystrophin staining to identify the revertant fibers was performed in TA muscle sections. Hoechst nuclear counterstain was used to help visualizing the total number of myofibers present in each section. Revertant fibers were manually enumerated and reported as percentage of total myofibers.

Western blotting

Total proteins from frozen TA muscles were extracted by crushing samples with a mortar and pestle under liquid nitrogen and further homogenization in the extraction buffer: 100 mg of muscle powder were homogenized in 500 μl of complete lysis M reagent (Sigma-Aldrich) enriched with protease inhibitor cocktail 1X and phosphatase inhibitor cocktail 2X (all Roche). All samples were centrifuged at 800 g for 3 min at 4 °C, and protein concentrations were determined using a Bicinchoninic Acid Kit (Sigma-Aldrich). 50 μg of protein was mixed at 1:1 $^{v}/_{v}$ ratio with Laemmli buffer 2X with 5% $^{v}/_{v}$ β-mercaptoethanol, heated for 5 min at 95 °C and chilled on ice. Proteins were then resolved on 6%–12% $^{w}/_{v}$ SDS-polyacrylamide gels and transferred onto Hybond PVDF membranes (Amersham). Membranes were blocked in 5% $^{w}/_{v}$ non-fat milk powder in 1× TBST with 0.01% $^{v}/_{v}$ Tween 20 (Sigma-Aldrich) for 1 h, then probed overnight at 4 °C with primary antibody diluted in the same blocking buffer, and finally incubated with the appropriate horseradish-peroxidase-conjugated secondary antibody (Sigma-Aldrich) for 1 h at room temperature. Specific protein bands were visualized using Laminata Western HRP Substre (Millipore) and images were obtained using a ChemiDoc MP system (BioRad). All densitometric analyses of protein bands were made using exposure times within the linear range and the integrated density measurement function of the imaging software. The CD11b antibody, clone M1/70 rabbit (Abcam) was used at a 1:1000 dilution and GAPDH (Santa Cruz) goat polyclonal antibody was used at 1:500 and served as the protein-loading control.

RT-qPCR

Total RNA was extracted from muscles using RNeasy Mini Kit (Qiagen) according to the manufacturer's protocol. Total RNA, containing miRNA was also extracted from sera of AZT- and PBS-treated *mdx* mice after 2 weeks of treatment according to the manufacturer's protocol for the miRNeasy Serum/Plasma kit (Qiagen). Quality and quantity was assessed using a NanoDrop spectrophotometer.

1 μg of RNA was reverse transcribed using a SuperScriptTM VILO cDNA Synthesis Kit (Invitrogen). For the RT-qPCR amplification, 25 ng and 12.5 ng of cDNA (respectively for the target genes and for GAPDH control) were used in 20 μl reaction volume prepared with TaqMan Universal Master MIX II (Applied Biosystem) or SYBR Green PrecisionPLUS qPCR MasterMix (Primer Design). Each sample was run in duplicate using a ViiA7 Real Time PCR Detection System (Applied Biosystems, USA). The expression of target genes relative to GAPDH was determined by using the △CT method [57] The primers used were as follows:

Taqman probe NCBI accession numbers: CD68: NM_001291058.1, CD163: NM_001170395.1, P2X4: NM_011026, CD4: NM_013488.2, CD8a: NM_001081110.2, Foxp3: NM_001199347.1, LY6G: NM_023463.3, TNF-a: NM_001278601.1, IL6: NM_031168.1, IL 10: NM_010548.2, IL-12a: NM_001159424.1, COX2: NC_005089.1, Bmp7: NM_007557.3, Mir206: NR_029593.1, Mfn2: NM_001285921.1, GAPDH: NM_008084.2.

SybrGreen primer sequences:

TGFb: Fwd 5'-CTCCACCTGCAAGACCAT-3′; Rev 5'-CTTAGTTTGGACAGGATCTGG-3'
IL33: Fwd TCCTTGCTTGGCAGTATCCA, Rev TGCTCAATGTGTCAACAGACG
iNOS: Fwd CAGTTCCGAGCGTCAAAGACCTGC-3′, Rev CAGCCCAACAATACAATACAAGATG.
IL1b: Fwd TCTGATGGGCAACCACTTAC, Rev GTTGACAGCTAGGTTCTGTTCT
Nlrp3: Fwd TGAATCGGAACAACCTGAC, Rev CCACCAGCAAGAAGAAGC
NF-kb: Fwd ACACGAGGCTACAACTCTGC, Rev GGTACCCCCAGAGACCTCAT

MtDNA copy number analysis

The qPCR (absolute quantification) was performed on total DNA isolated from snap-frozen GC muscle isolated from AZT- and PBS-treated *mdx* mice after 4 weeks of treatment tissue and externally generated standards using Sybr green (BioRad) and primers specific for mitochondrial DNA (mtDNA): Fwd CAGTCTAATGCTTACTCAGC, Rev GGGCAGTTACGATAACATTG and GAPDH: FwD TCAAGCTCATTTCCTGGTATGAC, Rev CTTGCTCAG TGTCCTTGCTG. As two copies of GAPDH are present in every nucleus, GAPDH amplification data were divided by 2 to calculate the number of nuclei present in each sample. The number of mtDNA copies was then calculated by dividing the mtDNA amplification data by the number of nuclei [7, 49]. Measurements were made in duplicate. The analysis was carried out on 4 mice per experiment.

Statistical analysis

For statistical analysis of cell assays a one-way analysis of variance (ANOVA) was performed with the post- hoc Tukey's test (Microcal Origin 7.0). Results are reported as mean (+/-SD), where n refers to number of independent samples or individuals. Mann Whitney test was used for comparisons between the two data sets (PBS-*mdx* vs AZT-*mdx*). Two way- ANOVA with Bonferroni multiple comparisons were used to compare the PBS and AZT treatment in 2 and 4 weeks. For RTqPCR data sstatistical analysis was performed on the relative expression values with the Mann Whitney test and represented as Log2 fold change versus the mean PBS-*mdx*.

A p-value of < 0.05 was considered statistically significant, and the values are reported as follows in figures: $^{*}p < 0.05$, $^{**}p < 0.01$, $^{***}p < 0.001$.

Results

It has not been known whether NRTIs bind directly to P2RX7 and, if so, where or whether they have an indirect effect. To gain insights into these questions, we have used molecular modeling and the recently published mammalian P2RX7 crystal structure [31] to identify putative binding sites for AZT (Zidovudine), to the P2RX7 molecule. AZT is one of the most widely used NRTIs. Moreover, the mechanism of action of NRTIs at the P2RX7 is independent from the reverse transcriptase inhibition because their methyl derivatives retain the P2RX7 antagonism but not the NRTI activity [22]. Therefore, we used the same approach to compare the most likely binding sites for 2-Me-AZT as well as for d4T and its 5'-O-methyl-modified derivative me-d4T.

Modelling of AZT and its derivatives on P2RX7

Human and mouse P2RX7 peptide sequences from UniProt were aligned with the giant panda (Additional file 1: Figure S1) and showed 77% and 81% of residues to be entirely conserved between panda and mouse and human, respectively. Moreover, the key residues involved in binding specific P2RX7 antagonists (e.g. A804598) are also conserved, demonstrating that the panda structure represents the best current template for investigating the potential mode of action of AZT both in the mouse model and patients.

The AZT molecule was docked into all of the 29 unique docking sites identified by the Alpha Site Finder Tool in MOE. The optimized binding energies for the AZT at all these sites are summarized in the Additional file 2: Table S1. The lowest energy position for AZT (-89.3 kJ mol^{-1}) was found to be at the allosteric binding site identified by Karasawa and Kawate [31]. This is the position that several structurally distinct antagonists (A74003, A804598, AZ10606120, GW791343 and JNJ47965567) were found to occupy inside the P2X7 receptor (Fig. 1a). A comparison between the predicted location for AZT and the experimental location for A804598 is shown in Fig. 1b. It is clear that the AZT molecule is predicted to occupy the same region of space as A804598 and it fills the available space inside the allosteric binding site well (Fig. 1c).

The most favorable binding sites for both d4T and me-d4T were also found to be at the same allosteric site. Their optimized energies were -74.7 and -80.2 kJ mol^{-1} respectively, very similar to the value obtained for AZT. The potentially enhanced binding affinity of the methylated molecule to the P2RX7 is likely to be due to enhanced van der Waals' interaction between the ligand and the protein. The optimized locations of d4T, me-d4T and AZT are shown in Fig. 1d.

Docking 2-Me-AZT inside the receptor also finds the most favorable binding site to be at the allosteric one. The optimized energy is -87.4 kJ mol^{-1}. Although the addition of the methyl group means that a hydrogen bond interaction with the residue Ala91 is lost, this is compensated by an increase in the van der Waals' interaction, which results in a very similar binding

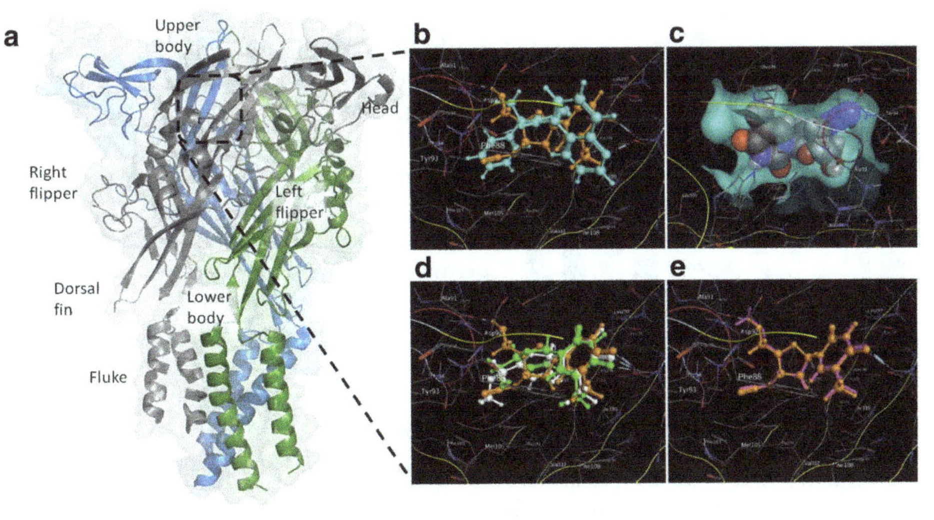

Fig. 1 AZT binds to the same allosteric site as canonical P2RX7 antagonists. **a** Surface representation of trimeric P2X7, combining the Giant panda [PDB:5U1V] shown in grey and two chicken monomers [PDB:5XW6] shown (for illustration only) in blue and green. The approximate location of the allosteric site formed by a groove between two of the adjacent monomers is highlighted by the black box. **b** The optimized location of AZT (orange) compared with the experimental location of A804598 (cyan). Both molecules occupy very similar regions of space. **c** The optimized location of the AZT molecule inside the allosteric pocket (light blue). **d** The optimized locations of AZT (orange), d4T (green) and d4T-me (white). **e** The optimized locations of AZT (orange) and me-AZT (magenta). H-bond interactions are shown via a dotted line

energy to the one obtained for AZT. The optimized locations for these molecules are shown in Fig. 1e.

AZT inhibits both the P2RX7 ion channel function and large pore formation in mdx myoblasts

The modelling data clearly points to AZT and 2-Me-AZT binding to the P2RX7 allosteric site. We tested whether these drugs inhibit this receptor in dystrophic muscle cells. P2RX7 functions as a Ca^{2+} permeable ion channel and, upon prolonged ATP stimulation, as a large pore. We have previously shown that A74003 can inhibit both of these functions in *mdx* cells [73, 75]. Pre-incubation of dystrophic myoblasts with AZT at 1, 5, 10 and 20 μM resulted in a concentration-dependent inhibition of the large pore opening measured by the EtBr uptake (Fig. 2a). While 1 μM AZT had no effect on channel or pore functions the inhibitory effect appeared to reach saturation at around 10–20 μM and, at these concentrations, AZT also blocked the Ca^{2+} influx (Fig. 2b). Furthermore, 20 μM me-AZT had the same inhibitory effect on the Ca^{2+} influx as equimolar AZT. Importantly, the ~50% inhibition evoked by AZT was comparable to the effects obtained previously using other antagonists [75]. Additionally, cells incubated with AZT or 2-Me-AZT were observed to retain a greater degree of elongation and adherence compared to cells exposed to the specific P2RX7 antagonist (data not shown), indicating that these drugs are better tolerated by muscle cells at inhibitory concentrations.

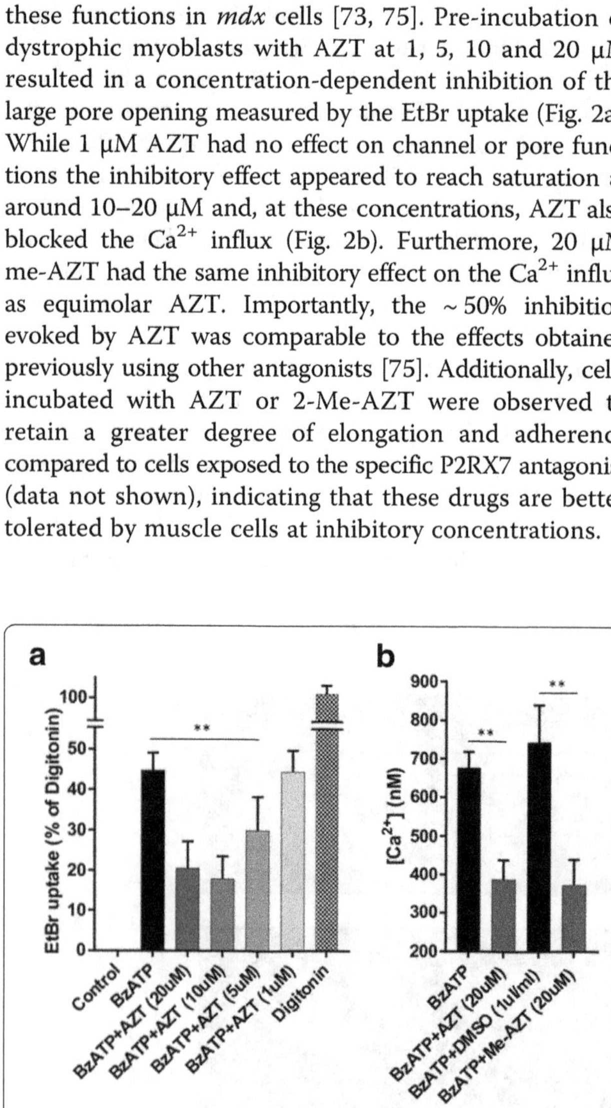

Fig. 2 AZT inhibits P2RX7 large pore and channel functions in *mdx* myoblasts **a** EtBr uptake (expressed as % permeabilization evoked by 50 μg/ml digitonin) following 30 min exposure to 1 mM BzATP with and without the specified concentrations of AZT. Note the concentration-dependent inhibition up to 20 μM of AZT. One-way ANOVA, df = 5, $n = 6$, $p = 0.008$. **b** 1 mM BzATP-stimulated Ca^{2+} influx was inhibited in the presence of 20 μM AZT or me-AZT. One-way ANOVA, df = 3, $n = 4$, $p = 0.001$. Error bars show mean ± SD, $^{**}p < 0.01$

AZT treatment reduces skeletal and heart muscle inflammation in mdx mice in vivo

To mimic the clinically relevant situation, treatment and analyses were performed at the age when *mdx* mice show the typical muscle degeneration and regeneration and the inflammatory cell infiltration pattern akin to human pathology. The 4 week old *mdx* males were injected i.p. with 50 mg/kg body weight AZT twice a day for 2 or 4 weeks. The weight gain profiles of mice treated with AZT showed no difference to the PBS-treated controls (Additional file 3: Figure S2). Inflammatory muscle infiltrates were evaluated in tibialis anterior (TA) muscles isolated from *mdx* mice injected with AZT or PBS for 4 weeks. H&E (Fig. 3a) and acid phosphatase (AP) staining (Fig. 3b) showed that AZT treatment significantly decreased the inflammatory infiltrations surrounding the necrotic muscle fibers. The morphometric AP analysis (Fig. 3c) revealed a statistically significant reduction in the AZT-treated mice (% of the inflammatory area in PBS-*mdx* = 0.68% vs. AZT-*mdx* = 0.35%; $p = 0.0121$; % reduction = 48,1%). Importantly, the reduction in inflammatory infiltrations was already clearly noticeable following 2 weeks of treatment. It involved significantly decreased levels of mRNAs for several inflammatory markers in both TA and GC muscles (TNFa: AZT-*mdx* vs PBS-*mdx* $p = 0.038$; IL12a: AZT-*mdx* vs PBS-*mdx* $p = 0.017$) (Additional file 4: Figure S3D).

Transcript levels of genes encoding inflammatory cell markers and associated with the innate and adaptive immune responses were quantified by RT-qPCR. Among the cell markers, the CD68 transcript (which predominates in macrophages) and the Ly6G neutrophil-specific transcript levels were all significantly reduced in the AZT-treated *mdx* mice (CD68;AZT-*mdx* vs PBS-*mdx* $p = 0.026$, LY6G;AZT-*mdx* vs PBS-*mdx* $p = 0.026$) (Fig. 4a). The ratio of pro-inflammatory to pro-regenerative macrophages (M1/M2), defined by the relative CD68 to CD163 expression was not altered significantly (Fig. 4b).

Subsequent immunofluorescence analysis of these cell markers in muscle sections both confirmed and extended these findings. It revealed that already after 2 weeks of AZT treatment the numbers of macrophages, identified by P2RX4 staining, were significantly decreased (Additional file 4: Figure S3 B and C) (PBS-*mdx* = 465 AU, AZT-*mdx* = 249 AU; $p = 0.038$; % reduction = 46,32%). At 4 weeks the CD68+ cell numbers were also reduced (PBS-*mdx* = 647,8 AU, AZT-*mdx* = 189,4 AU; $p = 0.015$; % reduction = 70%, Fig. 4c).

The AZT-evoked reduction of neutrophils was also confirmed in immunofluorescent analyses of the LY6G+ population in TA muscle samples collected following 4 weeks of treatment (PBS-*mdx* = 699 AU, AZT-*mdx* = 156 AU; $p = 0.015$; % reduction = 77%, Fig. 4d).

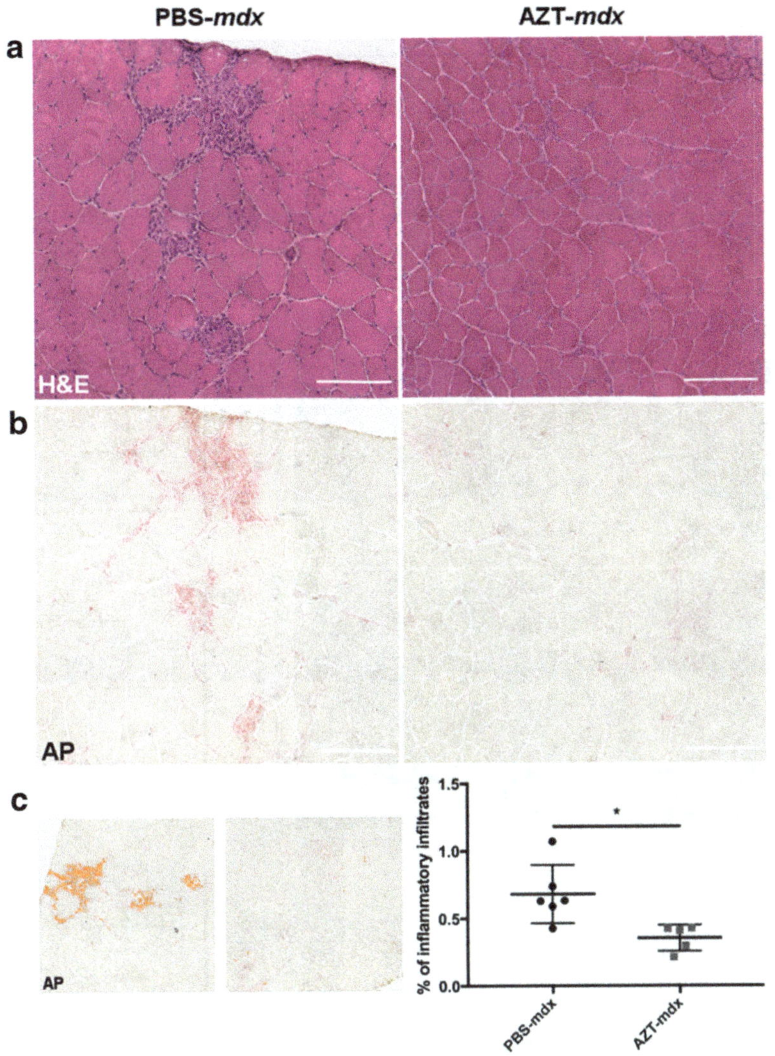

Fig. 3 AZT decreases inflammatory infiltrates in *mdx* muscle. Representative images of TA sections following 4 week treatment with PBS or AZT, stained with H&E (**a**) and AP (**b**). AZT-*mdx* shows smaller inflammatory infiltrate areas than PBS-*mdx*. Scale bar = 100 μm. The AP signal indicating inflammatory cells (**c**), was quantified using the automated image analysis system (Ariol) with the AP positive area calculated as % of the total cross-sectional area. Mann Whitney test, $n = 6$, $p = 0.012$. $^{*}p < 0.05$

Furthermore, levels of the CD11B leukocyte marker were analyzed by immunoblot in GC muscles collected after 2 weeks of treatment. This analysis demonstrated a significant, 58% reduction in CD11B protein levels in AZT-treated animals (PBS-*mdx* = 1.075, AZT-*mdx* = 0.446; $p = 0.003$; Fig. 4e).

Analysis of specific cytokine transcripts in muscles (Fig. 5) revealed that TNFa levels were significantly decreased in the AZT-treated *mdx* group, consistent with the functional link between TNFa and P2RX7 (TNFa: AZT-*mdx* vs PBS-*mdx* $p = 0.002$). Moreover, a significant reduction of the Nlrp3 transcript levels in AZT-*mdx* muscle confirmed the Fowler et al., [22] data that AZT suppresses the Nlrp3 inflammasome by blocking P2RX7activity (Nlrp3: AZT-*mdx* vs PBS-*mdx* $p = 0.03$). The IL1b and IL6 expressions did not differ between treated and control groups (Fig. 5). However, expression levels of the inducible forms of cyclooxygenase COX2 and the iNOS nitric oxide synthase genes were found significantly decreased in the AZT-treated *mdx* samples, confirming that the AZT treatment affects the inflammatory milieu of *mdx* muscles (COX2: AZT-*mdx* vs PBS-*mdx* $p = 0.032$; iNOS: AZT-*mdx* vs PBS-*mdx* $p = 0.03$). This was further confirmed by the decreased expression of NF-κb in AZT-treated muscles (NF-κb: AZT-*mdx* vs PBS-*mdx* $p = 0.03$). This short AZT treatment did not alter the expression levels of TGFb and BMP-7 transcripts used here as previously identified markers of the early fibrotic phenotype in *mdx* muscles [58].

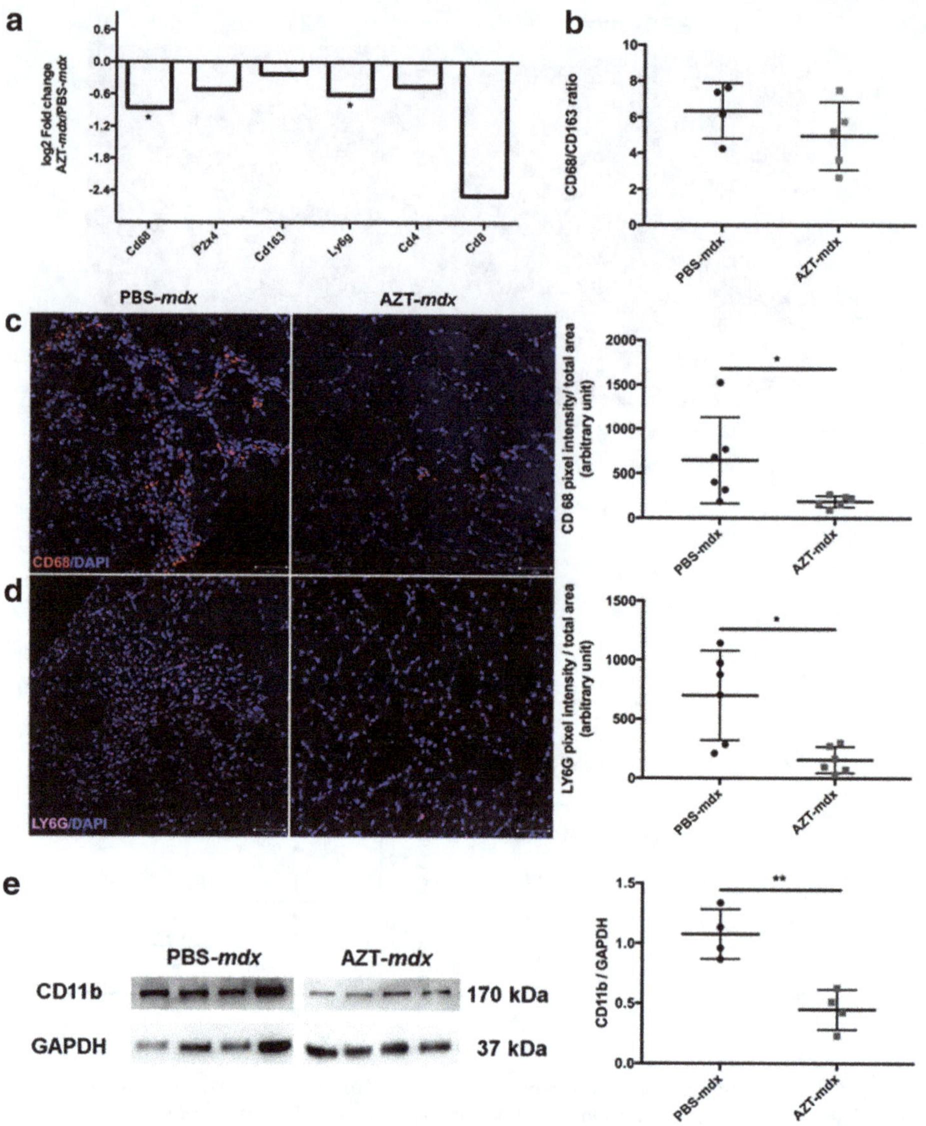

Fig. 4 AZT modulates the immune responses in *mdx* mouse muscle. Relative expression levels of inflammatory marker RNAs in gastrocnemii following 4 week AZT treatment (**a**). The data are expressed as Log2 fold change versus the mean PBS-*mdx*. Mann Whitney test, $n = 5–6$. CD68;AZT-*mdx* vs PBS-*mdx* $p = 0.026$, LY6G;AZT-*mdx* vs PBS-*mdx* $p = 0.03$. **b** Comparison of M1 to M2 macrophages calculated as the ratio between CD68 and CD163 expression. Error bars show mean ± SD. Mann Whitney test, $n = 4–6$. Immunofluorescent analysis of inflammatory cell subpopulations in TA sections following 4 week AZT treatment. Representative images of CD68 (**c**) and LY6G staining (**d**) are shown while scatter plots demonstrate individual values of immunofluorescent signal levels in respective AZT treated and control muscles expressed in arbitrary units: pixel intensity/total area. Error bars show mean ± SD, Mann Whitney test, $n = 6$. CD68; PBS-*mdx* vs AZT-*mdx* $p = 0.015$, LY6G; PBS-*mdx* vs AZT-*mdx* $p = 0.015$. **e** Western blot of CD11b in TA muscles following 2-week treatment with GAPDH used as the protein loading control. The graph shows the individual values of the CD11b protein normalized to GAPDH, error bars show mean ± SD. Mann Whitney test, $n = 4$, $p = 0.003$. *$p < 0.05$, **$p < 0.01$

Concerning the adaptive immune response markers following this short-term treatment with AZT in the *mdx* mice the reduction of the CD8 and CD4 T-cell transcripts did not reach statistical significance (Fig. 4a). While ablation of *P2RX7* gene and broad purinergic inhibition with ox-ATP has previously been shown to increase the level of T regulatory (T_{reg}) cells [24, 58], the AZT treatment applied here did not significantly increase the IL 12 but reduced the Foxp3 expression levels (Foxp3: AZT-*mdx* vs PBS-*mdx* $p = 0.002$). Expression of IL10 and IL 33 transcripts, the latter found important for muscle repair [36], was also unaltered (Fig. 5).

DMD patients who survive to their third decade present with cardiomyopathy and heart failure [11, 38]. Therefore, hearts were studied to investigate the impact of AZT treatment at an early stage of disease. H&E (Fig. 6a) and

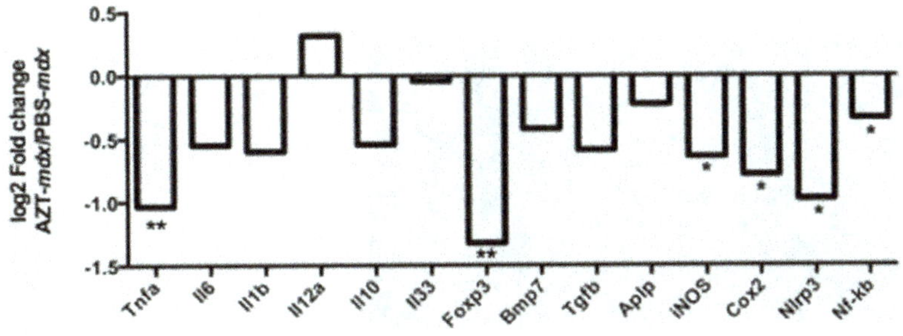

Fig. 5 AZT treatment impacts on cytokine and inflammasome pathway gene expressions. Results of qPCR expression analyses of indicated markers in GC muscles. The data are shown as Log2 fold change versus the PBS-*mdx* and statistical analysis was performed on the relative expression values with the Mann Whitney test, $n = 6$, TNFa;AZT-*mdx* vs PBS-*mdx* $p = 0.002$, Foxp3;AZT-*mdx* vs PBS-*mdx* $p = 0.002$, iNOS;AZT-*mdx* vs PBS-*mdx* $p = 0.03$, COX2;AZT-*mdx* vs PBS-*mdx* $p = 0.032$, Nlrp3;AZT-*mdx* vs PBS-*mdx* $p = 0.016$, NFkb;AZT-*mdx* vs PBS-*mdx* $p = 0.03$.. $n = 6$; $*p < 0.05$ $**p < 0.01$

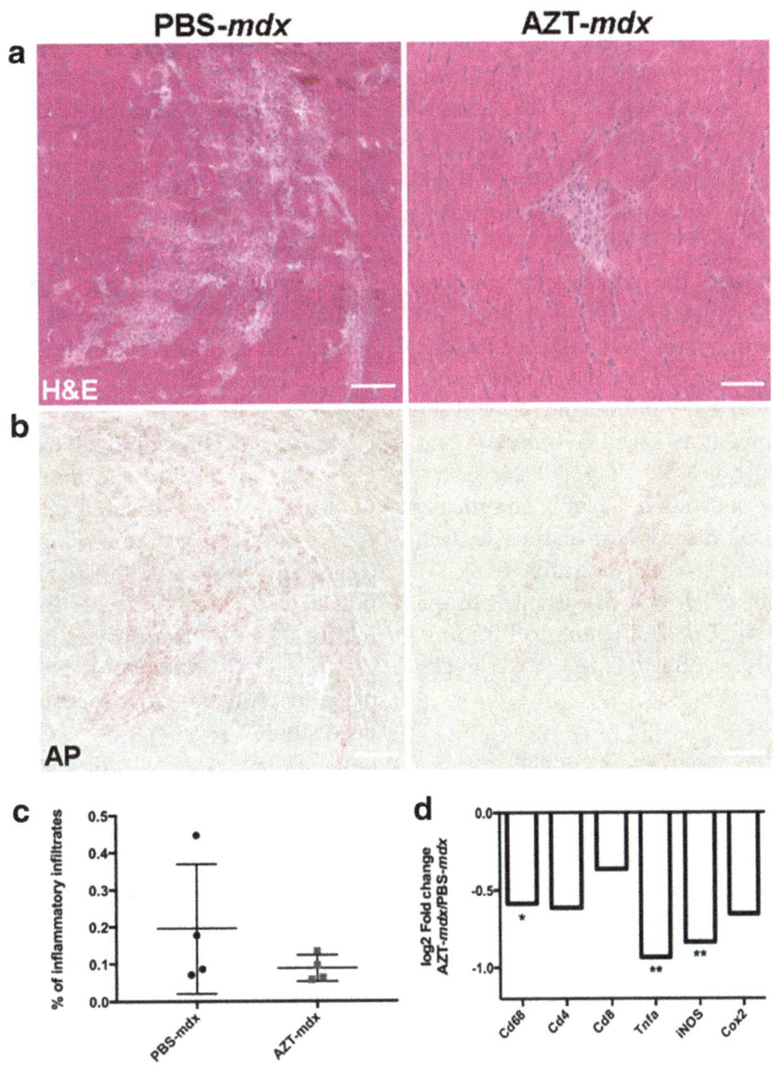

Fig. 6 AZT treatment reduces inflammatory infiltrates and expression of inflammatory markers in *mdx* hearts. Representative images of heart muscle sections following 4-week treatment with AZT or PBS stained with H&E (**a**) and AP (**b**). **c** The AP signal indicating inflammatory cell infiltration was quantified using the Ariol image analysis system with the AP positive area calculated as % of the total cross-sectional area. Error bars show mean ± SD, Mann Whitney test, $n = 4$. **d** qPCR analysis of specified transcript expressions in heart muscles in response to AZT treatment. Scale bar = 100 μm. Mann Whitney test, $n = 6$, CD68: AZT-*mdx* vs PBS-*mdx* $p = 0.029$; TNFa: AZT-*mdx* vs PBS-*mdx* $p = 0.008$; iNOS: AZT-*mdx* vs PBS-*mdx* $p = 0.009$. $*p < 0.05$; $**p < 0.01$

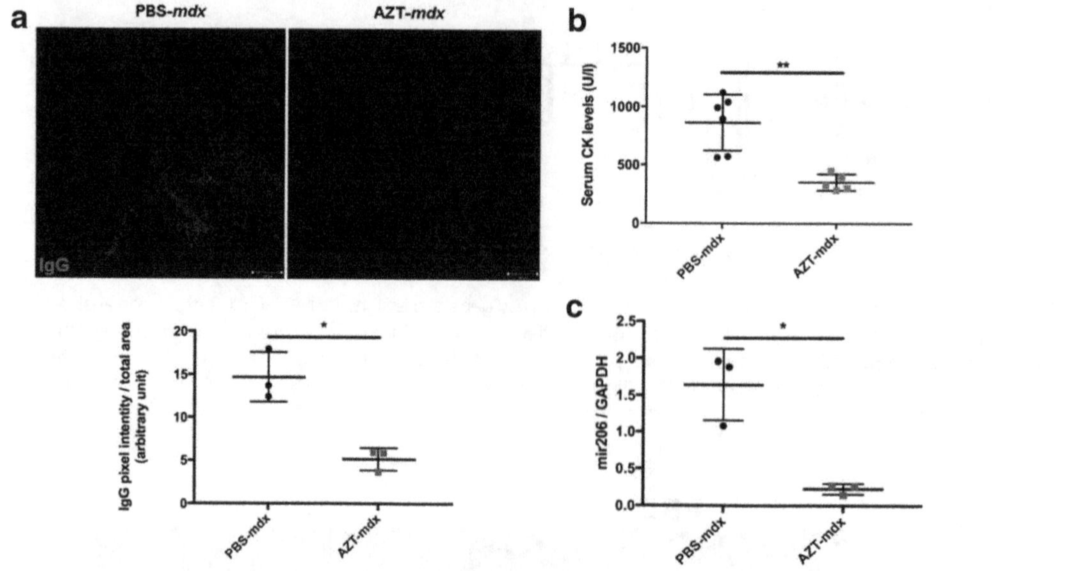

Fig. 7 AZT treatment increases sarcolemma stability in *mdx* muscle. **a** Representative images of IgG penetration into damaged TA muscle fibers from *mdx* mice treated for 2 weeks with AZT or PBS and the graph below shows enumeration of IgG penetration represented as pixel intensity/total unit of area. Error bars show mean ± SD, Mann Whitney test, $n = 3$, $p < 0.05$ **b** Serum CK levels in AZT-treated mice (4-week treatment) compared to controls. Error bars show mean ± SD, Mann Whitney test, $n = 5–6$, $p = 0.004$. **c** qPCR analysis of Mir206 in serum samples from PBS or AZT treated mice following 2-week treatment. Error bars show mean ± SD. Mann Whitney test, $n = 3$, $p = 0.029$. *$p < 0.05$, **$p < 0.01$

AP (Fig. 6b) staining showed the presence of reactive inflammatory infiltrates in heart muscles of 8 week old *mdx* mice. The inflammation area was reduced by the AZT treatment, albeit the values did not reach significance probably due to the high variability in the controls and the small sample size (% inflammatory area PBS-*mdx* = 0,19%, AZT-*mdx* = 0,08%; % reduction = 57%, Fig. 6c). Nevertheless, RTq-PCR analysis demonstrated a highly statistically significant decrease of CD68 macrophage marker as well as TNFa and iNOS transcript levels in hearts of AZT-treated *mdx* mice (Fig. 6d), which was consistent with the findings in skeletal muscles (CD68: AZT-*mdx* vs PBS-*mdx* $p = 0.029$; TNFa: AZT-*mdx* vs PBS-*mdx* $p = 0.008$; iNOS: AZT-*mdx* vs PBS-*mdx* $p = 0.009$).

The AZT treatment increases sarcolemma stability and impacts muscle strength in vivo

AZT treatment resulted in significantly improved sarcolemma integrity: An analysis of membrane permeability using IgG influx into TA muscle revealed a significant reduction in IgG-positive fibers already after 2 weeks of treatment (IgG pixel intensity PBS-*mdx* = 14.7 AU, AZT-*mdx* = 5.14 AU) (Fig. 7a). After 4 weeks of AZT treatment there was a significant, 60% reduction in serum CK level (Fig. 7b), indicative of less sarcolemma damage and therefore less leakage of this intracellular muscle enzyme (serum CK levels: PBS-*mdx* = 864.37 UI/l, AZT-*mdx* = 351.72 UI/l; $p = 0.004$). The serum levels of miR-206, dystroMir, in *mdx* mice have been found to be less affected by movement compared to CK [39] and therefore this dystroMir has been proposed as a stable molecular marker of muscle damage. Here, the serum levels of Mir-206 were significantly decreased in the AZT-treated *mdx* mice after 2 weeks of treatment (Fig. 7c).

Muscle morphological parameters such as the Minimum Feret's diameter and the number of fibers with central nucleation were evaluated in TA muscle sections from AZT- and PBS-treated *mdx* after both 2 and 4 weeks of treatment, but no statistically significant differences between the groups were observed (Additional file 5: Figure S4). Revertant fibers found in dystrophic muscle arise due to spontaneous exon skipping events, taking place in proliferating myogenic cells activated by muscle degeneration/regeneration cycles. Fewer revertant fibers have been used as an indicator that a muscle underwent fewer such cycles [47, 56]. The revertant fiber reduction was not statistically significant but no increase indicated that AZT treatment is not accelerating muscle damage (Additional file 5: Figure S4).

In order to establish if AZT would affect the muscle function in *mdx* mice, muscle strength and resistance were evaluated at 2 and 4 weeks of treatment using the forelimb grip strength and 30 min treadmill run tests. The single 30 min treadmill exercise session has previously been shown suitable for proof-of concept studies in adult *mdx* mice [51]. The 4 week AZT treatment improved grip strength compared to the 2 week one while no improvement with age was observed in the PBS-treated mice (Fig. 8a). Moreover, 50 and 75% of AZT-*mdx* mice in

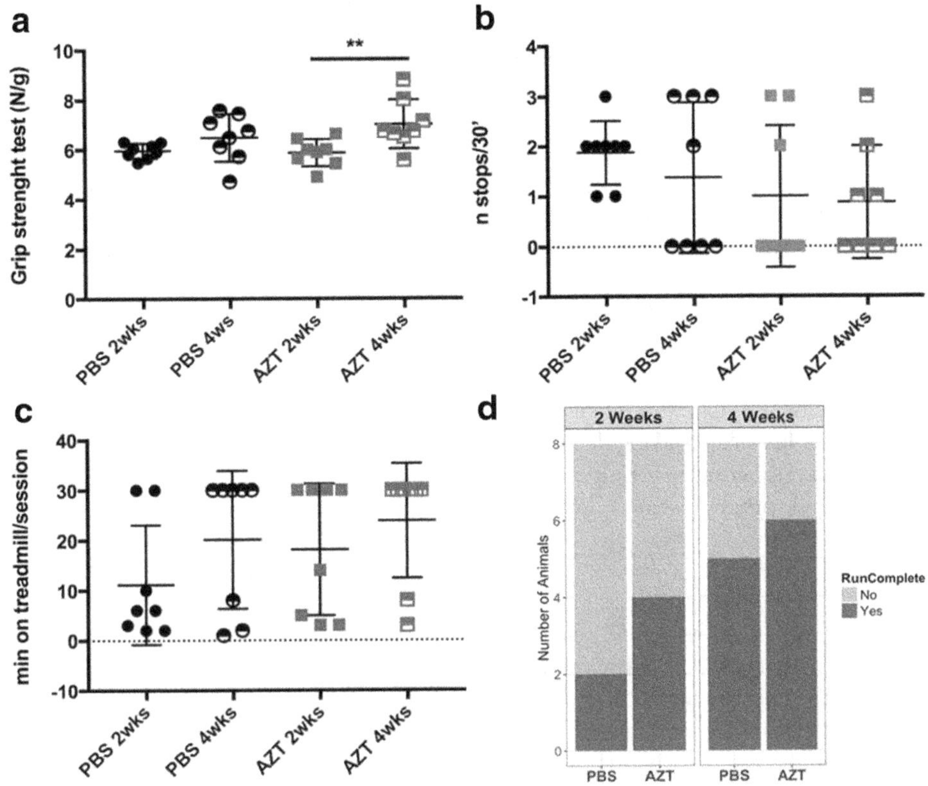

Fig. 8 AZT improves muscle strength in *mdx* mice. **a** Forelimb grip strength measurements in control and AZT-treated *mdx* mice at the end of the second and the fourth week of treatment showed a significant improvement in the AZT group (Error bars show mean ± SD, two way-ANOVA, df = 7, $n = 8$, Bonferroni's test, AZT:2wks vs AZT:4wks, $p = 0.0089$). **b** The number of stops per treadmill session in the analyses performed at the end of the second and fourth week of treatment. Error bars show mean ± SD, two way-ANOVA, df = 7, $n = 8$), **c** Time (in minutes) spent by individual mouse on the treadmill (Error bars show mean ± SD, two way-ANOVA, df = 7, $n = 8$) and **d** Number of PBS- or AZT-treated animals, which completed or not the 30 min treadmill session at the end of the second and fourth week of treatment (Pearson Chi-Square test, df = 2, $n = 8$). $^{**}p < 0.01$

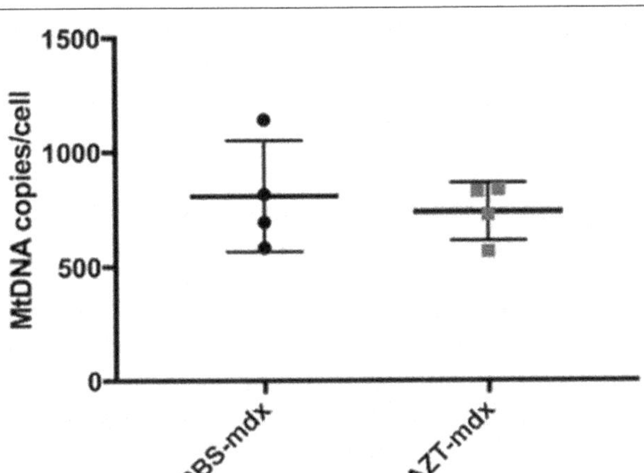

Fig. 9 AZT treatment did not induce mitochondrial toxicity in *mdx* mice. mtDNA copy number per cell determined using qPCR (absolute quantification method) in PBS- and AZT-treated mouse muscle. Error bars show mean ± SD, Mann Whitney test, $n = 4$

the 2 and 4-week treatment groups, respectively completed the 30 min treadmill run compared to only 25 and 62% of PBS-treated *mdx* mice, even though the result did not reach the statistical significance (Fig. 8b-d). The differences in the number of stops and the total time on the treadmill did not reach statistical significance following this short treatment regimen.

AZT had no acute detrimental effect on mitochondria and 2-Me-AZT retains anti-P2RX7 activity

It is known that NRTIs, including AZT, can affect mtDNA-specific polymerase (polymerase-gamma) activity, which can lead to deficiencies in mtDNA maintenance and transcription, and consequently mitochondrial abnormalities, especially in tissues requiring high energy, such as muscles. Notably, 100 mg/kg/day i.p. used here is somewhat higher than the equivalent human i.v. therapeutic dose (e.g. 8.1 vs. 6 mg/kg). Therefore, we analyzed the number of mtDNA copies in TA muscles from animals that received AZT treatment for 4 weeks. No differences in the amount of mtDNA copies were observed (Fig. 9), indicating that this AZT treatment had no immediate detrimental effect on the mitochondrial replication.

Nevertheless, appreciating the possibility of side effects caused by a chronic AZT treatment, we performed a preliminary study with 2-Me-AZT, a compound shown not to affect DNA polymerases [22, 44] but to retain its anti-P2RX7 activity (Fig. 2b). Following a 4-week treatment, RT-qPCR analysis of key inflammatory cell markers (CD68, PRX4, LY6G, Foxp3, TNFa) showed that this compound triggers a significant reduction of these inflammatory parameters in the treated *mdx* muscle (CD68: AZT-*mdx* vs PBS-*mdx* $p = 0.03$; LY6G: AZT-*mdx* vs PBS-*mdx* $p = 0.026$; TNFa: AZT-*mdx* vs PBS-*mdx* $p = 0.002$) (Additional file 6: Figure S5). This result confirms the observations of Fowler et al., [22] and indicates that this drug and/or derivatives of other NRTIs could be developed as safer alternatives for treatment of DMD and other diseases involving over-activation of P2RX7.

Discussion

Loss of dystrophin disrupts various downstream processes. Recent studies demonstrated that such abnormalities can be good targets for therapeutic interventions [24, 25, 35, 46, 58, 67, 68, 70, 72]. Unlike exon skipping or Ataluren, aimed at restoration of dystrophin, these treatments are not constrained by the causative DMD mutation. Therefore, all DMD patients rather than just a small subpopulation might benefit from these therapies. Moreover, these treatments may be effective in alleviating multiple abnormalities: muscle cell damage, inflammation, cognitive impairment and bone defects, which all make a substantial contribution to the clinical picture of DMD.

We demonstrated here that P2RX7 inhibition using a short treatment with AZT at the peak of disease severity in *mdx* mice attenuated the phenotype without any detectable side effects. The recovery was evident in key pathological parameters in treated leg and heart muscles such as reduced serum CK levels, decreased inflammatory markers and increased muscle strength in vivo.

The interest in P2RX7 as a therapeutic target in DMD results from the recent discovery that dystrophinopathy causes functional alterations of this purinoceptor and that the genetic ablation and pharmacological inhibition of P2RX7 in *mdx* mice produced significant improvements in key functional and molecular disease parameters [24, 58, 74]. In addition to the alleviation of muscle disease and decreased inflammation, reduced non-muscle symptoms (CNS and bones) were also evident [41, 58].

The wide therapeutic impact of P2RX7 inhibition reflects convergence of P2RX7 on multiple pathological mechanisms of DMD: P2RX7 inhibition reduces dystrophic muscle cell death directly [54, 73, 75], prevents the MMP-evoked damage [74] and also inhibits chronic inflammation [17, 24]. The association of P2RX7 with inflammation and immunity is long established. P2RX7 is involved in a range of responses including cytokine release, lymphocyte proliferation, intracellular pathogen killing, stimulation of gut mucosal immunity and even pain perception [15, 17, 43]. Not surprisingly, P2RX7 activation has been linked with a number of human diseases with an inflammatory component [22, 64, 66, 69, 71]. However, there is increasing evidence that P2RX7 also plays a pivotal role in central nervous system pathologies and in psychiatric disorders, where the link with inflammation is not always clear [61]. Indeed, the P2RX7 expression can be modulated in non-immune cells and it changes in disease states. For example, in addition to the aforementioned increased P2RX7 expression and function in dystrophic muscle [73–75], over-expression of this purinoceptor is evident in various human cancer cells [1, 16, 18].

Given the range of diseases involving this receptor, P2RX7 has attracted a lot of attention as a therapeutic target and specific antagonists have been developed. However, none of these are currently available as a drug. Moreover, each would need to undergo a lengthy and expensive evaluation process prior to use in a pediatric population such as for DMD.

Therefore, we studied AZT's potential to ameliorate DMD symptoms by blocking the P2RX7-evoked effects. We established, through molecular modelling, that both AZT and its methylated derivative could potentially bind with high affinity to the same allosteric site found to be occupied by the canonical antagonists. This site is distinct from the ATP-binding pocket and can accommodate structurally-similar but diverse molecules, mostly through hydrophobic interactions. Allosteric binding of these compounds prevents narrowing of the drug-binding pocket, a process crucial for opening the P2RX7 channel. Interestingly, the equivalent pocket in other P2X receptors is too narrow to accommodate the P2RX7 antagonist and therefore the size difference confers binding specificity of P2RX7 inhibitors [31]. In vitro assays confirmed that AZT could prevent the channel and the large pore opening in dystrophic myoblasts.

Using the most widely exploited animal model of DMD, we provided evidence that even a short (2 weeks) treatment with AZT causes P2RX7 inhibition in vivo. This was evidenced by the decreased TNFa levels, the production of which is P2RX7-dependent [10]. Given that pharmacological interference with TNFa has been shown to reduce DMD pathology [25], reduction of this inflammatory mediator is also clinically important. Indeed, AZT therapy improved muscle functions and sarcolemma stability measured by reduced CK and MiR206 serum levels and inhibited influx of IgG into muscle fibers. The most evident beneficial effect of AZT was a significant dampening of inflammation. AZT decreased the inflammatory *milieu* of dystrophic muscles chiefly by influencing the innate response. The inflammatory cell repertoire analysis in treated *mdx* skeletal and cardiac muscles showed that the treatment led to a reduction of markers for neutrophil and macrophage populations, which was noticeable just after 2 weeks of treatment and enhanced at 4 weeks.

Significantly reduced neutrophil marker Ly6G levels were found in AZT-treated samples, which corresponded with our previous findings in *mdx*/P2RX7 double mutant mice [58]. Hodgetts et al. [29] showed neutrophil depletion to be very effective in reducing myofibers necrosis in young *mdx* mice. Neutrophil-mediated skeletal muscle injury seems dependent on the free radical production and is tightly associated with the cytokines profile [29, 53]. Interestingly, in AZT-treated *mdx* we found remarkably reduced transcript levels of TNFa and of the inducible forms of COX and NOS (COX2 and iNOS). AZT may trigger neutrophil down-regulation and thus reduce inflammation by directly inhibiting P2RX7 in these cells: A recent study showed that both human and murine neutrophils express functional P2RX7, activation of which leads to NLRP3 inflammasome activation and IL-1b secretion [32]. Moreover, P2RX7 ablation has a widespread impact on the inflammatory cell migration, including neutrophils [33] and this might also explain the reduced neutrophil load in dystrophic muscles.

AZT treatment did not significantly reduce the levels of CD4+ or CD8+ T-cells and this short term treatment did not unequivocally affect expression levels of Foxp3 and IL12a, markers of the T_{reg} cells. Given that our previous studies demonstrating this enhancement of muscle T_{reg} involved the genetic ablation of P2RX7 or global purinergic inhibition [24, 58], further experiments are needed to establish whether sustained AZT treatment or different dosing regimen would result in a shift in T-cell responses.

The reduction of inflammatory cell infiltrations and inflammatory markers expression in cardiac muscles following AZT treatment was also in agreement with our previous data in mice with blocked P2RX7 receptors [24, 58]. This finding is of clinical importance because heart failure becomes the most common cause of death in DMD patients surviving longer due to advances in general care [11].

Taken together, these results demonstrate that AZT, targeting P2RX7 functions in both muscle and inflammatory cells, reduces the production of pro-inflammatory mediators thus leading to reduced inflammation with fewer lymphocytes, neutrophils and macrophages within *mdx* muscles. There is also reduced muscle membrane damage and slightly improved muscle strength in AZT-treated dystrophic mice. In experimental paradigms not inducing dystrophin exon skipping, such as one described here, fewer revertant fibers have been used as an indicator that a muscle underwent fewer degeneration/regeneration cycles [47, 56]. Not unexpectedly, given the short treatment period, no significant reduction in the revertant fiber count was found. However, this result indicated that AZT has no negative effect as any disease acceleration should be quickly reflected in muscles' degeneration/regeneration history.

AZT is a mainstay in the prevention of mother-to-child HIV transmission. A recent extensive survey on the safety of AZT in the pediatric population in the EU and Thailand has shown AZT to be a well-tolerated drug with few side effects [65], thus confirming earlier findings in the pediatric population [50] High NRTI dosage can interfere with the eukaryotic mtDNA-specific polymerase. However, these side-effects occur in long term treatment regimens and are reversible: Elimination half-life following i.v. administration is ~ 1.1 h [6, 23]. Notably, 100 mg/kg/day i.p. used here is higher than the equivalent human i.v. dose (8.1 vs. 6 mg/day). While this treatment had no detrimental effect on mitochondria, which are typically the most sensitive organelles in NRTIs therapy, a longer-term and different dosing regimen would help correlating the therapeutic impact and potential side-effects of AZT fully. Appreciating the possibility of side effects of a chronic AZT treatment, we also tested its methyl derivative (2-Me-AZT) not affecting DNA polymerases [22, 44] but found by us to bind the same allosteric site and to retain anti-P2RX7 activity. Following a 4-week treatment, we demonstrated that 2-Me-AZT caused a significant reduction of inflammatory parameters akin to the effects of AZT.

Conclusions

In conclusion, AZT emerges as a P2RX7 inhibitor effective in reducing harmful inflammation and potential to improve muscle function in dystrophic *mdx* mice. Given extensive safety and pharmacokinetic data available following decades of AZT use in humans, also in children and neonates, this drug should be considered for trials in DMD. Unlike other experimental drugs, it could be used from the very early stage of this debilitating and ultimately lethal disease, where any treatment is likely to be most effective.

Additional files

Additional file 1: Figure S1. Human, giant panda and mouse P2RX7 peptide sequence alignments. (PDF 779 kb)

Additional file 2: Table S1. Binding Energies for AZT at all of the sites in the 5U1V identified by the site finder in MOE. (DOCX 16 kb)

Additional file 3: Figure S2. Average weight gain of mice following AZT treatment. (TIFF 756 kb)

Additional file 4: Figure S3. Impact of the 2-week AZT treatment on key pathological parameters. (TIFF 6394 kb)

Additional file 5: Figure S4. Muscle fiber analysis following AZT administration in vivo. (TIFF 3875 kb)

Additional file 6: Figure S5. 2-Me-AZT treatment impact on the expression of selected inflammatory genes. (TIFF 900 kb)

Acknowledgements
RA-K was supported by the Higher Committee for Education Development in Iraq (HCED). This research was supported in parts by the National Science Centre, Poland according to the decision number DEC-2013/11/B/NZ3/01573 (KZ, JR, DCG). J.A. was supported by NIH grants (DP1GM114862, R01EY022238 and R01EY024068), the John Templeton Foundation and through a DuPont Guerry, III Professorship. Dr. S. Robson advice on statistical analyses of the data and the COST Action BM1406 are gratefully acknowledged.

Authors, contributions
Designed the experiments/the study: DCG, CNJY, KZ. Collected data/did experiments for the study: RA-K, CP, PC, NC, JR, CNJY, RMcG, DCG. Pharmacological inhibition studies: RA-K, CP, CNJY, JR, SA, KZ. 2Me-AZT synthesis and development: KA, JA. Drug modelling: PC, RMcG. Western blotting: RA-K, CP, NC, CNJY. Immunolocalization and histology: RA-K, CP, NC, CNJY. qPCR: RA-K, CP, NC. Muscle strength measurements in vivo: RA-K, CP. Mitochondrial DNA analysis: RMcG. Data analysis: RA-K, CP, PC, NC, JR, CNJY, RMcG, JA, KZ, EG, SA, CB, DCG. Wrote the first draft of the paper: CP, RA-K, PC, NC, JR, CNJY, RMcG. Contributed to the writing of the manuscript: RA-K, CP, PC, NC, JR, CNJY, RMcG, JA, KZ, EG, SA, CB, DCG. All authors agree with the manuscript's results and conclusions.

Competing interests
J.A. is a cofounder of iVeena Holdings, iVeena Delivery Systems and Inflammasome Therapeutics and has been a consultant for Allergan, Biogen, Olix Pharmaceuticals, and Saksin LifeSciences in a capacity unrelated to this work. J.A. and K.A. are named as inventors on patent applications on macular degeneration filed by the University of Kentucky or the University of Virginia.

Author details
[1]Molecular Medicine Laboratory, School of Pharmacy and Biomedical Sciences, University of Portsmouth, Portsmouth, UK. [2]Center of Myology and Neurodegenerative Disorders, Department of Neuroscience and Rehabilitation, Istituto Giannina Gaslini, Genoa, Italy. [3]Laboratory of Cellular Metabolism, Department of Biochemistry, Nencki Institute of Experimental Biology of the Polish Academy of Sciences, Warsaw, Poland. [4]Department of Ophthalmology & Center for Advanced Vision Science, University of Virginia, Charlottesville, VA, USA. [5]Department of Pathology, Microbiology, Immunology & Cancer Biology, University of Virginia, Charlottesville, VA, USA. [6]Present Address: Biotechnology Department, Faculty of Science, University of Baghdad, Baghdad, Iraq. [7]Present Address: School of Allied Health Sciences, Faculty of Health and Life Sciences, De Montfort University, Leicester, UK.

References

1. Adinolfi E, Raffaghello L, Giuliani AL, Cavazzini L, Capece M, Chiozzi P, Bianchi G, Kroemer G, Pistoia V, Di Virgilio F (2012) Expression of P2X7 receptor increases in vivo tumor growth. Cancer Res 72(12):2957–2969
2. Altamirano F, Valladares D, Henriquez-Olguin C, Casas M, Lopez JR, Allen PD, Jaimovich E (2013) Nifedipine treatment reduces resting calcium concentration, oxidative and apoptotic gene expression, and improves muscle function in dystrophic mdx mice. PLoS One 8(12):e81222
3. Banihani R, Smile S, Yoon G, Dupuis A, Mosleh M, Snider A, McAdam L (2015) Cognitive and neurobehavioral profile in boys with Duchenne muscular dystrophy. J Child Neurol 30(11):1472–1482
4. Barka T, Anderson PJ (1962) Histochemical methods for acid phosphatase using hexazonium pararosanalin as coupler. J Histochem Cytochem 10:741–753
5. Berman HM, Westbrook J, Feng Z, Gilliland G, Bhat TN, Weissig H, Shindyalov IN, Bourne PE (2000) The protein data bank. Nucleic Acids Res 28(1):235–242
6. Blümer RM, van Vonderen MG, Sutinen J, Hassink E, Ackermans M, van Agtmael MA, Yki-Jarvinen H, Danner SA, Reiss P, Sauerwein HP (2008) Zidovudine/lamivudine contributes to insulin resistance within 3 months of starting combination antiretroviral therapy. AIDS 22(2):227–236
7. Bowles EJ, Lee JH, Alberio R, Lloyd RE, Stekel D, Campbell KH, St John JC (2007) Contrasting effects of in vitro fertilization and nuclear transfer on the expression of mtDNA replication factors. Genetics 176(3):1511–1526
8. Buvinic S, Almarza G, Bustamante M, Casas M, López J, Riquelme M, Sáez JC, Huidobro-Toro JP, Jaimovich E (2009) ATP released by electrical stimuli elicits calcium transients and gene expression in skeletal muscle. J Biol Chem 284(50):34490–34505
9. Caseley EA, Muench SP, Fishwick CW, Jiang LH (2016) Structure-based identification and characterisation of structurally novel human P2X7 receptor antagonists. Biochem Pharmacol 116:130–139
10. Chessell IP, Hatcher JP, Bountra C, Michel AD, Hughes JP, Green P, Egerton J, Murfin M, Richardson J, Peck WL, Grahames CB, Casula MA, Yiangou Y, Birch R, Anand P, Buell GN (2005) Disruption of the P2X7 purinoceptor gene abolishes chronic inflammatory and neuropathic pain. Pain 114(3):386–396
11. D'Amario D, Amodeo A, Adorisio R, Tiziano FD, Leone AM, Perri G, Bruno P, Massetti M, Ferlini A, Pane M, Niccoli G, Porto I, D'Angelo GA, Borovac JA, Mercuri E, Crea F (2017) A current approach to heart failure in Duchenne muscular dystrophy. Heart 103:1770–1779
12. Daluge SM, Purifoy DJ, Savina PM, St Clair MH, Parry NR, Dev IK, Novak P, Ayers KM, Reardon JE, Roberts GB (1994) 5-Chloro-2',3'-dideoxy-3'-fluorouridine (935U83), a selective anti-human immunodeficiency virus agent with an improved metabolic and toxicological profile. Antimicrob Agents Chemother 38(7):1590–1603
13. De Luca A, Nico B, Liantonio A, Didonna MP, Fraysse B, Pierno S, Burdi R, Mangieri D, Rolland JF, Camerino C, Zallone A, Confalonieri P, Andreetta F, Arnoldi E, Courdier-Fruh I, Magyar JP, Frigeri A, Pisoni M, Svelto M, Conte Camerino D (2005) A multidisciplinary evaluation of the effectiveness of cyclosporine a in dystrophic mdx mice. Am J Pathol 166(2):477–489
14. Di Virgilio F (2007) Purinergic signalling in the immune system. A brief update. Purinergic Signal 3(1–2):1–3
15. Di Virgilio F (2015a) P2X receptors and inflammation. Curr Med Chem 22(7): 866–877
16. Di Virgilio F (2015b) P2RX7: a receptor with a split personality in inflammation and cancer. Mol Cell Oncol 3(2):e1010937
17. Di Virgilio F, Dal Ben D, Sarti AC, Giuliani AL, Falzoni S (2017) The P2X7 receptor in infection and inflammation. Immunity 47(1):15–31
18. Di Virgilio F, Ferrari D, Adinolfi E (2009) P2X(7): a growth-promoting receptor-implications for cancer. Purinergic Signal 5(2):251–256
19. Dumont NA, Wang YX, von Maltzahn J, Pasut A, Bentzinger CF, Brun CE, Rudnicki MA (2015) Dystrophin expression in muscle stem cells regulates their polarity and asymmetric division. Nat Med 21(12):1455–1463
20. Ermolova NV, Martinez L, Vetrone SA, Jordan MC, Roos KP, Sweeney HL, Spencer MJ (2014) Long-term administration of the TNF blocking drug Remicade (cV1q) to mdx mice reduces skeletal and cardiac muscle fibrosis, but negatively impacts cardiac function. Neuromuscul Disord 24(7):583–595
21. Eser A, Colombel JF, Rutgeerts P, Vermeire S, Vogelsang H, Braddock M, Persson T, Reinisch W (2015) Safety and efficacy of an oral inhibitor of the purinergic receptor P2X7 in adult patients with moderately to severely active Crohn's disease: a randomized placebo-controlled, double-blind, phase IIa study. Inflamm Bowel Dis 21(10):2247–2253
22. Fowler BJ, Gelfand BD, Kim Y, Kerur N, Tarallo V, Hirano Y, Amarnath S, Fowler DH, Radwan M, Young MT, Pittman K, Kubes P, Agarwal HK, Parang K, Hinton DR, Bastos-Carvalho A, Li S, Yasuma T, Mizutani T, Yasuma R, Wright C, Ambati J (2014) Nucleoside reverse transcriptase inhibitors possess intrinsic anti-inflammatory activity. Science 346(6212): 1000–1003
23. Gao RY, Mukhopadhyay P, Mohanraj R, Wang H, Horváth B, Yin S, Pacher P (2011) Resveratrol attenuates azidothymidine-induced cardiotoxicity by decreasing mitochondrial reactive oxygen species generation in human cardiomyocytes. Mol Med Rep 4(1):151–155
24. Gazzerro E, Baldassari S, Assereto S, Fruscione F, Pistorio A, Panicucci C, Volpi S, Perruzza L, Fiorillo C, Minetti C, Traggiai E, Grassi F, Bruno C (2015) Enhancement of muscle T regulatory cells and improvement of muscular dystrophic process in mdx mice by blockade of extracellular ATP/P2X Axis. Am J Pathol 185(12):3349–3360
25. Grounds MD, Torrisi J (2004) Anti-TNFalpha (Remicade) therapy protects dystrophic skeletal muscle from necrosis. FASEB J 18(6):676–682
26. Grynkiewicz G, Poenie M, Tsien RY (1985) A new generation of Ca2+ indicators with greatly improved fluorescent properties. J Biol Chem 260:3440–3450
27. Guile SD, Alcaraz L, Birkinshaw TN, Bowers KC, Ebden MR, Furber M, Stocks MJ (2009) Antagonists of the P2X(7) receptor. From lead identification to drug development. J Med Chem 52(10):3123–3141
28. Wehling M, Spencer MJ, Tidball JG (2001) A nitric oxide synthase transgene ameliorates muscular dystrophy in mdx mice. J Cell Biol 155:123–31.
29. Hodgetts S, Radley H, Davies M, Grounds MD (2006) Reduced necrosis of dystrophic muscle by depletion of host neutrophils, or blocking TNFalpha function with Etanercept in mdx mice. Neuromuscul Disord 16(9–10):591–602

30. Idzko M, Ferrari D, Eltzschig HK (2014) Nucleotide signalling during inflammation. Nature 509(7500):310–317
31. Karasawa A, Kawate T (2016) Structural basis for subtype-specific inhibition of the P2X7 receptor. elife 5:e22153
32. Karmakar M, Katsnelson MA, Dubyak GR, Pearlman E (2016) Neutrophil P2X7 receptors mediate NLRP3 inflammasome-dependent IL-1ß secretion in response to ATP. Nat Commun 7:10555
33. Kawamura H, Kawamura T, Kanda Y, Kobayashi T, Abo T (2012) Extracellular ATP-stimulated macrophages produce macrophage inflammatory protein-2 which is important for neutrophil migration. Immunology 136(4):448–458
34. Keystone EC, Wang MM, Layton M, Hollis S, McInnes IB, D1520C00001 Study Team (2012) Clinical evaluation of the efficacy of the P2X7 purinergic receptor antagonist AZD9056 on the signs and symptoms of rheumatoid arthritis in patients with active disease despite treatment with methotrexate or sulphasalazine. Ann Rheum Dis 71(10):1630–1635
35. Kuno A, Horio Y (2016) SIRT1: a novel target for the treatment of muscular dystrophies. Oxidative Med Cell Longev 2016:6714686
36. Kuswanto W, Burzyn D, Panduro M, Wang KK, Jang YC, Wagers AJ, Benoist C, Mathis D (2016) Poor repair of skeletal muscle in aging mice reflects a defect in local, Interleukin-33-dependent accumulation of regulatory T cells. Immunity 44(2):355–367
37. Lambertucci C, Dal Ben D, Buccioni M, Marucci G, Thomas A, Volpini R (2015) Medicinal chemistry of P2X receptors: agonists and orthosteric antagonists. Curr Med Chem 22(7):915–928
38. McNally EM (2007) New approaches in the therapy of cardiomyopathy in muscular dystrophy. Annu Rev Med 58:75–88
39. Mizuno H, Nakamura A, Aoki Y, Ito N, Kishi S, Yamamoto K, Sekiguchi M, Takeda S, Hashido K (2011) Identification of muscle-specific microRNAs in serum of muscular dystrophy animal models: promising novel blood-based markers for muscular dystrophy. PLoS One 6(3):e18388
40. Mizutani T, Fowler BJ, Kim Y, Yasuma R, Krueger LA, Gelfand BD, Ambati J (2015) Nucleoside reverse transcriptase inhibitors suppress laser-induced choroidal neovascularization in mice. Invest Ophthalmol Vis Sci 56(12):7122–7129
41. Mohamad NS, Sinadinos A, Górecki DC, Zioupos P, Tong J (2016) Impact of P2RX7 ablation on the morphological, mechanical and tissue properties of bones in a murine model of duchenne muscular dystrophy. J Biomech 49(14):3444–3451
42. Molecular Operating Environment (MOE). 2013.08; Chemical Computing Group ULC, Montreal, 2017. https://www.chemcomp.com/Research-Citing_MOE.htm.
43. North RA, Jarvis MF (2013) P2X receptors as drug targets. Mol Pharmacol 83(4):759–769
44. Ambati J, Fowler B, Ambati K (2016) Compositions and methods for treating retinal degradation. Patent Application No. PCT/US2016/019852
45. Pelosi L, Berardinelli MG, De Pasquale L, Nicoletti C, D'Amico A, Carvello F, Moneta GM, Catizone A, Bertini E, De Benedetti F, Musarò A (2015) Functional and morphological improvement of dystrophic muscle by interleukin 6 receptor blockade. EBioMedicine 2(4):285–293
46. Percival JM, Whitehead NP, Adams ME, Adamo CM, Beavo JA, Froehner SC (2012) Sildenafil reduces respiratory muscle weakness and fibrosis in the mdx mouse model of Duchenne muscular dystrophy. J Pathol 228(1):77–87
47. Pigozzo SR, Da Re L, Romualdi C, Mazzara PG, Galletta E, Fletcher S, Wilton SD, Vitiello L (2013) Revertant fibers in the mdx murine model of Duchenne muscular dystrophy: an age- and muscle-related reappraisal. PLoS One 8:e72147
48. Pizzirani C, Ferrari D, Chiozzi P, Adinolfi E, Sandonà D, Savaglio E, Di Virgilio F (2007) Stimulation of P2 receptors causes release of IL-1beta-loaded microvesicles from human dendritic cells. Blood 109(9):3856–3864
49. Ponchel F, Toomes C, Bransfield K, Leong FT, Douglas SH, Field SL, Bell SM, Combaret V, Puisieux A, Mighell AJ, Robinson PA, Inglehearn CF, Isaacs JD, Markham AF (2003) Real-time PCR based on SYBR-Green I fluorescence: an alternative to the TaqMan assay for a relative quantification of gene rearrangements, gene amplifications and micro gene deletions. BMC Biotechnol 3:18
50. Pryce C, Pierre RB, Steel-Duncan J, Evans-Gilbert T, Palmer P, Moore J, Rodriguez B, Christie CD (2008) Safety of antiretroviral drug therapy in Jamaican children with HIV/AIDS. West Indian Med J 57(3):238–245
51. Radley-Crabb H, Terrill J, Shavlakadze T, Tonkin J, Arthur P, Grounds M (2012) A single 30 min treadmill exercise session is suitable for 'proof-of concept studies' in adult mdx mice: a comparison of the early consequences of two different treadmill protocols. Neuromuscul Disord 22(2):170–182
52. Rando TA (2001a) The dystrophin-glycoprotein complex, cellular signaling, and the regulation of cell survival in muscular dystrophies. Muscle Nerve 24: 1575e1594
53. Rando TA (2001b) Role of nitric oxide in the pathogenesis of muscular dystrophies: a "two hit" hypothesis of the cause of muscle necrosis. Microsc Res Tech 55(4):223–235 Review
54. Rawat R, Cohen TV, Ampong B, Francia D, Henriques-Pons A, Hoffman EP, Nagaraju K (2010) Inflammasome up-regulation and activation in dysferlin-deficient skeletal muscle. Am J Pathol 176(6):2891–2900
55. Rufo A, Del Fattore A, Capulli M, Carvello F, De Pasquale L, Ferrari S, Pierroz D, Morandi L, De Simone M, Rucci N, Bertini E, Bianchi ML, De Benedetti F, Teti A (2011) Mechanisms inducing low bone density in Duchenne muscular dystrophy in mice and humans. J Bone Miner Res 26(8):1891–1903
56. Sacco A, Mourkioti F, Tran R, Choi J, Llewellyn M, Kraft P, Shkreli M, Delp S, Pomerantz JH, Artandi SE, Blau HM (2010) Short telomeres and stem cell exhaustion model Duchenne muscular dystrophy in mdx/mTR mice. Cell 143:1059–1071
57. Sch mittgen TD, Livak KJ (2008) Analyzing real-time PCR data by the comparative CT method. Nat Protoc 3(6):1101–1108
58. Sinadinos A, Young CN, Al-Khalidi R, Teti A, Kalinski P, Mohamad S, Floriot L, Henry T, Tozzi G, Jiang T, Wurtz O, Lefebvre A, Shugay M, Tong J, Vaudry D, Arkle S, doRego JC, Górecki DC (2015) sP2RX7 purinoceptor: a therapeutic target for ameliorating the symptoms of duchenne muscular dystrophy. PLoS Med 12(10):e1001888
59. Snow WM, Anderson JE, Jakobson LS (2013) Neuropsychological and neurobehavioral functioning in Duchenne muscular dystrophy: a review. Neurosci Biobehav Rev 37(5):743–752
60. Spencer MJ, Montecino-Rodriguez E, Dorshkind K, Tidball JG (2001) Helper (CD4(+)) and cytotoxic (CD8(+)) T cells promote the pathology of dystrophin-deficient muscle. Clin Immunol 98(2):235–243
61. Sperlágh B, Illes P (2014) P2X7 receptor: an emerging target in central nervous system diseases. Trends Pharmacol Sci 35(10):537–547
62. Stock TC, Bloom BJ, Wei N, Ishaq S, Park W, Wang X, Gupta P, Mebus CA (2012) Efficacy and safety of CE-224,535, an antagonist of P2X7 receptor, in treatment of patients with rheumatoid arthritis inadequately controlled by methotrexate. J Rheumatol 39(4):720–727
63. Subramanyam C, Duplantier AJ, Dombroski MA, Chang SP, Gabel CA, Whitney-Pickett C, Perregaux DG, Labasi JM, Yoon K, Shepard RM, Fisher M (2011) Discovery, synthesis and SAR of azinyl- and azolylbenzamides antagonists of the $P2X_7$ receptor. Bioorg Med Chem Lett 21(18):5475–5479
64. Sugiyama T, Lee SY, Horie T, Oku H, Takai S, Tanioka H, Kuriki Y, Kojima S, Ikeda T (2013) $P2X_7$ receptor activation may be involved in neuronal loss in the retinal ganglion cell layer after acute elevation of intraocular pressure in rats. Mol Vis 19:2080–2091
65. The European Pregnancy and Paediatric HIV Cohort Collaboration (EPPICC) study group in EuroCoord (2017) Safety of zidovudine/lamivudine scored tablets in children with HIV infection in Europe and Thailand. Eur J Clin Pharmacol 73(4):463–468
66. Vergani A, Tezza S, D'Addio F, Fotino C, Liu K, Niewczas M, Bassi R, Molano RD, Kleffel S, Petrelli A, Soleti A, Ammirati E, Frigerio M, Visner G, Grassi F, Ferrero ME, Corradi D, Abdi R, Ricordi C, Sayegh MH, Pileggi A, Fiorina P (2013) Long-term heart transplant survival by targeting the ionotropic purinergic receptor P2X7. Circulation 127(4): 463–475
67. Vidal B, Ardite E, Suelves M, Ruiz-Bonilla V, Janue A, Flick MJ, Degen JL, Serrano AL, Munoz-Canoves P (2012) Amelioration of Duchenne muscular dystrophy in mdx mice by elimination of matrix-associated fibrin-driven inflammation coupled to the alphaMbeta2 leukocyte integrin receptor. Hum Mol Genet 21(9):1989–2004
68. Vieira NM, Elvers I, Alexander MS, Moreira YB, Eran A, Gomes JP, Marshall JL, Karlsson EK, Verjovski-Almeida S, Lindblad-Toh K, Kunkel LM, Zatz M (2015) Jagged 1 rescues the Duchenne muscular dystrophy phenotype. Cell 163(5): 1204–1213
69. Wan P, Liu X, Xiong Y, Ren Y, Chen J, Lu N, Guo Y, Bai A (2016) Extracellular ATP mediates inflammatory responses in colitis via P2 × 7 receptor signaling. Sci Rep 6:19108
70. Wehling-Henricks M, Li Z, Lindsey C, Wang Y, Welc SS, Ramos JN, Khanlou N, Kuro-O M, Tidball JG (2016) Klotho gene silencing promotes pathology in the mdx mouse model of Duchenne muscular dystrophy. Hum Mol Genet 25(12):2465–2482

71. Wilhelm K, Ganesan J, Müller T, Dürr C, Grimm M, Beilhack A, Krempl CD, Sorichter S, Gerlach UV, Jüttner E, Zerweck A, Gärtner F, Pellegatti P, Di Virgilio F, Ferrari D, Kambham N, Fisch P, Finke J, Idzko M, Zeiser R (2010) Graft-versus-host disease is enhanced by extracellular ATP activating P2X7R. Nat Med 16(12):1434–1438
72. Xie X, Tsai SY, Tsai MJ (2016) COUP-TFII regulates satellite cell function and muscular dystrophy. J Clin Invest 126(10):3929–3941
73. Young CN, Brutkowski W, Lien CF, Arkle S, Lochmüller H, Zabłocki K, Górecki DC (2012) P2X7 purinoceptor alterations in dystrophic mdx mouse muscles: relationship to pathology and potential target for treatment. J Cell Mol Med 16(5):1026–1037
74. Young CN, Chira N, Róg J, Al-Khalidi R, Benard M, Galas L, Chan P, Vaudry D, Zabłocki K, Górecki DC (2017) Sustained activation of P2X7 induces MMP-2-evoked cleavage and functional purinoceptor inhibition. J Mol Cell Biol. https://doi.org/10.1093/jmcb/mjx030. Epub ahead of print.
75. Young CN, Sinadinos A, Lefebvre A, Chan P, Arkle S, Vaudry D, Gorecki DC (2015) A novel mechanism of autophagic cell death in dystrophic muscle regulated by P2RX7 receptor large-pore formation and HSP90. Autophagy 11(1):113–130

Permissions

All chapters in this book were first published in ANC, by BioMed Central; hereby published with permission under the Creative Commons Attribution License or equivalent. Every chapter published in this book has been scrutinized by our experts. Their significance has been extensively debated. The topics covered herein carry significant findings which will fuel the growth of the discipline. They may even be implemented as practical applications or may be referred to as a beginning point for another development.

The contributors of this book come from diverse backgrounds, making this book a truly international effort. This book will bring forth new frontiers with its revolutionizing research information and detailed analysis of the nascent developments around the world.

We would like to thank all the contributing authors for lending their expertise to make the book truly unique. They have played a crucial role in the development of this book. Without their invaluable contributions this book wouldn't have been possible. They have made vital efforts to compile up to date information on the varied aspects of this subject to make this book a valuable addition to the collection of many professionals and students.

This book was conceptualized with the vision of imparting up-to-date information and advanced data in this field. To ensure the same, a matchless editorial board was set up. Every individual on the board went through rigorous rounds of assessment to prove their worth. After which they invested a large part of their time researching and compiling the most relevant data for our readers.

The editorial board has been involved in producing this book since its inception. They have spent rigorous hours researching and exploring the diverse topics which have resulted in the successful publishing of this book. They have passed on their knowledge of decades through this book. To expedite this challenging task, the publisher supported the team at every step. A small team of assistant editors was also appointed to further simplify the editing procedure and attain best results for the readers.

Apart from the editorial board, the designing team has also invested a significant amount of their time in understanding the subject and creating the most relevant covers. They scrutinized every image to scout for the most suitable representation of the subject and create an appropriate cover for the book.

The publishing team has been an ardent support to the editorial, designing and production team. Their endless efforts to recruit the best for this project, has resulted in the accomplishment of this book. They are a veteran in the field of academics and their pool of knowledge is as vast as their experience in printing. Their expertise and guidance has proved useful at every step. Their uncompromising quality standards have made this book an exceptional effort. Their encouragement from time to time has been an inspiration for everyone.

The publisher and the editorial board hope that this book will prove to be a valuable piece of knowledge for researchers, students, practitioners and scholars across the globe.

List of Contributors

Ayako Nakamura and Toshiki Uchihara
Laboratory of Structural Neuropathology, Tokyo Metropolitan Institute of Medical Science, 2-1-6 Kamikitazawa, Setagaya-ku, Tokyo 156-8506, Japan

Ryosuke Takahashi
Department of Neurology, Kyoto University Graduate School of Medicine, Sakyo-ku, Kyoto, Japan

Miho Uematsu
The Japan Society for the Promotion of Science (JSPS), Chiyoda-ku, Tokyo, Japan
Department of Neurology, Kyoto University Graduate School of Medicine, Sakyo-ku, Kyoto, Japan
Laboratory of Structural Neuropathology, Tokyo Metropolitan Institute of Medical Science, 2-1-6 Kamikitazawa, Setagaya-ku, Tokyo 156-8506, Japan

Momoko Ebashi
Division of Neurology, Department of Medicine, Nihon University School of Medicine, Itabashi-ku, Tokyo, Japan
Laboratory of Structural Neuropathology, Tokyo Metropolitan Institute of Medical Science, 2-1-6 Kamikitazawa, Setagaya-ku, Tokyo 156-8506, Japan

Katsuiku Hirokawa
Department of Pathology, Nitobe-Memorial Nakano General Hospital, Nakano-ku, Tokyo, Japan

Nobutaka Sakae, Kevin F. Bieniek, Yong-Jie Zhang, Kelly Ross, Tania F. Gendron, Melissa E. Murray, Rosa Rademakers, Leonard Petrucelli and Dennis W. Dickson
Department of Neuroscience, Mayo Clinic, 4500 San Pablo Road, Jacksonville, FL 32224, USA

Megan Hayes, Jacob C. Zbesko and Jennifer B. Frye
Department of Immunobiology, University of Arizona, 1656 E. Mabel Street, Tucson, AZ 85719, USA

Thuy-Vi V. Nguyen
Department of Immunobiology, University of Arizona, 1656 E. Mabel Street, Tucson, AZ 85719, USA
Department of Neurology, University of Arizona, 1656 E. Mabel Street, Tucson, AZ 85719, USA

Kristian P. Doyle
Department of Immunobiology, University of Arizona, 1656 E. Mabel Street, Tucson, AZ 85719, USA
Department of Neurology, University of Arizona, 1656 E. Mabel Street, Tucson, AZ 85719, USA
Arizona Center on Aging, University of Arizona, 1656 E. Mabel Street, Tucson, AZ 85719, USA

Nicole R. Congrove and Brian S. McKay
Department of Ophthalmology and Vision Science, University of Arizona, Tucson, AZ, USA

Nadia P. Belichenko and Frank M. Longo
Department of Neurology and Neurological Sciences, Stanford University, Stanford, CA, USA

Joseph Buxbaum
Department of Psychiatry, Icahn School of Medicine at Mount Sinai, New York, NY 10029, USA
Mount Sinai Center for Transformative Disease Modeling, Icahn Institute of Genomics and Multiscale Biology, Icahn School of Medicine at Mount Sinai, New York, NY 10029, USA

Kristen J. Brennand
Department of Psychiatry, Icahn School of Medicine at Mount Sinai, New York, NY 10029, USA
Department of Genetics and Genomic Sciences, Icahn School of Medicine at Mount Sinai, New York, NY 10029, USA
Department of Neuroscience, Icahn School of Medicine at Mount Sinai, New York, NY 10029, USA
Friedman Brain Institute, Icahn School of Medicine at Mount Sinai, New York, NY 10029, USA

Erming Wang, Minghui Wang, Eric Schad and Bin Zhang
Department of Genetics and Genomic Sciences, Icahn School of Medicine at Mount Sinai, New York, NY 10029, USA
Mount Sinai Center for Transformative Disease Modeling, Icahn Institute of Genomics and Multiscale Biology, Icahn School of Medicine at Mount Sinai, New York, NY 10029, USA

Wun Chey Sin and Christian C. Naus
Department of Cellular and Physiological Sciences, University of British Columbia, Vancouver, British Columbia V6T 1Z3, Canada

Yuji Kajiwara
Denali Therapeutics South San Francisco CA 94080, USA
Department of Psychiatry, Icahn School of Medicine at Mount Sinai, New York, NY 10029, USA

Jeroen van Ameijde, Rosa Crespo, Roosmarijn Janson, Jarek Juraszek, Berdien Siregar, Hanneke Verveen, Imke Sprengers, Tariq Nahar, Wouter Koudstaal and Adrian Apetri
Janssen Prevention Center, Janssen Pharmaceutical Companies of Johnson and Johnson, Archimedesweg 6, 2333 Leiden, CN, the Netherlands

Jeroen J. Hoozemans
Department of Pathology, Amsterdam Neuroscience, VU University Medical Center, De Boelelaan 1117, 1081, HV, Amsterdam, the Netherlands

Stefan Steinbacher
Proteros Biostructures GmbH, Bunsenstraße 7a, 82152 Planegg, Germany

Roland Willems, Lore Delbroek, Marianne Borgers, Kristof Van Kolen and Marc Mercken
Janssen Neuroscience Discovery, Janssen Pharmaceutical Companies of Johnson and Johnson, Turnhoutseweg 30, 2340 Beerse, Belgium

Koen Dockx
Molecular and Cellular Pharmacology, Discovery Sciences, Janssen Pharmaceutical Companies of Johnson and Johnson, Turnhoutseweg 30, 2340 Beerse, Belgium

Gabriel Pascual
Janssen Prevention Center, Janssen Pharmaceutical Companies of Johnson and Johnson, 3210 Merryfield Row, San Diego, CA 92121, USA

Stephanie Ziegler-Waldkirch, Karin Marksteiner, Johannes Stoll, Paolo d'Errico, Denise Eiler, Lea Neudel, Verena Sturn, Isabel Opper, Moumita Datta, Marco Prinz and Melanie Meyer-Luehmann
Faculty of Medicine, University of Freiburg, Freiburg, Germany
Department of Neurology, Medical Center - University of Freiburg, Freiburg, Germany

Marina Friesen
Department of Neurology, Medical Center - University of Freiburg, Freiburg, Germany
Faculty of Biology, University of Freiburg, Freiburg, Germany
Institute of Neuropathology, Medical Center - University of Freiburg, Freiburg, Germany

Moumita Datta
Institute of Neuropathology, Medical Center - University of Freiburg, Freiburg, Germany

Marco Prinz
BIOSS Centre for Biological Signalling Studies, University of Freiburg, Freiburg, Germany
Institute of Neuropathology, Medical Center - University of Freiburg, Freiburg, Germany

Michael X. Henderson, Chao Peng, John Q. Trojanowski and Virginia M. Y. Lee
Department of Pathology and Laboratory Medicine, Institute on Aging and Center for Neurodegenerative Disease Research, University of Pennsylvania School of Medicine, 3600 Spruce St, 3rd Floor Maloney, Philadelphia, PA 19104-4283, USA

Aiko Ishiki, Naoki Tomita, Yukitsuka Kudo and Hiroyuki Arai
Department of Geriatrics and Gerontology, Division of Brain Science, Institute of Development, Aging and Cancer, Tohoku University, 4-1 Seiryo-machi, Aoba-ku, Sendai, Miyagi, Japan

Ryuichi Harada
Department of Pharmacology, Tohoku University School of Medicine, 2-1 Seiryo-machi, Aoba-ku, Sendai, Miyagi, Japan

Kazuhiko Yanai
Department of Pharmacology, Tohoku University School of Medicine, 2-1 Seiryo-machi, Aoba-ku, Sendai, Miyagi, Japan
Cyclotron and Radioisotope Center, Tohoku University, 6-3 Aoba, Aramaki, Aoba-ku, Sendai, Miyagi, Japan

Hideaki Kai and Tetsuyuki Kitamoto
Department of Neurological Science, Tohoku University School of Medicine, 2-1 Seiryo-machi, Aoba-ku, Sendai, Miyagi, Japan

Naomi Sato and Hironobu Sasano
Department of Pathology, Tohoku University School of Medicine, 4-1 Seiryo-machi, Aoba-ku, Sendai, Miyagi, Japan

Tomoko Totsune
Department of Nuclear Medicine and Radiology, Institute of Development, Aging and Cancer, Tohoku University, 4-1 Seiryo-machi, Aoba-ku, Sendai, Miyagi, Japan

Shoichi Watanuki, Kotaro Hiraoka, Yoichi Ishikawa, Yoshihito Funaki, Ren Iwata, Shozo Furumoto and Manabu Tashiro
Cyclotron and Radioisotope Center, Tohoku University, 6-3 Aoba, Aramaki, Aoba-ku, Sendai, Miyagi, Japan

Katsutoshi Furukawa
Division of Community Medicine, Faculty of Medicine, Tohoku Medical and Pharmaceutical University, 1-15-1 Fukumuro, Miyagino-ku, Sendai, Miyagi, Japan

Nobuyuki Okamura
Division of Pharmacology, Faculty of Medicine, Tohoku Medical and Pharmaceutical University, 1-15-1 Fukumuro, Miyagino-ku, Sendai, Miyagi, Japan
Department of Pharmacology, Tohoku University School of Medicine, 2-1 Seiryo-machi, Aoba-ku, Sendai, Miyagi, Japan
Cyclotron and Radioisotope Center, Tohoku University, 6-3 Aoba, Aramaki, Aoba-ku, Sendai, Miyagi, Japan

Ryuichi Harada
Department of Pharmacology, Tohoku University School of Medicine 2-1, Seiryo-machi, Aoba-ku, Sendai 9808575, Japan
Department of Geriatrics and Gerontology, Division of Brain Science, Institute of Development, Aging and Cancer, Tohoku University, 4-1 Seiryo-machi, Aoba-ku, Sendai, Miyagi, Japan

Andrea B. Ganz
Department of Molecular and Cellular Neuroscience, Center for Neurogenomics and Cognitive Research, Amsterdam Neuroscience, Vrije Universiteit Amsterdam, De Boelelaan 1085, 1081 HV Amsterdam, The Netherlands
Department of Pathology, Amsterdam Neuroscience, VU University Medical Center, MB Amsterdam, The Netherlands
Alzheimer Centre, Department of Neurology, Amsterdam Neuroscience, VU University Medical Center, Postbus 7057, 1007 MB Amsterdam, The Netherlands

August B. Smit
Department of Molecular and Cellular Neuroscience, Center for Neurogenomics and Cognitive Research, Amsterdam Neuroscience, Vrije Universiteit Amsterdam, De Boelelaan 1085, 1081 HV Amsterdam, The Netherlands

Annemieke J. M. Rozemuller and Jeroen J. M. Hoozemans
Department of Pathology, Amsterdam Neuroscience, VU University Medical Center, MB Amsterdam, The Netherlands

Nina Beker, Sietske Sikkes and Philip Scheltens
Alzheimer Centre, Department of Neurology, Amsterdam Neuroscience, VU University Medical Center, Postbus 7057, 1007 MB Amsterdam, The Netherlands

Marc Hulsman
Department of Clinical Genetics, Amsterdam Neuroscience, VU University Medical Center, de Boelelaan, 1118 1081 HV Amsterdam, The Netherlands

Henne Holstege
Department of Clinical Genetics, Amsterdam Neuroscience, VU University Medical Center, de Boelelaan, 1118 1081 HV Amsterdam, The Netherlands
Alzheimer Centre, Department of Neurology, Amsterdam Neuroscience, VU University Medical Center, Postbus 7057, 1007 MB Amsterdam, The Netherlands

Netherlands Brain Bank
Netherlands Institute for Neuroscience, Meibergdreef 47, 1105 BA Amsterdam, The Netherlands

Yvonne S. Davidson, Andrew Robinson and David M. A. Mann
Institute of Brain, Behaviour and Mental Health, Faculty of Medical and Human Sciences University of Manchester, Salford Royal Hospital, Stott Lane, Salford M6 8HD, England

Vee P. Prasher
South Birmingham Community NHS Trust, Birmingham, UK
Liverpool John Moores University, Liverpool, UK

Martin Timo Henrich, Fanni Fruzsina Geibl, Bolam Lee, Wei-Hua Chiu, Lars Timmermann and Wolfgang Hermann Oertel
Department of Neurology, Philipps University Marburg, Baldingerstraße 1, 35043 Marburg, Germany

James Benjamin Koprich and Jonathan Michael Brotchie
Krembil Research Institute, Toronto Western Hospital, University Health Network, Toronto, ON, Canada

Niels Decher and Lina Anita Matschke
Department of Physiology and Pathophysiology, Philipps University Marburg, 35043 Marburg, Germany

Heehong Hwang, Seulah Choi, Sang Ho Kwon, Suhyun Lee, Jae Hong Park and Sang Min Kim
Neuroregeneration and Stem Cell Programs, Institute for Cell Engineering, The Johns Hopkins University School of Medicine, Baltimore, MD 21205, USA

Donghoon Kim
Department of Neurology, The Johns Hopkins University School of Medicine, Baltimore, MD 21205, USA
Neuroregeneration and Stem Cell Programs, Institute for Cell Engineering, The Johns Hopkins University School of Medicine, Baltimore, MD 21205, USA

Han Seok Ko
Neuroregeneration and Stem Cell Programs, Institute for Cell Engineering, The Johns Hopkins University School of Medicine, Baltimore, MD 21205, USA
Department of Neurology, The Johns Hopkins University School of Medicine, Baltimore, MD 21205, USA
Diana Helis Henry Medical Research Foundation, New Orleans, Louisiana 70130, USA
Adrienne Helis Malvin Medical Research Foundation, New Orleans, Louisiana 70130, USA

Sukriti Nag
Departments of Pathology (Neuropathology), Rush University Medical Center, Chicago, IL, USA
Rush Alzheimer Disease Center, Rush University Medical Center, Suite 1000, 1750 W Harrison Street, Chicago, IL 60612, USA

Julie A. Schneider
Departments of Pathology (Neuropathology), Rush University Medical Center, Chicago, IL, USA
Departments of Neurological Sciences, Rush University Medical Center, Chicago, IL, USA

Lei Yu, Sue E. Leurgans and David A. Bennett
Departments of Neurological Sciences, Rush University Medical Center, Chicago, IL, USA
Rush Alzheimer Disease Center, Rush University Medical Center, Suite 1000, 1750 W Harrison Street, Chicago, IL 60612, USA

Patricia A. Boyle
Departments of Behavioral Sciences, Rush University Medical Center, Chicago, IL, USA
Rush Alzheimer Disease Center, Rush University Medical Center, Suite 1000, 1750 W Harrison Street, Chicago, IL 60612, USA

Ignazio Cali
Departments of Pathology, Case Western Reserve University, School of Medicine, Cleveland, OH 44106, USA
Department of Pathology, 4th floor, room 402C, Case Western Reserve University, 2085 Adelbert Road, Cleveland, OH 44106, USA

Mark L. Cohen
Departments of Pathology, Case Western Reserve University, School of Medicine, Cleveland, OH 44106, USA
National Prion Disease Pathology Surveillance Center, Case Western Reserve University, School of Medicine, Cleveland, OH 44106, USA

Stéphane Haïk
Inserm U1127, CNRS UMR 7225, Sorbonne Universités, UPMC Univ Paris VI UMR S 1127, Institut du Cerveau et de la Moelle épinière, Paris, France
AP-HP, Cellule Nationale de Référence des maladies de Creutzfeldt-Jakob, Groupe Hospitalier Pitié-Salpêtrière, Paris, France
AP-HP, Laboratoire de Neuropathologie R Escourolle, Groupe Hospitalier Pitié-Salpêtrière, Paris, France

Piero Parchi
Department of Experimental, Diagnostic and Specialty Medicine, University of Bologna, Bologna, Italy
IRCCS, Institute of Neurological Sciences, Bologna, Italy

Véronique Sazdovitch and Charles Duyckaerts
Inserm U1127, CNRS UMR 7225, Sorbonne Universités, UPMC Univ Paris VI UMR S 1127, Institut du Cerveau et de la Moelle épinière, Paris, France
AP-HP, Laboratoire de Neuropathologie R Escourolle, Groupe Hospitalier Pitié-Salpêtrière, Paris, France

Tetsuyuki Kitamoto
Department of Neurological Science, Tohoku University Graduate School of Medicine, Sendai, Japan

Ermias D. Belay and Lawrence B. Schonberger
Division of High-Consequence Pathogens and Pathology, National Center for Emerging and Zoonotic Infectious Diseases, Centers for Disease Control and Prevention, Atlanta, GA, USA

Pierluigi Gambetti
Departments of Pathology, Case Western Reserve University, School of Medicine, Cleveland, OH 44106, USA
Department of Pathology, 4th floor, room 419, Case Western Reserve University, 2085 Adelbert Road, Cleveland, OH 44106, USA

Rasha Al-Khalidi, Paul Cox, Natalia Chira, Rhiannon E. McGeehan and Dariusz C. Górecki
Molecular Medicine Laboratory, School of Pharmacy and Biomedical Sciences, University of Portsmouth, Portsmouth, UK

Chiara Panicucci
Center of Myology and Neurodegenerative Disorders, Department of Neuroscience and Rehabilitation, Istituto Giannina Gaslini, Genoa, Italy
Molecular Medicine Laboratory, School of Pharmacy and Biomedical Sciences, University of Portsmouth, Portsmouth, UK

Justyna Róg and Krzysztof Zabłocki
Laboratory of Cellular Metabolism, Department of Biochemistry, Nencki Institute of Experimental Biology of the Polish Academy of Sciences, Warsaw, Poland

Kameshwari Ambati
Department of Ophthalmology & Center for Advanced Vision Science, University of Virginia, Charlottesville, VA, USA

Jayakrishna Ambati
Department of Pathology, Microbiology, Immunology & Cancer Biology, University of Virginia, Charlottesville, VA, USA
Department of Ophthalmology & Center for Advanced Vision Science, University of Virginia, Charlottesville, VA, USA

Rasha Al-Khalidi
Biotechnology Department, Faculty of Science, University of Baghdad, Baghdad, Iraq

Christopher N. J. Young
School of Allied Health Sciences, Faculty of Health and Life Sciences, De Montfort University, Leicester, UKRush Alzheimer Disease Center, Rush University Medical Center, Suite 1000, 1750 W Harrison Street, Chicago, IL 60612, USA
Molecular Medicine Laboratory, School of Pharmacy and Biomedical Sciences, University of Portsmouth, Portsmouth, UK

Index

www.ingramcontent.com/pod-product-compliance
Lightning Source LLC
LaVergne TN
LVHW080724210926
848485LV00003B/516
9781639272914